HANDBOOK OF
OBESITY

HANDBOOK OF
OBESITY

Clinical Applications
Second Edition

edited by

GEORGE A. BRAY
CLAUDE BOUCHARD

Pennington Biomedical Research Center
Louisiana State University
Baton Rouge, Louisiana, U.S.A.

MARCEL DEKKER, INC.　　　　　　　　　　　　　NEW YORK • BASEL

The first edition of this book and its companion volume, *Handbook of Obesity: Etiology and Pathophysiology, Second Edition*, was published as *Handbook of Obesity*, edited by George A. Bray, Claude Bouchard, and W. P. T. James (Marcel Dekker, Inc., 1998).

Although great care has been taken to provide accurate and current information, neither the author(s) nor the publisher, nor anyone else associated with this publication, shall be liable for any loss, damage, or liability directly or indirectly caused or alleged to be caused by this book. The material contained herein is not intended to provide specific advice or recommendations for any specific situation.

Trademark notice: Product or corporate names may be trademarks or registered trademarks and are used only for identification and explanation without intent to infringe.

Library of Congress Cataloging-in-Publication Data
A catalog record for this book is available from the Library of Congress.

ISBN: 0-8247-4773-9

This book is printed on acid-free paper.

Headquarters
Marcel Dekker, Inc.
270 Madison Avenue, New York, NY 10016, U.S.A.
tel: 212-696-9000; fax: 212-685-4540

Distribution and Customer Service
Marcel Dekker, Inc.
Cimarron Road, Monticello, New York 12701, U.S.A.
tel: 800-228-1160; fax: 845-796-1772

Eastern Hemisphere Distribution
Marcel Dekker AG
Hutgasse 4, Postfach 812, CH-4001 Basel, Switzerland
tel: 41-61-260-6300; fax: 41-61-260-6333

World Wide Web
http://www.dekker.com

The publisher offers discounts on this book when ordered in bulk quantities. For more information, write to Special Sales/ Professional Marketing at the headquarters address above.

Current printing (last digit):

10 9 8 7 6 5 4 3 2

PRINTED IN THE UNITED STATES OF AMERICA

Preface to the Second Edition

The publication of the first edition of the *Handbook of Obesity* occurred just as the Food and Drug Administration requested the recall of fenfluramine and dexfenfluramine. Each drug alone and in combination with phentermine had been associated with a rash of valvular heart disease. These cases were similar to some seen with the carcinoid syndrome that secretes serotonin. There was an accumulation of material on the aortic valves in the heart that made them leaky. The good news is that many of these valvular lesions have been reversible when the drugs were discontinued, and there are no cases known to us of progression after the drugs were stopped.

Thus, at the time the first edition of the *Handbook of Obesity* was published, the chapters dealing with fenfluramine and combination therapy were already out of place. In addition, there were few drug treatments on the horizon.

In spite of this negative impact, the scientific advances preceding the publication of the first edition had been substantial. As we began to plan the second edition, we reviewed each of the 49 chapters in the first edition. The major changes were in the therapeutic area, where many new drugs were under evaluation and where new strategies for prevention of obesity were being evaluated.

Based on these advances in the therapeutic area, we have added 12 new chapters, which made a substantially

longer volume with 61 chapters. We have thus decided to divide the handbook into two separate volumes. The first deals with the prevalence, etiology, and consequences of obesity. In the second volume we have included the chapters dealing with evaluation, prevention and treatment.

This volume has been significantly expanded to cover the new important, growing areas. In addition to a chapter on evaluation that was included in the previous volume, we have added three new chapters dealing with the role of the primary care physician (Chap. 2), the impact of cultural influences (Chap. 3), and the stigmatization of obesity as reflected in bias, prejudice, and discrimination (Chap. 4).

We have also expanded the section on prevention. In addition to the initial chapter on prevention (Chap. 5), we have added a new chapter on environments that produce obesity (Chap. 6) and a new chapter on prevention and management of dyslipidemias (Chap. 7).

The section on treatment includes the largest number of new chapters, with new chapters on sympathomimetic drugs (Chap. 12), drugs affecting fat absorption (Chap. 13), a chapter on leptin (Chap. 14), and one on the new drugs on the horizon (Chap. 15). The chapter on surgical approach to obesity focuses on the data derived from the Swedish Obese Subjects Study (Chap. 18). Finally, we have added a new chapter on herbal and alternative approaches to obesity (Chap. 17).

We are indebted to a number of people for this volume. Ms. Nina Laidlaw and Ms. Heather Miller at the Pennington Biomedical Research Center have provided able assistance to the editors. At Marcel Dekker, Inc., Ms. Moraima Suarez has taken the principal role. We are both indebted to each of these three people. Without the excellent writing from each of the authors and their collaborators, we would not have the superb chapters that make up this volume. We thank all of them.

George A. Bray
Claude Bouchard

Preface to the First Edition

This volume has been designed to provide up-to-date coverage of the range of subjects that make up the field of obesity research. The chapters have been written by many of the leading scientists and clinicians in the field.

We have divided the book into four sections. Part one deals with the history, definitions, and prevalence of obesity. The first of these nine chapters outlines the history of obesity using a series of timelines to put the important events in the development of obesity research into the historical context. This is followed by a chapter written by the three editors on definitions that can be used to frame the subject matter of obesity. Chapters on the measurement of body composition follows. The global prevalence of obesity in children and in the elderly is then presented in three separate chapters. This section ends with a discussion of the behavioral and psychological correlates of obesity, and the cultural context in which obesity is viewed by different ethnic groups.

The second section focuses on the etiological factors involved in the development of this problem. The first chapter is a detailed presentation of the genetics of human obesity. A genetic approach has proved particularly important since the discovery of leptin and the rapid mapping of genetic loci that are associated with the development of obesity. A Great deal has been learned about obesity from the study of animals models, a variety of which are presented by two of the experts in the field. The third chapter deals with the rise of genetic approaches to obesity, which has been aided by advances in molecular biology. There follows three chapters on the intake of food. One of these deals with this problem in humans, the second with the problem in animals, and the third with the neural basis for the intake of food in both humans and animals. Together these chapters provide a vivid view of the current standing of the field of nutrient intake.

Our understanding of the importance of adipose tissue has steadily increased, from regarding it as a simple storage organ to recognizing it as a secretory organ as well. The important differences between white and brown adipose tissue have also been elucidated, and their role in the development and maintenance of human obesity defined. These concepts are developed in the next four chapters. The final group of chapters in the second section deals with energy expenditure. There is a chapter on energy expenditure and thermogenesis during test and one on physical activity and its relation to obesity and food intake. Finally, the roles of the endocrine system, the autonomic nervous system, and substrate handling are discussed. From this second section the reader should obtain a detailed understanding of the genetic basis of obesity; the role and control of food intake in the development of obesity; the way fat cells function as a storage, thermogenic, secretory organ; and, finally, the way in which energy expenditure is controlled and involved in the development of obesity.

The fourth section deals with the pathophysiology of obesity, that is, the mechanisms by which obesity produces damaging effects on health. The first two chapters in this section deal with the role of central fat and the metabolic syndrome. This is followed by a detailed discussion of the effects of obesity on a variety of individual organ systems. Three chapters are devoted to problems of the cardiovascular system and lipoprotein abnormalities, which are important consequences of obesity. Diabetes is one of the most frequent problems associated with obesity, as explained in one chapter. The ways in which obesity enhances the risk of gall bladder disease are developed in another chapter. This is followed by a clear discussion of the pulmonary problems arising from obesity, one of which (the Pickwickian syndrome, or sleep apnea) is named after the famous fat boy, Joe, in Dicken's *Pickwick Papers*. Obesity has important effects on the risk for gout and arthritis and this is discussed in a separate chapter. Two chapters in this section deal with the effects of obesity on endocrine function and pregnancy. Finally, the problem of weight cycling and the risk of intentional and unintensional weight loss are discussed in two chapters that have picked up important themes of obesity research and put them into a valuable perspective.

The final section deals with prevention and treatment. Since an ounce of prevention is worth a pound of cure, the section begins with a chapter on prevention. This is followed by a clinically useful set of guidances for the evaluation of the overweight patient. The cornerstones for treatment of obesity—behavior therapy, diet, and exercise—are presented in three separate chapters. These are followed by three important chapters on the management of diabetes, hypertension, and hyperlipidemia in the obese individual. Finally, there is a chapter on the current status of pharmacological treatment of obesity and the chapter on the surgical approaches that can be used for a individual for whom other approaches to treatment have failed.

The preparation of this volume has required the work of many people. First, we want to thank the authors and their secretarial assistants for submitting the chapters so promptly. This will make the entire volume timely. Several individuals in the editor's office have also played a key role in moving this forward. We want to thank especially Ms. Millie Cutrer and Terry Hodges in Baton Rouge, Ms. Karen Horth and Ms. Diane Drolet in Quebec City, and Ms. Jean James in Aberdeen. The guiding hand at Marcel Dekker, Inc., who has been so valuable in nudging and cajoling us along when we needed, is Ms. Lia Pelosi. We thank you all and hope that the readers appreciate the important role each of you, and others we have not mentioned, including especially our long-suffering families, has made to the success of this volume.

George A. Bray
Claude Bouchard

Contents

Contributors

Louis J. Aronne, M.D. Clinical Associate Professor, Department of Medicine, Weill Medical College of Cornell University, New York, New York, U.S.A.

Arne Astrup, M.D., Dr.Med.Sci. Director and Professor, Department of Human Nutrition, The Royal Veterinary and Agricultural University, Frederiksberg, Denmark

George A. Bray, M.D. Boyd Professor, Chronic Disease Prevention, Pennington Biomedical Research Center, Louisiana State University, Baton Rouge, Louisiana, U.S.A.

Kelly D. Brownell, Ph.D. Professor, Department of Psychology, and Director, Yale Center for Eating and Weight Disorders, Yale University, New Haven, Connecticut, U.S.A.

José F. Caro, M.D. Vice President, Endocrine Research and Clinical Investigation, Lilly Research Laboratories, Eli Lilly and Company, Indianapolis, Indiana, U.S.A.

Robert V. Considine, Ph.D. Assistant Professor, Department of Medicine, Indiana University School of Medicine, Indianapolis, Indiana, U.S.A.

Garry J. Egger, M.P.H., Ph.D. Adjunct Professor, Department of Public Health Nutrition, School of Health Sciences, Deakin University, Melbourne, Victoria, Australia

John P. Foreyt, Ph.D. Professor, Department of Medicine, Baylor College of Medicine, Houston, Texas, U.S.A.

Timothy P. Gill, Ph.D., R.P.H.Nutr. Director, New South Wales Centre for Public Health Nutrition, University of Sydney, Sydney, New South Wales, Australia

Frank L. Greenway, M.D. Medical Director, Clinical Trials, Pennington Biomedical Research Center, and Professor, Department of Human Ecology, Louisiana State University, Baton Rouge, Louisiana, U.S.A.

Scott M. Grundy, M.D., Ph.D. Center for Human Nutrition and Department of Internal Medicine, University of Texas Southwestern Medical Center at Dallas, Dallas, Texas, U.S.A.

David Heber, M.D., Ph.D., F.A.C.N., F.A.C.P. Professor of Medicine and Public Health, Division of Clinical Nutrition, Department of Medicine, David Geffen School of Medicine at UCLA, and Director,

UCLA Center for Human Nutrition, Los Angeles, California, U.S.A.

W. Philip T. James, M.D., D.Sc., F.R.C.P. Professor and Chairman, International Obesity TaskForce, London, England

Roland T. Jung, M.D., F.R.C.P.(Lond), F.R.C.P.(Edin) Professor of Medicine, Diabetes Centre, Ninewells Hospital and Medical School, Dundee, Scotland

Shiriki Kumanyika, Ph.D., M.P.H. Professor, Center for Clinical Epidemiology and Biostatistics, University of Pennsylvania School of Medicine, Philadelphia, Pennsylvania, U.S.A.

Robert F. Kushner, M.D. Professor, Department of Medicine, Northwestern University Feinberg School of Medicine, Chicago, Illinois, U.S.A.

Wayne C. Miller, Ph.D. Professor, Department of Exercise Science, The George Washington University, Washington, D.C., U.S.A.

Michael G. Perri, Ph.D., A.B.P.P. Professor, Department of Clinical and Health Psychology, University of Florida, Gainesville, Florida, U.S.A.

Rebecca M. Puhl, M.S., M.Phil. Department of Psychology, Yale University, New Haven, Connecticut, U.S.A.

Donna H. Ryan, M.D. Associate Executive Director and Professor, Department of Clinical Research, Pennington Biomedical Research Center, Louisiana State University, Baton Rouge, Louisiana, U.S.A.

Lars Sjöström, M.D., Ph.D. Professor, Department of Body Composition and Metabolism, Sahlgrenska University, and Sahlgrenska University Hospital, Göteborg, Sweden

Albert J. Stunkard, M.D. Professor, Department of Psychiatry, University of Pennsylvania School of Medicine, Philadelphia, Pennsylvania, U.S.A.

Boyd Anthony Swinburn, M.B., Ch.B., M.D., F.R.A.C.P. Professor, Department of Public Health Nutrition, School of Health Sciences, Deakin University, Melbourne, Victoria, Australia

Søren Toubro, M.D. Associate Professor, Department of Human Nutrition, The Royal Veterinary and Agricultural University, Frederiksberg, Denmark

Luc F. Van Gaal, M.D., Ph.D. Professor, Department of Diabetology, Metabolism, and Nutrition, University of Antwerp, and University Hospital Antwerp, Antwerp, Belgium

Thomas A. Wadden, Ph.D. Professor, Department of Psychiatry, University of Pennsylvania School of Medicine, Philadelphia, Pennsylvania, U.S.A.

Rena R. Wing, Ph.D. Professor, Department of Psychiatry and Human Behavior, Brown Medical School, Providence, Rhode Island, U.S.A.

Susan Z. Yanovski, M.D. Director, Obesity and Eating Disorders Program, Division of Digestive Diseases and Nutrition, National Institute of Diabetes and Digestive and Kidney Diseases, National Institutes of Health, Bethesda, Maryland, U.S.A.

1

Classification and Evaluation of the Overweight Patient

George A. Bray

Pennington Biomedical Research Center, Louisiana State University, Baton Rouge, Louisiana, U.S.A.

Obesity is now recognized as a risk factor for the development of diabetes, gallbladder disease, cardiovascular disease, hypertension, sleep apnea, osteoarthritis, and some forms of cancer. Since the major cause of death in the United States and most other countries is cardiovascular disease, the approach to obesity should be designed to reduce the risks of this problem. In this chapter, I will discuss a classification of obesity that is based on anatomic, etiologic, and functional considerations. I will then use the natural history for the development of obesity to identify the factors associated with its progression and to suggest a stepped approach to evaluation of the overweight patient.

I CLINICAL CLASSIFICATION

A Anatomic Characteristics of Adipose Tissue and Fat Distribution

Obesity is a disease whose pathology lies in the increased size and number of fat cells. An anatomic classification of obesity from which a pathologic classification arises is based on the number of adipocytes, on the regional distribution of body fat, or on the characteristics of localized fat deposits (1,2).

1 Size and Number of Fat Cells

The number of fat cells can be estimated from the total amount of body fat and the average size of a fat cell (3).

Because fat cells differ in size in different regions of the body, a reliable estimate of the total number of fat cells should be based on the average fat cell size from more than one location. In adults, the upper limits of the total of normal fat cells range from 40 to 60×10^9. The number of fat cells increases most rapidly during late childhood and puberty, but may increase even in adult life. The number of fat cells can increase three- to fivefold when obesity occurs in childhood or adolescence.

a. Hypertrophic Obesity

Enlarged fat cells are the pathologic sine qua non of obesity (3–5). Enlarged fat cells tend to correlate with an android or truncal fat distribution and are often associated with metabolic disorders such as glucose intolerance, dyslipidemia, hypertension, and coronary artery disease. These derangements occur because large fat cells secrete more of the many peptides and metabolites that they make.

b. Hypercellular Obesity

An increased number of fat cells usually occurs when obesity develops in childhood. Whether it begins in early or middle childhood, this type of obesity tends to be severe (6). Increased numbers of fat cells may also occur in adult life and this is to be expected when the body mass index (BMI) is $>40 \text{ kg/m}^2$ (7).

2   Fat Distribution

a.   Measurement

Measuring fat distribution in subcutaneous versus visceral compartments is important because visceral fat predicts development of health risks better than total body fat. The distribution of body fat can be estimated by a variety of techniques. The ratio of waist circumference divided by hip circumference waist-hip ratio; (WHR) was used in the pioneering studies that brought scientific recognition in the 1980s to the relationship of centrally located fat to the risk of developing heart disease, diabetes, and other chronic problems associated with obesity (8–10). This concept was originally suggested by Vague in 1948 (11) and is now widely accepted. The subscapular skinfold has also been valuable in estimating central fat in epidemiologic studies (12). The sagittal diameter, measured as the distance between the surface of the midabdominal skin and the table beneath a recumbent subject, has been used as an index of central fat (13). The only truly reliable estimates of visceral fat, however, are made by computed tomography (CT) (14) or magnetic resonance imaging (MRI). Using this technique and its association with dyslipidemia, Pouliot et al. (15) and Lean et al. (16) showed that waist circumference was as good as or better than WHR or sagittal diameter in estimating visceral fat. For practical purposes, waist circumference alone and/or WHR are used as one criterion for evaluating the contribution of fat distribution to the health risk from obesity.

b.   The Metabolic Syndrome

Central adiposity is one diagnostic criterion for the metabolic syndrome. This syndrome is a complex of traits that enhance the risk of cardiovascular disease and is discussed in more detail later in this chapter (17,18). The diagnosis requires three of the following five features: central obesity, hypertension, insulin resistance, dyslipidemia, or diabetes mellitus (17).

3   Lipomas and Lipodystrophy

a.   Lipomas

Localized fat accumulations include single lipomas, multiple lipomas, liposarcomas, and lipodystrophy (2). Lipomas vary in size from 1 cm to >15 cm. They can occur in any body region, and represent encapsulated accumulations of fat. Multiple lipomatosis is an inherited disease transmitted as an autosomal-dominant trait. Von Recklinghausen's syndrome, Maffucci's syndrome, and Madelung's deformity are lipomatous syndromes.

Liposarcomas are relatively rare, representing < 1% of lipomas. They tend to affect the lower extremities and consist of four types: well-differentiated myxoid; poorly differentiated myxoid; round cell or adenoid; and mixed (2).

Weber-Christian disease and Dercum's disease are idiopathic accumulations of fat. Dercum's disease, also called adiposis dolorosa, is named after the painful nodules in the subcutaneous fat of middle-aged women. Weber-Christian disease, on the other hand, is a relapsing febrile disease occurring in younger women. All of these forms of localized fat deposits are relatively rare (2).

b.   Lipodystrophy

Lipodystrophy is a loss of body fat in one or more regions of the body (19). It can have genetic causes or it can be acquired. Table 1 shows the various types of lipodystrophy. The clinical features include regional or general decrease in adipose tissue, severe insulin resistance, often with diabetes, markedly elevated triglycerides, and fatty liver. Acanthosis nigricans is also common. Animals with no body fat (20) show similarly marked insulin resistance that can be relieved when small amounts of fat are transplanted into the fat-deficient animals.

Familial partial lipodystrophy is a genetic defect due to an alternation in the laminin A/C gene. The protein

Table 1   Types of Lipodystrophy

Type of lipodystrophy	Syndrome name
Generalized congenital lipodystrophy	Berardinelli-Seip syndrome
Partial lipodystrophy	Dunnigan's syndrome
Acquired lipodystrophy	Lawrence syndrome
Acquired peripheral lipodystrophy	AIDS or protease lipodystrophy

normally produced by this gene is thought to be involved in the entry of molecules into the nucleus. When the aberrant base substitution in the DNA is in one end of the molecule, the disease manifests itself as muscular dystrophy or congestive heart failure. When the molecular substitution is at the other end of the molecule, lipodystrophy is the result.

Drug-induced lipodystrophies appeared when patients with human immunodeficiency virus (HIV) disease were treated with proteases. The proteases reduce the viral burden, but also cause a central distribution of body fat. The mechanism for this central location of fat is currently under intense study.

B Etiologic Classification

A number of specific etiologies that cause obesity are described below.

1 Neuroendocrine Obesity

a. Hypothalamic Obesity

Hypothalamic obesity is rare in humans (21). It can be regularly produced in animals by injuring the ventromedial or paraventricular region of the hypothalamus or the amygdala (22). These brain regions are responsible for integrating metabolic information on nutrient stores provided by leptin with afferent sensory information on food availability. When the ventromedial hypothalamus is damaged, hyperphagia develops, the response to leptin is eliminated, and obesity follows. Hypothalamic obesity in humans may be caused by trauma, tumor, inflammatory disease (22) (Table 2),

Table 2 Hypothalamic Obesity

Lesions causing hypothalamic obesity
    tumors
    inflammation
    trauma
Clinical features of hypothalamic obesity
  1. Endocrine disturbances
      amenorrhea/impotence
      impaired growth
      diabetes insipidus
      thyroid/adrenal insufficiency
  2. Intracranial pressure
      papilledema
      vomiting
  3. Neurologic disturbances
      thrist
      somnolence

surgery in the posterior fossa, or increased intracranial pressure (22). The symptoms usually present in one or more of three patterns: (1) headache, vomiting and diminished vision due to increased intracranial pressure; (2) impaired endocrine function affecting the reproductive system with amenorrhea or impotence, diabetes insipidus, and thyroid or adrenal insufficiency; or (3) neurologic and physiologic derangements, including convulsions, coma, somnolence, and hypothermia or hyperthermia (Table 2). The clinical presentation of one patient is shown in Figure 1. Weight gain occurred in the third year after the appearance of several endocrine and hypothalamic changes. The patient died with multiple tuberculomas in the hypothalamus despite triple-antibiotic therapy.

b. Cushing's Syndrome

Obesity is one of the cardinal features of Cushing's syndrome (Table 3) (23). Thus, the differential diagnosis of obesity from Cushing's syndrome and pseudo-Cushing's syndrome is clinically important for therapeutic decisions (23,24). Pseudo-Cushing's is a name used for a variety of conditions that distort the dynamics of the hypothalamic-pituitary-adrenal axis and can confuse the interpretations of biochemical tests for Cushing's syndrome. Pseudo-Cushing's includes such things as depression, anxiety disorder, obsessive-compulsive disorder, poorly controlled diabetes mellitus, and alcoholism. Four different biochemical tests can be used to separate these entities. The first is a urinary free cortisol, which is the initial screening test, and is considered abnormal if it is more than two times the upper limit of normal (25,26). Patients with pseudo-Cushing's syndrome can have values that are elevated by fourfold, so other tests may be needed. The next test is the overnight suppression of cortisol at 8 AM with a 1-mg dose of dexamethasone given orally at midnight. The dividing line is 3.6 μg/dL, but the lower the value the more likely it is to exclude Cushing's syndrome. If the overnight dexamethasone test is equivocal, a nighttime cortisol level may be drawn. This distinguishes Cushing's syndrome from pseudo-Cushing's syndrome with 95% accuracy if the value is <7.5 μg/dL. The final test is a dexamethasone-CRH test. This test can be helpful, but is also cumbersome to perform because of the timing. If tests are equivocal, then they may be repeated, but it may be advisable to wait for a few weeks in case the patient is an individual with intermittent Cushing's syndrome. For the differential diagnosis and treatment of Cushing's syndrome, the reader is referred elsewhere (24–26).

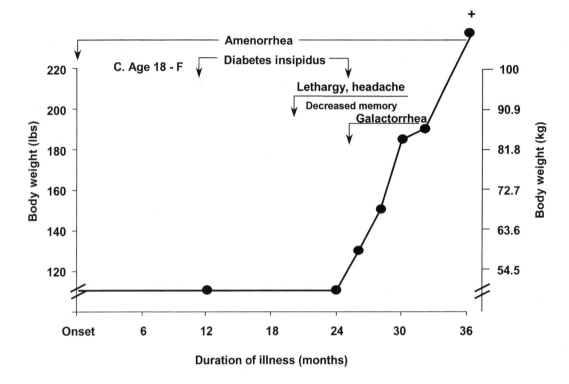

Figure 1 Symptomatic course of a patient with tuberculomas and hypothalamic obesity. Numerous symptoms developed in the first 2 years, followed by rapid weight gain in the third year.

c. Hypothyroidism

Patients with hypothyroidism frequently gain weight because of a generalized slowing of metabolic activity. Some of this gain is fat. However, the weight gain is usually modest, and marked obesity is uncommon. Hypothyroidism is common, particularly in older women. In this group, measurement of thyroid-stimulating hormone (TSH) is a valuable diagnostic tool (27).

d. Polycystic Ovary Syndrome

The definition of the polycystic ovary syndrome (PCOS) is based on a conference held at the National Institutes of health in April of 1990 and includes menstrual irregularity plus hyperandrogenism, excluding other pathology such as congenital adrenal hyperplasia and androgen-secreting tumors (28). The presence of these other diseases can be suspected from measurements of TSH, prolactin, follicle-stimulating hormone (FSH), plasma testosterone, dehydroepiandrosterone-sulfate (DHEA-S), and a morning 17-hydroxyprogesterone.

The features of the syndrome are summarized in Table 4. Obesity, particularly central obesity, is common in this syndrome. Similarly, insulin resistance is

Table 3 Clinical Findings with Cushing's Syndrome

Sign/symptom	Percent of 70 patients
Decreased libido (men/women)	100%
Obesity or weight gain	97%
Plethora	94%
Round face	88%
Menstrual changes	84%
Hirsutism	81%
Hypertension	74%
Ecchymoses	62%
Lethargy, depression	62%
Striae	56%
Weakness	56%
ECG changes/atherosclerosis	55%
Dodrsal fat pad	54%
Edema	50%
Abnormal glucose tolerance	50%
Osteopenia or fracture	50%
Headache	47%
Backache	43%
Recurrent infections	25%
Abdominal pain	21%
Acne	21%
Female balding	13%

Source: Refs. 23, 24.

Table 4 Features of the Polycystic Ovary Syndrome

Clinical and metabolic components of the polycystic ovary syndrome	
Menstrual abnormalities	Amenorrhea or oligomenorrhea
	Anovulation
	Infertility
	Increase risk of miscarriage
	Dysfunctional bleeding
Hyperandrogenism	Hirsutism
	Seborrhea and acne
	Male pattern of balding
	Elevated plasma androgens
Hypothalamic-pituitary abnormalities	Increased LH or LH/FSH ratio
	Increased prolactin
Metabolic abnormalities	Obesity (10–80%)
	Insulin resistance, even in nonobese women
	Acanthosis nigricans

present, even when obesity is minimal. The basis for the association of the hypothalamic-adrenal-gonadal problem and the obesity is unclear. Luteinizing hormone (LH) is usually increased, and the ovary is the source for the increased amounts of testosterone, possibly through stimulation by insulinlike growth factor-1 (IGF-1).

More than 50% of women with PCOS are obese (29). The cardinal features of this syndrome are oligomenorrhea, hirsutism, and polycystic ovaries. Although obesity is not always present, it occurs more often than not. Insulin resistance is present in both normal and overweight women with PCOS. LH is usually increased, and ovarian overproduction of testosterone, probably through ovarian stimulation by IGF-1, is a main source of the elevated testosterone. The factors responsible for this association are not understood.

e. Growth Hormone Deficiency

Lean body mass is decreased and fat mass is increased in adults and children who are deficient in growth hormone (GH), compared with those who have normal GH secretion. However, the increase in fat does not produce clinically significant obesity. Growth hormone replacement reduces body fat and visceral fat (30). Acromegaly produces the opposite effects with reduced body fat and particularly visceral fat. Treatment of acromegaly, which lowers GH, increases body fat and visceral fat. Growth hormone selectively decreases visceral fat. The gradual decline in GH with age may be one reason for the increase in visceral fat with age.

2 Drug-Induced Weight Gain

Several drugs can cause weight gain, including a variety of psychoactive agents (31) and hormones (Table 5).

The degree of weight gain is generally not sufficient to cause true obesity, except occasionally in patients treated with high-dose corticosteroid, some psychoactive drugs, or valproate.

Most antipsychotics (phenothiazines and butyrophenones) cause weight gain. One study found that men hospitalized for mental illness, many of whom were treated with phenothiazines, gained an average of 3.2 kg over a stay of 35 months. Phenothiazines and the "atypical" antipsychotics are particularly prominent in this weight gain. Antidepressants are a second group of drugs that can cause obesity. The tricyclic antidepressant amitriptyline (Elavil) is particularly likely to cause weight gain and to increase the preference for carbohydrates. Lithium also has been implicated in weight gain. Valproate (Depakote®) is an antiepileptic drug that acts on the NMDA (glutamate) receptor. It causes weight gain in up to 50% of patients. Glucocorticoids cause fat accumulation in particular areas, similar to that of Cushing's syndrome. These changes occur mostly in patients taking >10 mg/d of prednisone. Megestrol acetate (Megace) is a progestin used in women with breast cancer and in patients with AIDS to increase appetite and induce weight gain (32). The increase in weight is fat. The serotonin antagonist cyproheptadine (Periactin) is associated with weight gain. Insulin probably produces weight gain by stimulating appetite, with intermittent hypoglycemia as the most likely mechanism. Weight gain occurs in diabetic patients treated with insulin; with sulfonylureas, which enhance endogenous insulin release; and with thiazolidinediones, which act on the PPAR-γ receptor. In contrast, weight gain is not a problem with metformin (Glucophage). In the large UKPDS Trial diabetics treated conventionally or with metformin gained the same amount of weight

Table 5 Drugs That Produce Weight Gain and Alternatives

Category	Drugs that cause weight gain	Possible alternatives
Neuroleptics	Thioridazine; olanzepine; quetiapine; resperidone; clozapine	Molindone; haloperidol; ziprasodone
Antidepressants		
Tricyclics		
Monoamine oxidase inhibitors	Amitriptyline; nortriptyline imipramine; mitrazapine; paroxetine	Protriptyline Bupropion; nefazadone
Selective serotonin reuptake inhibitors		Fluoxetine; sertraline
Anticonvulsants	Valproate; carbamazepine; gabapentin	Topiramate; lamotrigine; zonisamide
Antidiabetic drugs	Insulin	
	Sulfonylureas	Miglitol; sibutramine
	Thiazolidinediones	Metformin; orlistat
Antiserotonin	Pizotifen	
Antihistamines	Cyproheptidine	Inhalers; decongestants
Adrenergic blockers	Propranolol	ACE inhibitors; calcium channel blockers
Adrenergic blockers	Terazosin	
Steroid hormones	Contraceptives	Barrier methods
	Glucocorticoids	Nonsteroidal anti-inflammatory agents
	Progestational steroids	

(3.1 kg in 10 years). Patients treated with chlorpropamide gained 5.7 kg, patients treated with glibenclamide gained 4.8 kg, and patients treated with insulin gained 7.1 kg (33). The effect of insulin was dose dependent. In the Diabetes Control and Complications Trial, the mean increase in weight in patients with insulin-dependent diabetes was 5.1 kg with intensive insulin therapy and 2.4 kg with conventional therapy (34).

3   Cessation of Smoking

Weight gain is very common when people stop smoking and is at least partly mediated by nicotine withdrawal. Weight gain of 1–2 kg in the first few weeks is often followed by an additional 2- to 3-kg weight gain over the next 4–6 months. Average weight gain is 4–5 kg, but can be much greater (35). Researchers have estimated that smoking cessation increases the odds ratio of obesity 2.4-fold in men and 2.0-fold in women, compared with nonsmokers.

The effects of smoking and smoking cessation on body weight have also been evaluated by comparing pairs of identical twins to control for genetic and certain environmental factors. Light, moderate, and heavy-smoking twins were an average of 3.2, 2.4, and 4.0 kg lighter than their nonsmoking twin. On the other hand, past smokers had a significantly higher incidence of obesity (27%) than their currently smoking siblings.

Because of the substantial predictability of weight gain after smoking cessation, an exercise program and decreased caloric intake and the possible use of bupropion (Zyban) are recommended for all patients who plan to stop smoking.

4   Sedentary Lifestyle

A sedentary lifestyle lowers energy expenditure and promotes weight gain in both animals and humans. Restriction of physical activity in rats causes weight gain, and animals in zoos tend to be heavier than those in the wild. In an affluent society, energy-sparing devices in the workplace and at home reduce energy expenditure and may enhance the tendency to gain weight (36). In children there is a graded increase in BMI as the number of hours of television watching increases (37).

A number of additional observations illustrate the importance of decreased energy expenditure in the pathogenesis of weight gain. The highest frequency of overweight occurs in men in sedentary occupations. Estimates of energy intake and energy expenditure in Great Britain suggest that reduced energy expenditure is more important than increased food intake in causing obesity (36). A study of middle-aged men in the Netherlands found that the decline in energy expenditure accounted for almost all the weight gain (38). According to the Surgeon General's Report on Physical Activity (39), the percentage of adult Americans participating in physical activity decreases steadily with age, and reduced energy expenditure in adults and children predicts weight gain. In the United States, and possibly other countries, the amount of time spent watching television is related to the degree of obesity in children; the number of automobiles is related to the degree of obesity in adults. Finally, the fatness of men in several affluent countries (the Seven Countries Study) was inversely related to levels of physical activity (40).

5 Diet

The amount of energy intake relative to energy expenditure is the central reason for the development of obesity. However, diet composition also may be variably important in its pathogenesis. Dietary factors become important in a variety of settings.

a. Breastfeeding

Several recent papers have suggested that breastfeeding may reduce the prevalence of obesity in later life. In a large German study of more than 11,000 children, Von Kries et al. (41) showed that the duration of breastfeeding as the sole source of nutrition was inversely related to the incidence of obesity, defined as a weight above the 95th centile, when children entered the first grade. In this study, the incidence was 4.8% in children with no breastfeeding, falling in a graded fashion to 0.8% in children were were solely fed from the breast for 12 months or more. A second large report (42) also showed that breastfeeding reduced the incidence of overweight, but not obese, adolescents. The third report, with fewer subjects and more ethnic heterogeneity, failed to show this effect (43). However, the potential that breastfeeding can reduce the future risk of obesity is another reason to recommend breastfeeding for at least 6–12 months.

b. Overeating

Voluntary overeating (repeated ingestion of energy exceeding daily energy needs) can increase body weight in normal-weight men and women. When these subjects stop overeating, they invariably lose most or all of the excess weight. The use of overeating protocols to study the consequences of food ingestion has shown the importance of genetic factors in the pattern of weight gain (44).

Progressive hyperphagic obesity is one clinical form of overeating (2). A small number of patients begin to be overweight in childhood and then have unrelenting weight gain, usually surpassing 140 kg (300 lb) by 30 years of age. The recent death of a 13-year-old weighing 310 kg (680 lb) illustrates a nearly maximal rate of weight gain of 25 kg/year. These patients gain about the same amount of weight year after year. Because ~ 22 kcal/kg is required to maintain an extra kilogram of body weight in an obese individual, the energy requirements in these patients must increase year by year, with the weight gain being driven by excess energy intake.

Japanese sumo wrestlers who eat large quantities of food twice a day for many years, and who have a very active training schedule, have low visceral fat relative to total weight during training. When their active career ends, however, the wrestlers tend to remain overweight and have a high probability of developing diabetes mellitus (45).

c. Dietary Fat Intake

Epidemiologic data suggest that a high-fat diet is associated with obesity. The relative weight in several populations, for example, is directly related to the percentage of dietary fat in the diet (46–48). A high-fat diet introduces palatable, often high-fat foods into the diet, with a corresponding increase in energy density (i.e., lesser weight of food for the same number of calories). This makes overconsumption more likely. Differences in the storage capacity for various macronutrients may also be involved. The capacity to store glucose as glycogen in liver and muscle is limited, and needs to be replenished frequently. This contrasts with fat stores, which are more than 100 times the daily intake of fat. This difference in storage capacity makes eating carbohydrates a more important physiologic need that may lead to overeating when dietary carbohydrate is limited and carbohydrate oxidation cannot be reduced sufficiently.

d. Dietary Carbohydrate and Fiber

When the consumption of sugar and body weight are examined there is usually an inverse relationship. However, there are recent data to suggest that the consumption of sugar-sweetened beverages in children may enhance the risk of more rapid weight gain. Both the baseline consumption and the change in consumption over 2 years were positively related to the increase in BMI over 2 years. That is, children who drank more sugar-sweetened beverages gained more weight, and those who increased their beverage consumption had an even greater increase (49).

A second relationship between obesity and carbohydrate intake may be through the glycemic index. In a review of six studies, Roberts documented that the consumption of higher glycemic index foods was associated with higher energy intake than when the foods had a lower glycemic index. This means that the higher-fiber foods that release carbohydrate more slowly stimulate food intake less than the food in which the glucose is rapidly released, as it is in the high glycemic index foods (50).

The glycemic index is a way of describing the ease with which starches are digested in the intestine with the release of glucose that can be readily absorbed (53). A high glycemic index food is one that is readily digested and produces a large and rapid rise in plasma glucose. A low glycemic index food, on the other hand, is more slowly digested and is associated with a slower and lower rise in glucose. Comparative studies show that feeding high-glycemic index food suppresses food intake less than low-glycemic index foods. The low-glycemic foods are the fruits and vegetables that tend to have fiber. Potatoes, white rice, and white bread are high-glycemic foods. Legumes, whole wheat, etc., are low-glycemic foods.

In addition to the relation of energy intake and glycemic index, there are recent data to support the idea that diets with higher fiber intake are associated with lower weight. The Seven Countries Study initiated by Keys and associates more than 20 years ago has been a fertile source for epidemiologic data (40). A recent reexamination of this group has shown that the fiber intake within each of the participating countries was inversely related to the body weight. Men eating more fiber had lower body weight. Epidemiological data suggest that countries that have a higher fiber consumption have a lower prevalence of obesity (40). Fiber intake may also be inversely related to the development of heart disease (51) and diabetes (52).

e. Dietary Calcium

Nearly 20 years ago, McCarron et al. (54) reported that there was a negative relationship between BMI and dietary calcium intake in the data collected by the National Center for Health Statistics. More recently, Zemel et al. (55) found that there was a strong inverse relationship between calcium intake and the risk of being in the highest quartile of BMI. These studies have prompted a reevaluation of studies measuring calcium intake or giving calcium orally. In the prospective trials, subjects receiving calcium had a greater weight loss than those who were receiving placebos. Increasing calcium

from 0 to nearly 2000 g/d was associated with a reduction in BMI of ~5 BMI units (56). These data might suggest that low calcium intake is playing a role in the current epidemic of obesity.

f. Frequency of Eating

The relationship between the frequency of meals and the development of obesity is unsettled. Many anecdotal reports argue that overweight persons eat less often than normal-weight persons, but documentation is scanty. However, frequency of eating does change lipid and glucose metabolism. When normal subjects eat several small meals a day, serum cholesterol concentrations are lower than when they eat a few large meals a day. Similarly, mean blood glucose concentrations are lower when meals are frequent (57). One explanation for the effects of frequent small meals compared with a few large meals could be the greater insulin secretion associated with larger meals.

g. Restrained Eating

A pattern of conscious limitation of food intake is called "restrained" eating (58). It is common in many, if not most, middle-aged women of "normal weight." It also may account for the inverse relationship of body weight to social class; women of upper socioeconomic status often use restrained eating to maintain their weight. In a weight loss clinic, higher restraint scores were associated with lower body weights (59). Weight loss was associated with a significant increase in restraint, indicating that higher levels of conscious control maintain lower weight. Greater increases in restraint correlate with greater weight loss, but also with higher risk of "lapse" or loss of control and overeating.

h. Binge-Eating Disorder

Binge-eating disorder is a psychiatric illness characterized by uncontrolled episodes of eating, usually in the evening (60). The patient may respond to treatment with drugs that modulate serotonin.

i. Night-Eating Syndrome

The night-eating syndrome is the consumption of at least 25% (and usually >50%) of daily energy intake between the evening meal and the next morning (61,62). It is one pattern of disturbed eating in the obese. It is related to sleep disturbances and may be a component of sleep apnea, in which daytime somnolence and nocturnal wakefulness are often found.

6 Psychological and Social Factors

Psychological factors in the development of obesity are widely recognized, although attempts to define a specific personality type that causes obesity have been unsuccessful. One condition linked to weight gain is seasonal affective disorder (SAD), which refers to the depression that occurs during the winter season in some people living in the North, where days are short. These patients tend to increase body weight in winter. This can be effectively treated by providing higher-intensity artificial lighting in the winter (63).

7 Socioeconomic and Ethnic Factors

Obesity is more prevalent in lower socioeconomic groups in the United States and elsewhere. The inverse relationship of socioeconomic status (SES) and overweight is found in both adults and children. In the Minnesota Heart Study (64), for example, the SES and BMI were inversely related. People of higher SES were more concerned with healthy weight control practices, including exercise, and tended to eat less fat. In the National Heart, Lung and Blood Institute Growth and Health Study (65), SES and overweight were strongly associated in Caucasian 9- and 10-year-old girls and their mothers, but not in African-American girls. The association of SES and overweight is much stronger in Caucasian women than in African-American women. African-American women of all ages are more obese than are Caucasian women. African-American men are less obese than white men, and socioeconomic factors are much less evident in men. The prevalence of obesity in Hispanic men and women is higher than in Caucasians. The basis for these ethnic differences is unclear. In men, the socioeconomic effects of obesity are weak or absent. This gender difference, and the higher prevalence of overweight in women, suggests important interactions of gender with many factors that influence body fat and fat distribution. The reason for this association is not known.

8 Genetic and Congenital Disorders

Discovery of the basis for the five single-gene defects that produce obesity in animals was followed by the recognition that these same defects, though rare, also produce human obesity. Table 6 summarizes the clinical features of 25 cases caused by seven genetic defects.

The rare humans with leptin deficiency correspond to the obese (ob/ob) mouse animal model (66–68). Leptin is a 167–amino acid protein produced in adipose tissue, the placenta, and possibly other tissues that signals the brain through leptin receptors about the size of adipose stores. In three families, consanguineous marriages led to expression of the recessive leptin-deficient state. These very fat children are hypogonadal, but are not hypothermic or endocrine deficient. They lose weight when treated with leptin. A defect in the leptin receptor

Table 6 Cases of Human Obesity Caused by Single-Gene Mutations

Gene	Location	Mutation	Case no.	Sex	Age	Weight (kg)	BMI kg/m^2	Ref.
LEPR	1p31	G to A (exon 16)	1	F	19	166	65.5	Clément et al. (69)
			2	F	13	159	71.5	
			3	F	19	133	52.5	
POMC	2p23	G7013T and C deletion at nt 7133 exon 3; C3804A exon 2	4	F	3	30	NA	Krude et al. (73)
			5	M	7	50	NA	
THRB	3p42.1–p22	Cys434Stop C to v A exon 10	6	F	15	46	26.3	Behr et al. 1997 (73a)
PPARG	3p25	Pro115Gln	7	M	65	NA	47.3	Ristow et al. (74)
			8	F	32	NA	38.5	
			9	M	54	NA	43.8	
			10	M	75	NA	37.9	
PCSK1	5q15–q21	Gly483Arg A to C^{+1} intron 5	11	F	3	36	NA	Jackson et al. (75)
LEP	7q31	G398Δ (codon 133) C to T (codon 105) (exon 3)	12	F	8	86	45.8	Montague et al. (66)
			13	M	2	29	36.6	
			14	F	6	NA	32.5	Strobel et al. (67)
			15	M	22	NA	55.8	
			16	F	34	NA	46.9	
			17	F	30	130	54.9	Ozata et al. (68)

(69) has also been described, and these patients are very fat, just as are the leptin-deficient children. Also, they do not respond to leptin because they lack the leptin receptor.

A third defect results from mutations in the melanocortin receptor (70–72) (Table 6). Several forms of this receptor transmit signals for activation of the adrenal gland by ACTH (melanocortin 1-receptor), activation of the melanocyte (melanocortin 2-receptor), and suppression of food intake by α-MSH (melanocortin 3-receptor and melanocortin 4-receptor). Genetic engineering to eliminate the MC4R in the mouse brain produces massive obesity. Several reports claim a genetic defect in this receptor is the culprit in some humans with obesity. These individuals of either sex are also massively obese. A much rarer form of human obesity has been reported when production of proopiomelanocortin (POMC), the precursor for peptides that act on the melanocortin receptors, is defective (73). These people have red hair and endocrine defects and are moderately obese.

The peroxisome proliferator–activated receptor-γ (PPAR-γ) is important in the control of fat cell differentiation (74). Defects in the PPAR-γ receptor in humans have been reported to produce modest degrees of obesity that begin later in life. The activation of this receptor by thiazolidinediones, a class of antidiabetic drugs, is also a cause for an increase in body fat (see Table 5).

The final human defect that has been described is in prohormone convertase 1 (75,76). In one family a defect in this gene and in a second gene was associated with obesity. Members of the family with only the PC-1 defect were not obese, suggesting that it was the interaction of two genes that lead to obesity.

Several congenital forms of obesity exist, which are more abundant than most of the single-gene defects. The Prader-Willi syndrome results from an abnormality on chromosome 15q11.2 that is transmitted paternally (77). This chromosomal defect produces a "floppy" baby who usually has trouble feeding. Obesity in these children begins at about age 2 and is associated with overeating, hypogonadism, and mental retardation (77).

The Bardet-Biedl syndrome (78,79) is a rare variety of congenital obesity. It is named after the two physicians who described it in separated publications in the 1920s. It is a recessively inherited disorder that can be diagnosed when four of the six cardinal features are present. These six cardinal features are: (1) progressive tapetoretinal degeneration; (2) distal limb abnormalities; (3) obesity; (4) renal involvement

(80); (5) hypogenitalism in men; and (6) mental retardation (Table 7).

The genetic defect in one form of the Bardet-Biedl syndrome (BBS6) has been identified on chromosome 20q12 as a "chaperonin-like" protein that is involved in folding proteins (81). It is allelic with the McKusick-Kaplan syndrome (MKKS). This latter syndrome is characterized by polydactyly, hydrometrocolpus, and heart problems, but without obesity. When obesity is present, however, it must enter into the differential diagnosis (see below).

When the diagnosis of the **Bardet-Biedl syndrome** is suspected, it needs to be distinguished from a group of rare genetically transmitted forms of obesity. These include the **Prader-Willi syndrome** (77), which is transmitted sporadically through chromosomal abnormalities in the paternal chromosome. Intrauterine movement is reduced and at birth the infants are "floppy" babies that have trouble breathing and feeding. The obesity begins at age 1–3 years, and these children tend to be short. There are mild to moderate mental retardation and characteristic facies (narrow bifrontal diameter, strabismus, and V-shaped mouth), and they have hypogonadism. **Alstrom syndrome** (82) is an autosomal-recessive disorder with abdominal obesity beginning at age 2–5 years. Intelligence and stature are normal. The retinal problem is severe with progressive infantile retinal cone-rod dystrophy. Males are

Table 7 Features of the Bardet-Biedl Syndrome[a]

Features of the syndrome	
Tapetoretinal degeneration (retinal dystrophy)	100%
Renal abnormalities	100%
Obesity (grossly obese = 56%)	98%
Dysmorphic extremities	50%
Bachydactyly	100%
Polydactyly-feet	89%
hands	50%
Hypogenitalism in men (small genitalia in 7/8)	88%
Menstrual irregularities (11/11 women)	100%
Mental retardation	41%
Diabetes (9/20)	45%
Macrocephaly	17%

[a] Diagnosis required presence of four of the six cardinal features indicated by *italics*.
Source: Ref. xxx.

hypogonadal. There are hearing disorders that may lead to deafness. There are also kidney disease and diabetes mellitus. **Cohen's syndrome** is an autosomal-recessive disorder characterized by abdominal obesity beginning before age 5. Stature can be normal, short, or tall. There are craniofacial disorders with cleft lip, arched palate, and dysplastic ears. Hypodonadism is present along with mild mental regardation. **Carpenter's syndrome** is also an autosomal-recessive disorder. Stature is normal. There is acrocephaly, gynoid obesity, hypogonadism, and slight mental retardation. The presence of polydactyly or syndactyly make this closest to the Bardet-Biedl syndrome. **Type 2 Biemond syndrome** (83) is a very rare disease closely related to the Bardet-Biedl syndrome. Obesity is not always present, but there are mental retardation, short stature, coloboma of the iris, polydactyly, hypogonadism, hydrocephalus, and facial dysostosis. Finally, the **McKusick-Kaplan syndrome** must be considered since one author has reported a group of children diagnosed with the MKKS in infancy who were later classified as Bardet-Biedl syndrome when obesity and retinal dystrophy developed (84).

In one study (85) the prevalence of obesity in heterozygotic fathers was examined and found to be 27%, compared to 9% in white males of comparable age. If the BBS gene is present at a frequency of 1% in the population, then it could account for 2.9% of all severely overweight males. However, Reed et al. (86) did not find a relation between markers in the vicinity of the BBS genes and obesity in markedly obese humans.

II NATURAL HISTORY OF OBESITY

Individuals can become overweight at any age, but this is more common at certain ages. At birth, those who will and those who will not become obese later in life can rarely be distinguished by weight (87), except for the infants of diabetic mothers, for whom the likelihood of obesity later in life is increased (88). Thus, at birth, a large pool of individuals will eventually become overweight, and a smaller group will never become overweight. I have labeled these pools "preoverweight" (Fig. 2) and "never overweight," using the NCHS data for prevalence of BMI >25 kg/m^2 as the solid line.

Several surveys suggest that one-third of overweight adults become overweight before age 20, and two-thirds do so after that (2). Thus, 75–80% of adults will become overweight at some time. Between 20% and 25% of the population will display their overweight before age 20, and 50% will do so after age 20. Some of these overweight individuals will develop clinically significant

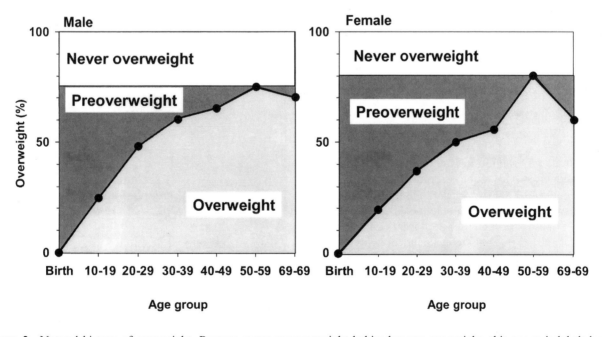

Figure 2 Natural history of overweight. Because many nonoverweight babies become overweight, this group is labeled preoverweight. About one-third of those who become overweight do so before age 20, and two-thirds do so after. The remainder are not overweight.

Table 8   Predictors of Weight Gain

Parental overweight
Lower socioeconomic status
Smoking cessation
Low level of physical activity
Low metabolic rate
Childhood overweight
Heavy babies
Lack of maternal knowledge of child's sweet-eating habits
Recent marriage
Multiple birth

problems such as diabetes, hypertension, gallbladder disease, or the metabolic syndrome. These are the overweight people that I call "clinically overweight."

Because most preoverweight people will become overweight, it is important to have as much insight as possible into the risk factors. Table 8 lists a number of predictors for overweight. These predictors fall into two broad groups: demographic and metabolic. When an individual becomes overweight (i.e., BMI >25 kg/m^2) without clinically significant problems, they manifest "overweight" or "preclinical overweight." With the passage of time or a further increase in weight, they may show clinical signs of diabetes, hypertension, gallbladder disease, or dyslipidemia. I call this group "clinical overweight." The relationship of one to the other may be depicted as a pyramid (Fig. 3).

At the base is the reservoir of never-overweight and preoverweight individuals, many of whom will become overweight in their adult life. Some of these will in turn show signs of clinical disease and become clinically overweight.

A   Overweight Developing Before Age 10

1   Prenatal Factors

Caloric intake by the mother may influence body size, shape, and later body composition. Birth weights of identical and fraternal twins have the same correlation ($r = .63$), indicating that birth weight is a poor predictor of future obesity (87). In the first years of life, the correlation of body weight among identical twins begins to converge, rapidly becoming much closer together ($r = .9$), whereas dizygotic twins diverge during this same period ($r = .5$). Infants born to diabetic mothers have a higher risk of being overweight as children and adults (88). Infants who are small-for-dates, are short, or have a small head circumference are at higher risk of developing abdominal fatness and other comorbidities associated with obesity later in life (89).

2   Infancy Through Age 3

Body weight triples and body fat normally doubles in the first year of life. This increase in body fat and how long the infant was breastfed in the first year of life are important predictors of overweight later in life in infants and young children with overweight parents. An infant above the 85th centile at age 1–3 years has a fourfold increased risk of adult overweight if either parent is overweight, compared with nonoverweight infants. If neither parent is overweight, this infantile overweight does not predict overweight in early adult life (Fig. 4) (90). These observations are similar to the older observations suggesting that the risk for adult obesity was 80% for children with two overweight parents, 40% for those with one overweight parent, and <10% if neither parent was overweight (2).

3   Childhood Obesity from Age 3 to Age 10

Ages between 3 and 10 are high-risk years for developing obesity. Adiposity rebound describes the inflection point between a declining BMI and an increasing BMI that occurs between age 5 and 7 years. The earlier this rebound occurs, the greater the risk of overweight later in life. About half of the overweight grade school children remain overweight as adults. Moreover, the risk of overweight in adulthood was at least twice as great for overweight children as for nonoverweight

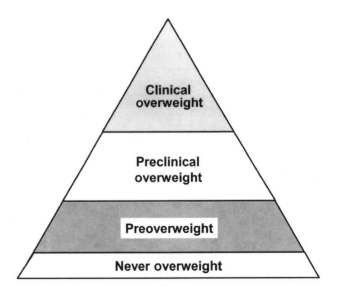

Figure 3   Pyramid of overweight. Many individuals who become overweight do not have diabetes, hypertension, or other diseases. These are called preclinical overweight. Those who develop clinical disease are clinically overweight.

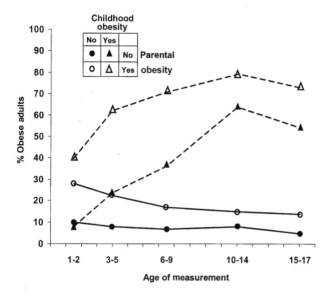

Figure 4 Effect of parental and childhood weight on weight status during early adulthood. Percentage of overweight adults are plotted in relation to whether the child was overweight at each age and whether the child had one or both overweight parents at the same time. When one parent was overweight, nonoverweight 1- to 2-year-old children had a much greater risk of becoming overweight as adults than children with no overweight parents. This effect of parental weight status was no longer evident by age 7–9. The effect of parental overweight declined as children entered adolescence, and the tracking of adolescent overweight into early adulthood became much stronger. (From Ref. 12.)

children. The risk is three to 10 times higher if the child's weight is above the 95th centile for age. Parental overweight plays a strong role in this group as well. Nearly 75% of overweight children age 3–10 remained overweight in early adulthood if they had one or more overweight parents, compared with 25–50% if neither parent was overweight. Overweight 3- to 10-year-olds with an overweight parent thus constitutes an ideal group for behavioral therapy. When body weight progressively deviates from the upper limits of normal in this age group, I label it "progressive obesity" (2); this is usually severe and lifelong, and is associated with an increase in the number of fat cells.

B Overweight Developing in Adolescence and Adult Life

1 Adolescence

Weight in adolescence becomes a progressively better predictor of adult weight status (Fig. 4). In a 55-year follow-up of adolescents, the weight status in adolescence predicted later adverse health events (91). Adolescents above the 95th centile had a five- to 20-fold greater likelihood of overweight in adulthood. In contrast with younger ages, parental overweight is less important, or has already had its effect. While 70–80% of overweight adolescents with an overweight parent were overweight as young adults, the numbers were only modestly lower (54–60%) for overweight adolescents without overweight parents. Despite the importance of childhood and adolescent weight status, however, it remains clear that most overweight individuals develop their problem in adult life (2).

2 Adult Women

Most overweight women gain their excess weight after puberty. This weight gain may be precipitated by a number of events, including pregnancy, oral contraceptive therapy, and the menopause.

a. Pregnancy

Weight gain during pregnancy, and the effect of pregnancy on subsequent weight gain, are important events in the weight gain history of women (92). A few women gain considerable weight during pregnancy, occasionally >50 kg. The pregnancy itself may leave a legacy of increased weight, as suggested by one study that evaluated women prospectively between the ages of 18 and 30 years (93). Women who remained nulliparous (n = 925) were compared with women who had a single pregnancy of 28 weeks' duration during that period and who were at least 12 months postpartum. The primiparas gained 2–3 kg more weight and had a greater increase in WHR than with the nulliparous women during this period. The overall risk of weight gain associated with childbearing after age 25, however, is quite modest for most American women (94).

b. Oral Contraceptives

Oral contraceptive use may initiate weight gain in some women, although this effect is diminished with the low-dose estrogen pills. One study evaluated 49 healthy women initiating treatment with a low-dose oral contraceptive (30 mg ethinyl estradiol plus 75 mg gestodene). Anthropometric measurements before and after the initiation of this formulation were used to compare 31 age- and weight-matched women (95). Baseline BMI, percent fat, percent water, and WHR did not change significantly after six cycles in the birth control pill users. A similar number of women gained weight in both groups (30.6% of users, 35.4% of controls). The typical weight gain in the pill user group was only 0.5 kg, but the small weight gain in these women was attributable to the accumulation of fat, not body water. Approximately 20% of women in both groups lost weight.

c. Menopause

Weight gain and changes in fat distribution occur after the menopause. The decline in estrogen and progesterone secretion alters fat cell biology so that central fat deposition increases.

Estrogen replacement therapy does not prevent the weight gain, although it may minimize fat redistribution (96). A prospective study of 63 early postmenopausal women compared 34 who initiated continuous estrogen and progesterone therapy to the remaining women who refused it. Body weight and fat mass increased significantly in both the treatment (71.5–73.5 kg) and the control groups (73.2–75.6 kg). However, WHR increased significantly only in the control group (0.80–0.85). Caloric and macronutrient intake did not change in either group. A 2-year trial with estrogen in postmenopausal women also showed an increase in body fat (97).

3 Adult Men

The transition from an active lifestyle during the teens and early 20s to a more sedentary lifestyle thereafter is associated with weight gain in many men. The rise in body weight continues through the adult years until the sixth decade (see Fig. 2). After ages 55–64, relative weight remains stable and then begins to decline. Evidence from the Framingham Study and studies of men in the armed services suggests that men became progressively heavier for height during the 20th century.

C Weight Stability and Weight Cycling

Body weight varies throughout the day as food is eaten and then metabolized. Body weight also varies from day to day, from week to week, and over longer intervals. Understanding these fluctuations and their relationship to more significant weight cycling related to dieting and regain (yo-yo dieting) is important in understanding obesity (98). Adults under age 55 tend to gain weight, and those over 55 tend to lose it (99). The youngest adults gain the most weight, and the oldest adults lose the most. Women have significantly greater variation in their weight over 10 years than do men. A 25% weight

gain was found in 2.9% of men aged 25–44, compared with 6.5% of women in the same age group. In the middle-age range, the numbers with weight gain of 25% had dropped by nearly half: 1.8% of men age 45–64, compared with 2.9% of women in the same age group. Weight loss of 25% or more in Americans age 65–74 was higher in women (6.5%) than in men (2.2%). The likelihood of a significant weight gain was substantially higher in the overweight than in those of normal weight in the younger age groups (99). Because the incidence of significant weight gain is more common in young adults, these are a prime target for preventive measures.

Weight cycling associated with dieting is popularly known as yo-yo dieting (98). Weight cycling refers to the downs and ups in weight that often happen to people who diet, lose weight, stop dieting, and regain the weight they lost and sometimes more. The possibility that the cycle of loss and regain is more detrimental than staying heavy has been hotly debated. In a review of the literature between 1964 and 1994, a group of experts concluded that most studies did not support any adverse effects on metabolism associated with weight cycling. Also, few or no data supported the contention that it is more difficult to lose weight a second time after regaining weight from a previous therapeutic approach. Most researchers agree that weight cycling neither necessarily increases body fat nor adversely affects blood pressure, glucose metabolism, or lipid concentrations.

III CLINICAL EVALUATION OF OVERWEIGHT PATIENTS

Overweight is now recognized as a risk factor for cardiovascular disease and as a contributing factor in the development of other diseases, most notably diabetes and gallbladder disease. In this context, it is important to evaluate and treat the obesity and other risk factors so as to reduce the overall likelihood for developing disease and to reduce the social consequence of being obese.

The section addresses the clinical evaluation of the overweight patients (1,100,101). It then reviews criteria for successful outcomes of treatment and goals of preventing progression from being at risk for overweight to becoming overweight, then developing the clinical sequelae of overweight (clinical overweight). Both clinical and laboratory information are needed for this evaluation. To make this evaluation effective, it must be done in the context of a sympathetic office practice concerned with the care and treatment of overweight patients. For additional insights into Care of the

Obese Patient in a Primary Care Setting, the reader is referred to the chapter by Kushner and Aronne.

A   Information from the Clinical Interview

The clinician or therapist who sees an overweight patient needs to obtain certain basic information which is relevant to assessing its risk (Table 9) (100–108). This includes an understanding of the events that led to the development of obesity, what patients have done to deal with the problem, and how successful and unsuccessful they were in these efforts. Several of these items are listed in Table 10. The family constellation is important for identifying attitudes about obesity and the possibility of finding rare genetic causes. Information about the amount of weight gain (>20 lb or >10 kg) since age 18–20 and the rate of weight gain is important because this is related to the risk of developing complications from obesity (109). The type and regularity of physical activity are also important since physical inactivity increases cardiovascular risk, particularly in overweight individuals (110). Information about comorbid conditions such as diabetes, hypertension, heart disease, sleep apnea, and gallbladder disease also needs to be elicited. Since a number of drugs can cause significant weight gain, a history of medication use for mental health problems, depression, convulsive disorders, diabetes, and for the use of steroids for asthma should be elicited as well. Information about whether the patient/client is "ready" to put in the effort needed to lose weight can help you decide with the patient whether this is the right time to proceed with treatment. Information about possible etiologies for obesity also needs to be obtained, for example, altered menstrual history in women suggesting

polycystic ovary syndrome, purplish abdominal striae suggesting Cushing's disease.

B   Clinical Evaluation

1   Step 1: Physical Measurements

a.   *Vital Signs*

As part of any clinical encounter, the nurse or physician should measure several so-called vital signs including height, weight (BMI), pulse, blood pressure, waist circumference, and if indicated by the patient's complaints, temperature.

b.   *Body Mass Index*

Accurate measurement of height and weight which are used to calculate the BMI is the initial step in the clinical assessment of overweight (107,111). This index is calculated as the body weight (kg) divided by the stature (height [m]) squared (wt/ht^2), or body weight (lb) $\times$ 703 divided by the height (stature) squared $(\text{Wt(lb)} \times 703/[\text{Ht(in)}]^2$. Table 10 lists BMI values for height in centimeters or inches and weight in kilograms or pounds. BMI correlates well with body fat, and is relatively unaffected by height.

This is the first step in assessing risk. Current classifications of obesity are based on BMI and waist circumference. The one recommended by the World Health Organization (105) and the National Heart, Lung and Blood Institute (100) is shown in Table 11.

BMI has a curvilinear relationship to risk (Fig. 5). Several levels of risk can be identified using the BMI. These cut-points are derived from data collected on Caucasians. It is now clear that different ethnic groups

Table 9   Clinical Information from Interview

	Yes	No
Are members of your family overweight?		
Do your parents or grandparents have diabetes?		
Do you have diabetes?		
Do you have high blood pressure?		
Do you take thyroid hormone?		
Have you gained 20 or more lb (10 kg) since age 20?		
Do you fall asleep easily during the day?		
Do you exercise regularly?		
Do you have gallstone or gallbladder disease		
Do you take medications regularly? If so, specify		
Are you depressed?		
For women: Do you have normal menstrual periods?		

Table 10 Body Mass Index[a] (Using Either Pounds and Inches or Kilograms and Centimeters)

	Body mass index (kg/m²)																						
Inches	19	20	21	22	23	24	25	26	27	28	29	30	31	32	33	34	35	36	37	38	39	40	
58	91	95	100	105	110	115	119	124	129	134	138	143	148	153	158	162	167	172	177	181	186	191	Cm
	41	43	45	48	50	52	54	56	58	61	63	65	67	69	71	73	76	78	80	82	84	86	147
59	94	99	104	109	114	119	124	128	133	138	143	148	153	158	163	168	173	178	183	188	193	198	
	43	45	47	50	52	54	56	59	61	63	65	68	70	72	74	77	79	81	83	86	88	90	150
60	97	102	107	112	118	123	128	133	138	143	148	153	158	164	169	174	179	184	189	194	199	204	
	44	46	49	51	53	55	58	60	62	65	67	69	72	74	76	79	81	83	85	88	90	92	152
61	100	106	111	116	121	127	132	137	143	148	153	158	164	169	174	180	185	190	195	201	206	211	
	46	48	50	53	55	58	60	62	65	67	70	72	74	77	79	82	84	86	89	91	94	96	155
62	104	109	115	120	125	131	136	142	147	153	158	164	169	175	180	186	191	196	202	207	213	218	
	47	50	52	55	57	60	62	65	67	70	72	75	77	80	82	85	87	90	92	95	97	100	158
63	107	113	118	124	130	135	141	146	152	158	163	169	175	180	186	192	197	203	208	214	220	225	
	49	51	54	56	59	61	64	67	69	72	74	77	79	82	84	87	90	92	95	97	100	102	160
64	110	116	122	128	134	140	145	151	157	163	169	174	180	186	192	198	203	209	215	221	227	233	
	50	52	55	58	60	63	66	68	71	73	76	79	81	84	87	89	92	94	97	100	102	105	162
65	114	120	126	132	138	144	150	156	162	168	174	180	186	192	198	204	210	216	222	228	234	240	
	52	54	57	60	63	65	68	71	74	76	79	82	84	87	90	93	95	98	101	103	106	109	165
66	117	124	130	136	142	148	155	161	167	173	179	185	192	198	204	210	216	223	229	235	241	247	
	54	56	59	62	65	68	71	73	76	79	82	85	87	90	93	96	99	102	104	107	110	113	168
67	121	127	134	140	147	153	159	166	172	178	185	191	198	204	210	217	223	229	236	242	248	255	
	55	58	61	64	66	69	72	75	78	81	84	87	90	92	95	98	101	104	107	110	113	116	170
68	125	131	138	144	151	158	164	171	177	184	190	197	203	210	217	223	230	236	243	249	256	263	
	57	60	63	66	69	72	75	78	81	84	87	90	93	96	99	102	105	108	111	114	117	120	173
69	128	135	142	149	155	162	169	176	182	189	196	203	209	216	223	230	237	243	250	257	264	270	
	58	61	64	67	70	74	77	80	83	86	89	92	95	98	101	104	107	110	113	116	119	123	175
70	132	139	146	153	160	167	174	181	188	195	202	209	216	223	230	236	243	250	257	264	271	278	
	60	63	67	70	73	76	79	82	86	89	92	95	98	101	105	108	111	114	117	120	124	127	178
71	136	143	150	157	165	172	179	186	193	200	207	215	222	229	236	243	250	258	265	272	279	286	
	62	65	68	71	75	78	81	84	87	91	94	97	100	104	107	110	113	117	120	123	126	130	180
72	140	147	155	162	169	177	184	191	199	206	213	221	228	235	243	250	258	265	272	280	287	294	
	64	67	70	74	77	80	84	87	90	94	97	100	104	107	111	114	117	121	124	127	131	134	183
73	144	151	159	166	174	182	189	197	204	212	219	227	234	242	250	257	265	272	280	287	295	303	
	65	68	72	75	79	82	86	89	92	96	99	103	106	110	113	116	120	123	127	130	133	137	185
74	148	155	163	171	179	187	194	202	210	218	225	233	241	249	256	264	272	280	288	295	303	311	
	67	71	74	78	81	85	88	92	95	99	102	106	110	113	117	120	124	127	131	134	138	141	188
75	152	160	168	176	184	192	200	208	216	224	232	240	247	255	263	271	279	287	295	303	311	319	
	69	72	76	79	83	87	90	94	97	101	105	108	112	116	119	123	126	130	134	137	141	144	190
76	156	164	172	180	189	197	205	213	221	230	238	246	254	262	271	279	287	295	303	312	320	328	
	71	74	78	82	86	89	93	97	101	104	108	112	115	119	123	127	130	134	138	142	145	149	193
BMI	19	20	21	22	23	24	25	26	27	28	29	30	31	32	33	34	35	36	37	38	39	40	BMI

[a] The Body Mass Index is shown as **bold underlined** numbers at the top and bottom. To determine your BMI, select your height in either inches or cm and move across the row until you find your weight in pounds or inches. Your BMI can be read at the top or bottom. *The Italics are for pounds and inches*; **The bold is for kilograms and centimeters.**
Copyright 1999 George A. Bray.

have different percentages of body fat for the same BMI. Thus, the same BMI presumably carries a different risk in each of these populations. The BMI needs to be adjusted for ethnicity. The variations in percent body fat for Caucasians, African Americans, Asians and Latinos for the same BMI and age is shown in Table 12 (112). For Japanese, a BMI of 23 or 24 kg/m² has the same % fat as that of a BMI of 25 in Caucasians or 28–29 in African-Americans (see Deurenberg, Chap. 3). Based on these differences and the observations that the risk for diabetes and hypertension had doubled when the BMI was 25 kg/m², a task force from the Asia-

Table 11 Classification of Overweight and Obesity as Recommended by the NHLBI Guidelines

| | BMI (kg/m²) | Obesity class | Disease risk[a] relative to normal weight and waist circumference | |
			Men <102 cm Women <88 cm	>102 cm >88 cm
Underweight	<18.5		—	—
Normal[b]	18.5–24.9		—	—
Overweight	25.0–29.9		Increased	High
Obesity	30.0–34.9	1	High	Very high
	35.0–39.9	2	Very high	Very high
Extreme obesity	≥40.0	3	Extremely high	Extremely high

[a] Disease risk for type 2 diabetes, hypertension; and CVD.
[b] Increased waist can also be a marker for increased risk in normal-weight individuals.
Source: Refs. 100, 105.

Oceania section of the International Association for the Study of Obesity has proposed an alternative table where obesity is defined as a BMI >25 kg/m² and high-risk waist circumference at >90 cm for men and >80 cm for women (Table 13).

Data from Hispanics and African-Americans suggest that increased body fat carries a greater risk of diabetes, but has less impact on heart disease. Figure 5 also identifies cut-points to separate preoverweight from overweight and clinical overweight or obesity, using BMI alone. After treatment begins, regular measurement of body weight is one important way to follow the progress of any treatment program.

2 Step 2: Measure Waist Circumference

The most accurate measurement of visceral or central fat is obtained from a computed tomogram or with

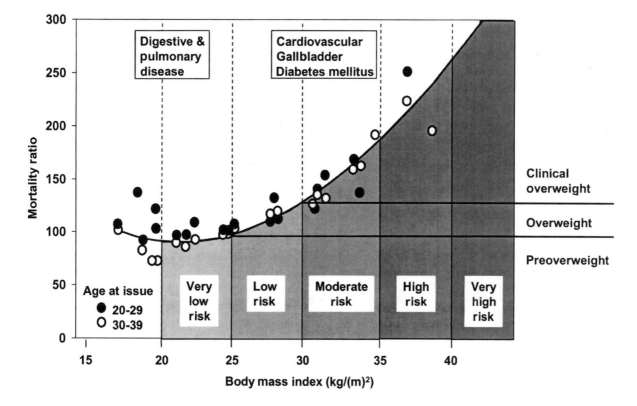

Figure 5 Relation of health risk to BMI and definitions of preoverweight, preclinical overweight, and clinical overweight.

Table 12 Variations in % Body Fat for African-Americans, Asian, and Caucasians

	Females			Males		
	African-American	Asian	Caucasian	African-American	Asian	Caucasian
Age–20–39						
18.5	20	25	21	8	13	8
25	32	35	33	20	23	21
30	38	40	39	26	28	26
Age–40–59						
18.5	21	25	23	9	13	11
25	34	36	35	22	24	23
30	39	41	41	27	29	29

Source: Ref. 112.

MRI, but these are expensive and not generally available for this purpose. Waist circumference is the most practical clinical alternative. Waist circumference is measured with a flexible tape placed horizontally at the level of the natural waist line or narrowest part of the torso as seen anteriorly (107,111).

Measuring the change in waist circumference is another good tool for following the progress of weight loss. It is particularly valuable when patients become more physically active. Physical activity may slow loss of muscle mass and thus slow weight loss while fat continues to be mobilized. Changes in waist circumference can help in making this distinction. As with BMI, the relationship of central fat to risk factors for health varies among populations as well as within them.

a. The Metabolic Syndrome

The metabolic syndrome is a complex of traits that enhance the risk of cardiovascular disease. It includes a variety of factors, including central obesity, hypertension, insulin resistance, dyslipidemia, and diabetes mellitus. In an effort to provide a definition of this syndrome, the Adult Treatment Panel III of the National Cholesterol Education Program (17,18) has provided the following defining features (Table 14). The syndrome is associated with abdominal obesity, measured in this definition by waist circumference. The recognition that the differences in ethnic populations have different relations of abdominal fat and its risks indicates that these definitions, like BMI itself, may need ethnic sensitivity in its interpretation. For example, measurements of insulin resistance suggest that individuals of Asian descent (Chinese, Japanese, and South Indians) may have more abdominal fat for a given BMI and body fat than Caucasians.

b. Other Physical Aspects of Obesity

A number of physical features of an obese individual may help identify a specific cause for their problem. Features of the hypothalamic syndrome were presented

Table 13 Classification of Obesity as Recommended by the Asia-Pacific Task Force

		Risk of comorbidities	
		Waist circumference	
Classification	BMI (kg/m^2)	<90 cm (men) <80 cm (women)	≥90 cm (men) ≥80 cm (women)
Underweight	<18.5	Low (but increased risk of other clinical problems)	Average
Normal range	18.5–22.9	Average	Increased
Overweight	≥23		
At risk	23–24.9	Increased	Moderate
Obese I	25–25.9	Moderate	Severe
Obese II	≥30	Severe	Very severe

Table 14 Clinical Features of the Metabolic Syndrome

Risk factor abdominal obesity (waist circumference)	Defining level
Men	>102 cm (>40 in.)
Women	> 88 cm (>35 in.)
HDL cholesterol	
Men	< 40 mg/dL
Women	< 50 mg/dL
Triglycerides	≥150 mg/dL
Fasting glucose	≥110 mg/dL
Blood pressure (SBP/DBP)	≥130/≥85 mm Hg

in Table 2. Cushing's syndrome has been described in Table 3. Polycystic ovarian disease is a common cause of obesity in younger women, and its features are shown in Table 4. Among the various genetic diseases that produce obesity, the Prader-Willi syndrome is the most common. It includes hypotonia, mental retaradation, and sexual immaturity, and can usually be recognized clinically. The Bardet-Biedl syndrome with its polydactyly and retinal disease is distinctive. A child with obesity and red hair might suggest a defect in the processing of pro-opiomelanocortin. Detection of acanthosis nigricans should suggest significant insulin resistance. This is a clinical finding of increased very dark pigmentation in the folds of the neck, along the exterior surface of the distal extremities, and over the knuckles. It may signify increased insulin resistance or malignancy, and these possibilities should be evaluated.

C Laboratory Tests and the Metabolic Syndrome

The third part of the evaluation is the laboratory tests. At the present time, laboratory tests often come in "batteries" that provide a larger number of tests than may be needed, but where unbundling these tests is more expensive than any benefits it gains. It is thus important to focus attention on the laboratory tests that are most relevant to decision making about the overweight patient. Because diabetes, gallbladder disease, heart disease, sleep apnea, and cancer have a relationship to obesity, these are important tests to evaluate with laboratory tests.

1 Plasma Glucose

With over 7% of the adult American population having diabetes and in the face of an epidemic, measurement and, if needed, confirmation of a high glucose or a 2-hr

value in a glucose tolerance test is the first order of business (Table 15).

2 Plasma Lipids

A low HDL cholesterol and a high triglycerides provides one combination of laboratory values that are included in the diagnosis of the metabolic syndrome. These are thus important values to determine. LDL cholesterol is the pivotal lipoprotein in decisions about prevention and treatment of coronary heart disease and other vascular diseases. In the presence of diabetes these values are lowered (Table 16).

3 TSH

TSH is important as an index of hypothyroidism, which can occur in up to 4% of older women and may be a factor in weight gain at this time in life.

4 Prostate-Specific Antigen (PSA)

Prostate cancer is one of the cancers associated with obesity. Although PSA is a common screening test in men, the relationship of obesity to prostate cancer highlights its value when screening overweight men.

5 Mammography

Breast cancer is increased in obese women. The presence of obesity may suggest the need for mammography on a regular basis.

6 Ultrasound of the Gallbladder

The high prevalence of gallstones in obese men and women would suggest the desirability of an ultrasound, especially if there any abdominal complaints of indigestion.

D Clinical Plan

Once the workup for etiologic and complicating factors is complete, the risk associated with elevated BMI, fat

Table 15 Diagnostic Criteria for Diabetes

	Fasting glucose	2-hr Value from glucose tolerance test
Diagnostic category	mg/dL	mg/dL
Normal	<110	>140
Impaired glucose tolerance (IGT)	110–125	140–199
Diabetes	≤126	>200

Table 16 LDL Cholesterol Goals and Cutpoints for Therapeutic Lifestyle Changes and Drug Therapy

Risk category	LDL goal	LDL level at which to initiate therapeutic lifestyle changes	LDL level at which to consider drug therapy
CHD or CHD risk Equivalents (10-year risk >20%	< 100 mg/dL	100 mg/dL	130 mg/dL (100–129 mg/dL: drug optional)
2+ Risk factors (10-year risk 20%)	< 130 mg/dL	130 mg/dL	10-year risk 10–20% 130 mg/dL; 10-year risk <10% 160 mg/dL
0–1 Risk factors	< 160 mg/dL	> 160 mg/dL	190 mg/dL (160–189 mg/dL: LDL-lowering drugs optional)

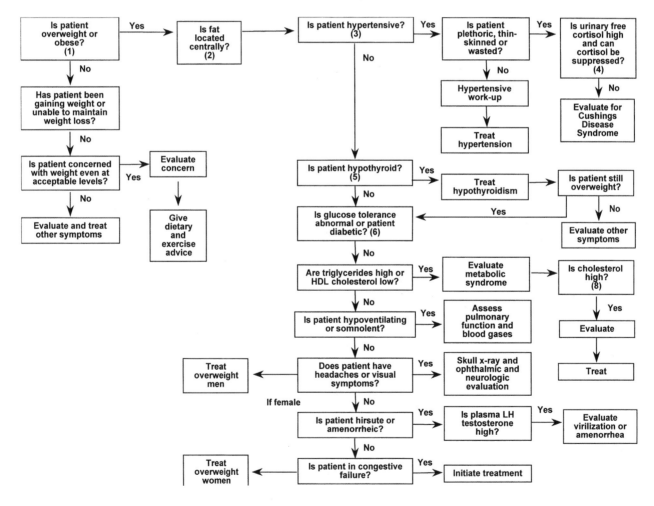

Figure 6 An algorithm for evaluating when laboratory and clinical testing may be needed and for approaching treatment strategies. (From Ref. 113.)

distribution, weight gain, and level of physical activity can be evaluated. Several algorithms have been developed for this purpose) (100,102,105,109). One of the earliest nomograms based on the BMI is shown in Figure 7 (102).

The BMI is divided into five unit intervals and modified by the presence or absence of complicating factors. Figure 8 shows a modification of this nomogram that was adopted in the World Health Organization monograph (105).

An early disease-oriented algorithm was published by Bray et al. (113) and updated in Figure 6. The one developed by the National Heart, Lung and Blood Institute (NHLBI) for The Practical Guide: Identification, Evaluation, and Treatment of Overweight and Obesity in Adults, is presented in Figure 9 (100).

The BMI provides the first assessment of risk. Individuals with a BMI <25 kg/m^2 are at very low risk but, nonetheless, nearly half of those in this category at age 20–25 will become overweight by age 60–69. Thus, a large group of preoverweight individuals need to prevent further weight gain. Risk rises with a BMI >25 kg/m^2 (Fig. 5). The presence of complicating factors further increases this risk. Thus, an attempt at a quantitative estimate of these complicating factors is important.

Treatments for obesity can be risky, as evidenced by the results from the past 100 years (Table 17). In many cases treatment for obesity needs to be chronic, hence

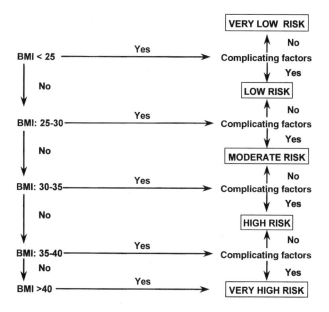

Figure 7 First algorithm using the BMI and "complicating factors" to develop a risk-based treatment plan. (Copyright 1987 Bray and Gray.)

the emphasis on risk-benefit and safety. Each treatment listed in Table 16 has been associated with a therapeutic disaster. This must temper enthusiasm for new treatments unless the risk is very low. Because obesity is stigmatized, any treatment approved by the FDA will be used for cosmetic purposes by preoverweight people who suffer the stigma of obesity. Thus, drugs to treat obesity must have very high safety profiles.

With a risk score based on BMI and waist circumference, treatment goals can be dilineated. The BMI is divided into five-unit intervals, just as in Figure 5. Risk, goals, and potential treatment strategies are noted opposite each of these intervals. Low levels of associated risks reduce the impact of any BMI, whereas high levels of these risk factors augment the effect of a given BMI. Using the BMI, selection of treatments can be more rational.

1 Is the Patient Ready to Lose Weight?

Before initiating any treatment, it is important to know that the patient's ready to make changes is important. A series of questions developed by Brownell (114) in the Dieting Readiness Test can be used to assess this.

When counseling patients who are ready to lose weight, accommodation of their individual needs, as well as ethnic factors, age, and other differences, is essential. The approach outlined above is not rigid and must be used to help guide clinical decision making, and not serve as an alternative to considering individual factors in developing a treatment plan. Because of increasing complications of obesity, more aggressive efforts at therapy should be directed at people in each of the successively higher risk classifications.

2 Do Patient and Doctor Have Realistic Expectations?

The doctor and his or her assistant who sees an elevated BMI in an overweight or obese patient should take a moment to make sure the patient knows his or her BMI and waist circumference and how to interpret them. If the patient know his or her BMI, it means that the physician or assistant also knows what the BMI and its adjustments mean. However, a recent survey showed that only 42% of obese patients seen for a routine checkup were told they needed to lose weight (115). We need to do better for our patients. The realities of treatment for obesity are often at odds with a patients' expectations. Patients were asked to give the weights they wanted to achieve in several categories, from their dream weight to a weight loss that would leave them disappointed (Fig. 9). These can be grouped as in Table

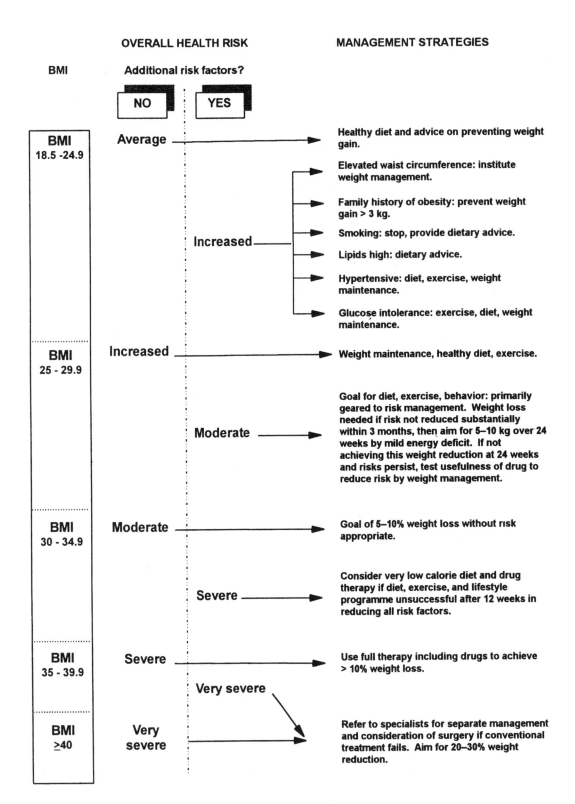

OVERALL HEALTH RISK   MANAGEMENT STRATEGIES

BMI   Additional risk factors?

NO   **YES**

BMI   Average   Healthy diet and advice on preventing weight
18.5 -24.9   gain.

Increased   Elevated waist circumference: institute
            weight management.

            Family history of obesity: prevent weight
            gain > 3 kg.

            Smoking: stop, provide dietary advice.

            Lipids high: dietary advice.

            Hypertensive: diet, exercise, weight
            maintenance.

            Glucose intolerance: exercise, diet, weight
            maintenance.

BMI   Increased   Weight maintenance, healthy diet, exercise.
25 - 29.9

            Moderate   Goal for diet, exercise, behavior: primarily
                        geared to risk management. Weight loss
                        needed if risk not reduced substantially
                        within 3 months, then aim for 5–10 kg over 24
                        weeks by mild energy deficit. If not
                        achieving this weight reduction at 24 weeks
                        and risks persist, test usefulness of drug to
                        reduce risk by weight management.

BMI   Moderate   Goal of 5–10% weight loss without risk
30 - 34.9   appropriate.

            Severe   Consider very low calorie diet and drug
                      therapy if diet, exercise, and lifestyle
                      programme unsuccessful after 12 weeks in
                      reducing all risk factors.

BMI   Severe   Use full therapy including drugs to achieve
35 - 39.9   > 10% weight loss.

            Very severe

BMI   Very   Refer to specialists for separate management
≥40   severe   and consideration of surgery if conventional
                    treatment fails. Aim for 20–30% weight
                    reduction.

Figure 8   WHO algorithm expands on the model with graded BMI and complicating factors and adds the appropriate treatment options.

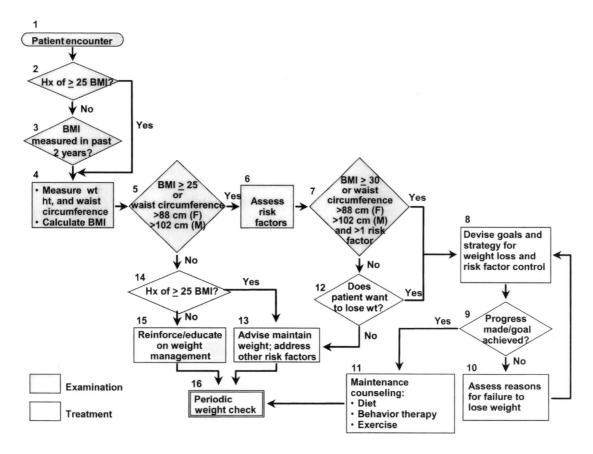

Figure 9 An algorithm for the assessment of overweight and obesity and subsequent decisions based on that assessment. (From Ref. 100.)

18 (116). When we compare the goals for these patients with the reported outcomes we find that many treatments will leave patients disappointed (Figure 9). The lines show the weight loss over time with a variety of different treatments (117–121). Note that only the surgical intervention produced a "dream" weight loss. None of the other treatments produced weight loss that would allow patients to achieve their dream weight,

Table 17 Disasters with Drug Treatments for Obesity

Date	Drug	Outcome
1893	Thyroid	Hyperthyroidism
1933	Dinitrophenol	Cataracts, neuropathy
1937	Amphetamine	Addiction
1967	Rainbow pills (digitalis, diuretics)	Death
1971	Aminorex	Pulmonary hypertension
1997	Fenfluramine/ phentermine	Valvular insufficiency

which was on average 38% below baseline. Nearly half failed to achieve even a weight loss outcome that would disappoint them. The desire to lose weight from a cosmetic standpoint almost always conflicts with the reality of weight loss. This mismatch between patient expectations and the realities of weight loss provides clinicians and their patients with an important challenge as they begin treatment. A weight loss goal of 5–15% can be achieved by most patients and will improve many of the risk factors associated with obesity (123).

One complaint about treatments for obesity is that they frequently fail. By this patients mean that weight loss stops well short of their desired level. An alternative interpretation may be better (122). Overweight is not curable. However, it can be treated in many ways, but in all cases weight loss reaches a "plateau" (see Fig. 10). When treatment is stopped, weight is regained. This is similar to what happens in patients with hypertension who stop taking their antihypertensive drugs, and in patients with high cholesterol who stop taking their hypocholesterolemic drugs. In each case, blood pressure

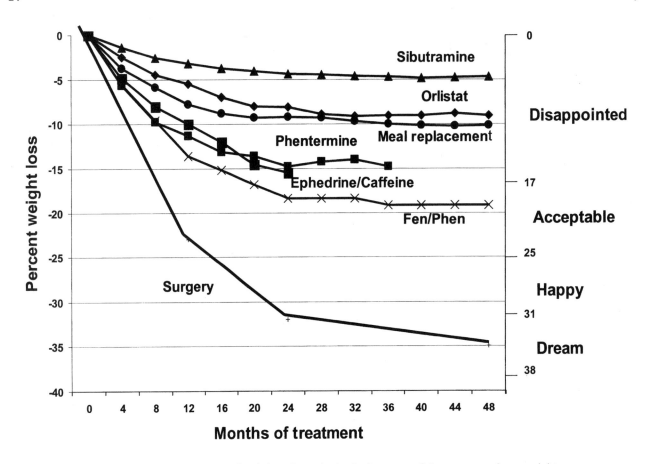

Figure 10   Natural history of weight gain and criteria for successful treatment of overweight.

or cholesterol rises. Like overweight, these chronic diseases have not been cured, but rather palliated. When treatment is stopped, the risk factor recurs.

A weight decrease of 5–15% from baseline improves most comorbidities associated with overweight (108). Patients who are ready to lose weight and have a reasonable expectation for their weight loss goals are ready to begin. An ideal outcome is a return of body weight to normal range with no weight gain thereafter (123) (Fig. 10).

However, this is rarely achieved and is unrealistic for most patients. Rather, they need guidance in accepting a realistic goal, usually a loss of 5–15% (108). A satisfactory outcome is a maintenance of body weight over the ensuing years. A good outcome would be a loss of 5–15% of initial body weight and regain no faster than the increase in body weight of the population (123). Patients who achieve this should be applauded. An excellent outcome would be weight loss of >15% of body weight. An unsatisfactory outcome is a loss of <5% with regain above the population weight.

E   Treatment Strategies by Age Group

After evaluating a patient and deciding that he or she is ready to lose weight, the patient can be placed in one of the categories based on the risk-adjusted BMI. The basic approaches to prevention and treatment are based on this characterization and the patient's age.

1   Age 1–10

Table 19 shows the strategies available for overweight children. A variety of genetic factors can enhance obesity in this age group (see chapter by Bouchard et al.). This age group also contains a high percentage of preoverweight individuals. Identifying individuals at highest risk for becoming overweight in adult life allows us to focus on preventive strategies. Among these strategies are the need to develop patterns of physical activity and good eating habits, including a lower fat intake and a lower energy density diet. Table 8 lists some predictors for developing overweight. Some of these are

Table 18 Weight Goals of 60 Overweight Women

Imagined goal (kg)	Weight loss in kg (%) to achieve goal	% of subjects achieving goal
Baseline weight (99.1)	—	—
Dream weight	37.7 (38)	0
Happy weight	31.1 (31)	9%
Acceptable weight (81.3)	24.9 (25)	24%
Disappointed weight	17.2 (17)	20%
Below disappointed weight	—	47%

evident in children; others are not evident until adult life. For growing children, medications should be used to treat the comorbidities directly. Drugs for weight loss are generally inappropriate until the patient reaches adult height, and surgical intervention should only be considered after consultation with medical and surgical experts.

2 Age 11–50

Table 20 outlines the available strategies for overweight and obese adults. Since nearly two-thirds of preoverweight individuals move into the overweight and obese categories in this age range, this age is quantitatively the most important. Preventive strategies should be used for patients with predictors of weight gain (Table 8). These should include advice on lifestyle changes, including increased physical activity, which would benefit almost all adults, and good dietary practices, including a diet lower in saturated fat.

For patients in the overweight category, behavior strategies should be added to these lifestyle strategies. This is particularly important for overweight adolescents, because good 10-year data show that intervention for this group can reduce the degree of overweight in adult life (124). Data on the efficacy of behavior pro-

grams carried out in controlled settings show that weight losses average nearly 10% in trials lasting more than 16 weeks (see chapters by Wing and by Perri and Foreyt). The limitation is the likelihood of regaining weight once the behavior treatment ends, although a long-term behavior therapy study did provide long-term weight loss (125).

Medication should be seriously considered for clinically overweight individuals in this group. Two strategies can be used. The first is to use drugs to treat each comorbidity, i.e., individually treating diabetes, hypertension, dyslipidemia, and sleep apnea. Alternatively, or in addition, patients with a BMI >30 kg/m^2 could be treated with antiobesity drugs (see chapters by Bray and Ryan and by Jung and Bray). Current drugs include appetite suppressants that act on the central nervous system and orlistat, which blocks pancreatic lipase (see chapter by Van Gaal and Bray). The availability of these agents differs from country to country, and any physician planning to use them should be familiar with the local regulations. Most of the drugs on the market were reviewed and approved more than 20 years ago, and are approved for short-term use only (122). The basis for the short-term use is twofold. First, almost all the studies of these agents are short term. Second, the regulatory agencies are concerned about the potential

Table 19 Therapeutic Strategies, Age 1–10

Predictors of overweight	Therapeutic strategies		
	Preoverweight at risk	Preclinical overweight	Clinical overweight
Positive family history Genetic defects	Family counseling	Family behavior therapy	Treat comorbidities
(dysmorphic-PWS; Bardet-Biedl; Cohen)	Reduce inactivity	Exercise Low-fat/low-energy-dense diet	Exercise Low-fat/low-energy-dense diet
Hypothalamic injury Low metabolic rate Diabetic mother			

Table 20 Therapeutic Strategies, Age 11–50

| | Therapeutic strategies | | |
Predictors of overweight	Preoverweight at risk	Preclinical overweight	Clinical overweight
Positive family history of diabetes or obesity Endocrine disorders (PCO) Multiple pregnancies Marriage Smoking cessation Medication	Reduce sedentary lifestyle Low-fat/low-energy-dense diet Portion control	Behavior therapy Low-fat/low-energy-dense diet Reduce sedentary lifestyle	Treat comorbidities Drug treatment for overweight Reduce sedentary lifestyle Low-fat-low-energy-dense diet Behavior therapy Surgery

for abuse, and thus have restricted most of them to prescription use with limitations. The withdrawal of fenfluramine and dexfenfluramine from the market in 1997 following in the development of valvular heart disease further compounds the concern of health authorities about the safety of those drugs. Because of the regulatory limitations and the lack of longer-term data on safety and efficacy, the use of the drugs approved for short-term treatment must be carefully justified. They may be useful in initiating treatment and in helping a patient who is relapsing.

Sibutramine (Meridia®; Reductil®) is approved in most countries for long-term use. The evidence shows that weight loss of 10% or more can be produced with this drug. The side-effects profile includes dry mouth, asthenia, insomnia, and constipation. It also produces a small increase in heart rate of between 2 and 5 beats a minute, and a small rise in blood pressure of between 2 and 4 mm Hg. Clinical data show no evidence of valvulopathy. Blood pressure should be followed carefully, and the drug may be inappropriate in patients with stroke, congestive heart failure, or recent myocardial infarction. It should not be used with other serotonergic drugs or drugs that inhibit monoamine oxidase (see chapter by Bray and Ryan).

Orlistat (Xenical), a drug that blocks intestinal lipase, has been approved for long-term use in most countries. In clinical trials lasting up to 2 years, orlistat was associated with a mean weight loss of up to 10% at the end of 1 year in patients who were prescribed a 30% fat diet. As might be expected, because the drug blocks pancreatic lipase in the intestine, fecal fat loss is increased. Major side effects reported early were markedly reduced over time, implying that patients learned to use the drug effectively in relation to dietary intake of fat. The effective use of this medication requires that physicians and their staffs provide good dietary control counseling to patients (see chapter by Van Gaal and Bray).

3 Age Over 51

Table 21 shows the proposed treatments for this age group. By age 60, almost all of the people who become overweight have done so. Thus, preventive strategies are no longer important, and the focus is on treatment for those who are overweight or obese. The basic treatments and treatment considerations are similar to those of the younger group. However, in this age group, the argument may be stronger for directly treating comorbidities

Table 21 Therapeutic Strategies for Ages over 61

| | Therapeutic strategies | | |
Predictors of overweight	Preoverweight at risk	Preclinical overweight	Clinical overweight
Menopause Declining GH Declining testosterone Smoking cessation Medication	Few individuals remain in this subgroup	Behavior therapy Low-fat/low-energy-dense diet Reduce sedentary lifestyle	Treat comorbidities Drug treatment for overweight Reduce sedentary lifestyle Low-fat/low-energy-dense diet Behavior therapy Surgery

and paying less attention to treating the clinically over-weight by weight loss. For patients in this group who wish to lose weight, however, the considerations for patients between age 11 and 50 still apply. Surgery should only be considered for individuals with class II or III obesity, or who are severely overweight. This form of treatment requires skilled surgical intervention, and should only be carried out in specialized centers.

F Quality of Life

Quality of life is important for all patients. This has effects in many areas. From the health care perspective, a reduction in comorbidities is a significant improve-ment. Remission of type 2 diabetes or hypertension can reduce costs of treating these conditions, as well as delay or prevent the development of disease. Weight loss can reduce the wear and tear on joints and slow the develop-ment of osteoarthritis. Sleep apnea usually resolves.

Psychosocial improvement is of great importance to patients. Studies of patients who achieved long-term weight loss from surgical intervention comment on the improved social and economic function of previously disabled overweight patients. Loss of 5% or more of initial weight almost always translates into improved mobility, improvement in sleep disturbances, increased exercise tolerance, and heightened self-esteem. A focus on these, rather than cosmetic outcomes, is essential.

IV THE REALITIES OF OVERWEIGHT

Overweight is a chronic, stigmatized disease that is increasing in prevalence with more than 60% of the American population who are now overweight (BMI >25 kg/m^2). This represents more than 100 million people. The prevalence of obesity (BMI >30 kg/m^2) has risen >50% in the past 15 years and continues to increase. The social disapproval of obesity and the lengths people go to prevent or reverse it fuel a $70 billion a year set of industries. Nearly 65% of American women consider themselves overweight, and even more (66–75%) want to weigh less. The figures for men are somewhat less. More than 50% of the women with a BMI <21 kg/m^2 (normal weight) want to weigh less. This individual perception of a "desirable" weight for them indicates the degree of both the stigmatization for those who are not "thin" and the drive to lose weight.

The cultural expectations for thinness are evident in the decreasing weight of the Miss America contestants from 1950 to 1980, and in the centerfolds of Playboy magazine. This has now leveled off with quite thin con-testants. The stigma of obesity is also evident in the general public disapproval of corpulence, and in the dis-approving moral attitudes of many health care profes-sionals. For example, mental health workers are more likely to assign negative psychological symptoms to the obese than to normal-weight people. Nursing, medical, and ancillary health care personnel also carry these negative stereotypes. Sensitivity training for health pro-fessionals dealing with overweight patients is important in any office or clinic offering treatment for obesity.

Overweight has many causes. The natural history of obesity indicates that it occurs gradually. Although overweight in childhood carries a serious adverse prog-nosis, particularly if the parents are overweight, nearly two-thirds of overweight adults developed their prob-lem in adult life. The risk for obesity with advancing age is illustrated in Figure 2, which shows the proportion of American men and women with BMI >25 kg/m^2 at various decades of life. Because the proportion increases until the sixth decade, those whose BMI is <25 kg/m^2 are considered preoverweight; those with BMI >25 kg/m^2 and <30 kg/m^2 are considered overweight; and those with BMI >30 kg/m^2 are considered clinically over-weight, or obese.

Results from most long-term clinical studies of treat-ment for overweight patients show a high prevalence of weight regain. In the Institute of Medicine report Weighing the Options (108), for those who achieved weight loss, more than one-third of the weight was

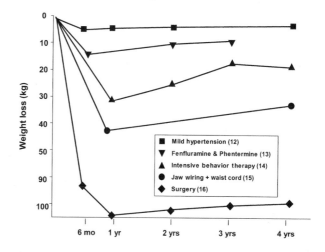

Figure 11 Comparison of 3- to 4-year weight losses. Each line represents a single study showing that weight loss varies greatly among treatments, and that maximum weight loss usually occurs in the first year. Long-term weight reduction is possible when the treatment is continuous, as in all of these studies.

typically regained within 1 year, and nearly all within 5 years. Despite this gloomy report, many long-term successes have occurred. A study of secondary prevention in successful weight maintainers showed no differences between those who regained weight in reported level of energy expenditure from exercise. However, those who successfully maintained weight loss showed greater control of fat intake, which included avoiding fried foods and substituting low-fat foods for high-fat foods. Several other programs have also reported long-term weight loss or prevention, especially in children (116).

The largest weight loss with the greatest maintenance was in individuals who underwent surgery (117). Behavior therapy produced modest weight loss while actively continued (see chapter by Wing). Pharmacologic therapy produced an 11% weight loss over 3.5 years (126). Most intriguingly, the second-best weight loss was produced by a nylon waist cord after initial weight loss was produced by jaw wiring (127). Diet alone in a treatment program for high blood pressure produced only a small effect.

Overweight, central or abdominal fat, weight gain after age 20, and a sedentary lifestyle all increase health risks and increase economic costs of obesity. Intentional weight loss by overweight individuals, on the other hand, reduces these risks. Although data are not yet available, researchers widely believe that long-term intentional weight loss lowers overall mortality, particularly from diabetes, gallbladder disease, hypertension, heart disease, and some types of cancer.

REFERENCES

1. Bray GA. Contemporary Diagnosis and Management of Obesity. Newtown, PA: Handbooks in Healthcare, 1998.
2. Bray GA. The Obese Patient: Major Problems in Internal Medicine. 9th ed. Philadelphia: W.B. Saunders, 1976.
3. Salans LB, Cushman SW, Weismann RE. Studies of human adipose tissue. Adipose cell size and number in nonobese and obese patients. J Clin Invest 1973; 52(4): 924–929.
4. Bjurlf P. Atherosclerosis and body build with special reference to size and number of subcutaneous fat cells. Acta Med Scand 1959; 166(suppl 349):99.
5. Bjorntorp P, Sjostrom L. Number and size of adipose tissue fat cells in relation to metabolism in human obesity. Metabolism 1971; 20:703–713.
6. Knittle JL, Timmers K, Ginsberg-Fellner F, Brown RE, Katz DP. The growth of adipose tissue in children and adolescents. Cross-sectional and longitudinal studies of adipose cell number and size. J Clin Invest 1979; 63(2):239–246.
7. Hirsch J, Batchelor B. Adipose tissue cellularity in human obesity. Clin Endocrinol Metab 1976; 5(2):299–311.
8. Kissebah AH, Vydelingum N, Murray, et al. Relation of body fat distribution to metabolic complications of obesity. J Clin Endocrinol Metab 1982; 54(2):254–260.
9. Lapidus L, Bengtsson C, Larsson B, Pennert K, Rybo E, Sjostrom L. Distribution of adipose tissue and risk of cardiovascular disease and death: a 12 year follow up of participants in the population study of women in Gothenburg. Sweden. Br Med J (Clin Res Educ) 1984; 289:1257–1261.
10. Larsson B, Svardsudd K, Welin L, Wilhelmsen L, Bjorntorp P, Tibblin G. Abdominal adipose tissue distribution, obesity, and risk of cardiovascular disease and death: 13 year follow up of participants in the study of men born in 1913. BMJ (Clin Res Educ) 1984; 288: 1404.
11. Vague J. The degree of masculine differentiation of obesities. Am J Clin Nutr 1956; 4:20–34.
12. Stokes J III, Kannel WB, Wolf PA, Cupples LA, D'Agostino RB. The relative importance of selected risk factors for various manifestations of cardiovascular disease among men and women from 35 to 64 years old: 30 year of follow-up in the Framingham Study. Circulation 1987; 75(6 Pt 2):V65–V73.
13. Sjostrom CD, Lissner L, Sjostrom L. Relationships between changes in body composition and changes in cardiovascular risk factors: the SOS Intervention Study. Swedish Obese Subjects. Obes Res 1997; 5(6): 519–530.
14. Sjostrom L, Kvist H, Cederblad A, et al. Determination of total adipose tissue and body fat in women by computed tomography, 40K, and tritium. Am J Physiol 1986; 250(6 Pt 1):E736–E745.
15. Pouliot MC, Despres JP, Lemieux S, Moorjani S, Bouchard C, Tremblay A, Nadeau A, Lupien PJ. Waist circumference and abdominal sagittal diameter: best simple anthropometric indexes of abdominal visceral adipose tissue accumulation and related cardiovascular risk in men and women. Am J Cardiol 1994; 1;73(7): 460–468.
16. Lean ME, Han TS, Morrison CE. Waist circumference as a measure for indicating need for weight management. BMJ 1995; 15;311(6998):158–161.
17. Expert Panel on Detection, Evaluation, and Tratament of High Blood Cholesterol in Adults. Executive Summary of the Third Report of the National Cholesterol Education Program (NCEP) Expert Panel on Detection, Evaluation and Treatment of High Blood Cholesterol in Adults (Adult Treatament Panel III). JAMA 2001; 285:2486–2497.

18. Wajchenberg BL. Subcutaneous and visceral adipose tissue: their relation to the metabolic syndrome. Endocr Rev 2000; 21(6):697–738 (Review).

19. Reitman ML, Gavrilova O. A-ZIP/F-1 mice lacking white fat: a model for understanding lipoatrophic diabetes. Int J Obes Relat Metab Disord 2000; 24(suppl 4): S11–S14 (Review.).

20. Garg A. Lipodystrophies. Am J Med 2000; 108(2):143–152. (Review)

21. Bray GA, Gallagher TF Jr. Manifestations of hypothalamic obesity in man: a comprehensive investigation of eight patients and a review of the literature. Medicine (Baltimore) 1975; 54:301–330.

22. Bray GA, York DA. The MONA LISA hypothesis in the time of leptin. Recent Prog Horm Res 1998; 53:95–118.

23. Plotz CM, Knowlton AI, Ragan C. The natural history of Cushing's syndrome. Am J Med 1952; 13:597–614.

24. Orth DN. Cushing's syndrome. N Engl J Med 1995; 332:791–803.

25. Papanicolaus DA, Yanovski JA, Cutler GB Jr, Chrousos GP, Nieman LK. A single midnight serum cortisol measurement distinguishes Cushing's syndrome from pseudo-Cushing states. J Clin Endocrinol Metab 1998; 83:1163–1167.

26. Newell-Price J, Trainer P, Besser M, Grossman A. The diagnosis and differential diagnosis of Cushing's syndrome and pseudo-Cushing's states. Endocr Rev 1998; 19:647–672.

27. Doucet J, Trivalle C, Chassagne P, Perol MB, Vuillermet P, Manchon ND, Menard JF, Bercoff E. Does age play a role in clinical presentation of hypothyroidism? J Am Geriatr Soc 1994; 42(9):984–986.

28. Dunaif A. Polycystic ovary syndrome. Polycystic ovary syndrome. Health News 1998; 4(9):4.

29. Kiddy DS, Sharp PS, White DM, et al. Differences in clinical and endocrine features between obese and non-obese subjects with polycystic ovary syndrome: an analysis of 263 consecutive cases. Clin Endocrinol (Oxf) 1990; 32:213–220.

30. Lonn L, Johansson G, Sjostrom L, et al. Body composition and tissue distributions in growth hormone deficient adults before and after growth hormone treatment. Obes Res 1996; 4:45–54.

31. Allison DB, Mentore JL, Heo M, Chandler LP, Cappelleri JC, Infante MC, Weiden PJ. Antipsychotic-induced weight gain: a comprehensive research synthesis. Am J Psychiatry 1999; 156(11):1686–1696. (Review.)

32. Loprinzi CL, Schaid DJ, Dose AM, et al. Body-composition changes in patients who gain weight while receiving megestrol acetate. J Clin Oncol 1993; 11:152–154.

33. United Kingdom Prospective Diabetes Study Group. Intensive blood glucose control with sulfonylureas or insulin compared with conventional treatment and risk of complications in patients with type 11 diabetes. Lancet 1998; 352:837–853.

34. Diabetes Control and Complications Trial Research Group. Weight gain associated with intensive therapy in the diabetes control and complications trial. Diabetes Care 1988; 11:567–573.

35. Flegal KM, Troiano RP, Pamuk ER, et al. The influence of smoking cessation on the prevalence of overweight in the United States. N Engl J Med 1995; 333: 1165–1170.

36. Prentice AM, Jebb SA. Obesity in Britain: gluttony or sloth? BMJ 1995; 311:437–439.

37. Crespo CJ, Smit E, Troiano RP, Bartlett SJ, Macera CA, Andersen RE. Television watching, energy intake, and obesity in US children: results from the third National Health and Nutrition Examination Survey, 1988–1994. Arch Pediatr Adolesc Med 2001; 155(3): 360–365.

38. Kromhout D. Changes in energy and macronutrients in 871 middle-aged men during 10 years of follow-up (the Zutphen study). Am J Clin Nutr 1983; 37:287–294.

39. U.S. Department of Health and Human Services. Physical Activity and Health: A Report of the Surgeon General. Atlanta: Centers for Disease Control and Prevention, 1996.

40. Kromhout D, Bloemberg B, Seidell JC, Nissinen A, Menotti A. Physical activity and dietary fiber determine population body fat levels: the Seven Countries Study. Int J Obes Relat Metab Disord 2001; 25(3):301–306.

41. Von Kries R, Koletzko B, Sauerwald T, Von Mutius E, Barnert D, Grunert V, Von Voss H. Breast feeding and obesity: cross sectional study. BMJ 1999; 319(7203): 147–150.

42. Gillman MW, Rifas-Shiman SL, Camargo CA Jr, Berkey CS, Frazier AL, Rockett HR, Field AE, Colditz GA. Risk of overweight among adolescents who were breastfed as infants. JAMA 2001; 285(19):2461–2467.

43. Hediger ML, Overpeck MD, Kuczmarski RJ, Ruan WJ. Association between infant breastfeeding and overweight in young children. JAMA 2001; 285(19): 2453–2460.

44. Bouchard CA, Tremblay A, Despres JP, et al. The response to long-term overfeeding in identical twins. N Engl J Med 1990; 322:1477–1482.

45. Nishizawa T, Akaoka I, Nishida Y, Kawaguchi Y, Hayashi E. Some factors related to obesity in the Japanese sumo wrestler. Am J Clin Nutr 1976; 29(10): 1167–1174.

46. Bray GA, Popkin BM. Dietary fat intake does affect obesity! Am J Clin Nutr 1998; 68:1157–1173.

47. Yu-Poth S, Zhao G, Etherton T, et al. Effects of the National Cholesterol Education Program's Step I and Step II dietary intervention programs on cardiovascular disease risk factors: a meta-analysis. Am J Clin Nutr 1999; 69(4):632–634.

48. Astrup A. The role of dietary fat in the prevention and treatment of obesity. Efficacy and safety of low-fat diets. Int J Obes Relat Metab Disord 2001; 25(suppl 1):S46–S50.

49. Ludwig DS, Peterson KE, Gortmaker SL. Relation between consumption of sugar-sweetened drinks and childhood obesity: a prospective, observational analysis. Lancet 2001; 357(9255):505–508.

50. Roberts SB, Pi-Sunyer FX, Dreher M, Hahn R, Hill JO, Kleinman RE, Peters JC, Ravussin E, Rolls BJ, Yetley E, Booth SL. Physiology of fat replacement and fat reduction: effects of dietary fat and fat substitutes on energy regulation. Nutr Rev 1998; 56(5 Pt 2):S29–S4; discussion S41–S49. (Review)

51. Wolk A, Manson JE, Stampfer MJ, Colditz GA, Hu FB, Speizer FE, Hennekens CH, Willett WC. Long-term intake of dietary fiber and decreased risk of coronary heart disease among women. JAMA 1999; 281(21): 1998–2004.

52. Salmeron J, Manson JE, Stampfer MJ, Colditz GA, Wing AL, Willett WC. Dietary fiber, glycemic load, and risk of non-insulin-dependent diabetes mellitus in women. JAMA 1997; 277(6):472–477.

53. Jenkins DJ, Jenkins AL, Wolever TM, Vuksan V, Rao AV, Thompson LU, Josse RG. Low glycemic index: lente carbohydrates and physiological effects of altered food frequency. Am J Clin Nutr 1994; 59(3 suppl): 706S–709S. (Review)

54. McCarron DA, Morris CD, Henry HJ, Stanton JL. Blood pressure and nutrient intake in the United States. Science 1984; 224(4656):1392–1398.

55. Zemel MB, Shi H, Greer B, Dirienzo D, Zemel PC. Regulation of adiposity by dietary calcium. FASEB J 2000; 14(9):1132–1138.

56. Davies KM, Heaney RP, Recker RR, Lappe JM, Barger-Lux MJ, Rafferty K, Hinders S. Calcium intake and body weight. J Clin Endocrinol Metab 2000; 85(12):4635–4638.

57. Jenkins DJ, Wolever TM, Vuksan V, et al. Nibbling versus gorging: metabolic advantages of increased meal frequency. N Engl J Med 1989; 321:929–934.

58. Lawson OJ, Williamson DA, Champagne CM, et al. The association of body weight, dietary intake, and energy expenditure with dietary restraint and disinhibition. Obes Res 1995; 3:153–161.

59. Williamson DA, Lawson OJ, Brooks ER, et al. Association of body mass with dietary restraint and disinhibition. Appetite 1995; 25:31–41.

60. Yanovski SZ, Gormally JF, Leser MS, et al. Binge eating disorder affects outcome of comprehensive very-low-calorie diet treatment. Obes Res 1994; 2:205–212.

61. Stunkard A. Two eating disorders: binge eating disorder and the night eating syndrome. Appetite 2000; 34(3):333–334.

62. Birketvedt GS, Florholmen J, Sundsfjord J, Osterud B, Dinges D, Bilker W, Stunkard A. Behavioral and neuro-endocrine characteristics of the night-eating syndrome. JAMA 1999; 282(7):657–663.

63. Partonen T, Lonnqvist J. Seasonal affective disorder. Lancet 1998; 352(9137):1369–1374. (Review.)

64. Jeffery RW, Forster JL, Folsom AR, et al. The relationship between social status and body mass index in the Minnesota Heart Health Program. Int J Obes 1989; 13(1):59–67.

65. Obarzanek E, Schreiber GB, Crawford PB, Goldman SR, Barrier PM, Frederick MM, Lakatos E. Energy intake and physical activity in relation to indexes of body fat: the National Heart, Lung and Blood Institute Growth and Health Study. Am J Clin Nutr 1994; 60(1):15–22.

66. Montague CT, Farooqi IS, Whitehead JP, et al. Congenital leptin deficiency is associated with severe early-onset obesity in humans. Nature 1997; 387:903–908.

67. Strobel A, Issad T, Camoin L, et al. A leptin missense mutation associated with hypogonadism and morbid obesity. Nat Genet 1998; 18:213–215.

68. Ozata M, Ozdemir IC, Licinio J. Human leptin deficiency caused by a missense mutation: multiple endocrine defects, decreased sympathetic tone, and immune system dysfunction indicate new targets for leptin action, greater central than peripheral resistance to the effects of leptin, and spontaneous correction of leptin-mediated defects. J Clin Endocrinol Metab 1999; 84:3686–3695.

69. Clement K, Vaisse C, Lahlou N, et al. A mutation in the human leptin receptor gene cause obesity and pituitary dysfunction. Nature 1998; 392:398–401.

70. Yeo GS, Farooqi IS, Aminian S, et al. A frameshift mutation in MC4R associated with dominantly inherited human obesity. Nat Genet 1998; 20:111–112.

71. Vaisse C, Clement K, Guy-Grand B, et al. A frameshift mutation in human MC4R is associated with a dominant form of obesity. Nat Genet 1998; 20:113–114.

72. Hinney A, Schmidt A, Nottebom K, et al. Several mutations in the melanocortin-4 receptor gene including a nonsense and a frameshift mutation associated with dominantly inherited obesity in humans. J Clin Endocrinol Metab 1999; 84:1483–1486.

73. Krude H, Biebermann H, Luck W, et al. Severe early-onset obesity adrenal insufficiency, and red hair pigmentation caused by POMC mutations in humans. Nat Genet 1998; 19:1555–1557.

73a. Behr M, Ramsden DB, Loos U. Deoxyribonucleic acid binding and transcriptional silencing by a truncated c-erbA beta 1 thyroid hormone receptor identified in a severely retarded patient with resistance to thyroid hormone. J Clin Endocrinol Metab 1997; 82:1081–1087.

74. Ristow M, Muller-Wieland D, Pfeiffer A, et al. Obesity associated with a mutation in a genetic regulator of adipocyte differentiation. N Engl J Med 1998; 339:953–959.

75. Jackson RS, Creemers JWM, Ohagi S, et al. Obesity

and impaired prohormone processing associated with mutations in the human prohormone convertase I gene. Nat Genet 1997; 16:303–306.

76. Perusse L, Chagnon YC, Weisnagel SJ, Rankinen T, Snyder E, Sands J, Bouchard C. The human obesity gene map: the 2000 update. Obes Res 2001; 9(2):135–169.

77. Gunay Agun M, Cassidy SB, Nicholls RD. Prader-Willi and other dynromes associated with obesity and mental regtardation. Behav Genet 1997; 27:307–324.

78. Green JS, Parfrey PS, Harnett JD, Farid NR, Cramer BC, Johnson G, Heath O, McManamon PJ, O'Leary E, Pryse Phillips W. The cardinal manifestations of Bardet-Biedl syndrome, a form of Laurence-Moon-Biedl syndrome. N Engl J Med 1989; 321:1002–1009.

79. Grace C, Beales P, Summerbell C, Kopelman P. The effect of Bardet-Biedl syndrom in the components on energy balance. Int J Obes Relat Metab Disord 2001; 25(suppl 2):S42 (abstract).

80. O'Dea D, Parfrey PS, Harnett JD, Hefferton D, Cramer BC, Green J. The importance of renal impairment in the natural history of Bardet-Biedl syndrome. Am J Kidney Dis 1996; 27:776–783.

81. Katsanis N, Beales PL, Woods MO, et al. Mutations in MKKS cause obesity, retinal dystrophy and renal malformations associated with Bardet-Biedl syndrome. Nat Genet 2000; 26:67–70.

82. Russell Eggitt IM, Clayton PT, Coffey R, Kriss A, Taylor DS, Taylor JG. Alstrom syndrome. Report of 22 cases and literature review. Ophthalmology 1998; 105: 1274–1280.

83. Verloes A, Temple IK, Bonnet S, Bottani A. Coloboma, mental retardation, hypogonadism and obesity: critical review of the so-called Biemond syndrome type 2, updated nosology, and dileneation of three "new" syndromes. Am J Med Genet 1997; 69:370–379.

84. David A, Bitoun P, Lacombe D, Lambert JC, Nivelon A, Vigneron J, Verloes A. Hydrometrocolpos and polydactyly: a common neonatal presentation of the Bardet-Biedl and McKusick-Kaufman syndromes. J Med Genet 1999; 36:599–603.

85. Croft JB, Morrell D, Chase CL, Swift M. Obesity in heterozygous carriers of the gene for Bardet-Bield syndrome. Am J Med Genet 1995; 55:12–15.

86. Reed DR, Ding Y, Xu W, Cather C, Price RA. Human obesity does not segregate with the chromosomal regions of Prader-Willi, Bardet-Biedl, Dohen, Borjeson or Wilson-Turner syndromes. Int J Obes Relat Metab Disord 1995; 19:599–603.

87. Wilson RS. Twin growth: initial deficit, recovery, and trends in concordance from birth to nine years. Ann Hum Biol 1979; 6(3):205–220.

88. Blank A, Grave GD, Metzger BE. Effects of gestational diabetes on perinatal morbidity reassessed. Report of the International Workshop on Adverse Perinatal Outcomes of Gestational Diabetes Mellitus, December 3–4, 1992. Diabetes Care 1995; 18(1):127–129.

89. Barker DJ, Hales CN, Fall CH, et al. Type 2 (non-insulin-dependent) diabetes mellitus, hypertension and hyperlipidaernia (syndrome X): relation to reduced fetal growth. Diabetologia 1993; 36:62–67.

90. Whitaker RC, Wright JA, Pepe MS, et al. Predicting obesity in young adulthood from childhood and parental obesity. N Engl J Med 1997; 337:869–873.

91. Must A, Jacques PF, Dallal GE, et al. Long-term morbidity and mortality of overweight adolescents. A follow-up of the Harvard Growth Study of 1922 to 1935. N Engl J Med 1992; 327:1350–1355.

92. Smith DE, Lewis CE, Caveny JL, et al. Longitudinal changes in adiposity associated with pregnancy. Coronary Artery Risk Development in Young Adults Study. JAMA 1994; 271:1747–1751.

93. Brown JE, Kaye SA, Folsom AR. Parity-related weight change in women. Int J Obes Relat Metab Disord 1992; 16:627–631.

94. Williamson DF, Madan SJ, Pamuk E, et al. A prospective study of childbearing and 10-year weight gain in US white women 25 to 45 years of age. Int J Obes Relat Metab Disord 1994; 18:561–569.

95. Reubinoff BE, Grubstein A, Meirow D, et al. Effects of lowdose estrogen oral contraceptives on weight, body composition, and fat distribution in young women. Fertil Steril 1995; 63:516–521.

96. Aloia JF, Vaswani A, Russo L, et al. The influence of menopause and hormonal replacement therapy on body cell mass and body fat mass. Am J Obstet Gynecol 1995; 172:896–900.

97. Haarbo J, Christiansen C. Treatment-induced cyclic variations in serum lipids, lipoproteins, and apolipoproteins after 2 years of combined hormone replacement therapy: exaggerated cyclic variations in smokers. Obstet Gynecol 1992; 80:639–644.

98. National Task Force on the Prevention and Treatment of Obesity. Weight cycling. JAMA 1994; 272:1196–1202.

99. Williamson DF. Descriptive epidemiology of body weight and weight change in U.S. adults. Ann Intern Med 1993; 119:646–649.

100. NHLBI Obesity Education Initiative Expert Panel on the Identification, Evaluation, and Treatment of Overweight and Obesity in Adults. Clinical guidelines on the identification, evaluation, and treatment of overweight and obesity in adults-the evidence report. Obes Res 1998; 6(suppl 2):51S–209S. (Review.)

101. National Institutes of Health, National Heart Lung and Blood Institute, North American Association for the Study of Obesity. The Practical Guide. Identification, Evaluation, and Treatment of Overweight and Obesity in Adults. Bethesda: National Institutes of Health, 2000. (NIH Publication No. 00-4084.)

102. Bray GA, Gray DS. Obesity. Part II—treatment. West J Med 1988; 149(5):555–571. (Review.)

103. U.S. Department of Health and Human Services.

Screening for obesity. Guide to Clinical Preventive Services 2nd ed. Bethesda: NIH, 1989:219–229.

104. American Obesity Association and Shape Up America! Guidance for treatment of adult obesity. Available at: http://www.shapeup.org/sua/bmi/guidance/ Accessed July 16, 1998.

105. World Health Organization. Obesity: Preventing and Managing the Global Epidemic. Geneva: World Health Organization, 1998.

106. AACE/ACE Obesity Task Force. AACE/ACE position statement on the prevention, diagnosis, and treatment of obesity. Endcro Prac 1997; 3:162–208.

107. U.S. Department of Health and Human Services. Body measurements. In: Clinician's Handbook of Preventive Services: Put Prevention into Family Practice. 1994: 141–146.

108. Thomas P, ed. Weighing the Options. Washington: National Academy Press, 1995.

109. Willett WC, Manson JE, Stampfer MJ, Colditz GA, Rosner B, Speizer FE, Hennekens CH. Weight, weight change, and coronary heart disease in women. Risk within the 'normal' weight range. JAMA 1995; 273(6): 461–465.

110. Blair SN, Kohl HW III. Physical fitness and all-cause mortality. A prospective study of healthy men and women. JAMA 1989; 262(17):2395–2401.

111. Roche A, Heymsfield SB, Lohman T. Human Body Composition. Champaign, IL: Human Kinetics, 1996.

112. Gallagher D, Heymsfield SB, Heo M, et al. Healthy percentage body fat ranges: an approach for developing guidelines based on body mass index. Am J Clin Nutr 2000; 72(3):694–701.

113. Bray GA, Jordan HA, Sims EA. Evaluation of the obese patient. 1. An algorithm. JAMA 1976; 235(14): 1487–1491.

114. Brownell KD. Dieting readiness. Weight Control Dig 1990; 1:1–9.

115. Galuska DA, Willi JC, Serdula MK, et al. Are health care professionals advising obese patients to lose weight? JAMA 1999; 282(16):1576–1578.

116. Foster GD, Wadden TA, Vogt RA, et al. What is a reasonable weight loss? Patients' expectations and evaluations of obesity treatment outcomes. J Consult Clin Psychol 1997; 65(1):79–85.

117. Sjostrom CD, Lissner L, Sjostrom L. Relationships between changes in body composition and changes in cardiovascular risk factors: the SOS Intervention Study. Swedish Obese Subjects. Obes Res 1997; 5(6): 519–530.

118. Flechtner-Mors M, Ditschuneit HH, Johnson TD, Suchard MA, Adler G. Metabolic and weight loss effects of long-term dietary intervention in obese patients: four-year results. Obes Res 2000; 8(5):399–402.

119. Finer N, Bloom SR, Frost GS, Banks LM, Griffiths J. Sibutramine is effective for weight loss and diabetic control in obesity with type 2 diabetes: a randomised, double-blind, placebo-controlled study. Diabetes Obes Metab 2000; 2(2):105–112.

120. McMahon FG, Fujioka K, Singh BN, Mendel CM, Rowe E, Rolston K, Johnson F, Mooradian AD. Efficacy and safety of sibutramine in obese white and African American patients with hypertension: a 1-year, double-blind, placebo-controlled, multicenter trial. Arch Intern Med 2000; 160(14):2185–2191.

121. Munro JF, MacCuish AC, Wilson EM, Duncan LJP. Comparison of continuous and intermittent anorectic therapy in obesity. BMJ 1968; 1:352–356.

122. Bray GA. Drug treatment of obesity: don't throw the baby out with the bath water. Am J Clin Nutr 1998; 67(1):1–2.

123. Rossner S. Factors determining the long-term outcome of obesity treatment. In: Bjorntorp P, Brodoff BN, eds. Obesity. Philadelphia: J.B. Lippincott, 1992:712–719.

124. Epstein LH, Valoski A, Wing RR, et al. Ten-year follow-up of behavioral, family-based treatment for obese children. JAMA 1990; 264(19):2519–2523.

125. Bjorvell H, Rossner S. A ten-year follow-up of weight change in severely obese subjects treated in a combined behavioural modification programme. Int J Obes Relat Metab Disord 1992; 16(8):623–625.

126. Weintraub M. Long-term weight control: the National Heart, Lung, and Blood Institute funded multimodal intervention study. Clin Pharmacol Ther 1992; 51(5): 581–646.

127. Garrow JS, Gardiner GT. Maintenance of weight loss in obese patients after jaw wiring. BMJ (Clin Res Educ) 1981; 282(6267):858–860.

2

Obesity and the Primary Care Physician

Robert F. Kushner

Northwestern University Feinberg School of Medicine, Chicago, Illinois, U.S.A.

Louis J. Aronne

Weill Medical College of Cornell University, New York, New York, U.S.A.

I INTRODUCTION

With nearly 60% of U.S. adults currently categorized as overweight or obese, this condition represents one of the most common chronic medical problems seen by the primary care physician. Since obesity is associated with an increased risk of multiple health problems, these patients are also more likely to present with silent diseases, e.g., hypertension, dyslipidemia, type 2 diabetes, or with a variety of complaints requiring further medical attention. For this reason, the U.S. Preventive Services Task Force recommends periodic height and weight measurements for all patients along with appropriate counseling to promote physical activity and a healthy diet (1). In practice, however, fewer than half of obese adults report being advised to lose weight by health care professionals (2,3). Futhermore, analysis of over 55,000 adult physician office visits sampled in the 1995–96 National Ambulatory Medical Care Survey revealed that physicians reported obesity in only 8.6% of all patient visits, a rate significantly lower than the 22.7% prevalence figures from the same time period (4). The low rates of identification and treatment of obesity are thought to be due to multiple factors, including lack of reimbursement, limited time during office visits, lack of training in counseling, or low confidence in ability to treat and change patient behaviors. This chapter is divided into two sections. The first provides an overview of the general issues and concerns related to treating overweight and obese patients in the primary care setting, and the second provides a practical review of the obesity evaluation and treatment process that should be incorporated into the care of all patients.

II OFFICE-BASED OBESITY CARE

One of the most significant obstacles to patient counseling during a routine office visit is availability of time. Two 1998 national surveys found that the average office patient visit length was 21.5 min and 18.3 min, respectively (5). The Direct Observation of Primary Care (DOPC) study found that the average duration of direct physician-patient contact during an office visit was actually only 10 min (6). Within the confines of this time, the physician typically elicits a brief history, performs a limited physical examination, reviews and interprets pertinent laboratory and diagnostic tests, and provides recommendations that may include ordering further tests, writing prescriptions, and conducting counseling. Accordingly, care of the obese patient (and all patients) would be greatly facilitated by incorporating efficient and effective office-based systems. Put Prevention into Practice (PPIP), a national campaign by the Agency for Health Care Policy and Research (AHCPR) to improve the delivery of clinical preventive services such as counseling for health behavior change, provides a useful framework for analyzing the office systems designed to deliver patient care (7). PPIC identifies key components that can either expedite or hinder the care of patients in the office. They include organizational commitment, clinicians' attitudes, staff support, establishing policies and protocols, using simple office tools, and delegating tasks, among others. This section reviews the office-based systems that are uniquely geared to the care of the obese patient (Table 1). Collectively, they address a need for heightened sensitivity and thoroughness throughout all office systems.

A   The Physical Environment

Accessibility to the office is critical for the obese patient. Facility limitations include difficult access from the parking lot or stairs, narrow doors and hallways, and cramped restrooms. These are the same problems that face other patients with disabilities, and are covered under the regulations of the Americans with Disabilities Act of 1990. One of the first concerns obese patients have upon entering the waiting room is where they can safely sit. Office chairs of standard width and side arm rests will not comfortably accommodate moderately to severely obese patients. Ideal chairs have no arms so that patients do not have to squeeze themselves

Table 1   Office-Based Obesity Care

The physical environment
   Accessibility and comfort: stairs, doorways, hallways, restrooms, waiting room chairs and space, reading materials and other educational materials
Equipment
   Large adult and thigh blood pressure cuffs, large gowns, step stools, weight and height scales, tape measure
Materials
   Educational and behavior promoting handouts on diet, exercise, medications, surgery, BMI, obesity-associated diseases
Tools
   Previsit questionnaires, BMI stamps, food and activity diaries, pedometers
Protocols
   Patient care treatment protocols for return visit schedule, medications, referrals to dietitians and psychologists
Staffing
   Team approach to include office nurse, physician assistant, nurse practitioner, health advocate

into predefined "normal" dimensions. Although often thought insignificant, hanging artwork and magazines in the waiting and examination rooms can convey misinterpreted messages to patients. Magazines, newspapers, television, movies, and billboards constantly remind overweight individuals of society's beauty ideals. Magazines, newsletters, and artwork can be chosen that don't contribute to these unattainable images.

B   Equipment

Measurement of an accurate height and weight is paramount to treating patients with obesity. All too often, the physicians' office has a scale that does not measure above 350 pounds, or the foot platform is too narrow to securely balance the overweight individual. Although a wall-mounted sliding statiometer is the most accurate instrument, a sturdy height meter attached to the scale will suffice. The weight scale should preferably have a wide base with a nearby handlebar for support if necessary. Depending on the patient population, it is reasonable to select a scale that measures in excess of 350 pounds. To protect privacy, the scale should be located in a private area of the office to avoid unnecessary embarrassment.

Examination rooms should have large gowns available to wear as well as a step stool to mount the examination tables. Each room should be equipped with large adult and thigh blood pressure cuffs for measurement of blood pressure. A bladder cuff that is not the appropriate width for the patient's arm circumference will cause a systematic error in blood pressure measurement; if the bladder is too narrow, the pressure will be overestimated and lead to a false diagnosis of hypertension. To avoid errors, the bladder width should be 40–50% of upper-arm circumference. Therefore, a large adult cuff (15 cm wide) should be chosen for patients with mild to moderate obesity, while a thigh cuff (18 cm wide) will need to be used for patients whose arm circumferences are > 16 inches. Lastly, a cloth or metal tape should be available for measurement of waist circumference as per the NHLBI Practical Guide for obesity classification (8).

C   Using an Integrated Team Approach

How practices operate on a day-to-day basis is extremely important for the provision of effective obesity care. Several key office-based strategies have been shown to improve practice performance in relation to goals for primary care. Two of the most successful features are use of a multidisciplinary or interdisciplinary team and incorporation of protocols and procedures (9). Current therapies for obesity may be best provided using an integrative team approach (10,11). Because of limited time, physicians are generally unable to provide all of the care necessary for treatment. Moreover, other personnel are often better qualified to deliver the dietary, physical activity, and behavioral counseling. Accordingly, there is an opportunity for other office staff to play a greater role in the care of obese patients. A sense of "groupness," defined as the degree to which the group practice identifies itself and functions as a team, will enhance the quality and efficiency of care (12).

The optimal team composition and management structure will vary among practices. However, as an example of an integrative model, receptionists can provide useful information about the program, including general philosophy, staffing, fee schedules, and other written materials; registered nurses can obtain vital measurements including height and weight (for body mass index) and waist circumference; instruct on and review food and activity journals and other educational materials; and physician assistants can monitor the progress of treatment and assume many of the other responsibilities of care. A new position of health advocate, whose role is to serve as a resource to the physician and to patients by providing additional information and assisting in arranging recommended follow-up, may be particularly useful (13). Regardless of how the work load is delegated, the power of the physician's voice should not be underestimated. The physician should be perceived as the team leader and source of common philosophy of care (14).

D Protocols and Procedures

A significant portion of the time spent in the evaluation and treatment of the obese patient can be expedited by use of protocols and procedures. A self-administered medical history questionnaire can be either mailed to the patient prior to the initial visit or completed in the waiting room. In addition to standard questions, sections of the form should inquire about past obesity treatment programs, a body weight history, current diet and physical activity levels, social support, and goals and expectations. The review-of-systems section can include medical prompts that are more commonly seen among the obese, such as snoring, morning headaches and daytime sleepiness (for obstructive sleep apnea), urinary incontinence, intertrigo, and sexual dysfunction, among others.

Identifying the body mass index (BMI) as a fifth vital sign may also increase physician awareness and prompt counseling. This method was successfully used in a recent study where a smoking status stamp was placed on the patient chart, alongside blood pressure, pulse, temperature, and respiratory rate (15). Use of prompts, alerts, or other reminders has been shown to significantly increase physician performance of other health maintenance activities as well (9,16). Once the patient is identified as overweight or obese, printed food and activity diaries and patient information sheets on a variety of topics such as the food guide pyramid, deciphering food labels, healthy snacking, dietary fiber, aerobic exercise and resistance training, and dealing with stress can be used to support behavior change and facilitate patient education. Ready-to-copy materials can be obtained from a variety of sources free of charge such as those found in the Practical Guide, or for a minimal fee from other public sites and commercial companies.

Based on the health promotion literature, use of written materials and counseling protocols should lead to more effective and efficient obesity care. In a study of community-based family medicine physicians, Kreuter et al. (17) showed that patients were more likely to reduce smoking, increase physical activity, and limit dairy fat consumption when physician advice is supported by health education materials. In another randomized intervention study by Swinburn et al. (18), a written goal-oriented exercise prescription, in addition to verbal advice, was more effective than verbal advice alone in increasing the physical activity level of sedentary individuals over a 6-week period. Several exercise assessment and counseling protocols have been developed that can be easily incorporated into obesity care. These include Project PACE (Provider-based Assessment and Counseling for Exercise) (19), ACT (the Activity Counseling Trial) (20), and STEP (the Step Test Exercise Prescription) (21). Finally, protocols and procedures for various treatment pathways can be established for obtaining periodic laboratory monitoring and referral to allied health professionals, such as registered dietitians, exercise specialists, and clinical psychologists.

E The Patient-Physician Encounter

Although all of the office-based systems reviewed above are important, the cornerstone of effective treatment for obesity is grounded in skillful and empathetic physician-patient communication. This vital interaction is affirmed by Balint's assertion that "the most frequently used drug in medical practice is the doctor himself" (22). From the patient's perspective, a caring physician is compassionate, supportive, trustworthy, open-minded, and nonjudgmental. He or she takes into account the patient's needs, values, beliefs, goals, personality traits, and fears (23). In a review of the literature, Stewart found that the quality of communication between the physician and patient directly influenced patient health outcomes (24). A large body of literature has described key elements of communication that foster behavior change. Since the primary aim of obesity counseling is to influence what the patient does *outside* the office, the time spent *in* the office needs to be structured and effective.

Effective counseling begins with establishing rapport and soliciting the patient's agenda. Attentively listening to the patient to understand his or her goals and expectations is the first essential step. Asking the patient, "How do you hope that I can help you?" is an information-gathering open-ended question that directly addresses his or her concerns. Among 28 identified elements of care that were inquired about with patients before the office visit, Kravitz found that "discussion of own ideas about how to manage condition" was ranked as the highest previsit physician expectation (25). Interestingly, this is not always done in the primary care office. In a survey of 264 patient-physician interviews, patients completed their statement of concern only 28% of the time, being interrupted by the physician after an average duration of 23 sec (26). Physicians were found to redirect the patient and focus the clinical interviews before giving patients the opportunity to complete their statement of concern. Obesity interviewing and counseling should be patient centered, allowing the patient to be an active participant in setting the agenda and having his or her concerns heard. This requires skillful management by the physician to structure the interview within the time allocated.

The style of communication used by the physician refers to the approach taken when interacting with and counseling patients. Emanuel and Emanuel (27) describe four models of the physician-patient relationship: paternalistic—the physician acts as the patient's guardian, articulating and implementing what is best for the patient; informative—the physician is a purveyor of technical expertise, providing the patient with the means to exercise control; interpretive—the physician is a counselor, supplying relevant information and engaging the patient in a joint process of understanding; and deliberative–the physician acts as a teacher or friend, engaging the patient in dialogue on what course of action would be best.

Roter et al. (28) define four similar prototypes of doctor-patient relationships using a "power" balance sheet. In this model, power relates to who sets the agenda, whether the patient's values are expressed and considered, and what role the physician assumes. As illustrated in Table 2, high physician and high patient power (upper left) depicts a relationship of mutuality, balance, and shared decision making. High physician and low patient power (lower left) is consistent with Emanuel's paternalistic model where the doctor sets the agenda and prescribes the treatment. In the low physician and high patient power relationship (upper right), the patient sets the agenda and takes sole responsibility for decision making. Roter et al. (28) call this interaction consumerism. Lastly, in a low physician and low patient power relationship (lower right), the role of the doctor and patient is unclear and undefined. This is a dysfunctional relationship. According to Roter et al., the optimal relationship is that of mutuality or what they call "relationship-centered medicine." In the course of providing obesity care, it is likely that more than one of these relationships is used among patients. The important point is that the encounter should be functional, informative, respectful, and supportive.

Depending on the patient's course of treatment and response, various strategies and techniques are used during the visit. The traditional therapeutic role of the physician is to address concerns, build trust, give advice, and be supportive (29). Novack (30) describes four therapeutic interventions that support patient behavior change. Each of the therapeutic strategies listed in Table 3 is directed toward keeping the patient motivated and providing a sense of control. Among the components of effective counseling, empathy is perhaps the most important. The feeling of being understood is intrinsically therapeutic. Patients with obesity typically provide emotionally laden testimony about the frustration, anger, and shame of losing (and gaining) weight, the discrimination they feel in the workplace and society for being overweight, and the ridicule they may have experienced with other health care providers. Recogniz-

Table 2 Patient-Physician Communication Relationships

		Physician power	
Patient power		High	Low
	High	mutuality	consumerism
	Low	Paternalism	Dysfunctional

Source: Ref. 28.

Table 3 Therapeutic Aspects of the Clinical Encounter

Cognitive strategies
    Negotiation of priorities
    Giving an explanation
    Suggestion
    Patient education
    Giving a prognosis
Affective strategies
    Empathy
    Encouragement of emotional expression
    Encouragement
    Offering hope
    Touch
    Reassurance
Behavioral strategies
    Emphasizing patient's active role
    Praising desired behaviors
    Suggesting alternative behaviors
    Attending to compliance
Social strategies
    Use of family and social supports
    Use of community agencies and other health care providers

Source: Ref. 30.

ing and acknowledging the patient's concerns and experiences is an extremely important element in communication (31). In sum, it is important for patients to have the opportunity to tell the story of their weight journey in their own words and for the physician to validate the patients' experience.

Regardless of whether a good therapeutic and supportive relationship is established, many patients will not achieve their behavioral and weight loss goals. In this case, it is extremely important not to label these patients as noncompliant. The word "compliance" suggests that a submissive patient should obey the authoritative physicians' instructions. "Noncompliance" then denotes failure or refusal to cooperate. This description is consistent with the paternalistic physician-patient relationship model discussed above. Some authors have suggested that the word "adherence" is a better alternative to compliance, emphasizing the patient's role as an active decision making (32,33). Still others have abandoned both terms because they exaggerate the importance of the clinician and do not aid in helping the patient overcome behavioral obstacles (34). Simply asking the patient what is hard about a particular behavioral change is more productive in problem solving than giving them purposeless labels.

This brief review of the office environment and office systems that facilitate provision of obesity care is intended to provide a backdrop for the section that follows in this chapter. Herein we review the process of assessment, classification, and treatment of the overweight and obese adult patient in the primary care setting. Other chapters in the book address each of these processes in detail. Our focus is on the practical implementation of obesity care, highlighting the key elements of each step and the associated decision making that occurs in the process.

III ASSESSMENT, CLASSIFICATION, AND TREATMENT

The clinical approach to the patient follows three steps used in the care of any patient with a multifactorial, chronic disease: assessment, classification, and treatment (8). Assessment includes determining the degree of obesity using BMI and waist circumference, and evaluating the overall health status of the patient. Information collected during the assessment is then used to classify the severity of obesity and related health problems. Decisions about treatment can be made based on the results of the assessment and classification. Treatment includes not only acute treatment of obesity but maintenance of weight loss as well as management of comorbid conditions. An obesity-specific approach is outlined in Table 4.

Table 4 Assessment and Management of the Overweight and Obese Patient

Measure height and weight; estimate BMI.
Measure waist circumference.
Review the patient's medical condition; assess comorbidities:
    How many are present, and how severe are they?
    Do they need to be treated in addition to the effort at
      weight loss?
Look for causes of obesity including the use of medications
    known to cause weight gain.
Assess the risk of this patient's obesity using Table 7.
Is the patient ready and motivated to lose weight?
If the patient is not ready to lose weight, urge weight
    maintenance and manage the complications.
If the patient is ready, agree with the patient on reasonable
    weight and activity goals and write them down.
Use the information you have gathered to develop a
    treatment plan based on Table 8.
Involve other professionals, if necessary.
Don't forget that a supportive, empathetic approach is
    necessary throughout treatment.

Source: Ref. 8.

A Assessment

1 History and Physical Examination

The history is important for evaluating risk and deciding upon treatment. Questions should address age of onset of obesity, minimum weight as an adult, events associated with weight gain, recent weight loss attempts, and previous weight loss modalities used successfully and unsuccessfully and their complications. For example, loss of weight to below a patient's minimum weight as an adult is unusual, and an earlier age of onset of obesity often, but not always, predicts a less successful outcome. A treatment modality that was previously unsuccessful or during which the patient experienced adverse complications should generally be avoided. A history of eating disorders, bingeing, and purging by vomiting or laxative abuse are relative contraindications to treatment, and referral to a specialist in these areas should be considered. Alcohol and substance abuse require specific treatment that should take precedence over obesity treatment. Cigarette smoking can complicate treatment history because weight is often gained upon stopping smoking. While smoking cessation is of paramount importance, implementing a diet and exercise program on or before stopping can minimize weight gain.

The patient's current level of physical activity is important to determine the starting point for exercise recommendations. Some individuals may be completely sedentary while others are vigorously active. Providing the same recommendation to both patients would be inappropriate. Similarly, the patient's level of understanding of nutrition will determine whether a basic or more sophisticated level of nutrition education should be taught. This is crucial toward helping the patient get the most out of each session. Material that is too advanced won't be retained, and material that is too basic will be boring to the patient.

Diseases that may affect weight, such as polycystic ovarian syndrome and hypothyroidism, require specific treatment even though that treatment alone may not result in weight loss. In addition, patients may also exhibit substantial weight gain in the months or years before developing overt type 2 diabetes.

The clinician should search for complications of obesity, such as hypertension, type 2 diabetes, hyperlipidemia, coronary heart disease, osteoarthritis of the lower extremities, gallbladder disease, gout, and some forms of cancer. In men, obesity is associated with colorectal and prostate cancer; in women, it is associated with endometrial, gallbladder, cervical, ovarian, and breast cancer. Signs and symptoms of these disorders, such as vaginal or rectal bleeding, may have been overlooked by the patient and should be carefully reviewed by the physician.

Obstructive sleep apnea is a disorder often overlooked in obese patients. Symptoms and signs include very loud snoring, cessation of breathing during sleep followed by a loud clearing breath, nighttime awakening, daytime fatigue with episodes of sleepiness at inappropriate times, and morning headaches. Associated findings on examination may include hypertension, narrowing of the upper airway, scleral injection, and leg edema. Laboratory studies may show polycythemia. If signs of sleep apnea are present, the patient should have a diagnostic sleep study performed. The onset of sleep apnea is sometimes associated with further weight gain, and management of sleep apnea may assist with weight loss.

A number of medications are known to cause weight gain in some patients (Table 5). These include antidepressants, anitepileptics, phenothiazines, lithium, glucocorticoids, progestational hormones, antihistamines, sulfonylureas, insulin, thiazolidinediones, and beta-blockers, among others (35). If possible, medications should be changed to those that do not cause weight gain or may even induce weight loss. The use of medications that may interact with planned treatment, such as monoamine oxidase (MAO) inhibitors and other antidepressants should be reviewed. In addition, some patients take over-the-counter weight control products and cold remedies that may cause side effects and interactions with medications that may be prescribed. Examples include pseudoephedrine, which may be found in cold remedies and over-the-counter diet products, and ephedra (ma huang) a nonspecific beta agonist found in diet products. Both are contraindicated if prescribing a sympathomimetic appetite suppressant.

Clinical manifestations of the causes and complications of obesity should be particularly sought during the physical exam. Height and weight should be measured and the BMI calculated in order to categorize the severity and risk of obesity. Waist circumference should be assessed using a tape measure (Fig. 1). Blood pressure should be checked with an appropriately sized cuff. Other key features include examining the thyroid and looking for manifestations of hypothyroidism; looking for skin tags and acanthosis nigricans around the neck and axilla, which suggest hyperinsulinemia; and identifying leg edema, cellulitis, and intertriginous rashes with signs of skin breakdown. Leg edema may be secondary to right heart failure or direct compression by an abdominal pannus in the very obese patient.

Table 5 Drugs That May Promote Weight Gain and Alternatives

Category	Drugs that may promote weight gain	Alternatives
Psychiatric/neurologic	Phenothiazines	
	Antidepressants	Buproprion, Nefazadone
	Lithium	
	Neuroleptics	Ziprasidone, Aripiprazole
	Antiepileptics	Topiramate, Zonisamide, Lamotrigine
Steroid hormones	Hormonal contraceptives	Barrier methods of contraception
	Corticosteroids	Nonsteroidal anti-inflammatory drugs
	Progestational steroids	Weight loss for menometrorrhagia
Diabetes treatments	Insulin	Metformin
	Sulfonylureas	Acarbose, miglitol
	Thiazolidinediones	Orlistat, sibutramine
Antihistamines	Diphenhydramine, others	Decongestants, inhaled steroids
β-Adrenergic blockers	Propranolol, others	ACE inhibitors, Ca-channel blockers

Source: Modified from Ref. 35.

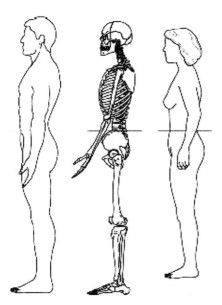

Figure 1 Measuring waist circumference. To measure waist circumference, locate the upper hip bone and the top of the right iliac crest. Place a measuring tape in a horizontal plane around the abdomen at the level of the iliac crest. Before reading the tape measure, ensure that the tape is snug, but does not compress the skin, and is parallel to the floor. The measurement is made at the end of a normal expiration. Men with a waist circumferences >40 inches (>102 cm) and women with a waist circumferences >35 inches (>88 cm) are at higher risk because of excess abdominal fat and should be considered one risk category above that defined by their BMI. (From Ref. 8.)

Look for the common disorders seen in the obese: type 2 diabetes, hyperlipidemia, coronary heart disease, osteoarthritis of the lower extremities, gallbladder disease, gout, colorectal and prostate cancer in men, and endometrial, gallbladder, cervical, ovarian, and breast cancer in women. Type 2 diabetes, gout, hyperlipidemia, and hepatic steatosis are the disorders most often discovered by laboratory evaluation (Table 6). Other labs may indicate disorders that may be involved in the induction of obesity and require specific treatment, such as hypothyroidism and hyperinsulinemia. Complete laboratory evaluation might include blood glucose, uric acid, BUN, creatinine, uric acid, ALT, AST, total and direct bilirubin, alkaline phosphatase, total cholesterol, HDL, LDL, triglycerides, complete blood count, TSH, and urinalysis. In some cases, a 2-hr postprandial insulin level is of value in diagnosing hyperinsulinemia. Measurements of body composition utilizing methods such as bioelectrical impedence, while motivating to some patients, are not necessary for treating the average patient.

Before beginning treatment, results of the physical examination and laboratory tests should be shared with the patient. Emphasis should be placed on any new findings, particularly those associated with obesity that would be expected to improve with weight loss. The patient should focus on improvements in these health parameters, rather than focus on achieving an ideal body weight or a similarly large weight loss that may not be attainable. Improvements in health complica-

Table 6 Laboratory and Diagnostic Evaluation of the Obese Patient Based on Presentation of Symptoms, Risk Factors, and Index of Suspicion

If there is a suspicion of . . .	Consider . . .
Alveolar hypoventilation (Pickwickian) syndrome (hypersomnolence, possible right-sided heart failure)	CBC (to rule out polycythemia); pulmonary function tests (reduced lung volume), blood gases (pCO_2 often elevated); ECG (to rule out right heart strain)
Cushing's syndrome	Screen with 24-hr urine for free cortisol (>150 μg/24 hr considered abnormal) and overnight dexamathasone suppression test: 1 mg ρo at 11 PM. At precisely 8 AM next morning, draw serum cortisol (<5 is normal suppression; axis intact). Failure of suppression indicates dysregulation, possibly Cushing's syndrome
Gallstones	Utrasonography of gallbladder
Hepatomegaly/nonalcoholic steatohepatitis	Liver function tests
Hypothyroidism	Serum TSH (normal generally <5 μU/mL)
Insulinoma	Elevated levels of insulin and C-peptide in absence of sulfonylurea in plasma, especially during hypoglycemic episode.
Sleep apnea	Sleep studies for oxygen desaturation; apneic and hypopneic events; ENT examination for upper airway obstruction
Polycystic ovarian syndrome (PCOS) (oligomenorrhea, hirsuitism, probable obesity, enlarged ovaries may be palpable)	Increase in LH:FSH ratio, often >2.5. (Cycle of increased LH, stimulating increased testosterone and androstenedione in ovarian stroma, which is converted to estrone in adipose tissue, leading in turn to increased LH)

CBC, complete blood count; ECG, electrocardiogram; TSH, thyroid-stimulating hormine; ENT, ear, nose, and throat; LH, leuteinizing hormone; FSH, follicle-stimulating hormone.
Source: Ref. 38.

tions should be discussed on an ongoing basis. Many patients find this a helpful motivator because, at some point, weight is likely to stabilize at a level above their own "ideal" weight. By focusing patients on the medical rather than the cosmetic benefits of weight loss, they may be more satisfied and better able to attain their goals and succeed long term.

The relative risk associated with a given degree of overweight and obesity can be estimated from Table 7.

2 Contraindications to Treatment

Obesity treatment is contraindicated in patients who are pregnant, have anorexia nervosa, or have terminal illness. Medical or psychiatric illnesses must be stable before weight reduction begins. Furthermore, patients with cholelithiasis and osteoporosis should be warned that these conditions might be aggravated by weight loss.

3 Consider the Patient's Readiness to Lose Weight

The decision to attempt weight-loss treatment should consider the patient's readiness to make lifestyle changes. Evaluation of readiness should include the following: (1) reasons and motivation for weight loss; (2) previous attempts at weight loss; (3) support expected from family and friends; (4) an understanding of risks and benefits; (5) attitudes toward physical activity; (6) time availability; and (7) potential barriers, including financial limitations.

For the patient to succeed, he or she must be ready to make the effort to lose weight. An unwilling patient rarely if ever succeeds, frustrating both the patient and the practitioner. If the patient does not wish to lose weight and is not at high risk, weight maintenance should be encouraged. If the patient is at high risk as a

Table 7 Classification of Overweight and Obesity by BMI, Waist Circumference, and Associated Disease Risk[a]

	BMI (kg/m^2)	Obesity class	Disease risk[a] (relative to normal weight and waist circumference)	
			Men ≤40 in. (≤102 cm) Women ≤35 in. (≤88 cm)	>40 in. (>102 cm) >35 in. (>88 cm)
Underweight	<18.5		—	—
Normal[b]	18.5–24.9		—	—
Overweight	25.0–29.9		Increased	High
Obesity	30.0–34.9	I	High	Very high
	35.0–39.9	II	Very high	Very high
Extreme obesity	≥40	III	Extremely high	Extremely high

[a] Disease risk for type 2 diabetes mellitus, hypertension, and CVD.
[b] Increased waist circumference can also be a marker for increased risk even in persons of normal weight.
Source: Ref. 8.

result of obesity, the clinician should make an effort to motivate the patient by discussing the medical consequences related to the patient's case. However, negative and pejorative statements should be avoided since they are of no therapeutic value and tend to be demoralizing.

B Classification and Treatment

While healthy eating and an increase in activity should be encouraged in every patient, the primary targets for treatment should be those individuals at health risk because of increased weight. This includes overweight patients with a BMI >25, and obese patients with a BMI >30, especially if complications are present. Table 8 outlines a guide to selecting the appropriate treatment based on BMI. Individuals at lesser risk should be counseled about effective lifestyle changes. Goals of therapy are to reduce body weight and maintain a lower body weight for the long term; the prevention of further weight gain is the minimum goal. An

initial weight loss of 10% of body weight achieved over 6 months is a recommended target. Even more modest weight loss can reduce visceral fat and improve comorbid conditions. The rate of weight loss should be 1–2 pounds each week but will vary from patient to patient. Greater rates of weight loss do not achieve better long-term results. Weight maintenance, achieved through the combined changes in diet, physical activity, and behavior, should be the priority after the first 6 months of weight loss.

Given our current state of knowledge and the treatments currently available, the goal of obesity treatment should be the lowest weight the patient can comfortably maintain, which in the average patient is about 5–10% of total body weight or 2 BMI units. Attaining "ideal" body weight, or a loss of 20–30% or more of total body weight, is not possible for the vast majority of overweight and obese people. Loss of 5–10% of body weight can significantly improve risk factors associated with obesity (36) even though many patients may be disappointed with not reaching their "dream weight." Coun-

Table 8 A Guide to Selecting Treatment

Treatment	BMI category				
	25–26.9	27–29.9	30–34.9	35–39.9	≥40
Diet, exercise, behavior therapy	With comorbidities	With comorbidities	+	+	+
Pharmacotherapy		With comorbidities	+	+	+
Surgery				With comorbidities	+

Prevention of weight gain with lifestyle therapy is indicated in any patient with a BMI > 25, even without comorbidities, while weight loss is not necessarily recommended for those with a BMI of 25–29.9 kg/m^2 or a high waist circumference, unless they have two or more comorbidities. Combined intervention with a low-calorie diet, increased physical activity, and behavior therapy provide the most successful therapy for weight loss and weight maintenance.
Source: Ref. 8.

seling about achievable goals and alternative goals such as an improvement in lipids or glucose, improved mobility, reduced waist circumference, or simply compliance with the regimen are worthy alternative goals. Prevention of weight gain is another important treatment goal, particularly for patients not ready to initiate an active weight loss program.

Patients on a weight loss regimen should be seen in the office within approximately 2–4 weeks of starting treatment in order to monitor both the treatment's effectiveness and its side effects. Visits every 4 weeks are adequate during the first 3 months if the patient has a favorable weight loss and few side effects. More frequent visits may be required based on clinical judgment, particularly if the patient has comorbid conditions. The patient should be weighed each visit, with waist circumference measured less often. Blood pressure and pulse should be monitored if the patient is taking an appetite suppressant. The visit should be used to monitor compliance with the program, provide encouragement, and set new goals. This can be accomplished by reviewing food and exercise records, discussing progress or lack therefore, and solving problems which the patient has encountered. Less frequent follow-up is required after the first 6 months.

C Available Treatments

1 Treatment

There are a number of available treatments that can be used for obesity. The backbone of conventional therapy includes behavior and lifestyle change, exercise, and diet. These are discussed in detail in the Practical Guide from NIH/NAASO (8) and in Chapters 53–55. Medications can also be used as an adjunct to treatment programs using lifestyle change, diet, and exercise. Orlistat, noradrenergic drugs including sibutramine, newer drugs, and thermogenic drugs are discussed in Chapters 14–18. Finally, surgical treatments may be considered for individuals with a BMI ≥ 40 kg/m^2 or BMI ≥ 35 kg/m^2 if they have comorbidities. Further details on this therapy are available in Chapter 18.

2 Resources Available to the Health Care Practitioner

The use of other health care providers with an interest in obesity treatment including dietitians, psychologists, nurses, and nurse practitioners is an efficient way to manage the obese patient. For example, while many physicians feel uncomfortable prescribing a diet, community- or hospital-based dietitians are available in most communities to assist with patient education and support. For the clinician interested in treating obesity in the office, important educational information including sample diets and other patient material may be found in the NIH publication, the Practical Guide: Identification, Evaluation, and Treatment of Overweight and Obesity in Adults (NIH Pub. No. 00-4084) (8) or on the NIH/NHLBI website at *http://www.nhlbi. nih.gov/nhlbi/cardio/obes/prof/guidelns/ob home.htm*. A comprehensive program for patient education can be found in the *LEARN* manual (37). Two recent review articles may also be helpful to the practitioner in crafting an approach to the overweight and obese patient (38,39). In some cases patients may choose to utilize commercial weight loss programs such as Weight Watchers, TOPS (Take Off Pounds Sensibly), or groups such as Overeaters Anonymous for support in addition to the efforts made by the health care provider. These groups can be a helpful addition to the support mechanism required for long-term success. Internet-based support may also be of value as an adjunct for some individuals. Information from the *Practical Guide* is available through the NIH *Aim for a Healthy Weight* website at www.nhlbi.nih.gov/health/public/heart/obesity/lose wt/index.htm. Interactive support is available at low cost ($10–15/month) through websites such as eDiets.com and weight-watchers.com. For patients who have serious problems that are beyond the scope of what can be comfortably managed in the primary care office, referral to an obesity specialist or endocrinologist with an interest in obesity would be appropriate. NAASO, the North American Society for the Study of Obesity, lists its members on its website, http://www.naaso.org.

REFERENCES

1. Guide to Clinical Preventive Services. Report of the U.S. Preventive Services Task Force. 2d ed. Baltimore: Williams & Wilkins, 1996.
2. Galuska DA, Will JC, Serdula MK, Ford ES. Are health care professionals advising obese patients to lose weight? JAMA 1999; 282:1576–1578.
3. Sciamanna CN, Tate DF, Lang W, Wing RR. Who reports receiving advice to lose weight? Results from a multistate survey. Arch Intern Med 2000; 160:2334–2339.
4. Stafford RS, Farhat JH, Misra B, Schoenfeld DA. National patterns of physician activities to obesity management. Arch Fam Med 2000; 9:631–638.
5. Mechanic D, McAlpine DD, Rosenthal M. Are patients' office visits with physicians getting shorter? N Engl J Med 2001; 344:198–204.

6. Stange KC, Zyzanski SJ, Jaen CR, Callahan EJ, Kelly RB, Gillanders WR. Illuminating the 'black box'. A description of 4454 patient visits to 138 family physicians. J Fam Prac 1998; 46:377–389.

7. 10 Steps: Implementation Guide. Put Prevention into Practice. Adapted from The Clinicians' Handbook of Preventive Services. 2d ed, Publication No. 98–0025, Rockville, MD: Agency for Healthcare Research and Quality, 1998. http://www.ahrq.gov/ppip/impsteps.htm

8. The Practical Guide: Identification, Evaluation, and Treatment of Overweight and Obesity in Adults. U.S. Department of Health and Human Services, Public Health Service, National Institutes of Health, National Heart, Lung, and Blood Institute. NIH Publication No. 00-4084, October 2000.

9. Yano EM, Fink A, Hirsch SH, Robbins AS, Rubenstein LV. Helping practices reach primary care goals. Lessons from the literature. Arch Intern Med 1995; 155:1146–1156.

10. Kushner R, Pendarvis L. An integrated approach to obesity care. Nutr Clin Care 1999; 2:285–291.

11. Frank A. A multidisciplinary approach to obesity management: the physician's role and team care alternatives. J Am Diet Assoc 1998; 98(suppl 2):S44–S48.

12. Crabtree BF, Miller WL, Aita VA, Flocke SA, Stange KC. Primary care practice organization and preventive services delivery: a qualitative analysis. J Fam Pract 1998; 46:404–409.

13. Scholle SH, Agatisa PK, Krohn MA, Johnson J, McLaughlin MK. Locating a health advocate in a private obstetrics/gynecology office increases patient's receipt of preventive recommendations. J Womens Health Gender-Based Med 2000; 9:161–165.

14. Dickey L, Frame P, Rafferty M, Wender RC. Providing more-and better—preventive care. Patient Care 1999; Nov 15:198–210.

15. Ahluwalia JS, Gibson CA, Kenney E, Wallace DD, Resnicow K. Smoking status as a vital sign. J Gen Intern Med 1999; 14:402–408.

16. Balas EA, Weingarten S, Garb CT, Blumenthal D, Boren SA, Brown GD. Improving preventive care by prompting physicians. Arch Intern Med 2000; 160:301–308.

17. Kreuter MW, Chheda SG, Bull FC. How does physician advice influence patient behavior? Evidence for a priming effect. Arch Fam Med 2000; 9:426–433.

18. Swinburn BA, Walter LG, Arroll B, Tilyard MW, Russell DG. The green prescription study: a randomized controlled trial of written advice provided by general practitioners. Am J Public Health 1998; 88:288–291.

19. Calfas KJ, Long BJ, Sallis JF, Wooten WJ, Fratt M, Patrick K. A controlled trial of physician counseling to promote the adoption of physical activity. Prev Med 1996; 25:225–233.

20. Albright CL, Cohen S, Gibbons L, Miller S, Marcus B, Sallis J. Incorporating physical activity advice into primary care. Physician-delivered advice within the activity counseling trial. Am J Prev Med 2000; 18:225–234.

21. Petrella RJ, Wight D. An office-based instrument for exercise counseling and prescription in primary care. The Step Test Exercise Prescription (STEP). Arch Fam Prac 2000; 9:339–344.

22. Balint M. The Doctor, His Patient, and the Illness New York: International University Press, 1972.

23. Groopman JE, Kunkel EJ, Platt FW, White MK. Sharing decision making with patients. Patient Care 2001; April 15:21–35.

24. Stewart MA. Effective physician-patient communication and health outcomes: a review. Can Med Assoc J 1995; 152:1423–1433.

25. Kravitz RL. Measuring patients' expectations and requests. Ann Intern Med 2001; 134:881–888.

26. Marvel MK, Epstein RM, Flowers K, Beckman HB. Soliciting the patient's agenda. Have we improved? JAMA 1999; 281:283–287.

27. Emanuel EJ, Emanuel LL. Four models of the physician-patient relationship. JAMA 1992; 267:2221–2226.

28. Roter D. The enduring and evolving nature of the patient-physician relationship. Patient Educ Counseling 2000; 39:5–15.

29. Branch WT, Malik TK. Using 'windows of opportunities' in brief interviews to understand patients' concerns. JAMA 1993; 269:1667–1668.

30. Novack DH. Therapeutic aspects of the clinical encounter. J Gen Intern Med 1987; 2:346–355.

31. Suchman AL, Markakis K, Beckman HB, Frankel R. A model of empathic communication in the medical interview. JAMA 1997; 277:678–682.

32. Luftey KE, Wishner WJ. Beyond "compliance" is "adherence." Improving the prospect of diabetes care. Diabetes Care 1999; 22:635–639.

33. Jaret P. 10 ways to improve patient compliance. Hippocrates 2001; Feb/Mar:22–28.

34. Steiner JF, Earnest MA. The language of medication-taking. Ann Intern Med 2000; 132:926–930.

35. World Health Organization. Preventing and Managing the Global Epidemic of Obesity. Report of the WHO Consultation on Obesity. Geneva: WHO, 1997:926.

36. Blackburn G. Effect of degree of weight loss on health benefits. Obesity Research 1995; 3:211–216S.

37. Brownell KD, Wadden TA. The LEARN Program for Weight Control—Medication Edition. Dallas: American Health Publishing Company, 1998.

38. Kushner RF, Weinsier RL. Evaluation of the obese patient. Practical considerations. Med Clin North Am 2000; 84:387–399.

39. Anderson DA, Wadden TA. Treating the obese patient. Suggestions for primary care practice. Arch Fam Med 1999; 8:156–167.

3

Cultural Differences as Influences on Approaches to Obesity Treatment

Shiriki Kumanyika

University of Pennsylvania School of Medicine, Philadelphia, Pennsylvania, U.S.A.

I INTRODUCTION

The significance of cultural influences in the etiology of obesity has been well documented, particularly with respect to societal standards of female attractiveness (1–3). Among the major chronic conditions that affect morbidity and mortality, obesity is unique in having a sociocultural significance unrelated to its presumed effects on long-term health, and biomedical definitions of obesity compete with sociocultural definitions (4). This chapter addresses the related issue of the potential influence of cultural factors on obesity treatment approaches and outcomes. The spectrum of cultural influences on obesity treatment goes far beyond body image or physical attractiveness variables. From the client perspective, this spectrum also includes perceptions and priorities in the domains of general health, food and eating, and physical activity as well as behavioral change variables. The latter include how food, activity, and weight interrelate with mechanisms for coping with stress, attitudes toward health professionals, and a host of contextual variables in which these attitudes and behaviors are anchored. From the programmatic perspective, cultural influences affect treatment models, professional orientations, program content and form, and provider attitudes and behaviors. The respective intersections of these types of cultural influences on obesity treatment are shown in Figure 1.

This figure also serves as a conceptual outline of the issues addressed in this chapter.

The goal of this chapter is to facilitate understanding of how the incorporation of cultural considerations into program design and implementation might improve obesity treatment outcomes, particularly long-term treatment outcomes. The term "obesity treatment" is defined broadly to refer to the various types of health behavior change programs that focus on weight reduction or weight control (5). The discussion is framed primarily in terms of the U.S. obesity treatment settings where the providers and clients have different ethnic backgrounds and where the clients are members of ethnic minority populations. The concepts are, however, applicable to cross-cultural settings more generally. An underlying theme is that all obesity treatment situations are "cross-cultural" to the extent that obesity treatment paradigms are not aligned with the cultural context of obesity and weight control in the general population.

Section II of the chapter provides some background on what is meant by culture and cross-cultural differences and on why these considerations are of increasing interest to the field of obesity treatment. This section describes differences in obesity prevalence and determinants in U.S. ethnic minority groups compared to the majority U.S. population. Section III examines the status of cultural considerations in relevant health and

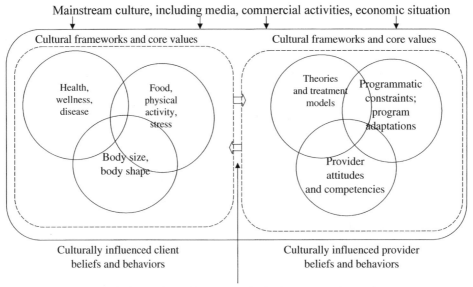

Mainstream culture, including media, commercial activities, economic situation

Cultural frameworks and core values

Health, wellness, disease

Food, physical activity, stress

Body size, body shape

Cultural frameworks and core values

Theories and treatment models

Programmatic constraints; program adaptations

Provider attitudes and competencies

Culturally influenced client
beliefs and behaviors

Culturally influenced provider
beliefs and behaviors

Congruencies and incongruencies in the treatment interaction

Figure 1 Schematic representation of the cultural influences in obesity treatment.

behavior change paradigms. Section IV focuses on the cultural variables that influence those who provide obesity treatment. Sections V and VI highlight ways that cultural factors have been addressed in obesity treatment programs and comment on future directions for the field.

II CULTURAL DETERMINANTS OF OBESITY

A A Culture and Cultural Differences

Culture influences all human behavior and dialectically shapes social institutions and social interactions among populations groups and individuals. Culture has many definitions, but all embody the underlying concept of implicit and explicit guidelines that are inherited and shared by members of a particular society or societal subgroup (6,7). These guidelines define "how to view the world, how to experience it emotionally, and how to behave in it in relation to other people, to supernatural forces or gods, and to the natural environment" (7). These cultural perspectives are identifiable and transmitted from one generation to the next through distinctive symbols, language, and rituals. Of particular relevance to cross-cultural treatment issues, cultural influences on behavior tend to be relatively invisible. Certain types of behavior seem universal, natural, and nonnegotiable to those influenced by a given culture (7). In fact, the influence of culture often becomes evident

only when cultural differences are encountered, e.g., in interactions between individuals or groups that have contrasting beliefs, expectations, or values related to a particular issue; that is, one might not perceive that one is operating within a culture until one has to operate outside of it.

Table 1 lists examples of culturally determined values and beliefs (8–14). Some of these variables, such as worldview or spirituality, are overarching and form the context for other elements. Differences between cultures on specific topics, sometimes termed "cultural distance," are often a matter of degree or emphasis. However, the sum total of cultural differences may result in qualitatively different ways of approaching life and day-to-day transactions. Furthermore, cultural norms, e.g., what is considered usual, expected, or appropriate, result from the interaction of cultural values and beliefs with environmental variables such as the social structure and the availability of commodities such as food and health care.

B The Obesity-Promoting Environment

There is a general concern within the field of behavior change that the available methods are not sufficient to produce long-term improvements in lifestyle risk factors related to diet and physical activity, including obesity, as well as cigarette smoking (15). The need for effective long-term weight control strategies has become especially urgent in light of recent increases in obesity

Table 1 Examples of Culturally Determined Values and Beliefs

1. Worldview—how person views himself or herself in relation to the environment; the types of explanatory models used to understand day to day occurrences and to make sense of life experiences
2. Spirituality—beliefs in God, belief in the supernatural, sense of destiny and control over one's life; view of life, death and afterlife
3. Harmony—view of oneself as interdependent with the environment; desire to dominate the environment; responsibility of the individual to humanity; sense of interconnectedness or discreteness of the various aspects of one's life; consumption and sharing of resources
4. Health and reproduction—concepts of wellness and optimal performance; disease and illness; food and sustenance; procreation
5. Interdependence—of people, individuals' freedoms and responsibilities, social orientation vs. individualistic orientation; definition of family (e.g., nuclear family; extended family; biologic vs. socially defined kinship); definitions of self-reliance; expectations for caregiving; gender roles
6. Rhythm—sense of rhythmic nature to life; role of seasons; orientation to rhythms, music, dance in behavior and overall approach to life.
7. Affect and cognition—importance of rationality; importance of emotion; degree to which emotion and thinking are considered separate; role of emotions and rationality in social relations
8. Individualism and communalism—separateness of self; uniqueness of individuals; social conformity; importance of individual expression; degree of interdependence with others
9. Linearity—value of order and step-by-step progression; acceptance of chaos and unpredictability
10. Vitality—energy of living; fullness of participation in all aspects of life
11. Interpersonal relationships—views about conflict and aggression; value for cooperation; ways of conveying approval/disapproval or social support
12. Status orientation—value of education and material possessions
13. Work orientation—work ethic; industriousness; work as self-definition; work as economic necessity
14. Approaches to technology—attitudes toward computers; attraction to new inventions; support of research and development activities
15. Communication styles—relative value of oral and written communication; directness of communication; body language
16. Time perspective—orientation to clock time or to events; future orientation or present orientation; history as a basis for reflection

Sources: Refs. 8–11,14.

prevalence (16,17). At the ecological level, this upward trend in prevalence can be directly linked to cultural norms and social structural factors that encourage and maintain chronic overconsumption of calories and physically inactive lifestyles (17,18). The most obvious trends are those related to food portion sizes (e.g., supersizing of food packaging and restaurant portions), use of automobiles, television watching, use of computers, and sedentary forms of recreation (19,20). These trends are embedded in a synergism between cultural values (e.g., for individual choice, free-market activity, and consumerism) and the social structure (e.g., production, availability, and aggressive marketing of large quantities of high-calorie foods and technological advances resulting in labor-saving devices and electronic communications that have economic benefits for society) (21). Thus, in the United States and in other countries where similar societal trends and cultural shifts have occurred, obesity treatment occurs in a context where there are strong societal forces promoting weight gain and potentially counteracting individual attempts to lose weight or maintain weight loss (22).

Thus, we are now attempting to treat obesity in a situation in which both being overweight and the eating and activity behaviors that lead to being overweight, although not normal in a physiologic sense, are normative; that is, those who do not maintain adequate weight control now outnumber those who do. The difficulty of maintaining self-control of behaviors related to eating and physical activity has increased from prior times partly because people are bombarded with consumption stimuli via the mass media, and partly because they are receiving mixed signals about eating, physical activity, and weight. Both the social structure and many current cultural norms favor day-to-day (e.g., not just on occasional holidays and at celebrations) behaviors that are highly obesity promoting, whereas obesity itself is still viewed as problematic.

C Obesity in Ethnic Minority Populations in the United States

1 Minority Populations

Last (23) defines an ethnic group as follows:

A social group characterized by a distinctive social and cultural tradition, maintained within the group from generation to generation, a common history and origin, and a sense of identification with the group. Members of the group have distinctive features in their way of life, shared experiences, and often a common genetic heritage. These features may be reflected in their health and disease experience (23:44).

Ethnicity is often a more appropriate designation than "race," which purports to describe a biologically homogeneous group (24). Variations in cultural perspectives of different ethnic groups have always been of some interest for biomedicine in comparisons across societies (25,26). Cultural issues are receiving more attention in the United States as the population becomes more diverse (24,27). There is considerable ethnic, socioeconomic, and sociocultural diversity within the broad minority population categories used by the U.S. Census Bureau. From a sociopolitical perspective, what these groups have in common is being "nonwhite" or "Hispanic," whereas the majority population is defined as whites who do not indicate Hispanic ethnicity. Stated from a behavioral intervention perspective, minority populations encompass those subgroups that are viewed as sufficiently different from the U.S. mainstream population and are therefore potentially less well served by programs designed with the majority in mind (28). The more distinct the language and cultural characteristics of the population from the mainstream, the greater the implied need for special considerations. However, if only by virtue of residence in the U.S. society, members of ethnic minority populations are also—to varying degrees—participants in the mainstream U.S. culture and influenced by mainstream cultural variables through media, workplace interactions, and other forms of social exchange. Thus, ethnicity and "minority" status are addional rather than necessarily alternative cultural influences. There are many cultural similarities among minority populations. Both the similarities and the differences must be considered.

Not all social and behavioral differences among ethnic minority populations and the majority are attributable to cultural values and beliefs. There are also differences in sociodemographic indicators such as: the percentage who are foreign born, fertility rates, life expectancy, household and family structure, educational achievement, occupations, neighborhood characteristics, income distribution, health insurance coverage, and interactions with the health system (24,27,29). It is therefore difficult to separate ethnic differences that are culturally determined from those due to sociodemographic factors, particularly those related to social structural factors such as poverty or discrimination that differentially affect minority populations. Moreover, there are culturally determined differences in attitudes and behaviors according to factors such as gender, age, geographic region, religious affiliation, and occupation within all populations. Each individual is, therefore, potentially influenced by a range of interrelated cultural and social structural variables. Behaviors of individuals in ethnic minority populations reflect a blend of the cultural perspectives to which they are exposed.

2 Obesity Prevalence and Determinants

The prevalence of obesity is higher among black, Hispanic, American Indian, and Pacific Islander populations in the United States than among non-Hispanic whites, especially among women (16,30,31) (see Fig. 2), and this high prevalence is associated with a high burden of diabetes and other obesity-related diseases (32–37). Data for children in these minority populations also suggest trends of increasing prevalence of obesity (38,39) and type 2 diabetes beginning early in life (40). Excess obesity in minority populations has led to explicit concerns about ethnic group differences in the factors that predispose to obesity and in the ability to effectively prevent and treat obesity in these populations. It is possible that the prevalence of a biological predisposition to gain weight is higher in the ethnic groups that exhibit such a high prevalence of obesity. However, to date this has not been established (3,41). What has been established, for example, from comparisons of Pima Indians and of African-descent individuals living in different environments (42,43), is that the predisposition to obesity is only expressed under permissive environmental circumstances.

Table 2 lists examples of culturally influenced variables that are specifically relevant to obesity treatment (44). As shown, these include variables that determine underlying or usual eating and physical activity patterns and assumptions about how food and activity relate to health as well as those that are specific to weight. As discussed elsewhere (3), cultural attitudes that favor a larger body image or at least do not support a strong drive to become thin can be documented for several ethnic minority populations (45). Overweight and obesity are especially normative in those minority populations where it affects half or two-thirds of adults and where the link between obesity and poor health outcomes is not always recognized (46,47). That illnesses associated with thinness or wasting (e.g., cancer, tuberculosis, or AIDS) are prominent in the health profiles of minority populations (29) may perpetuate the sense that

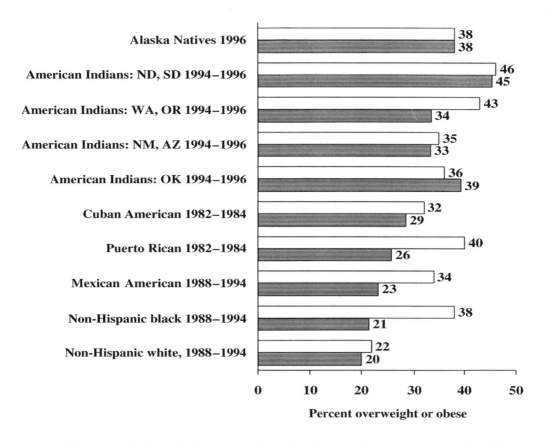

Figure 2 Prevalence of obesity in U.S. ethnic minority populations. BMI 30 +, or BMI 27.8 + for men (shaded bars) and 27.3 + for women (open bars); data for American Indians are based on self-report. (From Refs. 16,31.)

Table 2 Examples of General and Weight-Specific, Culturally Influenced Attitudes and Perceptions Relevant to Weight Management

Food, activity, and health in general	Related to body size and weight
Medicinal or health promoting properties of food; health-related food restrictions	Ideal, acceptable, and undesirable body sizes and shapes
Symbolic meanings and social uses of food	Definitions of thinness and fatness
Food and flavor preferences and aversions	Perceived determinants of weight status
Fasting and food deprivation	Importance of personal body size and shape and relationship to self-concept
Food portions; leaving food on plate; satiety	Functional and health effects (positive and negative) of being at a given weight
Overeating; food and coping style	Priority given to weight management
Physiological effects and health benefits of physical activity, exercise, and rest	Ways to lose or gain weight or influence body shape, including role of diet and exercise
Food-related social roles	Standards of personal attractiveness
Role constraints related to gender, age, social position, and work	Perceived social pressure to lose or gain weight
Preferred types of leisure time activity	Inclination toward low-fat diets, diet pills, or purging

Source: Ref. 44.

being heavy is healthier than being thin, particularly among low-income women (47,48).

Several aspects of body image, dieting, and dieting motivations appear to differ by ethnicity (49,50). However, there are also striking similarities in the prevalence of dieting across ethnic groups (51–54). That is, although there are clearly body image differences that alter the motivation and context for obesity treatment, there is substantial diversity in these attitudes within minority communities as well as substantial evidence of strong weight loss motivations—even if of a differential quality than in the white population (54–56). For example, in the analysis of national survey data reported by Serdula et al. (54), Hispanic men and women were significantly more likely than white men and women to be trying to lose weight. Body image may be the most dissimilar across ethnic groups in women who are not overweight or obese. In most or all populations and even where there are positive cultural values for large body size, those who are overweight or obese seems to be less satisfied with their weight than those who are lean (55,56). Wolfe (57) has criticized the amount of attention given to cultural attitudes of black women, suggesting that it detracts attention from the many societal factors that predispose black women to gain weight and the need to address these in an attempt to control obesity.

As shown in Table 2, there are many culturally influenced attitudes and behaviors related to food and activity that have implications for weight but that are not driven primarily by body image or weight concerns. Norms about food, activity, and health are defined and continually reinforced within cultures—for example, the concept of what constitutes having enough food or feasting when food is abundant to anticipate possible food shortages, how food should be flavored, what combinations of food can be eaten together, what physical activities are appropriate for children but not for adults or for males but not females, the importance of inactivity (e.g., rest), or how one should cope with stress and restore physical and mental balance (45,58–60). The cultural embeddedness of food and the role of food as a carrier of ethnic identity and vehicle for social expression and social interactions is the subject of a large anthropological literature (45,61–63) that, if taken seriously, can be very daunting to anyone who seeks to change food habits. Nevertheless, weight and health risk reduction considerations can only be viewed logically as superimposed onto these more basic attitudes and as competing with other day-to-day survival and quality-of-life priorities. Priority on weight reduction relative to other health or survival concerns may be lower for the medically obese in ethnic or socioeconomic status groups for which body size and shape are less central to self-image or social acceptance or where some aspects of large body size (shapeliness, muscularity, strength) improve social acceptance or status. As discussed below, there may also be less congruency between basic attitudes and beliefs related to food and activity in minority populations and those advised for weight management.

Compared to the U.S. white population, minority populations are experiencing social and economic transitions from relative poverty, food shortages, and lifestyles that involved significant physical labor to circumstances in which there are more than sufficient amounts of food readily available to even the poorest segment of society and limited demand for physical work (64–67). Although cultural perspectives change, they tend to follow societal changes after a considerable time lag. Thus, the food and activity-related cultural perspectives of ethnic minority populations may still be primed to promote survival under prior circumstances—simplistically, to feasting and resting from hard work rather than restricting food and seeking extra physical work. Such perspectives would heighten the vulnerability to obesity in the current environment in which food and activity-related survival needs have been reversed from prior times. For example, poor food security—defined as worrying about having access to sufficient food—has been associated with an excess of overweight in women, and the prevalence of overweight was generally highest among women in the lowest income categories (68).

National surveys do not necessarily show higher energy intakes in minority populations compared to whites (69). One reason for this may be a differentially high level of energy underreporting in ethnic minority populations compared to whites. Conclusive evidence of differences in energy balance requires data on both energy intake and energy expenditure. Data for minority populations are strongly indicative of higher than average levels of physical inactivity (70–72). Excess obesity could, therefore, result even if energy intakes in minority populations were not high in comparison to those of less obese populations. Physical activity questionnaires may have differential validity in populations with different leisure time and occupational activity lifestyles. However, in black women, for example, the finding of lower activity compared to white women has been corroborated in studies using objective measures of physical activity (73,74).

Those with the least latitude in personal choices have the greatest lifestyle constraints (75). Thus, when the society at large has an overabundance of obesity-promoting forces, the potential deleterious effects may be intensified in minority populations. U.S. communities continue to be ethnically segregated (27). Most individuals in minority populations live in communities where the other residents are also minorities, whereas most non-Hispanic whites live in predominantly white communities. Constraints of particular importance in minority communities may include too few supermarkets and neighborhood or workplace physical fitness facilities, too many fast food establishments or food vendors selling high-fat foods at low prices, and high neighborhood crime rates that discourage outdoor activities (71,76–78). Media exposure may also be particularly detrimental (79,80). For example, a recent analysis of food advertising on prime-time television found that the shows oriented to blacks had significantly more food commercials per 30-min segment and that more of these commercials were for high calorie-low nutrient density foods (80). These authors also noted that more of the characters on the black-oriented shows were overweight—perhaps reflecting the prevalence of obesity in the community but also reinforcing the concept that obesity is normative. That is, the high prevalence of obesity in minority populations is in itself an important contextual factor potentially influencing obesity treatment.

Finally, the reproductive and health status profiles of minority populations may predispose to weight gain and physical inactivity. Fertility rates are higher in minority women than white women (24), predisposing to pregnancy-related weight gain. The amount of weight that is gained and retained with each pregnancy may also be higher (81). In addition, the high prevalence of obesity-related health problems such as diabetes or osteoarthritis may interact with age-related social role perceptions to limit, or be perceived as limiting, participation in physical activity.

In summary, living circumstances, eating and activity practices, and related attitudes vary among ethnic groups, leading to potential differences in weight loss motivations and in the way that obesity treatment programs will be received and adhered to. Relevant factors include the psychosocial receptivity to food restriction, body image issues, the congruency between behavior change recommendations and accustomed habits, feasibility of recommended changes, and social network and community support for lower calorie eating or increased physical activity.

III BEHAVIOR CHANGE PARADIGMS

All paradigms reflect and are grounded in culture. However, the currently dominant biomedical paradigm in the United States is allopathic, technology centered,

and clinical (25,82). As such, it does not readily incorporate cultural considerations in its explanatory framework, at least not directly, even for conditions such as obesity that are clearly culture bound in many respects (4). However, the awareness of cultural issues in U.S. health care generally has increased with ongoing globalization and population diversity and with the resulting interactions and overlap among cultures (82–84). This general phenomenon, together with the particularly high burden of obesity and related disease in minorities and some evidence that obesity treatments are less effective in minority populations than in whites, has led to some acknowledgment of the importance of attention to cultural influences in obesity treatment (85). It is therefore useful to examine the extent to which current obesity treatment or lifestyle change theories and treatment models, which are still grounded in the dominant paradigm, accommodate cross-cultural issues.

The relevant conceptualizations for these paradigms relate primarily to theories of long-term maintenance of behavior and involve two related themes. One theme is that individual behavior and, consequently, behavior change, occur within contexts that constitute critical influences on treatment outcomes. Cultural variables are implicit and explicit elements of these contexts. The other theme is that the client's adherence perspectives, including cultural norms and values and social-structural constraints, should be used to tailor behavioral change programs for greater effectiveness with subgroups and individuals. Both themes are discussed in more detail in the following text.

A Contextualization of Learning and Behavior

1 Social Cognitive Theory

Bandura, whose theoretical guidance has been a critical underpinning of obesity treatment, has commented on the relationship of cultural factors to Social Cognitive Theory (SCT) (86). In a recent text, he is critical of the apparent divergence between microanalytic and macroanalytic inquiry into the processes of human functioning. The microanalysts focus on "the inner workings of the mind in processing, representing, retrieving, and using the coded information to manage various task demands, and locating where the brain activity for these events occurs...[with] these cognitive processes generally studied disembodied from interpersonal life, purposeful pursuits, and self-reflectiveness" (86:5). In contrast, the macroanalysts focus on the "workings of socially situated factors in human development, adaptation, and change...[and] human functioning is analyzed as socially interdependent, richly contextualized, and conditionally orchestrated within the dynamics of various societal subsystems and their complex interplay" (86:5). He observes that because sociostructural influences operate through psychological mechanisms to produce behavioral effects, "comprehensive theory must merge the analytic dualism by integrating personal and social foci of causation within a unified causal structure" (86:5).

In an attempt to make this link, Bandura promotes the notion of "human agency," which embodies the endowments, belief systems, self-regulatory capacities, and distributed structures and functions through which personal influence is exercised. In short, he introduces a theoretical view of the human being as an agent who can intentionally make things happen by his or her actions. For example, he proposes that efficacy beliefs are the foundation of human agency, and that cross-cultural research attests to their universal functional value. Bandura also notes that "cultural embeddedness shapes the ways in which efficacy beliefs are developed, the purposes to which they are put, and the sociostructural arrangements through which they are best exercised" (86:16). People from cultures that are individualistic "feel most efficacious and perform best under an individually oriented system, whereas those from collectivistic cultures judge themselves most efficacious and work most productively under a group-oriented system." (86:16). Congruency between the person's psychological orientation and the structure of the social system is thought to provide for the greatest personal efficacy (86). If that is true, it follows then that attention to cultural issues in obesity treatment programs has as its goal the fostering of such congruency. However, providers from the individualistic, U.S. mainstream culture, may have difficulty in understanding the efficacy orientations of ethnic minority participants who are grounded in a collectivistic culture. Fisher et al. suggest that the tendency of those with an individualistic perspective to view social support as "a 'crutch' that psychologically mature individuals do not need" (87:54), in itself a value judgment, may interfere with appropriate programming in minority communities.

2   Social Ecologic Theory

Stokols, a proponent of Social Ecological Theory, emphasizes the critical influence of the context in which behaviors occur on the potential for behavior change (88). Referring to cardiovascular risk reduction programs such as the Multiple Risk Factor Intervention Trial (MRFIT) and the Minnesota Heart Health Program, he suggests that the "modest impact of these interventions reveals some potential limitations that are inherent in behavior change models of health pro-

motion" (88:284). These limitations center around insufficient attention to economic, social, and cultural constraints that may impede a person's efforts to modify his/her health practices. Strategies to enhance the health promoting capacity of the environment are advised in conjunction with those that are geared to facilitating behavior change at the individual level, that is, strategies that "enhance the fit between people and their surroundings." Similar to the concepts discussed by Bandura, Stokols notes that "instances of people-environment fit occur in settings where participants enjoy a high degree of control over their surroundings and are free to initiate goal-directed efforts to modify the environment in accord with their preferences and plans" (88:290).

Social Ecologic Theory may be viewed by some as relating primarily to community-based treatment programs, whereas obesity treatment paradigms are dominated by practice in clinical settings. However, as Bandura's analysis (86) reminds us, the concept of enhancing person-environment fit as a goal of treatment applies generally. If one accepts that effective human functioning depends on a level of efficacy that requires a reasonable person-environment fit, the result of a mismatch between a treatment program and the needs and perspectives of the client will be either psychological stress (because of the high psycho-social cost of adherence) or nonadherence (to avoid the stress).

3   Context Dependency of Learning

Bouton (89) offers some insights as to how context influences behavioral adoption and long-term maintenance, drawing on both human and animal experiments, as follows. All learned behaviors, both old and new, are dependent upon the context in which they are learned, and the cues that lead to a given behavioral response are associated with that context. Consistent with the discussion above, Bouton points out that context can be defined broadly, to include physical and psychosocial stimuli and presumably—although not mentioned by Bouton—cultural forces. Furthermore, when behaviors are unlearned or relearned, this "extinction" or "counterconditioning" does not involve permanent removal of a prior behavior or habit. Rather, both old and new behaviors persist as possible responses to a given cue or set of cues, and the context is what "selects" or determines the response that occurs. Bouton's elaboration on this theoretical perspective offers a plausible explanation for the problem of lapse and relapse in the treatment of obesity as well as for other areas of lifestyle change. For example, he points out that the second response learned to a given stimulus seems to be more context dependent than the original learning, rendering the old or first-learned behaviors likely to occur and reoccur whenever the context does not preclude their occurrence. Relapse can then be thought of not as failure of the new behaviors but as success of the old ones. Using this logic, eating and physical activity behaviors targeted in obesity treatment can be viewed as strongly cued and reinforced by the conditions under which they were initially learned. This learning presumably takes place in family and community settings. The behaviors can, therefore, be expected to respond to reference group cultural values and norms. In contrast, new behaviors developed during treatment would be viewed as secondary learning, inherently weaker responses, and tied to cues present only in association with treatment and the associated values and norms. Leaving the treatment setting ("returning home," physically or psychologically) would then clearly favor the original behaviors, leading to lapses and, potentially, to continued reinforcement of the original behavior (relapses) (89).

Bouton extends this reasoning to a discussion of how one might prevent lapses and relapses (89). One approach would be to avoid contexts that will retrieve the original behavior. Although this may be advised, such cue avoidance is almost always impossible—especially in the long term—given that the context in question includes, for example, a person's deep-seated cultural values and beliefs related to eating as well as day-to-day social- or work-related behaviors and interactions within which eating occasions and activities occur. The other approaches suggested by Bouton involve providing a broader contextualization of the new learning, for example: placing cues to the treatment context in the larger environment (phone calls at home; mailings) or actually conducting the therapy in multiple environments, or extending the temporal context of treatment over a longer period of time. Bouton also suggests that deliberately switching contexts during treatment may ultimately lead to more robust learning, although the initial effect may be to make learning more difficult. As will be discussed, the strategies that are used increasingly in tailoring treatment and cultural adaptation are very consistent with the realization that a person's usual context of daily living cannot be avoided and may be counter to the treatment context.

Bouton's perspective on context is consistent with Bandura's discussion of human agency in SCT (86) and with Social Ecologic Theory (88), as discussed above, in expressing the principle that elicited changes must by definition be linked to the person's usual operational cultural context in order to be maintained over the long term. Several major SCT constructs are indicative of the need to contextualize learning, both physically and affectively (89,90). However, those who design and implement SCT-based programs may not emphasize these cultural aspects. Culturally based provider attitudes may promote the belief that potentially problematic contextual cues can be overcome by sheer self-control.

B Tailoring Treatment Programs

1 "Focal points" for Intervention

"Tailoring" refers to deliberate attempts to account for important individual or subgroup variables when developing program messages or intervention strategies (91). The concept of tailoring has particular relevance to theories that incorporate contextual factors as primary intervention variables as opposed to those that tend to subordinate the importance of contextual issues in favor of greater emphasis on self-control. As reviewed by Rakowski (91), the concept of tailoring has evolved to a high level of specificity with respect to how tailoring can be approached and why it might work where other approaches have failed (91). Many of the relevant variables are culturally determined, although this is implicit rather than directly argued. According to Rakowski, key principles are the need for prior knowledge of the constellation of variables that predict individual variation in a given behavior, and the context specificity of these variables to the interaction of behavior, population, and setting. He designates the particular combination of these three elements as "focal points" for intervention, giving as an example, "blood pressure control [behavioral focus] among blue collar smokers [population focus] in a worksite intervention [setting]" (91:285).

Rakowski's discussion of tailoring highlights the importance of needs assessment and process evaluation in the development and conduct of interventions. This approach is at the other extreme from one in which professionals design a program and then expect clients to fit into it. Defining an initial focal point is one stage of tailoring; the second stage would involve further tailoring to individuals within this focal point based on additional variables. The definition of the focal points themselves is dynamic to the extent that subgroups initially thought to be relatively homogeneous on certain broad characteristics might subsequently be found to comprise several focal points, for example, the increasingly recognized heterogeneity within the major ethnic minority populations. Similarly, increasing levels of differentiation are also possible for behavioral foci and settings. Evaluation of intervention process variables and assessments of the relationship of process to outcome can ultimately inform tailoring to refine program strategies and improve effectiveness.

Table 3 lists variables identified by Rakowski as potentially important for tailoring within a given focal point, selected to illustrate the multiple types of cultural influences that are relevant. The selected variables relate either to characteristics of target populations or to the performance demand characteristics of the behavior. Rakowski stresses the importance of basing both the selection and refinement of focal points and the tailoring of intervention strategies on theoretical frameworks, and cites an array of available theories, including SCT and the Transtheoretical Model. However, he cautions that formal theories may not have incorporated key relevant considerations. For example, current theoretical frameworks that do not include culturally based explanatory models of disease causation would provide inadequate guidance for tailoring interventions in situations where a health problem is attributed to irreversible aging.

2   Cultural Sensitivity

a.   "Surface Structure" and "Deep Structure"

Resnicow et al. define "cultural sensitivity" as "the extent to which ethnic/cultural characteristics, experiences, norms, values, behavioral patterns and beliefs of a target population as well as relevant historical, environmental, and social forces are incorporated in the design, delivery, and evaluation of targeted health promotion materials and programs" (92:11). These authors differentiate between "culturally tailored" interventions, which may involve adaptation of existing materials and programs for racial/ethnic subpopulations, and "culturally based" interventions. Culturally based intervention—a relatively recent term—refers to "programs and messages that combine culture, history, and core values as a medium to motivate behavior change" (92:11), for example, programs for American Indians that focus on ancestral spiritual systems.

Resnicow et al. conceptualize cultural sensitivity in two primary dimensions using the terminology, from sociology and linguistics, of "surface structure" and "deep structure." Cultural sensitivity at the level of surface structure involves attention to relatively superficial characteristics, e.g., depicting people from the same ethnic group in illustrations, incorporating preferences for settings, brands, clothing, or music, or having ethnically matched staff. These superficial characteristics are viewed as important for improving program fit with the culture or experience of the population served and can increase the face validity of the program. Deep structure is much more difficult to characterize and grasp. Sensitivity at this level requires an understanding of a range of contextual variables, including core cultural values, historical factors, and others. Resnicow et al. (92) comment that cultural sensitivity at these different levels has different effects on outcome—deep structure relates more to the salience of the program, whereas surface structure relates more to receptivity to the program.

Resnicow et al. emphasize the importance of focus groups and pretesting in the early stages of implementation of culturally tailored or culturally based programs. Focus groups provide for elicitation of surface structure variables as well as a potential opportunity for exploration of deep structure. Pretesting to assess the actual responses of members of the proposed audience to the materials or messages is particularly critical, because cultural content and cultural tailoring are highly vulnerable to nuances of connotation or context that can cause a well-intended message to be received negatively rather than positively.

Table 3 Culturally Relevant Variables Important for Tailoring Behavioral Interventions

Client or population characteristics
    Age, race/ethnicity, gender and socioeconomic variables
    Risk perception/perceived threat of illness
    Readiness for change; stage of change
    Self-efficacy perceptions
    Attitudes about the health practice or illness
    Information processing style
    Attribution of causality for illness
    Availability of family/friend support; social support systems
    Reliance on medical professionals to determine one's health actions
    Tendency to avoid (approach) the health care system
    Level of acculturation to mainstream
Required Psychosocial Resources and Performance Demands
    Holding a positive self-image
    Social support to assist the change process
    Optimism/long-range time perspective
    Sense of timing/scheduling
    Tolerance of discomfort

Source: Ref. 91.

b.   Pen-3 Model

Airhihenbuwa's PEN-3 Model provides a conceptual framework for designing health programs in which cultural considerations are at the core of rather than peripheral or latent considerations in program design (12). In the terminology of Resnicow et al. (92), this would refer to "culturally based" programming. Airhihenbuwa's premise is that "it is more effective to adapt preventive health programs to fit community needs and cultural contexts than the reverse..." (12:26) This, again, expresses the principle of client-program fit and attention to context but in a completely client-centered tone.

The PEN-3 model is shown schematically in Figure 3. The three domains of the model relate to the foci of health education, the understanding of health-related beliefs, and the classification of relevant cultural influences in ways that can guide the selection of program emphases and strategies. In the health education domain, Airhihenbuwa suggests that a central focus on cultural variables cannot be achieved by focusing only on individuals; rather, extended family and neighborhood foci should be included. One could argue that even in individually focused, clinic-based programs it is more efficient to include the family and community in the treatment perspective to the greatest extent possible because of their relationship to the contextual cues of culturally defined behaviors of the primary client. This is particularly true for ethnic groups in which individuals consider themselves to be very interdependent with others and have a communal orientation. One can also argue—using obesity as a case in point—that behavioral programs restricted to clinical environments become increasingly less culturally appropriate as the relevance of culture to the focal points of intervention (to use Rakowski's term) increases.

The second domain for consideration in PEN-3 is educational diagnosis, i.e., the identification of factors that influence health actions of the individual, family, or community. Airhihenbuwa notes that this dimension of PEN-3 evolved from the confluence of three of the principal theoretical frameworks in the health behavior change field: the Health Belief Model, the Theory of Reasoned Action, and the PRECEDE framework (12). Culture does not have a central role in educational diagnosis in these models, but PEN-3 identified cultural elements that are implied in these other models, as follows:

> Perceptions comprise the knowledge, attitudes, values, and beliefs, within a cultural context, that may facilitate or hinder personal, family, and community motivation to change.... Enablers are cultural, societal, systematic, or structural influences or forces that may enhance or be barriers to change, such as the availability of resources, accessibility, referrals, employers, government officials, skills, and types of services (e.g., traditional medicine)... (12:31–32).

Nurturers reflect the "degree to which health beliefs, attitudes, and actions are influenced and mediated, or nurtured, by extended family, kin, friends, peers, and the community" (12:33).

The third dimension of PEN-3 provides specific guidance for the development of culturally appropriate health programs by offering a schema in which culturally based beliefs, norms, and actions can be classified as positive (known to be beneficial to health), existential (exotic to the outside observer but having no harmful health consequences), and negative (known to be harmful to health). Airhihenbuwa notes that the designation given to a particular belief or practice will vary depending on the targeted behavioral outcome. That is, a belief could be positive in relation to one behavior and negative or existential in relation to another. This aspect of the PEN-3 framework can help health professionals, particularly if from outside of the community or culture in question, to avoid overemphasizing negative behaviors without sufficient reinforcement of positive behaviors, to avoid viewing behaviors that are existential or neutral as harmful simply because they are unusual, and to avoid underestimating the cultural anchoring of certain behaviors. Airhihenbuwa recommends segmentation of beliefs and practices with respect to whether they are historically rooted in cultural traditions over the long term or are more recent and short term. For example, the home setting may be most appropriate for addressing either traditional or relatively recent beliefs and practices, whereas media strategies may only work for those beliefs and practices that are not traditionally entrenched.

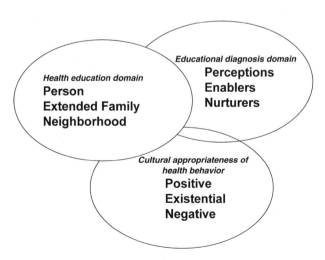

Figure 3 The PEN-3 model. (From Ref. 12.)

IV TREATMENT PROVIDERS

Obesity treatment is ultimately a social exchange between one or more clients and one or more providers who are usually health care professionals. From the foregoing discussion, it is clear that cultural variables and related contextual factors are highly relevant to lifestyle change from the client's perspective. This section addresses cultural influences from the provider perspective. For example, what factors support or limit the receptivity of those who provide obesity treatment to recognizing the importance of cultural variables in treatment? What does professional competence in this domain require?

A Cultural Competence

The topic of cultural competence, i.e., "the ability of a system, agency, or professional to work effectively in cross cultural situations" (83), has become prominent in the health care literature as the challenge of delivering effective health care to an increasingly diverse population has emerged (11,83,93–95). Unlike the terms "compliance" and "adherence," which emphasize client variables as potential barriers to the success of treatment, "cultural competence" puts the focus on what the provider brings to the treatment relationship and requires self-reflection among health professionals. Providers vary in age (e.g., reflecting both generation effects and life stage), ethnicity, regional background, disciplines, language skills, and gender. There are also wide variations in socioeconomic status, political opinions, values, moral codes, and world views among health professionals. These culturally influenced attributes are not eliminated by professional training, and they influence the treatment process. Moreover, because of the social stigma that has been attached to it, obesity constitutes a special case with respect to potential providers; that is, in treating obesity, professionals have the additional challenge of managing their own culturally influenced attitudes about obesity and obese people (96). This does not apply to conditions such as diabetes or hypertension, for example.

The three critical domains of cultural competence are awareness of one's own cultural values and biases, knowledge of client views and perspectives, and skills for designing and delivering culturally appropriate interventions (83). Examples of specific competencies within each of these domains as they relate to nutrition counseling are presented in Table 4. The steps in developing cultural competence follow directly from the nature of the competencies themselves, e.g., increasing one's personal readiness to engage in cross-cultural interactions through self-reflection and learning how to value and be comfortable with differences; learning about other cultures, how one is viewed by people from other cultures, and how to find common ground with people from other cultures; improving both verbal and nonverbal communication styles in cross-cultural interactions, and overcoming associated fears; and learning how to maintain alertness to cross-cultural issues and information (97).

A workshop conducted within the Clinical Trials component of the Women's Health Initiative (WHI) is an example of the increased recognition of the need for cultural competence among health professionals involved in behavioral change interventions (98). The WHI is a 15-year study involving ~ 68,000 older women (ages 50–79) recruited from throughout the United States and including nearly 28,000 from ethnic minority populations. Participant adherence to lifestyle change or medication regimens is of paramount importance to the scientific integrity of this large-scale and costly study. The workshop curriculum was designed to increase knowledge of the demographic and cultural characteristics among and within the diverse groups of women in the WHI, to increase awareness of how diversity affects the interpersonal interactions with study staff, including the potential effect of staff behavior on participant adherence and retention, and to improve effective listening and communication skills. Five cultural domains identified as particularly relevant to the conduct of the WHI were explored during this workshop.

B Professional Culture

As cultures are least visible to those who operate within them, it may be especially difficult for providers to recognize that their professional and organizational cultures have a significant impact on the treatment interaction. Professions create cultures (99) that may act as barriers to both the motivation and ability to provide services in a culturally competent manner. Professional cultures define the ethics of professional conduct, expectations that professionals have about each other and about clients, and systems of rewards and sanctions that help them to gain and maintain public confidence and trust (100,101). Professionals place a high premium on lifelong commitment (102), invest heavily in their training, and incorporate their identity as professionals into their self-concept. Professionals also develop jargon and learn a communication style that makes them at ease with each other, often in a

Table 4 Multicultural Nutrition Counseling Competencies

Domain	Competencies
Self-awareness	Know how personal cultural background and experiences and attitudes, values, and biases influence nutrition counseling
	Know limits of one's own cultural competencies and abilities
	Be aware of and sensitive to one's own cultural heritage and also value and respect differences
	Be comfortable with differences between self and clients related to ethnicity, culture, beliefs, and food practices
	Value personal cultural heritage and world view as a significant starting point for understanding those who are culturally different
	Believe that cultural differences do not have to affect interactions negatively
	Be aware of personally held stereotypes and preconceived notions toward culturally different groups
	Be knowledgeable about cultural differences in communication styles and able to anticipate how one's own style might influence the counseling process
Food and nutrition counseling knowledge	Understand cultural influences on food selection, preparation, and storage
	Have knowledge about cultural eating patterns and family traditions, e.g., core foods
	Be familiar with latest research findings about food practices and related health problems of various ethnic groups
	Have specific knowledge of cultural values, beliefs, and eating practices of population served, including culturally different clients
	Have knowledge of diversity in food practices within ethnic groups
	Use the principle of "starting where the client is" with respect to recommending changes in eating patterns
Nutrition counseling skills	Be able to evaluate new techniques, research, and knowledge for validity and applicability in working with culturally diverse populations
	Take responsibility for orienting the client to the counseling process with respect to goals and expectations
	Have an explicit knowledge of the general characteristics of counseling and how they may clash with expectations of different cultural groups
	Have ability to gain trust and respect of individuals who are culturally different
	Be aware of institutional or agency factors that may be barriers to accessing treatment
	Be able to identify additional resources that may be useful to the client
	Understand how ethnicity, culture, and economics may affect food practices, related health problems, and the appropriateness of various counseling strategies.

Source: Ref. 83.

way that excludes or creates discomfort for others, including their clients (103). These styles are not easy to change. Professionals embrace paradigms to help make sense of their domain, the nature of their knowledge, and the directions of their research agendas (104). Thus, a given type of professional will use and defend a dominant paradigm, often blocking other venues for treatment and understanding.

Professionals, by definition, rely on expert knowledge to claim authority for their roles in diagnosis and treatment and tend to minimize the importance of possible causal factors that fall outside of their areas of expertise (101). Relevant here, to the extent that obesity has been claimed by the domains of clinical medicine and psychology (105,106), the importance of social-contextual factors in obesity causation and treatment will be deemphasized even where acknowledged. "Medicalization" of obesity has also led to a preference for using treatment approaches that have been tried and tested for other medical conditions and to comparing the costs and benefits of obesity treatment with those for other conditions. These professional biases may limit the ability to understand and manage obesity as a unique entity. The training of professionals to keep an appropriate emotional distance in the treatment encounter is also relevant, since—in a cross-cultural interaction—expression of emotion may be necessary for establishing trust and rapport (93).

Understanding the cultural perspective that the provider brings to the treatment encounter also requires an understanding of the culture of the organization in which the professional works (107). Organizations work hard to create a distinctive culture, viewing this as contributing to higher effectiveness (108). For example, organizational culture may be expressed in the form of preferred communications (109), hierarchical structures, and decision-making processes (110) as well as in time horizons, market approaches, and style of teamwork (111). Organizations have bureaucratic rules and processes and legal requirements (112,113). In addition, to survive financially, they must attain goals that have very little to do with any specific treatment and use methods that have a high level of productivity. To be successful within an organization, providers must be able to absorb and function within the culture of their organization. For example they master and abide by the administrative processes and show productivity by organizational standards. These elements directly or indirectly influence the way the provider views obesity as a condition, the treatment options, and the clients themselves (i.e., as potential "treatment successes" or "treatment failures").

The intersection of these personal, professional (including paradigmatic), and organizational elements culminates in expectations about patient/client "compliance" or "adherence." Providers have guidance to offer, and the goal of treatment is for patients to follow that guidance. However, Anderson and Funnell (114) argue that adherence is a dysfunctional concept in relation to the treatment of a chronic disease such as diabetes, because it takes the value of following the health professional's advice as the central value apart from the context in which the patient must follow the advice. Their arguments, summarized in Table 5, are relevant to obesity treatment, as follows: the health professional has needs, expectations, and values with respect to adherence that are inappropriate, because health professionals have no control over the client behaviors in question. These professional expectations and needs may be carryovers from the model of acute-illness care in which it makes sense to expect a patient to give short-term priority to following, directly, a health professional's life-saving advice. In contrast, chronic disease management, and particularly management of conditions such as obesity that may not even be considered by the client to be "diseases," is primarily a function of day-to-day decisions made by the patient. As noted previously, these decisions are, of necessity, made in the context of other life decisions, regardless of the provider's expectations about adherence.

Table 5 Problematic Aspects of the Concept of Adherence or Compliance

Professional expectations
   High investment made to develop helping skills to improve patients' health
   Expectation, from training, that patients should follow advice directly
   Awareness of potential health consequences to individuals of their failure to adopt or refrain from certain health practices
   Awareness of societal costs in health care costs and lost productivity if disease is not controlled
   Need to feel competent and effective in chosen profession
Strongly held beliefs
   Strong belief that patients should strive to prevent disease progression and complications
   Strong belief that patients who do not comply will later regret this
   Perceived obligation to convey seriousness of disease
Limited control over what patients do on a day-to-day basis
   Sense of responsibility for outcome without leverage to affect outcome
   Inadvertent frustration with patients who do not maximize their adherence
   Blaming patients to compensate for feelings of ineffectiveness (e.g., labeling those who are noncompliant as "disobedient")
   Patients may blame provider for not appreciating the impact of recommendations on their lives

Source: Ref. 114.

Thus, in the social interaction that is obesity treatment, several forces are at work that tend to be incompatible, and it is within the realm of the professional, not the client, to find solutions for bridging these forces and creating "win-win" scenarios. This implies that the professional not only grasps the contextual limitations and possibilities of the clients, but also can negotiate substantial amounts of flexibility within his or her own professional and social contexts (115). To use Bandura's conceptualization (86), professionals have to learn the art of human agency as well.

V CULTURAL ADAPTATION STRATEGIES

A Overview

To be theoretically sound, cultural adaptation strategies should link culturally influenced variables to specific aspects of treatment process and outcomes. Examples of such possible links from the client and provider per-

Table 6 Potential Links Between Culturally Influenced Client Variables and Treatment Process and Outcomes[a]

Influences from and interactions between primary reference culture(s) and mainstream culture	Relevant treatment process and outcome variables
Body image	Motivation to seek treatment
Social pressure to lose weight	Enrollment in treatment
Weight-related health concern	Remaining in treatment (vs. dropping out)
Perceived appeal of program	Quality of participation in treatment program
Reactions to treatment setting	Regular attendance
Interactions with provider	Ability to establish trust and rapport
Interactions with other participants	Active engagement in program (passive participation)
Preferred language	Adoption of weight management behaviors
Baseline knowledge, attitudes, and practices	Learning and skill acquisition while in program
Prior relevant experience	Adherence to recommended short-term behavior changes
Perceived relevance of program content	Achievement of short-term weight reduction (vs. no loss, or gain)
Experience of program	Long-term behavior change
Worldview	Motivation for long-term behavior change
Health lifestyle	Feasibility of long-term behavior change
Contextual congruence	Maintenance of long-term behavior changes
Perceived benefits of weight loss	Continued or maintained weight loss (vs. relapse and regain)

[a] Cultural influences on these pathways may be magnified or reduced by other relevant variables that influence feasibility or appropriateness of the program (see text).
Source: Ref. 44. Adapted with permission from Dalton, S. ed. Overweight and Weight Management. Chapter 3: Cultural appropriateness of weight management programs. Gaithersburg, MD: Aspen Publishers; 1997; 69–106.

spective are presented in Table 6. For example, body image and other attitudes may have an influence primarily through effects on the motivation to seek treatment initially or to continue with treatment. Outreach to increase enrollment in a program might then employ persuasive strategies to increase awareness of the possible health or functional status benefits of modest weight loss (e.g., on blood pressure, breathing difficulties, or knee problems) as separate from potentially less salient social or physical attractiveness issues. Cultural sensitivity in the way treatment is delivered would be helpful in ensuring that participants fully engage in the process (quality of participation). The distinction between factors affecting initial adoption versus long-term behavior changes is informed by Rothman's proposition that different theoretical models are needed to explain initial adoption and maintenance (116). For example, whereas initial adoption is related primarily to a desire to achieve a favorable outcome and expectations that these outcomes will be achieved, once adopted, behaviors may be maintained by satisfaction with the outcomes that result.

Thus, offering behavior change content in ways that are relevant to the patient's lifestyle issues and accessible from the perspective of language and learning style would be expected to facilitate short-term behavior changes. Contextual factors such as the world view, the general salience of health considerations in making lifestyle choices, and the structural constraints would be most relevant at the level of maintaining long-term change. Ultimately then, the rewards of having lost weight must be sufficiently reinforcing (positively) within the applicable context to motivate continued practice of the altered eating and activity patterns or, rather, according to Bouton, to drown out the inherently strong reinforcement for the prior, original, and culturally embedded behavior pattern. Clinical programs may be able to maintain changes by providing continued reinforcement through continued treatment. On the other hand, given the nature of obesity and its determinants, a better alternative might be to reframe obesity treatment within health promotion paradigms. Health promotion paradigms are broader than clinical paradigms, are more inclusive of contextual issues, and are ahead of clinical paradigms in articulating specific frameworks for addressing cultural variables (88,117).

B Examples of Cultural Adaptations

Table 7 lists variables within each of several aspects of program design or implementation that might be foci for adaptations to improve cultural relevance or sensitivity. Examples from culturally adapted programs reported in the literature are described in the Appendix. Each of the studies in the Appendix focused on a single ethnic minority population, e.g., African-Americans

Table 7 Culturally Influenced Programmatic Variables as Possible Targets for Cultural Adaptation

Selection and interpretation of theoretical framework
    Emphasis on contextual factors
    Emphasis on cognition over emotion
    Conceptualization of obesity
Provider behavior
    Type of provider
    Role perception, expectations, and needs in the treatment
      setting
    Perception of the ideal client
    Cultural competency (see Table 3)
    Cultural distance from clients
Delivery system and setting
    Research, clinical, or commercial setting
    Emphasis on functionality or familiarity
    Psychological and physical accessibility
    Resources available
Focus of treatment
    Individual
    Family unit
    Community
Treatment goals
    Expected amount and rate of weight loss
    Inclusion of treatment goals other than weight loss
    Protocol or client-driven goal setting
Program content
    Food selections and recipes
    Activity choices
    Assumptions and messages about body size and shape
    Attention to emotions and spirituality
    Language used
Format and mode of contact
    Group, individual, or both
    Didactic or interactive process
    Program duration
    Sequencing of information
    "School culture" (see text)
    Face to face, telephone, mail

(118–127), Mexican-Americans (128,129), Caribbean Latinos (46), Pima Indians (130), or Native Hawaiians (131).

One strategy for increasing the cultural sensitivity of those providing treatment is to involve peer counselors (122,125,130) instead of or in addition to professional counselors. Some studies provide for explicit attention to family issues through home visits (118) or by framing treatment as for families rather than individuals (123, 128). Changing the setting in which treatment is offered is another common strategy. Churches may be used as the physical setting for program delivery (119,122,129) or as both a physical setting and psychosocial setting (126) through the direct incorporation of spiritual con-

tent. A strong "process orientation" is also evident in some programs, e.g., a deliberate attempt to be flexible and incorporate participant suggestions during the course of the program (118,127). The most commonly reported change in program format cited in programs described as culturally adapted is the use of active discovery learning and nondidactic methods (46,120–122). Two studies were identified as culturally based in that core cultural traditions or values were used as the basis for the intervention. In one case, the cultural tradition was a very low-fat, high-carbohydrate diet based on traditional foods of ethnic groups in Hawaii (131). The other example, "Pima Pride," involved discussion focused on attitudes about current lifestyle in the community and invited local speakers to address Pima Indian culture and history (130). This intervention was used as the control condition for comparison with a conventional structured lifestyle change program but had comparable if not better effects than the active intervention.

The reference in Table 7 to "school culture" is taken from the Wilcox et al. (98) WHI workshop summary. Participation in clinical trials was viewed as involving skills that are usually learned in school, including "self-discipline, observing and reporting events, setting long-term goals, and reading and completing forms" (98:285). The WHI authors noted that these demands may be stressful for study participants who lack these skills. This may also apply to clients who have a strong cultural preference for a different style of learning. The emphasis on active discovery learning and nondidactic approaches in programs that have been culturally adapted for ethnic minority populations may reflect the recognition of the need to minimize the "school culture" that is common in conventional programs.

The focus here is on the types of cultural adaptations that have been implemented from a conceptual perspective, i.e., not with respect to the weight losses achieved. As reviewed elsewhere (85), the culturally adapted programs reported in the literature have generally been of relatively low intensity and short duration. These approaches would not necessarily be expected to lead to large initial weight changes, but they were often not continued long enough to determine whether larger effects would have resulted with continued counseling.

VI SUMMARY AND CONCLUSION

Cultural issues arise in conjunction with health programs in general, including weight management programs, because of the belief that attending to cultural factors will allow for services that are better aligned with the client's needs and circumstances and thus more sensitive and effective. In addition, cultural influences on obesity treatment are of particular interest because of the disproportionate prevalence of obesity in U.S. ethnic minority populations. Culture influences obesity and weight change through several attitudinal and behavioral pathways that converge in food intake and energy output. Differences in weight related attitudes and practices can be readily documented among U.S. ethnic groups. In particular, compared to middle-class whites, some population groups with a higher prevalence of obesity have more tolerant views about obesity.

Cultural perspectives on obesity treatment should be viewed along all relevant dimensions, such as age, gender, and socioeconomic status. Moreover, both clients and providers bring cultural issues to the treatment setting, and the cultural competence of providers is a critical element of cultural sensitivity. Inasmuch as the treatment setting is the professional's domain, so should the building of cultural bridges be considered a primary responsibility of the treatment provider. However, there is a sense that addressing cultural influences adequately will ultimately require a paradigm expansion in the obesity treatment—away from more narrowly conceived clinical treatment models to broader health promotion paradigms—or at least a stronger and clearer articulation of the existing paradigmatic guidance on this issue.

The validity of attending to cultural and contextual influences in the design and delivery of obesity treatment can be established on a theoretical basis. However, success in cultural adaptations is inherently difficult to define and evaluate. We do not yet have many examples of scientifically rigorous models of culturally adapted weight management programs and are far from knowing whether these will improve overall treatment outcomes in specific populations. Some components of possible cultural adaptations have been outlined, and these can be formatively evaluated. Other salient cultural influences may be difficult to articulate and assess because they are tied to subtle symbolic meanings learned through affective rather than rational mechanisms. Finally, if a certain level of cultural appropriateness is a minimum standard for any program, then it is difficult to justify the conduct of studies in ethnic minority populations in which no cultural adaptations have been made. Finally, the time course for effectiveness of cultural adaptations may be long, that is, far out into the maintenance phase of behavior change rather than observable in the short term.

Appendix Examples of Culturally Adapted Weight Loss or Lifestyle Change Programs

First author and year (ref.)	Program description highlighting components of cultural adaptation
Lasco, 1989 (118)	Community Health Assesment and Promotion Project (CHAPP) was a 10-week nutrition and exercise program designed by a community coalition on the basis of data from a needs assessment
	Numerous supports were provided, e.g., child care, transportation, and a home visit to build family support
	Ancillary topics and activities were included in response to participants' requests (e.g., a class on makeup, a wardrobe and fashion analysis, and a theater party)
	Participant feedback and suggestions were solicited and incorporated
Kumanyika, 1992 (119)	Church-based program for African-American women (8-week group program)
	Built on an existing church-based high blood pressure screening, referral, and monitoring program
	Adapted a State Health Department weight loss curriculum
	Program conducted in churches and aligned with church program schedule and policies
	Project director was actively involved and often attended sessions
	Individual and team competitions (pooling $1.00 per week fees to give prizes to three participants who were most successful in meeting their goals); teams for mutual support
Cousins, 1992 (128)	*Cuidando el Corazon* was a 1-year weight loss program for Mexican-American women who were married with at least one preschool child
	Bilingual manual with nutrition, exercise, and behavior information and modified to reflect cultural values of the population; family condition included content on parenting skills to encourage healthful eating
	Cookbook with fat-modified traditional Mexican-American foods
	Behavior modification strategies illustrated in simple terms
	Spouses were encouraged to attend classes; separate classes were held for preschool children
Domel, 1992 (120)	Weight control program for black women was offered at literacy program sites or recreation centers (11 weeks)
	Emphasized being able to lose weight at low cost and active learner participation

(*continued on next page*)

Appendix Continued

First author and year (ref.)	Program description highlighting components of cultural adaptation
Domel, 1992 (129)	Weight control for Hispanic women was adapted from program developed for low-income black women
	Program was held in churches in low-income communities
	Hispanic, bilingual dietitian was involved in making cultural adaptations such as translating information into Spanish, adding ethnic foods and recipes, stressing overall family health, and reformatting printed and audio materials to be applicable to Hispanic cultural preferences
Shintani, 1994 (131)	The Waianae Diet Program used a traditional Hawaiian diet (low in fat and very high in complex carbohydrates) to reduce weight and cardiovascular disease risk factors in Native Hawaiians
	Participants were encouraged to eat to satiety; calories were not restricted
	Program themes included family support, role modelling, and a whole-person approach
Fitzgibbon, 1995 (123)	Obesity prevention program for African-American girls and their mothers attending a tutoring program in an inner-city housing project
	6-Week program with 1-hr weekly meetings
	Didactic information kept to a minimum
	All activities involved mother-daughter dyads
	Topics addressed included health problems of African-American women and how to eat low fat in a fast-food restaurant
	Each group developed a "rap against fat" using program information which was put to music, taped, and played at the final session
Agurs-Collins, 1997 (121)	Weight loss and exercise program for older African-American adults with type 2 diabetes
	Program was offered at an African-American university hospital
	Program materials depicted African-American individuals, families, and community settings
	Program content was based on relevant language, social values, situations, foods, and flavorings
	Recipes used in dietary instruction were provided by participants
	Program format allowed time for participants to discuss and problem solve regarding social context issues such as church meals
Venkat-Narayan, 1997 (130)	Pima Pride was a lifestyle change program for Pima Indians in Arizona
	Main emphasis was self-directed learning through monthly small group meetings led by a member of the community
	Discussion focused on attitudes about current lifestyle in the community
	Local speakers were invited to address Pima culture and history
	Newsletters sometimes carried poetry, stories, and folklore contributed by group members
McNabb, 1997 (122)	PATHWAYS was a church-based weight loss program for African-American women with type 2 diabetes (14 weeks)
	Program was adapted from a successful clinical program for delivery in a community setting by trained lay volunteers
	Emphasized health rather than appearance motivations for weight loss
	Interactive, guided discovery approach to learning activities; small-group instruction
Vazquez, 1998 (46)	*Buena Alimentación, Buena Salud* (Good Eating, Good Health) was a nutrition intervention program designed for Carribean Latinos with type 2 diabetes (12 weeks)
	Intervention was developed by a multidisciplinary bilingual team of health professionals in collaboration with Latino community based on results of a planning survey and focus group interviews
	Intervention was designed for cultural sensitivity in relation to 12 concepts
	Resulting features included involving bilingual/bicultural staff; offering the program in Spanish; emphasis on health risks of obesity; using a group setting; using interactive rather than didactic sessions; recommending modifications to traditional recipes; making intervention sessions into social events; and introducing the concept of empowerment
Ard, 2000 (124)	Clinical program based on the Duke University Rice Diet, involving commonly available foods, daily dietary counselling, nutrition education, and an exercise prescription, with the following cultural adaptations for African-American patients;
	Costs of program were reduced
	Ethnic recipes were used in cooking classes
	Changes in ideas about exercise
	Open invitation to family members to attend weekly classes

Appendix Continued

First author and year (ref.)	Program description highlighting components of cultural adaptation
Keyserling, 2000 (125)	Most classes conducted by an African-American instructor
	New Leaf...Choices for Healthy Living with Diabetes was designed for African-American women with type 2 diabetes
	Cultural relevance and acceptability of program components were assessed in a series of focus groups
	Recipes build on positive aspects of the southern regional diet, e.g., the use of dry peas and beans
	Simplified counselling materials in both individually tailored and nontailored formats
	Telephone counselling provided by community diabetes advisers (African-American women with type 2 diabetes acting as peer counselors)
	Active discovery learning approach in group sessions
Oxemann, 2000 (126)	"Lighten Up," a church-based program for African-American men, women, and children (8-week group program)
	Developed and implemented in collaboration with local faith community
	Bible study combined with a health message
	Eight educational sessions based on the spiritual fruits of love, knowledge, peace, faith, kindness, joy, self-control, and Godliness
	All sessions were opened and closed with prayer
	Participants brought food items from home for practice in label-reading skills
Mayer-Davis, 2001 (127)	Feasibility study for POWER (Pounds Off with Empowerment), a program that adapted a state-of-the-art weight management research protocol for a primarily African-American men and women with type 2 diabetes served by a federally funded rural primary care clinic (8-week program that included two individual and six group sessions)
	Intervention materials included a "toolbox" with guidelines for monitoring and supporting adherence and problem solving
	Interventionists used "Continous Quality Programming." They obtained observational, conversational, and—in one arm—written feedback to make decisions about how to modify the program delivery/content to improve adherence

REFERENCES

1. Rodin J. Cultural and psychosocial determinants of weight concerns. Ann Intern Med 1993; 119:643–645.
2. Sobal J, Maurer D. Weighty Issues. Fatness and Thinness as Social Problems. Hawthorne, NY: Gruyter, 1999.
3. Brown PJ, Konner M. An anthropological perspective on obesity. Annals of the New York Academy of Sciences 1987; 499:29–46.
4. Ritenbaugh C. Obesity as a culture-bound syndrome. Culture Med Psychiatry 1982; 6:347–361.
5. Thomas PR, ed. Weighing the Options. Criteria for Evaluating Weight-Management Programs. Washington: National Academy Press, 1995.
6. Kuhn TS. The Structure of Scientific Revolutions Chicago: University of Chicago Press, 1970.
7. Helman CF. Culture, Health, and Illness. An Introduction for Health Professionals Boston: Wright, 1990.
8. Mithun JS. The role of the family in acculturation and assimilation in America. A psychocultural dimension. In: McCready WC, ed. Culture, Ethnicity, and Identity. Current Issues in Research New York: Academic Press, 1983:209–232.
9. Baldwin JA, Hopkins R. African-American and European-American cultural dfferences as assessed by the worldviews paradigm. An empirical analysis. Western J Black Studies 1990; 14:38–52.
10. Sue DW, Sue D. Counseling the Culturally Different: Theory and Practice. 2d ed. New York: John Wiley and Sons, 1990:27–48.
11. Leininger M. Becoming aware of types of health practitioners and cultural imposition. J Transcultural Nur 1991; 2:32–39.
12. Airhihenbuwa CO. Health and Culture. Beyond the Western Paradigm. Chap. 3: Developing culturally appropriate health programs. Thousand Oaks, CA: Sage Publications, 1995:25–43.
13. Huff RM, Kline MV, eds. Promoting Health in Multicultural Populations. A Handbook for Practitioners Thousand Oaks, CA: Sage, 1999.
14. Williams J, Tharp M. African Americans: ethnic roots, cultural diversity. In: Tharp M, ed. Marketing and

Consumer Identity in Multicultural America. Thousand Oaks, CA: Sag, 2001:161–211.

15. Wing RR, Vorhees CC, Hill DR. Maintenance of behavior change in cardiorespiratory risk reduction. Health Psychol 2000; 19(suppl 1):1–88.

16. National Heart, Lung, and Blood Institute Obesity Education Initiative. Clinical guidelines on the identification, evaluation, and treatment of overweight and obesity in adults. Obes Res 1998; 6(suppl 2).

17. World Health Organization. Obesity: Preventing and Managing the Global Epidemic. Report of a WHO consultation. Geneva World Health Organization, WHO Technical Report Series 894, 2000.

18. Egger G, Swinburn B. An 'ecological' approach to the obesity pandemic. BMJ 1997; 315:477–480.

19. Nestle M, Jacobson MF. Halting the obesity epidemic. A public health policy approach. Public Health Rep 2001; 115:12–24.

20. French SA, Story M, Jeffery RW. Environmental influences on eating and physical activity. Annu Rev Public Health 2001; 22:309–335.

21. Kumanyika SK. Minisymposium on obesity: overview and some strategic considerations. Annu Rev Public Health 2001; 22:293–308.

22. Ritenbaugh C, Kumanyika S, Antipatis V, Jeffery R, Morabia A. Caught in the causal web: a new perspective on social factors affecting obesity. Healthy Weight J 1999; 13:88–89.

23. Last J. A Dictionary of Epidemiology. 2d ed. New York: Oxford University Press, 1988.

24. Pollard K, O'Hare W. America's racial and ethnic minorities. Popul Bull 1999; 54:1–34.

25. Kleinman A, Eisenberg L, Good B. Culture, illness and care. Clinical lessons from anthropologic and cross-cultural research. Ann Intern Med 1978; 88:251–258.

26. McElroy A, Jezewski MA. Cultural variation in the experience of health and illness. In: Albrecht GL, Fitzpatrick R, Scrimshaw SC, eds. Handbook of Social Studies in Health and Medicine. Thousand Oaks CA: Sage Publications, 2000:191–209.

27. Kent MM, Pollard KM, Haaga J, Mather M. First glimpse from the 2000 U.S. Census. Popul Bull 2001; 56(2):1–38. Accessed at www.ameristat.org. Oct. 12, 2001.

28. Kumanyika SK. Minority populations. In: Burke LE, Ockene IS, eds. Compliance in Healthcare and Research. Armonk, NY: Futura, 2001:195–218.

29. Council on Economic Advisers for the President's Initiative on Race (1998). Changing America. Indicators of social and economic well-being by race and Hispanic origin. Available at: http://www.access.gpo.gov/eop/ca/index.html. Accessed Oct. 16, 2001.

30. Flegal KM, Carroll MD, Kuczmarski RJ, Johnson CL. Overweight and obesity in the United States. Prevalence and trends, 1960–1994. Int J Obes 1998; 22:39–47.

31. Will JC, Denny C, Serdula M, Muneta B. Trends in body weight among American Indians. Findings from a telephone survey, 1985-1996. Am J Public Health 1999; 89:395–398.

32. Ellis JL, Campos-Outcalt D. Cardiovascular disease risk factors in native Americans: a literature review. Am J Prev Med 1994; 10:295–307.

33. Howard BV, Lee ET, Cowan LD, Fabsitz RR, Joward WH, Oopik AJ, Robbins DC, Savage PJ, Yeh JL, Welty TK. Coronary heart disease prevalence and its relation to risk factors in American Indians. The Strong Heart Study. Am J Epidemiol 1995; 142:254–268.

34. Must A, Spadano J, Coakley EH, Field AE, Colditz G, Dietz WH. The disease burden associated with overweight and obesity. JAMA 1999; 282:1523–1529.

35. Sahyoun NR, Hochberg MC, Helmick CG, Harris T, Pamuk ER. Body mass index, weight change, and incidence of self-reported, physician diagnosed arthritis among women. Am J Public Health 1999; 89:391–394.

36. Ostir GV, Markides KS, Freeman DH, Goodwin JS. Obesity and health conditions in elderly Mexican Americans: the Hispanic EPESE. Ethn Dis 2000; 10:31–38.

37. Diabetes 2001. Vital Statistics. Alexandria, VA: American Diabetes Association, 2001.

38. Troiano RP, Flegal KM, Kuczmarski RJ, Campbell SM, Johnson CL. Overweight prevalence and trends for children and adolescents. The National Health and Nutrition Examination Surveys, 1963–1991. Arch Pediatr Adolesc Med 1995; 149:1085–1091.

39. Story M, Evans M, Fabsitz RR, Clay TE, Rock BH, Broussard B. The epidemic of obesity in American Indian communities and the need for childhood obesity-prevention programs. Am J Clin Nutr 1999; 69:747S–754S.

40. Rosenbloom AL, House DV, Winter WE. Non-insulin-dependent diabetes mellitus (NIDDM) in minority youth: research priorities and needs. Clin Pediatr (Phila) 1998; 37:143–152.

41. Goran MI, Weinsier RL. Role of environmental vs. metabolic factors in the etiology of obesity. Time to focus on the environment. Obes Res 2000; 8:407–409.

42. Ravussin E, Valencia ME, Esparza J, Bennett PH, Schulz LO. Effects of a traditional lifestyle on obesity in Pima Indians. Diabetes Care 1994; 17:1067–1074.

43. Kaufman JS, Durazo-Arvizu RA, Rotimi CN, McGee DL, Cooper RS. Obesity and hypertension prevalence in populations of African origin. The Investigators of the International Collaborative Study on Hypertension in Blacks. Epidemiology 1996; 7:398–405.

44. Kumanyika SK, Morssink CB. Cultural appropriateness of weight management programs. In: Dalton S, ed. Overweight and Weight Management Gaithersburg, MD: Aspen Publisher, 1997:69–106.

45. Counihan C, Van Esterik P, eds. Food and Culture. A Reader New York: Routledge, 1997.

46. Vazquez IM, Millen B, Bissett L, Levelnson SM, Chipkin SR. A preventive nutrition intervention in Caribbean Latinos with type 2 diabetes. Am J Health Promotion 1998; 13:116–119.

47. Allan JD, Mayo K, Michel Y. Body size values of white and black women. Res Nurs Health 1993; 16:323–333.

48. Jain A, Sherman SN, Chamberlin DL, Carter Y, Powers SW, Whitaker RC. Why don't low-income mothers worry about their preschoolers being overweight? Pediatrics 2001; 107:1138–1146.

49. Faith MS, Manibay E, Kravitz M, Griffith J, Allison DB. Relative body weight and self-esteem among African Americans in four nationally representative samples. Obes Res 1998; 6:430–437.

50. Flynn KJ, Fitzgibbon M. Body images and obesity risk among black females. Ann Behav Med 1998; 20:13–24.

51. Williamson DF, Serdula MK, Anda RF, Levy A, Byers T. Weight loss attempts in adults: goals, duration, and rate of weight loss. Am J Public Health 1992; 82(9): 1251–1257.

52. Serdula MK, Williamson DF, Anda RF, Levy A. Weight control practices in adults: results of a multistate telephone survey. Am J Public Health 1994; 84: 1821–1824.

53. Cachelin FM, Striegel-Moore R, Elder KA. Realistic weight perception and body size assessment in a racially diverse community sample of dieters. Obes Res 1998; 6:62–68.

54. Serdula MK, Mokdad AH, Williamson DF, Galuska DA, Mendlein JM, Heath GW. Prevalence of attempting weight loss and strategies for controlling weight. JAMA 1999; 13:1353–1358.

55. Smith DE, Thompson JK, Raczynski JM, Hilner JE. Body image among men and women in a biracial cohort. The CARDIA Study. Int J Eat Disor 1999; 25:71–82.

56. Sherwood NE, Harnack L, Story M. Weight-loss practices, nutrition beliefs, and weightloss program preferences of urban American Indian women. J Am Diet Assoc 2000; 100:442–446.

57. Wolfe WA. Obesity and the African-American woman. A cultural tolerance of fatness or other neglected factors? Ethn Dis 2000; 10:446–453.

58. Matthews HF. Rootwork. Description of an ethnomedical system in the American South. South Med J 1987; 80:885–891.

59. Airhihenbuwa CO, Kumanyika S, Agurs TD, Lowe A. Perceptions and beliefs about physical activity, exercise, and rest among African Americans. Am J Health Promotion 1995; 9:426–429.

60. Airhihenbuwa CO, Kumanyika S, Agurs TD, Lowe A, Saunders D, Morssink CB. Cultural aspects of African-American eating patterns. Ethn Health 1996; 1:245–260.

61. Murcott A. Sociological and social anthropological approaches to food and eating. World Rev Nutr Diet 1988; 55:1–40.

62. Mintz SW. Tasting Food, Tasting Freedom. Excursions into Eating, Culture, and the Past. Boston: Beacon Press, 1997.

63. Kittler PG, Sucher KP. Food and Culture in America: A Nutrition Handbook. 2nd ed. Washington: West/Wadsworth, 1998.

64. Sobal J, Stunkard AJ. Socioeconomic status and obesity: a review of the literature. Psychol Bull 1989; 105:260–275.

65. Kumanyika SK, Golden PM. Cross-sectional differences in health status in U.S. racial/ethnic minority groups. Potential influence of temporal changes, disease, and lifestyle transitions. Ethn Dis 1991; 1:50–59.

66. Kumanyika SK. Obesity in minority populations: an epidemiologic assessment. Obes Res 1994; 2:66–182.

67. Gillum RF. The epidemiology of cardiovascular disease in black Americans. N Engl J Med 1996; 335:1597–1599.

68. Townsend MS, Peerson J, Love B, Acherberg C, Murphy SP. Food insecurity is positively related to overweight in women. J Nutr 2001; 121:1738–1745.

69. Kumanyika SK, Krebs-Smith SM. Preventive nutrition issues in ethnic and socioeconomic groups in the United States. In: Bendich A, Deckelbaum RJ, eds. Preventive Nutrition. Vol 2 .Totowa, NJ: Humana Press, 2001: 325–356.

70. Winkelby MA, Kraemer HC, Ahn DK, Varady AN. Ethnic and socioeconomic differences in cardiovascular disease risk factors: findings for women from the Third National Health and Nutrition Examination Survey, 1988-1994. JAMA 1998; 280:356–362.

71. King AC, Castro C, Eyler AA, Wilcox S, Sallis J, Brownson RC. Personal and environmental factors associated with physical activity among different racial-ethnic groups of U.S. middle-aged and older-aged women. Health Psychol 2000; 19:354–364.

72. Ford ES, De Proost Ford MA, Will JC, Galuska DA, Ballew C. Achieving a healthy lifestyle among United States adults. A long way to go. Ethn Dis 2001; 11:224–231.

73. Kushner RF, Racette SB, Neil K, Schoeller DA. Measurement of physical activity among black and white obese women. Obes Res 1995; 3:261s–265s.

74. Hunter GR, Weinsier RL, Darnell BE, Zuckerman PA, Goran MI. Racial differences in energy expenditure and aerobic fitness in premenopausal women. Am J Clin Nutr 2000; 71:500–506.

75. Cockerham WC, Rütten A, Abel T. Conceptualizing contemporary health lifestyles: moving beyond Weber. Sociol Q 1997; 38(2):321–342.

76. Wechsler H, Basch CE, Zybertx CE, Lantigua R, Shea S. The availability of low-fat milk in an inner-city Latino community: implications for nutrition education. Am J Public Health 1995; 85:1690–1692.

77. Diez-Roux AV, Nieto FJ, Caulfield L, Tyroler HA, Watson RL, Szklo M. Neighborhood differences in diet: the atherosclerosis risk in communities (ARIC) study. J Epidemiol Community Health 1999; 53:55–63.

78. Freedman AM. Habit forming: fast-food chains' central role in diet of the inner-city poor. Wall Street Journal 1990; Dec 19, 1, A6.

79. Williams JD, Achterberg C, Pazzaglia Sylvester G. Target marketing of food products to ethnic minority youth. In: Williams CL, Kimml SYS, eds. Prevention and Treatment of Childhood Obesity. New York: New York Academy of Sciences, 1993:107–114.

80. Tirodkar MA, Jain A. Food messages on African American television shows. Pediatr Res 2001; 49(4 part 2 of 2):19A.

81. Smith DE, Lewis CE, Caveny JL, Perkins LL, Burke GL, Bild DE. Longitudinal changes in adiposity associated with pregnancy. The CARDIA Study. JAMA 1994; 271:1747–1751.

82. Pachter LM. Culture and clinical care. Folk illness beliefs and behaviors and their implications for health care delivery. JAMA 1994; 271:690–694.

83. Harris-Davis E, Haughton B. Model for multicultural nutrition counseling competencies. J Am Diet Assoc 2000; 100:1178–1185.

84. Office of Minority Health. Assuring cultural competence in health care. Recommendations for National Standards and an Outcomes-Focuse Research Agenda. http://www.omhrc.gov/cls/finalcultural1a.htm. Accessed Oct. 16, 2001.

85. Kumanyika SK. Obesity treatment in minorities. In: Wadden TA, Stunkard AJ, eds. Handbook of Obesity Treatment. New York: Guilford Publications, 2002: 416–446.

86. Bandura A. Social cognitive theory. An agentic perspective. Annu Rev Psychol 2001; 52:1–26.

87. Fisher EB, Auslander W, Sussman L, Owens N, Jackson-Thompson J. Community organization and health promotion in minority neighborhoods. In: Becker DM, Hill DR, Jackson JS, Levine DM, Stillman FA, Weiss SM, eds. Health Behavior Research in Minority Populations. Washington: U.S. Government Printing Office, 1992:53–72 NIH Publication No. 92-2965.

88. Stokols D. Translating social ecologic theory into guidelines for community health promotion. Am J Health Promotion 1996; 10:282–298.

89. Bouton ME. A learning theory perspective on lapse, relapse, and the maintenance of behavior change. Health Psychol 2000; 19(suppl to No. 1):57–63.

90. Baranowski T, Perry CL, Parcel GS. How individuals, environments, and health behavior interact. Social cognitive theory. In: Glanz K, Lewis FM, Rimer BK, eds. Health Behavior and Health Education: Theory, Research, and Practice. 2d ed. San Francisco: Jossey-Bass, 1997:153–178.

91. Rakowski W. The potential variances of tailoring in health behavior interventions. Ann Behav Med 1999; 21:284–289.

92. Resnicow K, Baranowski T, Ahluwalia JS, Braithwaite RL. Cultural sensitivity in public health. Defined and demystified. Ethn Dis 1999; 9:10–12.

93. Kavanagh KH, Kennedy PH. Promoting cultural diversity. Strategies for health care professionals. Newbury Park, CA: Sage Publications, 1992.

94. Huff RM. Cross cultural concepts of health and disease. In: Huff RM, Kline MV, eds. Promoting Health in Multicultural Populations. A Handbook For Practitioners Thousand. Oaks, CA: Sage, 1999:23–39.

95. Yutrenzka BA. Making a case for training in ethnic and cultural diversity in increasing treatment efficacy. J Consult Clin Psychol 1995; 63:197–206.

96. Harvey EL, Hill AJ. Health professionals' views of overweight people and smokers. Int J Obes Relat Metab Disord 2001; 25:1253–1261.

97. Kumanyika SK, Morssink CB. Working effectively in cross-cultural and multicultural settings. In: Owen AL, Splett PL, Owen GM, eds. Nutrition in the Community. The Art and Science of Delivering Services. 4th ed. New York: McGraw Hill, 1998:542–567.

98. Wilcox S, Shumaker SA, Bowen DJ, Naughton MJ, Rosal MC, Ludlam SE, Dugan E, Hunt JR, Stevens S. Promoting adherence and retention to clinical trials in special populations. A Women's Health Initiative workshop. Control Clin Trials 2001; 22:279–289.

99. Leicht KT, Fennell ML. The changing organizational context of professional work. Annu Rev Sociol 1997; 23:215–231.

100. Abbot A. The Systems of Professions; An Essay on the Division of Expert Labor. Chicago: University of Chicago Press, 1989.

101. Freidson E. Professionalism Reborn; Theory, Prophecy, and Policy. Chicago: University of Chicago Press, 1994.

102. Brierley J. The measurement of organizational commitment and professional commitment. J Soc Psychol 1996; 136:265–267.

103. Anderson JM, Dyck I, Lynam J. Health care professionals and women speaking; constraints in everyday life and the management of chronic illness. Health 1997; 1:57–79.

104. Glanz K, Lewis FM, Rimer BK, eds. Health Behavior and Health Education: Theory, Research, and Practice. 2 ed. San Francisco: Jossey-Bass, 1997.

105. Conrad P, Kern R, eds. The Sociology of Health and Illness; Critical Perspectives New York: St. Martin's Press, 1997.

106. Sobal J. The medicalization and demedicalization of obesity. In: Maurer D, Sobal J, eds. Eating Agendas: Food and Nutrition as Social Problems. Social Problems and Social Issues. Hawthorne, NY: Aldine de Gruyter, 1995:1:67–90.

107. Martin J. Cultures in Organizations: Three Perspectives. New York: Oxford University Press, 1992.

108. Peters T, Waterman R. In Search of Excellence. New York: Harper & Rowe, 1983.

109. Mohan M.L. Organizational Communication and Cultural Vision: Approaches for Analysis. Albany: State University of New York Press, 1993.

110. Mumby DK. Communication and Power in Organizations: Discourse, Ideology, and Domination. Norwood, NJ: Ablex Publishing Co., 1988.

111. Hofstede G. Culture's Consequences: International Differences in Work-Related Values. Newbury Park, CA: Sage Publications, 1980.

112. Downs A. Inside Bureaucracy Chicago: Waveland Press, 1994.

113. Caiden Gerald E. Excessive bureaucratization: The J-curve theory of bureaucracy and Max Weber through the looking glass. In: Farazmand Ali, ed. Handbook of Bureaucracy. New York: Marcel Dekker, 1994:66–72.

114. Anderson RM, Funnel M. Compliance and adherence are dysfunctional concepts in diabetes care. Diabetes Educator 2000; 26:597–601.

115. Kidd KE, Altman DG. Adherence in social context. Control Clin Trials 2000; 21:184S–187S.

116. Rothman AJ. Towards a theory-based analysis of behavioral maintenance. Health Psychol 2000; 191: 64–69.

117. Frankish JC, Lovato CY, Shannon WJ. Models, theories, and principles of health promotion with multicultural populations. In: Huff RM, Kline MV, eds. Promoting Health in Multicultural Populations. A Handbook for Practitioners Thousand. Oaks, CA: Sage, 1999:41–72.

118. Lasco RA, Curry RH, Dickson VJ, Powers J, Menes S, Merritt RK. Participation rates, weight loss, and blood pressure changes among obese women in a nutrition-exercise program. Public Health Rep 1989; 104:640–646.

119. Kumanyika SK, Charleston JB. Lose weight and win. A church-based weight loss program for blood pressure control among black women. Patient Educ Counseling 1992; 19:19–32.

120. Domel SB, Alford BB, Cattlett HN, Rodriguez ML, Gench BE. A pilot weight control program for Black women. J Am Diet Assoc 1992; 92:346–348.

121. Agurs-Collins TD, Kumanyika SK, TenHave TR, Adams-Campbell LL. A randomized controlled trial of weight reduction and exercise for diabetes management in older African American subjects. Diabetes Care 1997; 20:1503–1511.

122. McNabb W, Quinn M, Kerver J, Cook S, Karrison T. The Pathways church-based weight loss program for urban African Americans. Diabetes Care 1997; 20: 1518–1523.

123. Fitzgibbon ML, Stolley MR, Kirschenbaum DS. An obesity prevention pilot program for African American mothers and daughters. J Nutr Educ 1995; 27:93–99.

124. Ard J, Rosati R, Oddone EZ. Culturally-sensitive weight loss program produces significant reduction in weight, blood pressure, and cholesterol in eight weeks. J Natl Med Assoc 2000; 92:515–523.

125. Keyserling TC, Ammerman AS, Samuel-Hodge CD, Ingram A, Skellyx A, Elasy TA, Johnston LF, Cole AS, Henriquez-Roldaán CF. A diabetes management program for African American women with type 2 diabetes. Diabetes Educ 2000; 26:796–805.

126. Oexmann MJ, Thomas JC, Taylor KB, O'Neil PM, Garvey WT, Lackland DT, Egan BM. Short-term impact of a church-based approach to lifestyle change on cardiovascular risk in African Americans. Ethn Dis 2000; 10:17–23.

127. Mayer-Davis EJ, D'Antonio A, Martin M, Wandersman A, Parra-Medina D, Schulz R. Pilot study of strategies for effective weight management in type 2 diabetes. Pounds Off With Empowerment (POWER). Fam Community Health 2001; 24:27–35.

128. Cousins JH, Rubovits DS, Dunn JK, Reeves RS, Ramirez AG, Foreyt JP. Family versus individually-oriented intervention for weight loss in Mexican American women. Public Health Rep 1992; 107:549–555.

129. Domel SB, Alford BB, Cattlett HN, Rodriguez ML, Gench BE. A pilot weight control program for Hispanic women. J Am Diet Assoc 1992; 92:1270–1271.

130. Venkat-Narayan KM, Hoskin M, Kozak D, Kriska AM, Hanson RL, Pettitt DJ, Nagi DK, Bennett PH, Knowler WC. Randomized clinical trial of lifestyle interventions in Pima Indians: a pilot study. Diabet Med 1998; 15:66–72.

131. Shintani T, Beckham S, Kanawaliwali-O'Connor H, Hughes C, Sato A. The Waianae Diet Program. A culturally-sensitive, community-based obesity and clinical intervention program for the Native Hawaiian population. Hawaii Med J 1994; 53:136–147.

4

Bias, Prejudice, Discrimination, and Obesity

Rebecca M. Puhl and Kelly D. Brownell

Yale University, New Haven, Connecticut, U.S.A.

I INTRODUCTION

Research is clear in showing that obese individuals are highly stigmatized, and that bias and discrimination are often a consequence (1). Given that half the American population is overweight, the number of people potentially faced with discrimination and stigmatization is immense. The consequences of being denied jobs, disadvantaged in education, or marginalized by health care professionals because of one's weight can have a profound impact on family life, social status, and quality of life. Obese individuals can suffer terribly from this, both from direct discrimination and from other behaviors (e.g., teasing and social exclusion) that arise from weight-related stigma.

Discrimination has largely been ignored in the obesity field, despite discussion dating back at least 30 years (2). Perhaps because obesity research itself has been stigmatized, too few researchers have attended to weight discrimination, and as a result, it is not possible to define the exact pervasiveness of the problem and how many people are affected. Still, there is clear evidence of discrimination in areas of employment, education, and health care, thus painting a picture of obese persons as acceptable targets of discrimination (1). The purpose of this chapter is to summarize existing literature, introduce preliminary theories to explain weight stigma, and highlight stigma reduction strategies and research needs in this new area of study.

II EMPLOYMENT DISCRIMINATION

Both laboratory and field studies show widespread weight bias in all aspects of the employment process (3–7). Research addressing employer attitudes and hiring decisions suggests that overweight people face prejudice even prior to initial job interviews. Studies have manipulated participant perception of employee weight (through written vignettes, videos, or photographs), where subjects are randomly assigned to a condition in which they are asked to evaluate a fictional applicant's qualifications. Overweight employees are evaluated more negatively and are rated as less likely to be hired than average-weight employees, despite identical qualifications. Though this bias has been demonstrated within a variety of employment positions, it appears that overweight applicants are especially denigrated in sales positions and are perceived to be unfit for jobs involving face-to-face interactions (3,8,9).

Several recent reviews indicate that discrimination may continue once an overweight person is employed. Overweight employees are viewed as sloppy, lazy, less competent, poor role models, lacking in self-discipline, disagreeable, and emotionally unstable (10,11). These attitudes may be a primary reason for inequity faced by overweight employees in wages, promotions, and termination. For example, obese men are more likely to hold low-paying jobs and are underrepresented in professional positions compared to average-weight men (12). There is also evidence of lower wages for obese women doing the same work performed by average-weight counterparts (13). Overweight women are more likely to have low-paying jobs compared to thinner women (12). Other studies demonstrate lower promotion prospects for obese individuals than for average-weight employees with identical qualifications (14,15).

Finally, legal case documentation reveals a growing number of cases in which obese employees have been fired or suspended because of their weight (16–18). Many terminated employees held jobs in which body weight was unrelated to job responsibilities (computer analyst, office manager, lecturer, etc.) and received excellent job performance ratings, suggesting that prejudiced employers are responsible.

III MEDICAL AND HEALTH CARE DISCRIMINATION

Health care is an additional arena where weight discrimination appears to occur. Negative antifat attitudes have been reported among physicians, nurses, and medical students. Perceptions of obese patients include beliefs that they are unsuccessful, unpleasant, unintelligent, overindulgent, weak-willed, and lazy (19–23). Attributions about the cause of obesity may be partially responsible, and include assumptions that obesity can be prevented by self-control (22), that patient noncompliance explains failure at weight loss (24), and that obesity is caused by emotional problems (21). Two self-report studies of nurses showed that they felt uncomfortable caring for obese patients, that they would prefer not to care for an obese patient, that obese patients "repulsed" them, and that they would prefer not to touch an obese patient at all (22,25).

It is possible that such bias affects the quality of care provided to obese individuals. Though this has not been directly assessed, several studies have demonstrated poor obesity management practices by physicians, who report that they rarely discuss weight issues with overweight patients, that they feel weight loss counseling is inconvenient, and that they do not intervene as often as they should with obese patients (23,26). This parallels reports of obese individuals who claim to be dissatisfied with the care they receive for their weight and who report negative experiences with physicians when discussing weight issues (27). Other research shows that health care workers more frequently assign negative symptoms and more severe psychological

symptoms to obese patients than to average-weight clients (28).

It appears that such negative attitudes may increase patient resistance in seeking health care services. Several studies have documented delays in seeking pelvic exams and preventive services like breast and gynecological exams among obese women (29,30), and other research shows a positive relationship between body mass index (BMI) and appointment cancelations (27). Obese women report that negative body image, embarrassment about weight, and previous negative physician experiences are the reasons for their reluctance to seek medical care (27,29).

Finally, denial of medical coverage to obese individuals must be examined in more detail. Denying access to beneficial treatment is one such form of discrimination, and occurs often despite evidence showing improved health status with modest weight losses and increasing evidence of cost-effective weight loss methods like surgery and drugs (31–34). Factors underlying inadequate coverage may be widespread perceptions of obesity as a problem of willful behavior, the view that obese people get what they deserve, and unwillingness to accept data on effective treatments because the population is stigmatized.

IV EDUCATIONAL DISCRIMINATION

Multiple forms of weight discrimination occur in educational settings. Antifat attitudes have been demonstrated in preschool children (35), which likely sets the stage for later peer rejection and teasing. These types of negative attitudes are shown in studies in which obese children are rated as the least desirable friends by their peers when compared to photos of children varying in weight and physical disabilities (36). Indeed, peers appear to be the primary proponents of weight-related teasing, and the school seems to be the most frequent location where overweight children are harassed (37). Unfortunately, the shame surrounding obesity is also evident in overweight children themselves, who blame their weight as the reason for why they have few friends and are excluded by peers, and who believe that they would stop being teased and humiliated if they could lose weight (38). Any professional who asks obese patients about these experiences will hear wrenching stories of ridicule and humiliation.

Beyond peer harassment at school, educational discrimination appears to be a reality at the college level. There are cases of obese students being dismissed from college on the basis of weight despite good academic performance (39). Research shows that obese students receive poorer evaluations and lower college acceptances than average-weight students with comparable application rates and school performance (40). Some studies even suggest that parental biases may result in poorer educational outcomes for obese students. Studies by Crandall (41,42) have demonstrated a relationship between BMI and financial support for education, where parents were found to give more financial support to their average-weight children than to overweight children, who relied more on financial aid. These differences persisted even after controlling for income, family size, ethnicity, and education, and it appeared that politically conservative attitudes of parents predicted who gave parental support. These results have led to further research by Crandall and colleagues proposing that particular ideological beliefs are at the core of weight prejudice, as discussed below.

V THE LEGAL SYSTEM AND WEIGHT DISCRIMINATION

Given the apparent pervasiveness of weight prejudice, it is surprising that no federal laws prohibit this form of discrimination and that only a handful of states include body weight in their definitions of unlawful discrimination (16,43,44). Weight discrimination has most often been fought using the Rehabilitation Act and American Disabilities Act (45), though the success of this legislation for obese people has been inconsistent. Unreliable rulings result from differing court views of when or if obesity meets disability criteria, common assumptions that obesity is a voluntary and changeable condition, and ambiguities surrounding definitions of obesity and impairment (43,46). If these trends persist in the courts, rulings will likely produce mixed and unpredictable results.

VI BELIEFS UNDERLYING STIGMA

Discrimination is caused by negative attitudes and beliefs about obese persons, so an important question to address is why such negative attitudes exist. A number of studies by Crandall and colleagues have tested a social ideology model which suggests that antifat attitudes are the result of certain attributional tendencies of blame (47–49). Traditional, conservative American values of self-determination and individualism lead to stigmatization of obese people through beliefs that

people get what they deserve, and to the tendency to attribute the fates of others to internal and controllable factors (50). Thus, if an individual believes that obese people are responsible for their weight (e.g., through laziness, overeating, or low self-discipline), stigma is more likely to occur (47).

In addition to attributions of responsibility, research suggests that perceptions of causality and stability of obesity are also important factors contributing to stigmatizing attitudes. Obese people are more likely to be stigmatized if their overweight condition is perceived to be caused by controllable versus uncontrollable causes (e.g., overeating vs. a thyroid condition) and if the obesity is perceived to be personally changeable rather than an irreversible condition (51,52).

These studies are just a start in understanding stigma. Much more basic psychological research is needed on attitude formation, and the social roots of these attitudes must be defined. Relatively little such work is now occurring.

VII PREVENTION: THE NEED FOR STIGMA REDUCTION STRATEGIES

A central priority for research is to develop and test stigma reduction strategies. Very few studies have attempted this, but of those that have, there are promising findings. One randomized study attempted to reduce stigma toward obese patients among medical students. An educational course improved attitudes and beliefs about obesity in students compared to a control group (53). Another study reduced antifat attitudes among participants through education about the biological and genetic causes of obesity (47), and a third study improved attitudes and reduced weight-related teasing among children through a curriculum to promote size acceptance (54). Further studies examining the development of stigma reduction interventions will make important contributions to this area of research.

VIII FUTURE DIRECTIONS FOR RESEARCH

There is a clear and powerful indication of discrimination against obese persons in multiple areas of living. However, previous methodological limitations in the literature must be improved, and additional research questions must be addressed to more clearly understand the nature and consequences of weight discrimination.

Table 1 Summary of Research Needs to Be Addressed in Domains of Weight Discrimination

Domain	Research needs
General methodological issues	Inclusion of obese persons in study samples.
	Increased use of randomized designs and ecologically valid settings.
	Evaluation of reliability and validity of measures assessing weight discrimination.
	Development of assessment methods to examine discriminatory practices.
Theoretical issues	Evaluation of predictive power among obesity stigma models.
	Further exploration of why negative attitudes arise.
	Examination of psychological and social origins of weight prejudice.
	Experimental manipulation of proposed components of stigmatizing attributions.
	Assessment of attitudinal and behavioral expressions of weight bias.
	Cross-cultural examinations of antifat attitudes and weight-related attributions.
Legal questions	Clarification of definitions of disability and impairment relevant to obesity.
	Examination of legislative approaches used to counter discriminatory practices.
Employment	Increased attention to hiring, promotion and benefits discrimination against obese employees.
	Closer examination of which occupations are most vulnerable to weight bias.
Health care	Experimental assessment of physician/nurse attitudes toward obese patients.
	Examination of how negative professional attitudes influence health care.
	Examination of coverage practices by insurance providers to obese individuals.
	Evaluation of health care costs associated with small weight losses.
	Address cost-effectiveness of various weight loss treatments.
Education	Documentation of weight discrimination/bias among educators and peers.
	Development and testing of curricula to promote weight acceptance.
Unstudied topics	Documentation of weight discrimination in areas of public accommodations (seating in restaurants, theaters, planes, buses, trains), housing (raised rental fees for obese persons), adoption (weight-based criteria for parents), jury selection practices (biased against overweight jurors), health club memberships (raised fees for obese people), and others.
Prevention/intervention	Identification of theoretical components to guide stigma reduction strategies.
	Development and testing of stigma reduction strategies on antifat attitudes.
	Clarification of psychological/social consequences of weight discrimination.
	Examination of coping strategies used by obese persons to combat aversive stigma experiences.

Table 1 outlines areas of research which we believe are necessary directions in which to take these efforts.

IX CONCLUSION

The medical life of the obese person has received far more attention than the social and psychological life. As a field, we understand much more about the blood pressure, blood sugar regulation, and now genetics than we do about well-being, happiness, and position in society (examine the contents of this book as one example). It is likely that the social and psychological consequences of obesity are more troubling than its medical effects, and have a greater impact on quality of life, especially prior to the onset of chronic disease in midlife and later.

Negative beliefs about obese individuals, fueled by a culture that demeans and even disgraces people because of their weight, lead to prejudice, bias, and ultimately discrimination. Given the number of people affected, the inherent unfairness of prejudice, and the consequences of discrimination in key areas of living such as employment and education, much more needs to be done.

The obesity field can and must play a central role in this arena. Discrimination and related topics must be topics of discussion at professional meetings, must be represented in books and journals, and must be studied more as prominent figures in the field argue for more funding. The national obesity research agenda must now include these important social issues.

REFERENCES

1. Puhl R, Brownell KD. Obesity, bias, and discrimination. Obes Res 2001; 9:788–805.
2. Allon N. The stigma of overweight in everyday life. In: Woldman BB, ed. Psychological Aspects of Obesity. New York: Random House, 1982:130–174.
3. Bellizzi JA, Hasty RW. Territory assignment decisions and supervising unethical selling behavior: the effects of obesity and gender as moderated by job-related factors. J Personal Selling Sales Management 1998; XVIII(2): 35–49.
4. Decker WH. Attributions based on managers' self-presentation, sex, and weight. Psychol Rep 1987; 61:175–181.
5. Klassen ML, Jasper CR, Harris RJ. The role of physical appearance in managerial decisions. J Business Psychol 1993; 8:181–198.
6. Klesges RC, Haddock CK, Stein RJ, Klesges LM, Eck LH, Hanson CL. Relationship between psychosocial functioning and body fat in preschool children: a longitudinal investigation. Journal of Consulting & Clinical Psychology 1992; 60:793–796.
7. Rothblum ED, Miller CT, Garbutt B. Stereotypes of obese female job applicants. Int J Eating Disord 1988; 7:277–283.
8. Everett M. Let an overweight person call on your best customers? Fat chance. Sales Marketing Management 1990; 142:66–70.
9. Pingitoire R, Dugoni R, Tindale S, Spring B. Bias against overweight job applicants in a simulated employment interview. J Appl Psychol 1994; 79:909–917.
10. Roehling MV. Weight-based discrimination in employment: psychological and legal aspects. Personnel Psychol 1999; 52:969–1017.
11. Paul RJ, Townsend JB. Shape up or ship out? Employment discrimination against the overweight. Employee Responsibilities Rights J 1995; 8:133–145.
12. Pagan JA, Davila A. Obesity, occupational attainment, and earnings. Soc Sci Q 1997; 78:756–770.
13. Register CA, Williams DR. Wage effects of obesity among young workers. Soc Sci Q 1990; 71:130–141.
14. Bordieri JE, Drehmer DE, Taylor DW. Work life for employees with disabilities: recommendations for promotion. Rehab Counseling Bull 1997; 40:181–191.
15. Brink TL. Obesity and job discrimination: mediation via personality stereotypes? Perceptual Motor Skills 1988; 66:494.
16. Frisk AM. Obesity as a disability: an actual or perceived problem? Army Lawyer 1996; 3–19.
17. Perroni PJ. Cook v. Rhode Island, Department of Mental Health, Retardation, and Hospitals: the First Circuit tips the scales of justice to protect the overweight. N Engl Law Rev 1996; 30:993–1018.
18. Post R. Prejudicial appearances: the logic of American anti-discrimination. Calif Law Rev 2000; 88:1–40.
19. Blumberg P, Mellis LP. Medical students' attitudes toward the obese and morbidly obese. Int J Eating Disord 1980; 169–175.
20. Maddox GL, Liederman V. Overweight as a social disability with medical implications. J Med Educ 1969; 44:214–220.
21. Maiman LA, Wang VL, Becker MH, Finlay J, Simonson M. Attitudes toward obesity and the obese among professionals. J Am Diet Assoc 1979; 74:331–336.
22. Maroney D, Golub S. Nurses' attitudes toward obese persons and certain ethnic groups. Perceptual Motor Skills 1992; 75:387–391.
23. Price JH, Desmond SM, Krol RA, Snyder FF, O'Connell JK. Family practice physicians' beliefs, attitudes, and practices regarding obesity. Am J Prev Med 1987; 3:339–345.
24. Hoppe R, Ogden J. Practice nurses' beliefs about obesity and weight related interventions in primary care. Int J Obes 1997; 21:141–146.
25. Bagley CR, Conklin DN, Isherwood RT, Pechiulis DR, Watson LA. Attitudes of nurses toward obesity and obese patients. Perceptual Motor Skills 1989; 68:954.
26. Kristeller JL, Hoerr RA. Physician attitudes toward managing obesity: differences among six specialty groups. Prev Med 1997; 26:542–549.
27. Olson CL, Schumaker HD, Yawn BP. Overweight women delay medical care. Arch Fam Med 1994; 3:888–892.
28. Young LM, Powell B. The effects of obesity on the clinical judgements of mental health professionals. J Health Soc Behav 1985; 26:233–246.
29. Adams CH, Smith NJ, Wilbur DC, Grady KE. The relationship of obesity to the frequency of pelvic examinations: do physician and patient attitudes make a difference? Women Health 1993; 20:45–57.
30. Fontaine KR, Faith MS, Allison DB, Cheskin LJ. Body weight and health care among women in the general population. Arch Fam Med 1998; 7:381–384.
31. Greenway FL, Ryan DH, Bray GA, Rood JC, Tucker EW, Smith SR. Pharmaceutical cost savings of treating obesity with weight loss medications. Obes Res 1999; 7:523–531.
32. Martin LF, Tan TL, Horn JR, Bixler EO, Kauffman GL, Becker DA, Hunter SM. Comparison of the costs associated with medical and surgical treatment of obesity. Surgery 1995; 118:599–606.
33. Narbo K, Agren G, Jonnson E, Larsson B, Naslund I, Wedel H, Sjostrom L. Sick leave and disability pension before and after treatment for obesity: a report from the Swedish Obese Subjects (SOS) study. Int J Obes Relat Metab Disord 1999; 23:619–624.

34. Sjostrom CD, Lissner L, Wedel H, Sjostrom L. Reduction in incidence of diabetes and lipid disturbances after intentional weight loss induced by bariatric surgery: the SOS Intervention Study. Obes Res 1999; 7:477–484.

35. Cramer P, Steinwert T. Thin is good, fat is bad: how early does it begin? J Appl Dev Psychol 1998; 19:429–451.

36. Richardson SA, Goodman N, Hastorf AH, Dornbusch SM. Cultural uniformity in reaction to physical disabilities. Am Sociol Rev 1961;241–247.

37. Neumark-Sztainer D, Story M, Faibisch L. Perceived stigmatization among overweight African-American and Caucasian adolescent girls. J Adolesc Health 1998; 23: 264–270.

38. Pierce JW, Wardle J. Cause and effect beliefs and self-esteem of overweight children. J Child Psychol Psychiatry 1997; 38:645–650.

39. Weiler K, Helms LB. Responsibilities of nursing education: the lessons of Russell v Salve Regina. J Prof Nurs 1993; 9:131–138.

40. Canning H, Mayer J. Obesity-its possible effect on college acceptance. N Engl J Med 1966; 275:1172–1174.

41. Crandall CS. Do heavy-weight students have more difficulty paying for college? Pers Soc Psychol Bull 1991; 17:606–611.

42. Crandall CS. Do parents discriminate against their heavyweight daughters? Pers Soc Psychol Bull 1995; 21:724–735.

43. Adamitis EM. Appearance matters: a proposal to prohibit appearance discrimination in employment. Washington Law Rev 2000; 75:195–223.

44. Epstein E. Fat people get a positive hearing in San Francisco: supervisors set vote on protected status. San Francisco Chronicle 2000; May.

45. Ziolkowski SM. Case comment: the status of weight-based employment discrimination under the Americans with Disabilities Act after Cook v. Rhode Island Department of Mental Health, Retardation, and Hospitals. Boston Univ Law Rev 1994; 74:667–686.

46. Crossley M. The disability kaleidoscope. Notre Dame Law Rev 1999; 74:621–716.

47. Crandall CS. Prejudice against fat people: ideology and self-interest. J Pers Soc Psychol 1994; 66:882–894.

48. Crandall CS, Schiffhauer KL. Anti-fat prejudice: beliefs, values, and American culture. Obes Res 1998; 6: 458–460.

49. Crandall CS, D'Anello S, Sakalli N, Lazarus E, Wieczorkowska G, Feather NT. An attribution-value model of prejudice: anti-fat attitudes in six nations. Pers Soc Psychol Bull 2001; 27:30–37.

50. Crandall CS, Martinez R. Culture, ideology, and antifat attitudes. Pers Soc Psychol Bull 1996; 22:1165–1176.

51. Menec VH, Perry RP. Reactions to stigmas among Canadian students: testing an attributional-affect-help judgement model. J Soc Psychol 1998; 138:443–454.

52. Weiner B, Perry R, Magnusson J. An attributional analysis of reactions to stigmas. J Pers Soc Psychol 1988; 55:738–748.

53. Wiese HJ, Wilson JF, Jones RA, Neises M. Obesity stigma reduction in medical students. Int J Obes 1992; 16:859–868.

54. Irving L. Promoting size acceptance in elementary school children: the EDAP puppet program. Eating disorders. J Treatment Prev 2000; 8:221–232.

5

Prevention of Obesity

W. Philip T. James

International Obesity TaskForce, London, England

Timothy P. Gill

University of Sydney, Sydney, New South Wales, Australia

I INTRODUCTION

The importance of the prevention of obesity is apparent to anyone involved in coping with its consequences or struggling with the major difficulties associated with its management. However, few if any experts know how to proceed with a logical scheme for prevention. Most also assume that as scientists, or even as clinicians, the solution lies outside their domain. This chapter focuses on the principles of obesity prevention and takes account of the next chapter's contribution on public policy and the need to reengineer the environment. It also aims to explain why those concerned with obesity prevention need to broaden their perspective.

II IS OBESITY PREVENTABLE?

A number of chapters in this handbook have indicated that the rates of obesity throughout both the developed and the developing world are increasing at a dramatic rate. Indeed, the pandemic of overweight and obesity is now so advanced and so widespread that few regions of the world (with the possible exception of parts of sub-Saharan Africa) appear to have escaped the effects of this major public health problem. Previous chapters have highlighted the strong biological influences that

contribute to the creation and maintenance of a positive energy balance in humans; current attempts to abate the rapid increase in body weight at both an individual and a community level have been less than inspiring. This has led some people to question whether it is possible to prevent continued increases in population body weight (1–3).

Despite these concerns about the effectiveness of current obesity prevention approaches, there is indirect evidence from a range of sources that supports the view that prevention is not only feasible, but offers the only solution to controlling the worldwide epidemic of obesity. Bouchard (4) indicates that the heritability of obesity and body fat stores is only moderate and that recent increases in obesity rates have occurred at a rate too fast to be explained by changes in the frequency of obesity genes or susceptibility alleles. He concludes that the increase in obesity prevalence can only be due to the fact that a greater number of children and adults are in positive energy balance and that it should be possible to attend to this through influencing diet and physical activity patterns. This view is supported by studies of monozygotic (MZ) twins discordant for body mass index (BMI) which have shown that mean body weight can vary between the overweight and lean sibling by up to 16 kg in men and 19 kg in women, even though they have exactly the same genotype (5).

While the obesity epidemic appears to be affecting all regions of the world, there are some countries that appear to less affected than others. In the Netherlands, the rates of obesity for both men and women are only half of that experienced in the United Kingdom or neighboring Germany and are increasing at a much slower rate (6). In Brazil the prevalence of obesity within upper-income, urban women has actually decreased in recent times, although men continue to put on weight at a rapid rate (7). In addition, while rates of obesity continue to climb in Finland, men from higher education grades have shown only a marginal increase (8).

Attempts to reduce the rising rates of obesity and poor physical fitness in Singapore appear to have been successful, at least in the short term. Intensive programs of physical training and influence over dietary intake resulted in a significant reduction in the number of schoolchildren being classified as overweight between 1992 and 1995 (9). Studies of young men inducted into the Singapore army also showed improvements in mean BMI during their periods of service, which unfortunately are reversed when they are released from the military.

Although it may be possible to prevent obesity, organizations that have examined current obesity prevention initiatives (10–13) have come to a common conclusion that their impact has been very limited. However, they all conceded that, given the considerable health risks associated with obesity, the high rates of overweight and obesity in most countries, the cost implications, and the limited long-term success of current weight reduction methods, priority should be given to the prevention of obesity and weight maintenance over weight loss interventions. Jeffery and French (14) have also argued that the behavior change required to prevent small increments in weight with age is likely to be easier to sustain than the behavior change required to achieve and maintain large weight losses.

III TARGETING PREVENTIVE STRATEGIES

No country, regardless how wealthy, has unlimited resources to apply to health care. Although the chapter on the economics of obesity indicates the potential savings from the effective prevention and management of obesity, finite health resources will always mean making decisions about where to target interventions. The report of the WHO Consultation on Obesity (9) suggests that there are three different but equally valid and complementary levels of obesity prevention. These

are shown in Figure 1 with the inner circle representing the *targeted* prevention which is aimed at those with an existing weight problem while the second ring represents the selective approach directed at high-risk individuals and groups. The broad outside ring represents universal or public health prevention approaches, which are directed at all members of the community.

A Individuals or Populations?

The criteria chosen for the targeting of preventive strategies raise many issues. It might seem logical to consider identifying those who are on the borderline for becoming obese (i.e., adults with BMIs of perhaps 28–29) and attempting to prevent them from gaining further weight and thus entering the obese category (i.e. a $BMI \geq 30\,kg/m^2$). Success would relate to maintaining a maximum BMI of 29 for individual adults, with equivalent cutoff points being chosen on a sex- and age-specific basis for children (15). This targeted approach has the advantage that individuals could be selected and special efforts then focused on these obesity-susceptible individuals. In medical terms, this would seem to provide maximum benefit, and costs would be limited because a substantial part of the population would not have to be dealt with.

The effect of such a strategy in different societies is illustrated in Figure 2, which is taken from the quintile distribution curves found by Rose and his colleagues in

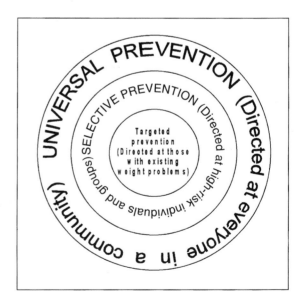

Figure 1 Levels of obesity prevention. (From Ref. 9.)

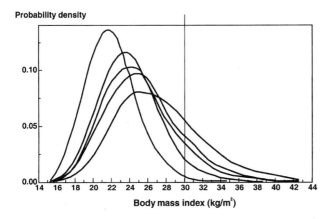

Figure 2 The shifting distributions of BMI of five population groups of men and women aged 20–59 years derived from 52 surveys in 32 countries. (From Ref. 16.)

the Intersalt Study concerned with monitoring age and sex-related differences in blood pressure in 52 surveys in 32 societies throughout the world (16). This shows that in some countries there would need to be a much bigger proportion of the population being targeted. In regions such as North America and Europe, with obesity rates of 20–30%, a substantial proportion of individuals would need to be identified if the aim is not only to prevent a further increase in obesity rates, but also to ensure that the obese reduce to a BMI <30 and then are prevented from weight regain.

Two flaws are evident in this approach. First, the shifting nature of the problem: the quintile distribution curves in Figure 2 reflect a dynamic process described as the global nutritional transition. As societies become more affluent, the BMI distribution shifts from quintile 1 toward quintile 5 so that more and more individuals will have to be targeted if the sole focus is on the prevention of individuals becoming frankly obese. In the SIGN Guidelines for the Primary Health Care approach to obesity management (12), it was estimated that a Scottish Health Centre with 10,000 children and adults and five doctors would have to cope with about 80 additional obese patients a year because of the growing obesity epidemic. Similar conclusions can be drawn for most countries, and thus the effort of this approach has to be progressively expanded as the obesity epidemic gathers pace. Second, Figure 2 also shows that the upper quintile curves simply reflect a shift in the whole societal pattern of body weights. Therefore the logic is to target the whole population rather than a smaller group with BMIs of 28–29. This is why obesity prevention has recently become very focused on population preventive strategies since both individuals and societies have to contend with the "obesogenic" environment.

The foregoing analysis presupposes a narrow definition of obesity prevention. In practice, it is well recognized (17–19) that the comorbidities of obesity are increasingly evident with increases of BMI from ~20.0 in adults. Thus diabetes, hypertension, and dyslipidemia rates are appreciably increased within the normal BMI range; adults who are already overweight should be seen as in need of immediate advice and help to prevent further weight gain. If possible, these overweight adults would also benefit from reducing their weight towards the normal BMI range of 18.5–24.9. The logic is therefore to consider the issue of preventing adult weight gain rather than just obesity per se.

B Higher-Risk Groups

A range of higher-risk groups can be defined for special attention based on their increased propensity to obesity or enhanced health hazards from obesity. Five key high-risk groups include: those with abdominal obesity; Asians and other susceptible ethnic groups; families with a history of obesity and/or type 2 diabetes; overweight adolescents; and obese pregnant women.

1 Abdominal Obesity

Abdominal obesity has now been clearly linked to an enhanced risk of comorbidities and is a key feature of Syndrome X, or the metabolic syndrome (20,21). Although no clear-cut definition has yet been agreed upon internationally, the syndrome includes a relative excess of abdominal fat, hypertension, insulin resistance, with glucose intolerance or diabetes, dyslipidemia, and microproteinuria. The additional health risk posed by abdominal obesity was highlighted by the WHO specification of two categories of increased risk based on sex-specific waist circumference measurements in its technical report on obesity (9). The WHO action points were based on the work of Lean et al. (22), who examined the association between waist circumference (as a marker of abdominal obesity) and comorbid risk factors in a sample of adults from the Netherlands. The U.S. National Institutes of Health (13) have also integrated waist circumference into their classification of risk associated with obesity, but for reasons of simplicity chose to include only the higher of the two action points proposed by WHO in the U.S. risk assessment system shown in Table 1. Recently a CDC-based working group (23) has reaffirmed the importance of

Table 1 NIH Classification of Overweight in Adults According to BMI, Waist Circumference, and Associated Disease Risk

| | BMI (kg/m^2) | Obesity class | Disease risk[a] relative to normal weight and waist circumference | |
			Men < 102 cm Women < 88 cm	> 102 cm > 88 cm
Underweight	< 18.5		—	—
Normal[b]	18.5–24.9		—	—
Overweight	25.0–29.9		Increased	High
Obesity	30.0–34.9	1	High	Very high
	35.0–39.9	2	Very high	Very high
Extreme obesity	≥40.0	3	Extremely high	Extremely high

[a] Disease risk for type 2 diabetes, hypertension, and CVD.
[b] Increased waist can also be a marker for increased risk in normal-weight individuals.
Source: Ref. 13.

addressing abdominal obesity, but the validity of identifying those with an elevated waist circumference as high risk now needs to be set out in a more integrated way in obesity prevention and management strategies.

2 Susceptible Ethnic Groups

A number of different ethnic groups have shown an increased propensity to develop obesity (particularly abdominal obesity) or to develop weight-related comorbidities at a lower BMI than Caucasians. For many years it has been apparent that emigrants from the Indian subcontinent are particularly susceptible to coronary heart disease (CHD) whether they live in South Africa, the Caribbean, or Europe (24). This susceptibility was apparent in McKeigue's observations of the enhanced diabetes rates linked to unusual degrees of

selective abdominal obesity with insulin resistance among migrants from the Indian subcontinent living in the United Kingdom (25). More recently, a WHO/IASO/IOTF (26) meeting in Hong Kong in 1999 proposed not only different BMI limits for Asians (see below) but also lower values for waist circumference based primarily on Hong Kong data for Chinese, who seem to have a much greater propensity for diabetes and lower waist values. These proposed cutoff points are included in Table 2.

Similarly, it has been noted that Australian Aborigines are also more likely to store fat abdominally and are more prone to diabetes, hypertension, and CHD at much lower levels of BMI than European-Australians (27). Aborigines who follow a traditional way of life remain very lean and suffer very little chronic disease, but once they become acculturated to a Western lifestyle

Table 2 Proposed Classification of Weight by BMI and Waist Circumference in Adult Asians

| Classification | BMI (kg/m^2) | Risk of comorbidities | |
| | | Waist circumference | |
		< 90 cm (men) < 80 cm (women)	≥90 cm (men) ≥80 cm (women)
Underweight	< 18.5	Low (but risk of other clinical problems increased)	Average
Normal range	18.5–24.9	Average	Increased
Overweight	≥ 23.0		
At risk	23.0–24.9	Increased	Moderate
Obese class I	25.0–29.9	Moderate	Severe
Obese class II	≥ 30.0	Severe	Very severe

Source: Ref. 26.

and begin to put on weight, their rates of comorbid illness increase rapidly (28). In the United States, Hispanics have disproportionately higher rates of obesity, diabetes, and hypertension when compared to non-Hispanic whites, although this does not translate into greater mortality from CHD (29).

Some researchers have attempted to explain these differences in obesity-related comorbidity risk on the basis of variations in the levels of body fat at any given BMI, with Asians, and particularly Indians, having much higher levels of body fat at lower levels of BMI when compared to Europeans (30). However, other studies have shown that the relationship between body fat and BMI is more dependent upon body proportions than on any genetic differences between ethnic groups (31,32).

3 Family History of Obesity and/or Diabetes

It has long been known that obesity runs in families, although the determinants of that heritability are not likely to be all genetic, with parental influence on dietary and physical activity patterns also playing a role (4,33). Whitaker et al. (34) examined the influence of parental obesity on the development of childhood obesity and its persistence into adulthood. They found that having at least one obese parent greatly increased one's risk of becoming obese as an adult. However, the risks of adult obesity were magnified in subjects who had an obese parent and who were also obese as children. In younger children this effect was small or nonexistent (OR = 1.3 for children aged 1–2 years) but was very pronounced in older children (OR = 17.5 in 15- to 17-year olds). Thus it would appear that identifying children with obese parents and intervening early to prevent unhealthy weight gain may allow the progression to adult obesity to be prevented.

It has also been well recognized for some time that the children of parents with type 2 diabetes are particularly susceptible themselves to type 2 diabetes should they gain weight. Recent studies have found that this susceptibility is much stronger in children whose mother, rather than father, had type 2 diabetes and have attributed this problem to the diabetic intrauterine environment (35). Therefore, preventive measures should properly be focused on the children of obese adults with or without a family history of diabetes and pregnant women with a history of type 2 diabetes.

4 Adolescent Obesity

A number of studies have attempted to track the relative weights of children throughout their lives to determine whether fatness in childhood leads to obesity in adult-

hood. These studies suggest that childhood obesity does not necessarily lead to adult obesity but that there is a reasonable level of tracking of fatness (36–38). The older the obese child, the higher the likelihood that he/she will be obese as an adult and the more likely he/she is to develop health consequences associated with weight in early adulthood (39). This is particularly true for females; around one-third of females who are obese in their mid-30s were obese as adolescents while for obese men this figure was only 10% (40). In addition, it has been shown that if adolescents enter adult life obese and increase their weight further, then they are extraordinarily susceptible to early type 2 diabetes (18). Adolescents are therefore a group deserving special attention in any obesity prevention strategy.

5 Obesity in Pregnancy

The problem of mothers accumulating excess weight and developing obesity during pregnancy has been described for over 50 years (41) and is a common reason given by obese women for their weight problem. Studies have shown that there is considerable variation in the amount of weight gained during gestation and that excess weight is often retained postpartum (42). Although the mean weight gain is quite small, some women experience extreme weight gains and others have cumulative increases in body weight after each pregnancy (43). Of equal concern is the potential impact upon the adiposity of a child born to an obese woman. Although only recently identified as of concern, the propensity of obese women to produce large babies, whether or not they display their increased susceptibility to gestational diabetes, is now linked to a much greater likelihood of these children becoming obese during childhood (44).

C Those with Existing Obesity or Weight-Related Comorbidities

Prevention of weight gain is an important strategy in people with existing obesity as a means of avoiding or delaying the onset of associated illness. It is also an important management strategy for those with existing weight-related comorbidities. However, perhaps the greatest impact of weight gain prevention can be achieved in those groups who are at high risk of comorbid illness. Those with existing impaired glucose tolerance have been shown to have less progression to full diabetes if they are able to maintain their weight when compared to those who continue to gain weight with age (see Sec. VII.C.2).

IV APPROPRIATE GOALS FOR OBESITY PREVENTION

Setting appropriate and achievable goals is an important component of the planning of any health promotion intervention. Past obesity prevention programs have been criticised for failing to adequately define a successful outcome (10). Jeffrey (45) believes that a failure to set specific weight-related goals was a contributing factor to the ineffectiveness of community CHD programs to prevent increases in the mean BMI of participants over time. Clear goals for obesity prevention not only provide outcome measures against which preventive programs can be evaluated, but they also guide the nature and the content of preventive efforts. Setting inappropriate goals, such as unattainable reductions in the prevalence of obesity in the community or reductions in the mean population BMI, are counterproductive and dangerous. Failure to achieve them will be taken as a measure of the weakness of an intervention and can often lead to the premature curtailment of potentially useful obesity prevention initiatives.

A Weight Gain Prevention in Individuals

The prevention of weight gain rather than a reduction in obesity prevalence is a goal that should apply equally to both populations and individuals and is appropriate to nearly all members of society regardless of their initial weight. Criteria have not been specifically set for obesity prevention, but it would seem appropriate to ensure that individuals avoid weight gain which has the potential to impact appreciably on their "well-being" and capacity to live a full life. However, this general definition leads to a plethora of issues because in affluent Western societies women, in particular, are striving to prevent even modest weight increases often when they are within the normal BMI range. The concept of well-being, therefore, involves recognition that the quality of life of children and adults is in part determined by their cultural setting and not just by whether or not they have symptoms relating to physical comorbidities. Prevention strategies could be defined for simplicity as strategies which (1) allow individuals to remain within the normal BMI range and restrict adult weight gain to < 5 kg, (2) prevent further weight gain in existing overweight and obese individuals, and (3) successfully prevent weight regain in overweight and obese patients who have lost a reasonable amount of weight (e.g., >5%). In the SIGN Guidelines, weight maintenance was defined as the weight regain of < 3 kg long term (i.e., >2 years)

(12). These three categories of successful prevention are chosen arbitrarily but demand very similar strategies.

B Optimum Population BMIs

If a general population approach to prevention is taken, then it is desirable to specify the appropriate mean BMI as well as the minimum expected prevalence of overweight and obesity. Figure 3 shows the relationships between the mean BMI of a male population and the prevalence of both overweight and obesity derived by IOTF from representative data from 26 countries. This analysis suggests that the mean BMI needs to be < 23.0 to ensure that obesity rates are close to zero, and the lower the mean BMI value, the smaller the proportion of overweight in the population. There are, however, disadvantages in having too low a mean BMI. Representative data obtained from relatively malnourished populations in Africa and Asia show that a median BMI

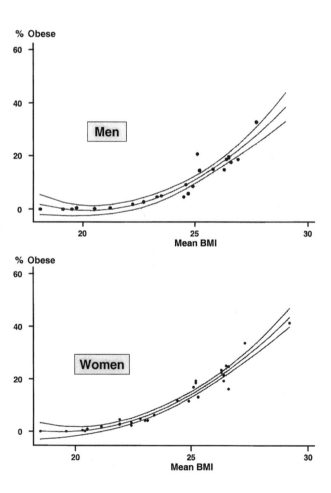

Figure 3 Relationship between mean BMI and prevalence of overweight and obesity. (From IOTF unpublished analysis.)

of ~22–23 is required if the prevalence of underweight women (i.e., with BMIs < 18.5) is to be kept low (46). Therefore it can be concluded that the optimum BMI for a society should be ~22.0. At this value, ~5–10% of adults are underweight, and a similar proportion are overweight. This is a theoretical, optimum mean BMI, which in practice is far removed from that seen in countries in affluent regions of the world where mean BMIs vary from 23.5 in the 18-to-29-year-olds up to 28.4 depending on the age group and region.

C Evaluating Interventions

Specific outcomes need to be set for any obesity prevention, intervention to enable a determination of the extent to which the objectives of the program have been met. Evaluation is an essential component of any program, but long-term goals can make it complex and costly to evaluate absolute outcomes that relate to shifts in population weight status. It has been suggested that intermediate-term or process evaluation measures which relate to appropriate dietary or physical activity behaviour change or changes in structures or environments may be a more useful guide to the success of a particular prevention program (47). This issue is taken up in more detail in the following chapter.

V KEY BEHAVIORS TO INFLUENCE IN OBESITY PREVENTION PROGRAMS

Many other chapters in this handbook have highlighted the complex, multifactorial nature of the etiology of obesity. Some of these factors are nonchangeable such as genetics, gender, and age, and others, such as physiological disturbances in hormonal regulatory systems, can only be dealt with at an individual level (if at all). However, this still leaves a large number of potential influences over energy intake or energy expenditure and thus body weight regulation which could be the focus of interventions to prevent obesity. Unfortunately, we have gained few insights into the most effective obesity prevention strategies from the limited number of programs that have attempted to address this issue in the past (see Sec. VII of this chapter). Thus it is necessary to speculate on what are the key behaviours to address that are most likely to support the attainment and maintenance of energy balance at both an individual and population level.

The prevention of obesity does not necessarily draw on the same strategies employed to treat obesity. The treatment of obesity requires the creation of a relatively large energy deficit, usually in excess of 500 kcal (2000 kJ) per day, which needs to be sustained for the period of weight loss. This usually involves moderate change in current diet and physical activity patterns, but is often achieved with more radical change. In contrast, the prevention of weight gain may only require very minor but long-term energy adjustments in the region of 50 kcal or less a day to avoid the accumulation of excess energy over time and prevent an increase in body fat stores. Thus the most effective prevention strategies may not necessarily be based on what makes the biggest contribution to the development of energy imbalance. Instead effective prevention strategies will need to focus on changes that are achievable, sustainable, simple, relevant to a large proportion of the target population, and capable of contributing to increased energy expenditure or decreased energy intake or both. Changes that may only result in a small reduction in energy intake or small increase in energy expenditure in an individual may be effective strategies when applied across the population. Additionally, given the level of concern expressed about eating disorders among certain susceptible subgroups of the population, it may be wise to ensure that prevention strategies are unlikely to contribute significantly to inappropriate eating behaviors.

A Select a Low-Fat, Low–Energy Dense Diet

1 The Importance of Low-Fat Diets in Preventing Weight Gain

The role of a high-fat diet in inducing weight gain was highlighted by the WHO Consultation on Obesity (9) and gained general acceptance as an appropriate strategy for the prevention of obesity until questioned by some authors who expressed doubts about the efficacy and safety of this approach (48–50). Their skepticism was based on the association of increasing levels of obesity with decreasing proportion of dietary energy from fat in the U.S. national diet, a belief that high-carbohydrate diets resulted in increased CHD risk and the variable and inconsistent outcome of trials of low-fat diets. However, a review of U.S. dietary patterns over the period 1970–1994 by the U.S. Department of Agriculture (51) revealed that, while there was a decrease in the percentage of energy from fat (from 42% to 38%), the absolute amount of fat in grams available for consumption actually increased by 3%. This apparent paradox is possible because over the same time period the energy available per capita increased by 15% (from 3300 kcal to 3800 kcal). Astrup et al. (52) have undertaken a meta-analysis of trials involving low-fat diets and shown that the lower the fat intake, the greater the weight loss, this loss being more marked in the more overweight subjects. In addition, recent detailed assessments on the matter (53–55) have all concluded that the balance of evidence supports an important role for dietary fat in the genesis of obesity and support the potential for weight gain prevention of reducing fat in the diet. This does not mean, however, that the other dietary components do not have an important role to play in the prevention of weight gain. There is some evidence that the source of dietary carbohydrate and the glycemic index may influence cardiovascular risk factors (56) and has the potential to amplify the risk of the metabolic syndrome in those who gain weight (57).

2   Food Eaten Away from Home

One of the most profound changes to affect the food supply in almost all developed and many developing countries has been the rapid increase in the proportion of food prepared away from home. The proportion of household budget spent on food eaten away from the home is as high as 40% in the United States (51) and ~25–30% in many other counties such as Australia and the United Kingdom (58,59). The spread of fast-food outlets across the world is responsible for the biggest proportion of food eaten away from home, with the number of outlets increasing from 30,000 to 140,000 in the United States between 1970 and 1980 and fast-food sales increasing 300% in the same period (60). Some analyses have linked the increase in fast food consumption to increasing rates of obesity (61). French et al. (62) have found that fast-food use was associated with increased energy and fat intake as well as higher body weight in females (but not males) in the subjects who participated in the "Pound of Prevention" study. The portion size of fast-food items has also been increasing rapidly in recent times and has been identified as a key issue in the consumption of dietary energy in excess of need (60). Evidence suggests that as portion size increases, the ability of consumers to estimate accurately their intake deteriorates (63). The sheer volume of sales achieved by fast food outlets and the association with increased fat and energy intake make them a useful target for obesity prevention efforts.

3   Sweetened Drinks

Evidence is accumulating from a range of sources that energy consumed as sweetened drinks is less well compensated for than when consumed as solid food (64,65). A recent longitudinal study has shown that children who consumed more soft drink at baseline were more likely to become obese and that every 1-serving increase

in soft drink consumption resulted in a 1.6-fold increase in the risk of obesity (66). Special trials in adult volunteers allowing plentiful soft drinks, with either sugars or sweeteners, for 10 weeks in double-blind trials also show progressive weight gain only in the sugar drink–consuming group (67). Market research data suggest that soft drink consumption is increasing worldwide at a rate faster than any other food group (68) and is replacing water and milk as the most popular drinks among children. The widespread availability of soft drinks from vending machines could be contributing to this trend (60).

B   Increase Physical Activity

Although it is difficult to accurately measure changes in physical activity, there can be little doubt that energy expenditure from activity has decreased substantially over the past 50 years. James (69) compared food intake data with population weight gain to estimate that it is likely that the average, adult energy expenditure in the United Kingdom decreased by ~800 kcal between 1970 and 1990. That this reduction in energy expenditure occurred in a period where surveys suggested that participation in leisure-time physical activity was increasing in the United Kingdom (70) supports the contention that the greatest contribution to this reduction in physical activity comes from the enormous changes in occupational and incidental activity. Prentice and Jebb (71) demonstrated the close association between increasing rates of obesity in the United Kingdom and two key indicators of inactivity (hours per week of television viewing and numbers of cars per household). Although there are few data to support the nature of this association, the extent of mechanization, computerization, and control systems imposed in the workplace and the shifting employment patterns away from manual to more sedentary occupations has markedly reduced the need for energy expenditure at work. In addition, the rapid increase in use of mechanized transport and labor-saving devices such as elevators has reduced the need to expend energy going about our daily lives.

A number of studies support the benefit of increasing physical activity in the prevention of weight gain, although it is not clear from current studies whether increased physical activity actually prevents or reverses age-related weight gain at the population level (72). Cohort studies in both Finland and the United States have shown that weight gain is less in those who are more active (73–75), and similar findings have emerged from assessments of a register of people who have been successful in losing and maintaining weight (76,77). It is also proving difficult to predict how much physical activity is required to prevent weight gain, with Schoeller et al. (78) estimating that an additional 80 min of moderate activity or 35 min of vigorous activity may need to be added to our usual sedentary lifestyle to prevent weight regain in subjects who have previously been obese. However, there are numerous health benefits to be gained from regular exercise regardless of the impact of physical activity on weight gain prevention (79,80).

C Decrease Sedentary Behaviors

Technological advances have allowed a reduction in hours spent at work and in undertaking household chores leading to a substantial increase in leisure time while at the same time spawning the development of numerous entertainment options to fill this time. Almost all of these new entertainment options such as television, video games, and computers are sedentary activities requiring little energy expenditure. In recent times these activities, which initially were used to complement existing forms of leisure activity, are occupying more hours in the day and displacing more active pursuits and games. This has raised concerns for both adults and children, and a number of studies have found association between the number of hours spent watching television and increased levels of BMI in children (81–83). Although small, these associations, have been relatively consistent but have not been demonstrated for other sedentary behaviors.

It is important to make a distinction between lack of physical activity and sedentary behavior as the mechanism for their impact on body weight may be different and a high level of sedentary behavior can coexist with a high level of physical activity. In the study of Andersen et al. (83), most of the children reported relatively high frequency of activity and although there was a strong association between TV watching and weight status, the association between physical activity and fatness was weak. Robinson (84) indicates that the mechanisms by which sedentary behavior influences body fatness are still to be elucidated. He suggests that a reduction in energy expenditure from a displacement of physical activity seems logical (although not clearly found) but television viewing may also be associated with an increased dietary intake, potentially driven by food advertising. It is interesting to note that studies of the treatment of overweight children have found that reinforcing decreased sedentary behavior leads to a greater weight loss than promoting increased physical activity. (85).

D Improve Infant Feeding and Maternal Nutrition

Infant feeding practices may have an important influence in the etiology of childhood overweight and obesity, and breastfeeding may assist with postpartum weight management in mothers. In addition, eating practices and food preferences developed in early childhood may persist throughout childhood and adolescence and contribute to the genesis of weight problems.

WHO has recently reevaluated the importance of breastfeeding in terms of subsequent health, but did not pay particular attention to the issue of obesity in later childhood. Breastfeeding induces faster longitudinal growth in newborn babies and results in babies that are thinner than bottle-fed babies. The choice of recommendation for exclusive breastfeeding until ~6 months is based on a series of small studies that reveal that the rate of growth of the breastfed child decelerates from soon after birth and crosses that of the NCHS standard group of predominantly bottle-fed babies at the age of ~6 months (86).

There has nevertheless been a renewed emphasis on the potential value of breastfeeding recently with a series of studies (see Table 3) (87), suggesting that breastfeeding may protect against the development of obesity in older children. However, not all studies have shown an association, and it was apparent that breastfeeding

Table 3 Recent Studies Examining the Impact of Breastfeeding on Later Obesity

Study (Ref.)	Sample	Age at follow-up	Breastfeeding (>6 months) effect on overweight and obesity rates odds ratio (95% CI)
Von Kries et al., 1999 (90)	9357 children	5–6 years	0.75 (0.57–0.98)
Gillman et al., 2001 (88)	8186 girls and 7155 boys	9–14 years	0.78 (0.66–0.91)
Hediger et al., 2001 (146)	2685 children	3–5 years	0.84 (0.62–1.13)

needs to be exclusive and sustained for at least 4 months to show any impact on weight in later childhood (88,89). The longer the breastfeeding period, the less likely the children are to become obese later. Von Kries et al. (90) found a dose-dependent protective effect of breastfeeding on the development of obesity with 3–5 months of exclusive breastfeeding being associated with a 35% reduction in obesity at age 5–6 years. However, Bute, in her recent analysis, highlights the difficulty in separating out the breastfeeding per se from confounding factors such as the socioeconomic status of the family, the educational level of the mother, and their degree of concern in modifying the children's subsequent diet (91). As Dietz (89) indicates in a recent editorial on the issue, the percentage of obesity cases preventable by breastfeeding may be small, with a maximum population attributable risk of 15–20%, but the numerous additional benefits, lack of potential risks and cheapness of breastfeeding, make it worth promoting vigorously.

Whether the effects of breast feeding on subsequent obesity levels are influenced by the fatty acid composition of the breast milk is unknown, but the diet of the pregnant woman influences the n-6 and n-3 supply to the fetus through the mechanisms of essential fatty acid (EFA) transport in the placenta (92) with the mother's diet also affecting her own body membrane lipid levels and the composition of the breast milk. The EFAs stimulate lipogenesis and cellular proliferation (93), and vegetarian mothers have reduced intakes of EFAs with an increase in the n-6/n-3 ratio (94). Insulin resistance limits the delta-9 desaturase responsible for the essential chain elongation of the EFAs, so overweight and obese mothers may also be influencing their babies' adipocyte proliferation depending on their own diet and whether or not they breastfeed.

The value of breastfeeding in promoting a faster return to prepregnancy weight is less clear. Sebire et al. (95) found in a retrospective analysis of 287,213 pregnancies in England that women who were breastfeeding their children on discharge from hospital were significantly less likely to be obese. However, this may be a consequence of the reluctance of overweight women to initiate and sustain breastfeeding (96) rather than a direct impact of breastfeeding on maternal weight. Studies of women who have breastfed in Brazil (97) and the United States (98) have shown that the long-term association between breastfeeding and maternal weight and fat stores is limited but does increase in strength when only women who exclusively breastfed are included in the analysis.

There is now a reasonable amount of evidence to suggest that low–birth weight infants are at increased risk of a combination of hypertension, dyslipidemia, and glucose intolerance (a cluster known as syndrome X) in adulthood (99). This condition is exacerbated in those who having been born small subsequently develop obesity in adulthood. However, the connection between low birth weight and the development of obesity appears slight at best (100), and these abnormalities are more likely to be mediated by catchup growth or abdominal obesity. Poor perinatal nutrition is only one of a number of factors, including age of parity, smoking, and sexually transmitted disease that influence birth weight, but the benefits of improving maternal nutrition are likely to be numerous.

VI MOVING BEYOND BEHAVIOR CHANGE STRATEGIES IN THE PREVENTION OF OBESITY

Changing eating and physical activity patterns that predispose to weight gain remains the key concern of obesity prevention strategies, as the prevention of weight gain is dependent upon balancing energy intake and expenditure. Until recently, interventions aimed at the population control of obesity have focused on improving the knowledge and skills of individuals within the community in the belief that large-scale individual change will have an impact on the population weight status. However, such programs have had only limited success because they have not engaged all sections of the community and because the environment in which eating and exercise behaviors are made is now so antagonistic to healthy lifestyle choices that even the most motivated individuals find it difficult to make and sustain appropriate changes (101). Recent analyses of the obesity problem have focused discussion on moving beyond strategies that focus solely on changing personal or community behaviors to tackling some of the underlying structural and environmental determinants that shape these behaviors (47,69,102,103).

The International Obesity Task Force produced a diagrammatic "causal web" to highlight the complex range of factors that have the potential to influence and constrain healthy choices in relation to weight (104). The web presents a "visual challenge" to the notion of free will by showing how such factors as global media and marketing, regional, national and local level policies relating to agriculture, urban design, education, and transport directly influence eating and physical activity in communities, homes, and schools (Fig. 4).

Tackling societal and environmental factors that underlie the development of obesity is covered in detail

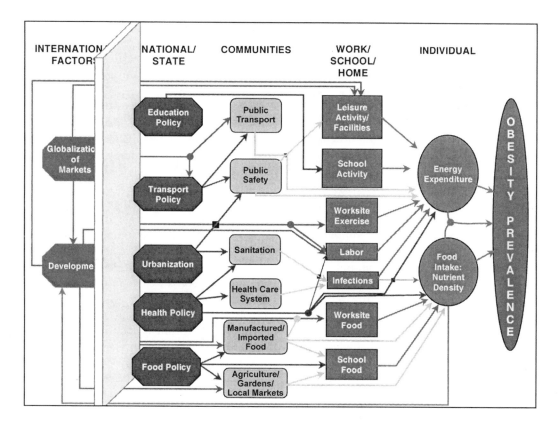

Figure 4 Causal web of societal influences on obesity prevalence. (From Ref. 104.)

in the following chapter. However, structural solutions and individual behavior change are not competing strategies in the prevention of weight gain. They are complementary and interdependent. The development of comprehensive programs of action to tackle obesity will require attention to both approaches. But, without structural change, individual-oriented behavior change strategies have the potential to worsen health disparities as the less advantaged members of the community have less latitude in physical activity and eating behaviors relating to obesity (47).

VII WEIGHT GAIN PREVENTION TRIALS

To date, there have only been a modest number of structured and evaluated interventions, which have had a primary objective of preventing or limiting weight gain. However, a broader range of projects have examined the most effective strategies for improving physical activity or encouraging specific dietary change or for combating allied chronic noncommunicable diseases such as CHD, hypertension, and diabetes. Examining the lessons

learned from these programs allows a preliminary perspective on the potentially most suitable approaches to supporting and encouraging the prevention of weight gain in the community.

A Preventing Childhood Overweight and Obesity

The longer-term benefits of limiting obesity rates in children are likely to be particularly important if the obesity persists into adult life. The persistence of excess weight in childhood into adult obesity appears to increase linearly with age from around 6 years and is particularly strong in adolescents (39). Parsons et al. (105) in their systematic review of childhood predictors of adult obesity found a range of factors including higher birth weight and earlier pubertal maturation consistently related to a greater risk of adult obesity. The issue of birth weights has already been addressed, but the causes of earlier pubertal maturation are more difficult to establish. Rapid early growth induced by high-protein and high energy-dense diets rich in fats and sugars may promote earlier maturation, but individual genetically related susceptibility to early puberty may also be involved. The review did not find a consistent relationship between physical activity or diet and childhood or adult obesity, but measures of habitual diet and activity are difficult to obtain accurately. The Amsterdam Growth and Health Longitudinal Study has suggested that high physical activities and lower protein intakes in adolescence were associated with lower fat masses and lower BMIs (106), but there are no known analyses of preventive initiatives that have focused specifically on reducing either total energy or protein intakes as a means of reducing adolescent obesity.

A recent Cochrane systematic review examined studies relating to the prevention of obesity in children and could only find seven trials that met their requirements (107). The review had intended originally to include only studies which lasted at least a year, but only three longer-term trials were found, and thus four short-term studies with a follow-up of at least 3 months were also included. Of these seven studies, two assessed physical activity interventions, one assessed reduction in sedentary behaviors, three assessed combined diet and physical activity interventions, and one involved a dietary intervention only. Although many of these studies produced promising results, the reviewers concluded that there are limited quality data on the effectiveness

of obesity prevention programs, and no generalizable conclusion could be drawn.

A recent systematic review sponsored by CDC examined community interventions in a range of different settings that aimed to increase physical activity (108). This review screened 6238 potential titles, assessed 849 abstracts and specialist reports, and reviewed 253 trials in detail and found firm evidence to recommend only six interventions, although many other approaches showed potential. The recommended list included a mix of educational, behavioral, and social approaches and environmental and policy change (see Table 4).

School-based physical education was one of the approaches strongly recommended by the review, and although the focus of the review was not weight control, nine of the 14 studies reviewed in this area examined markers of body weight/fatness as outcomes. These studies are presented in Table 5. The interventions involved changes in the way physical education classes were taught within a school setting, but additional policies involving comprehensive daily physical education were also assessed. The comparison groups usually received simply standard health education or changes in the physical education curriculum. The reviewers noted that physical education classes in schools usually

Table 4 Recommendations from the CDC Review of Interventions to Increase Physical Activity

Intervention	Recommendation
Informational approaches to increasing physical activity	
Communitywide campaigns	Strongly recommended
"Point-of-decision" prompts to encourage stair use	Recommended
Classroom-based health education focused on providing information	Insufficient evidence[a]
Mass media campaigns	Insufficient evidence[a]
Behavioral and social approaches to increasing physical activity	
School-based physical education (PE)	Strongly recommended
Social support interventions in community settings	Strongly recommended
Individually adapted health behavior change programs	Strongly recommended
Classroom-based health education focused on reducing television viewing and video game playing	Insufficient evidence[a]
College-age health education and PE	Insufficient evidence[a]
Family-based social support	Insufficient evidence[a]
Environmental and policy approaches to increasing physical activity	
Creation of or enhanced access to places for physical activity combined with informational outreach activities	Strongly recommended

[a] A determination that evidence is insufficient should not be confused with evidence of ineffectiveness. A determination of insufficient evidence assists in identifying (1) areas of uncertainty regarding an intervention's effectiveness, and (2) gaps in the evidence where future prevention research is needed. In contrast, evidence of ineffectiveness leads to a recommendation that the intervention not be used.
Source: Ref. 105.

Table 5 Controlled Trials of School-Based Physical Education BMI (10 arms; 10 measures)

Study (Ref.)	Measure	Comparison	Follow-up	Pre	Post	Net intervention effect	Sig
CATCH, 1996 (111a)	BMI	3rd Grade	2.5 yrs	NR	NR	NA	NS
Donnelly, 1996 (111b)	BMI	3–5 Grade	2 yrs	I: 17.9 C: 18.1	I: 18.9 C: 19.3	−1.0%	NS
Ewart, 1998 (111c)	BMI	9th Grade, girls	3 yrs	I: 24.8 C: 24.1	I: 25.1 C: 24.1	1.2%	NS
Manios, 1999 (111)	BMI	Cretan 1st graders	3 yrs	I: 16.2 C: 16.3	I: 17.0 C: 18.1	−6.1%	0.001
Dwyer, 1983 (111e)	Sum of 4 SF (mm)	5–6th Grade, boys	2 yrs	31.9	28.62	−10.3%	<0.05
Dywer, 1983 (111e)	Sum of 4 SF (mm)	5–6th Grade, girls	2 yrs	40.2	36.23	−10.3%	<0.05
SPARK, 1997 (111d)	Sum of 4 SF (mm)	PE specialist, boys	2.5 yrs	I: 26.9 C: 27.1	I: 26.4 C: 28.0	−5.2%	NS
SPARK, 1997 (111d)	Sum of 4 SF (mm)	Teacher-led, boys	2.5 yrs	I: 26.8 C: 27.1	I: 25.5 C: 28.0	−8.2%	NS
SPARK, 1997 (111d)	Sum of 4 SF (mm)	PE specialist, boys	2.5 yrs	I: 28.7 C: 31.2	I: 30.0 C: 30.1	8.1%	NS
SPARK, 1997 (111d)	Sum of 4 SF (mm)	Teacher-led, boys	2.5 yrs	I: 30.4 C: 31.2	I: 28.0 C: 30.1	−4.4%	NS
Manios, 1999 (111)	Bicep SF	Cretan 1st graders	3 yrs	I: 4.8 C: 5.5	I: 6.0 C: 6.4	8.6%	NS
	Tricep SF	Cretan 1st graders	3 yrs	I: 10.2 C: 11.9	I: 10.9 C: 11.5	10.2%	NS
	Suprailliac SF	Cretan 1st graders	3 yrs	I: 6.7 C: 7.0	I: 8.3 C: 9.6	−13.3%	<0.05
	Subscapular SF	Cretan 1st graders	3 yrs	I: 6.8 C: 7.4	I: 8.1 C: 8.4	5.6%	NS
Donnelly, 1996 (111b)	%BF	3–5	2 yrs	I: 16.3 C: 19.1	I: 18.1 C: 19.6	8.0%	NS

Source: Ref. 105.

involve very small amounts of time for moderate to vigorous physical activity, i.e., from 9% to 36% of the teaching time. The best-designed studies (e.g., 109–111) showed very significant effects on the amount of time spent in physical activity but did not induce significant changes in BMI or skinfold thicknesses. However, the longer-term studies, e.g., Manios (111) in Cretan first-graders monitored over 3 years, did show a highly significant restriction in the weight increase in the intervention group.

A recent careful study by Robinson (112) deserves attention because it evaluated a health education/TV turn-off approach to physical inactivity. In this study, the aim was to encourage children to reduce the time spent either watching television or playing video games. Body weight increases in children from the schools that provided 18 periods of intensive education and parental monitoring (through a special electronic device) of the time children spent sitting in front of a TV or computer were less than in the control schools where general health education only was provided. Another study, the Planet Health project, involved separate analyses of the response of boys and girls to a reduction in TV and video use from a base of about 3 hr/d in girls and 3.75 hr in boys. Girls responded better, with a 20% drop in viewing compared with a nonsignificant 9.5% reduction in boys (113). These approaches are quite different from routine classroom-based health education, which in the CDC analyses were found to be ineffective in influencing excess weight gain. The Robinson study lasted 6 months, but the Planet Health study was conducted for 2 years. Their data are shown in Table 6. However,

Table 6 Trials to Limit Sedentary Behavior by Reducing TV Viewing

Study (Ref.)	Measure	Comparison	Follow-up	Pre	Post	Net intervention effect	Sig
Robinson, 1999 (112)	BMI	I vs. C	6 months	I: 18.38 C: 18.10	I: 18.67 C: 18.81	−2.3%	.0002
	Skinfold	I vs. C	6 months	I: 14.55 C: 13.97	I: 15.47 C: 16.46	−11.5%	.002
Planet Health (113)	Obesity prevalence	Girls, I vs. C	2 academic years	I: 23.6 C: 21.5	I: 20.3 C: 23.7	−24.2% OR: 0.47	.03
	Obesity prevalence	Boys, I vs. C	2 academic years	I: 29.3 C: 34.7	I: 27.8 C: 31.8	3.2%	NS
	Obesity remission	Post only, girls	2 academic years	NA	I: 31.5 C: 19.1	64.9% OR: 2.16	.04
	Obesity remission	Post only, boys	2 academic years	NA	I: 23.7 C: 26.5	24.7%	NS

Source: Ref. 105.

the Task Force concluded that the results of these and other studies concerned with changing physical activity they reviewed were insufficient to produce firm conclusions.

There has been no systematic review of studies undertaken to induce selective dietary changes in children with the aim of limiting excess weight gain or combating obesity. The systematic review by Campbell et al. (107) could only identify one well-conducted study, which involved a school-based dietary intervention that assessed two levels of intensity of diet education over 12 months (114). In this study of 1320 boys and girls aged 3–9 years an intensive nutrition education program focused on energy reduction was able to show a 12% reduction in overweight and obesity. The Dietary Intervention Study in Children (DISC) compared the effect of a low-fat diet plan (28% energy from fat with 8% from saturated fat) against the standard U.S. diet in 660 8-to-10-year-old children with elevated LDL cholesterol (115). The intervention group showed modest reductions in LDL cholesterol over the 10-year trial and at the end of year 1, the lower-fat group also had a significantly lower adjusted BMI, but this effect disappeared later. Recently Resnicow and Robinson (116) reviewed 16 major school-based CVD prevention trials and found that measures of adiposity showed the worst rates of improvement from all the outcomes assessed.

In contrast, school-based interventions for the treatment of obesity have produced more promising results. In an assessment of such progams by Story (117), 11 out of the 12 studies reviewed showed a significant reduction in the percentage overweight within the intervention group when compared to the controls. All these programs were administered to overweight children only, with duration ranging from 6 weeks to 18 months and with the number of sessions ranging from once a week to five times a week. All contained diet and physical activity components, and nine included behavior modification strategies. The Kiel Obesity Prevention Study (KOPS) (118) is a comprehensive school-based intervention study with an 8-year follow-up which aims to build on existing prevention strategies. A cohort of 6000 children aged 5–7 years were recruited to the project in 1996. After a comprehensive baseline assessment, the children were assigned to different nutrition and physical activity interventions that involved their parents and teachers as well as the children. Follow-up measures will be assessed after 4 years and 8 years to compare changes in measures of adiposity.

The work of Epstein in defining the most effective approaches to the management of overweight children is also very informative. Working with small groups of obese children, he observed greater reductions and maintenance of weight after 10 years in children whose parents were involved in helping to produce a family-based approach to prevention (119). Simply dealing with the children on their own was insufficient, and suggests that the family environment is important if an individual is to cope with the problems of a general environment that is promoting a decline in physical activity and the unfettered consumption of high-fat and sugar-dense foods. The CDC analyses showed that many of these family-oriented strategies are given as an addition to the school program of behavioral change. In this context, the additional input of the parents did not produce additional benefits in terms of changes in the children's fatness or BMI (108). There was an inconsistent suggestion of a greater persistence with out-of-school hours physical activity if parents were involved.

By the time children move to college education in the United States, one might suppose that they would become more concerned for their individual welfare. However, the current evidence suggests that to use college-based physical education as a means of increasing physical activity is ineffective.

B Preventing Weight Gain in Adults

In the prevailing environment, where overweight and obesity are so common, the key issue in obesity prevention is how best to encourage and support individuals to change their behavior. Two recent systematic reviews of interventions to prevent obesity in adults could only identify four suitable controlled trials (10, 11). Not one of these trials, which lasted between 1 and 7 years, was able to show any reduction in the mean BMI of the intervention group. A range of education strategies was employed within each trial including mass media, seminars, literature, newsletters, and a restaurant program.

Mass media campaigns, sometimes developed at considerable expense, have generally been shown to have little impact on indices of weight status, although very few have specifically targeted obesity (108). The only study to assess the impact of the use of mass media over a reasonable time frame, e.g., 3 years (120), showed no significant effect on weight. In 1999, the British Broadcasting Corporation (BBC) ran a large-scale health education program to encourage people to eat a more healthy diet and to become more active with the explicit aim of helping them to control their weight. The Fighting Fat, Fighting Fit campaign ran for 7 weeks of peak and daytime programming across BBC television and radio. The campaign consisted of a series of programs and advertisements, with accompanying book, literature, and video (121). The community was encouraged to register for an additional support program, which involved returning three registration cards that charted their progress in weight loss, eating, and exercise behavior change over a 6-month period. An evaluation of the progress of 6000 people randomly selected from the 33,474 campaign registrants found significant self-reported reductions in weight and improvements in dietary and exercise behaviors (122). Although the authors of the evaluation point out the limitations of such a study and of mass media campaigns in general, they believed that such an approach could make a significant contribution to the management of population weight when combined with other strategies.

A variety of strategies were employed in the Minnesota Heart Program to improve the cardiovascular profile of the general population community based approaches to weight loss and control, worksite interventions, home correspondence to induce participation, and multimodal community strategies (123). Worksite interventions can be useful as they improve access to obese individuals, but the CDC systematic review (108) emphasizes the need for nonfamily social support if interventions are to be effective in preventing weight gain. In their analyses, primarily focusing on activity, only one longer-term study, on Samoan church members in New Zealand, assessed BMI changes over 2 years. This intervention, which included advice and support for exercising three or more times a week, prevented the increasing BMIs seen in the control group (124). Simple measures such as putting up notices encouraging the use of stairs at the point of decision making can increase stair climbing, and more of the obese than the nonobese will respond to this stimulus (125,126). The impact of such a small measure cannot be expected to have a discernible effect on weight but it will improve cardiovascular risk (79). There is, however, clear benefit in providing enhanced access to places for physical activity, e.g., by creating walk trails, activity facilities in community centers, and access to nearby fitness centers. This can lead to reductions in body fat or weight as assessed over 1-, 3- and 5-year periods in different studies involving naval personnel (127) company staff at high risk of CVD (128) and adults in Missouri (129). Shorter-term studies also show benefit but from the prevention point of view the 1-to-5-year studies are of more relevance. In successful studies, the emphasis has been on involving people in their workplaces or identifying the overweight or those at greater cardiovascular risk. Individually adapted interventions to induce behavior change can be particularly effective, but reductions were only achieved when individuals were trained by experts or given individual adapted advice for exercise with supervised walks and structured exercises (130,131) and followed for 18 months to 2 years.

C Prevention of Weight Gain in High-Risk Groups and Individuals

Prevention of weight gain and weight maintenance are important strategies for reducing or minimizing the expected complications associated with a number of common conditions, especially in those who have an existing weight problem. This is an area of clinical care that has received very little attention at present but that is potentially a much more efficacious and cost-effective approach for the management of a number of chronic diseases. However, it necessitates that clinicians adopt a much broader perspective on managing their patients health and requires the development of new skills and a willingness to provide long-term support and encouragement to patients to assist with effective weight maintenance.

1 Hypertension

It has been known for many years that it is possible to reduce the blood pressure of hypertensives by assisting them to lose and then maintain modest amounts of weight (132) and that these lifestyle effects on blood pressure can persist for 10 years (133). Recently, the Swedish Obese Subjects study (SOS) has revealed that hypertension resolved in 43% of extremely obese individuals who had lost an average of 28 kg ($\pm$15 kg) 2 years after surgery. However, after a 2-to-4-year period of maintained normotension, blood pressure began to rise again so that there was nearly as much hypertension evident after 8 years as before surgery (134). It would appear that the benefits of weight loss per se on blood pressure are not enduring unless they are accompanied by additional lifestyle change. In the 10-year follow-up studies of Stamler, weight loss was maintained at far more modest levels than in the Swedish surgical studies, but there are associated reductions in fat and salt intakes and increases in vegetable and fruit intakes. All three of these dietary changes have now been shown conclusively to lower blood pressure, particularly in hypertensive individuals (135).

2 Type 2 Diabetes

There is now clear evidence of the value and ability to engage individuals in longer-term weight reduction and weight maintenance if they are identified as at particular risk of serious comorbidities such as type 2 diabetes. Trials in Sweden (136) and China (137) were the first to demonstrate the effectiveness of weight maintenance in the prevention or delay in the progression of glucose intolerance to diabetes. Both these trials produced a reduction in the incidence of type 2 diabetes over a 6-year period when glucose-intolerant overweight and obese patients were explicitly advised to reduce the amount of fat in their diet and to take up modest increases in exercise. This education was reinforced through repeated investigator contact with the participants (every 3 months in the Chinese studies) and dietetic input. A more recent Finnish trial (138) involving over 500 overweight middle-aged men and women

also produced substantial benefits in terms of reduced diabetes incidence with very modest weight losses of ~5% of body weight when combined with improved physical activity. The latest and much larger U.S. trial, involving 3237 glucose-intolerant overweight and obese participants from 27 medical centers revealed the ability of patients with appropriate advice and help to lose 7% of their weight and maintain on average a 5% weight loss over a 3-year period. The intervention group reduced their diabetes incidence rate by 57% with those over 60 years of age showing nearly a 75% reduction (139). They were advised to eat a diet containing 25% of energy from fat (compared with the 35–40% energy from fat in the usual U.S. diet) and asked to engage in 150 min a week of moderate exercising such as brisk walking. Coaching classes over a 24-week period with follow-up meetings every 3 months with their coach backed up the process. The requested changes were not Draconian, which may explain why, with the coaching, 93% of the subjects completed the minimum 3 years in the programme.

3 Patients with Coronary Heart Disease

Most CHD prevention trials have concentrated on lowering LDL cholesterol levels by reducing saturated fatty acid intakes, with little emphasis on weight management and its role in reducing lipids and, especially, in improving HDL levels and addressing clotting problems (140,141). There is a clearly defined relationship between excess weight and the prevalence of low HDL cholesterol level, which is a powerful predictor of CHD risk. Weight reduction trials have also clearly shown a predictable increase in HDL levels (142), so it is surprising perhaps that little effort has been put into weight reduction as a means of contributing to lowering CHD rates particularly given the additional hypotensive effects of weight loss. Ornish has shown in 5-to-10-year trials that the atherosclerotic narrowing of the carotid arteries can be reversed if subjects totally change their lifestyles (143). The dietary and exercise changes within these trials were, however, drastic, with a 10% fat diet, marked reductions in salt intakes, a very modest meat consumption, and substantial exercise. These high-risk patients clearly had intense supervision, so it is not surprising that they lost substantial weight and maintained their lower weight indefinitely.

D Long-Term Prevention of Weight Regain

Recent studies with a liquid diet and meal replacement scheme have produced a better initial weight loss in obese patients than a standard, energy-restricted regimen. In addition, persisting with the replacement of a single meal together with an energy-restricted diet after a 3-month weight loss period allowed patients to both amplify their weight loss for a time and then maintain the reduced weight at 3 months for a further 4 years (144). Although this trial involved supervision, another 5-year trial with the same meal and snack replacement scheme but self-administered by obese patents achieved and maintained a 6% weight loss whereas their rural counterparts in Wisconsin gained ~7% (145). After the initial 3-month weight loss phase, the subjects were only seen twice a year. So it would appear that this dietary device was capable of allowing adjustments in intake to be maintained despite the lack of supervision and without the explicit advice and help to take more exercise, which has been a crucial part of maintaining longer-term weight loss in other programs.

VIII CONCLUSIONS

This chapter has shown the difficulties that past obesity prevention programs have faced, given the very disadvantageous environment which is so conducive to the inappropriate dietary and physical activity behaviors that underlie the emerging epidemic of obesity throughout the world. Current obesity prevention efforts may have been inhibited by a number of factors, including: a lack of acceptance of the importance of obesity as a serious health problem; the setting of inappropriate or unachievable goals; a lack of focus on weight gain prevention as the main outcome; a poor understanding of effective prevention strategies; underfunding of public health and obesity prevention research; problems identifying and targeting at risk individuals and groups; and inadequate public health and practical prevention skills within the health workforce.

Determining the most effective strategies for the prevention of obesity at the community level must be seen as a priority. There are some promising results from work with children, especially within the school setting, but limited success with adults. The prevention of obesity on an individual basis demands unusual commitment and seems most effective, given current techniques, when involving those who have a recognized comorbidity and are willing to commit themselves to sustained change. Too little has been done as yet, but it is clear that physicians and others involved in improving the health of overweight and obese patients and clients have to develop and apply individual, personally adapted strategies together with sustained

support. This is a major challenge without environmental changes.

REFERENCES

1. Foreyt J, Goodrick K. The ultimate triumph of obesity. Lancet 1995; 346:134–135.
2. Stunkard AJ. Prevention of obesity. In: Brownell K, Fairburn C, eds. Eating Disorders and Obesity: A Comprehensive Handbook. New York: Guilford Press, 1995:572–576.
3. Crawford D, Jeffery RW, French SA. Can anyone successfully control their weight? Findings of a three year community-based study of men and women. Int J Obes 2000; 24:1107–1110.
4. Bouchard C. Can obesity be prevented? Nutr Rev 1996; 54:S125–S130.
5. Rönnemaa T, Karonen SL, Rissanen A, Koskenvuo M, Koivisto VA. Relation between plasma leptin levels and measures of body fat in identical twins discordant for obesity. Ann Intern Med 1997; 126:26–31.
6. Seidell JC, Flegal KM. Assessing obesity: classification and epidemiology. Br Med Bull 1997; 53:238–252.
7. Monteiro CA, D'Abenicio MH, Conde WL, Popkin BM. Shifting obesity trends in Brazil. Eur J Clin Nutr 2000; 54(4):342–346.
8. Lahti-Koski M, Vartiainen E, Mannisto S, Pietinen P. Age, education and occupation as determinants of trends in body mass index in Finland from 1982 to 1997. Int J Obes Relat Metab Disord 2000; 24:1669–1676.
9. World Health Organization (WHO). Obesity: Preventing and Managing the Global Epidemic. Report of a WHO Consultation: WHO Technical Report Series 894. Geneva: World Health Organization, 2000.
10. Douketis JD, Feightner JW, Attia J, Feldman WF. Periodic health examination, 1999 update. 1. Detection, prevention and treatment of obesity. Canadian Task Force on Preventive Health Care. Can Med Assoc J 1999; 160:513–525.
11. Glenny AM, O'Meara S, Melville A, Sheldon TA, Wilson C. The treatment and prevention of obesity: a systematic review of the literature. Int J Obes 1997; 21:715–737.
12. Scottish Intercollegiate Guidelines Network (SIGN). Obesity in Scotland. Integrating Prevention and Weight Management. Edinburgh: SIGN, 1996.
13. National Institutes of Health. Clinical Guidelines on the Identification, Evaluation, and Treatment of Overweight and Obesity in Adults: The Evidence Report. Washington: U.S. Department of Health and Human Services, 1998.
14. Jeffery RW, French SA. Preventing weight gain in adults: design, methods and one year results from the

Pound of Prevention study. Int J Obes 1997; 21(6): 457–464.

15. Cole TJ, Bellizzi MC, Flegal KM, Dietz WH. Establishing a standard definition for child overweight and obesity worldwide: international survey. BMJ 2000; 320: 1240–1243.

16. Rose G. Population distributions of risk and disease. Nutr Metab Cardiovasc Dis 1991; 1:37–40.

17. Chan JM, Rimm EB, Colditz GA, Stampfer MJ, Willett WC. Obesity, fat distribution, and weight gain as risk factors for clinical diabetes in men. Diabetes Care 1994; 17:961–969.

18. Colditz GA, Willett WC, Rotnitzky A, Manson JE. Weight gain as a risk factor for clinical diabetes mellitus in women. Ann Intern Med 1995; 122:481–486.

19. Willett WC, Manson JE, Stampfer MJ, Colditz GA, Rosner B, Speizer FE, Hennekens CH. Weight, weight change, and coronary heart disease in women. Risk within the 'normal' weight range. JAMA 1995; 273(6): 461–465.

20. Després JP. The insulin resistance–dyslipidemic syndrome of visceral obesity: effect on patients' risk. Obes Res 1998; suppl 1:8S–17S.

21. Kopelman PG, Albon L. Obesity, non-insulin-dependent diabetes and the metabolic syndrome. Br Med Bull 1997; 53(2):322–340.

22. Lean ME, Han TS, Morrison CE. Waist circumference as a measure for indicating need for weight management. BMJ 1995; 311:158–161.

23. Seidell JC, Kahn HS, Williamson DF, Lissner L, Valdez R. Report from a Centers for Disease Control and Prevention Workshop on use of adult anthropometry for public health and primary health care. Am J Clin Nutr 2001; 73(1):123–126.

24. McKeigue PM, Miller GJ, Marmot MG. Coronary heart disease in South Asians overseas: a review. J Clin Epidemiol 1989; 42:597–609.

25. McKeigue PM, Shah B, Marmot MG. Relation of central obesity and insulin resistance with high diabetes prevalence and cardiovascular risk in South Asians. Lancet 1991; 337:382–386.

26. WHO/IASO/IOTF. The Asia-Pacific Perspective: Redefining Obesity and Its Treatment. Sydney: Health Communications, 2000. Full document available from: http://www.idi.org.au/obesity_report.htm.

27. O'Dea K, Patel M, Kubisch D, Hopper J, Traianedes K. Obesity, diabetes, and hyperlipidemia in a central Australian Aboriginal community with a long history of acculturation. Diabetes Care 1993; 16:1004–1010.

28. Rowley KG, Best JD, McDermott R, Green EA, Piers LS, O'Dea K. Insulin resistance syndrome in Australian Aboriginal people. Clin Exp Pharmacol Physiol 1997; 24:776–781.

29. Stern MP, Patterson JK, Mitchell BD, Haffner SM, Hazuda HP. Overweight and mortality in Mexican Americans. Int J Obes 1990; 14:623–629.

30. Deurenberg P, Yap M, Van Staveren WA. Body mass index and percent body fat: a meta analysis among different ethnic groups. Int J Obes 1998; 22:1164–1171.

31. Norgan NG. Interpretation of low body mass indices: Australian Aborigines. Am J Physical Anthropol 1994; 94:229–237.

32. Deurenberg P, Deurenberg-Yap M, Wang J, Lin Fu Po, Schmidt G. The impact of body build on the relationship between body mass index and body fat percent. Int J Obes 1999; 23:537–542.

33. Fogelholm M, Nuutinen O, Pasanen M, Myohanen E, Saatela T. Parent-child relationship of physical activity patterns and obesity. Int J Obes 1999; 23:1262–1268.

34. Whitaker RC, Wright JA, Pepe MS, Seidel KD, Dietz WH. Predicting obesity in young adulthood from childhood and parental obesity. N Engl J Med 1997; 337: 869–873.

35. Dabelea D, Pettitt DJ. Intrauterine diabetic environment confers risks for type 2 diabetes mellitus and obesity in the offspring, in addition to genetic susceptibility. J Pediatr Endocrinol Metab 2001; 14:1085–1091.

36. Garn SM, LaVelle M. Two-decade follow-up of fatness in early childhood. Am J Dis Child 1985; 139:181–185.

37. Rolland-Cachera MF, Deheeger M, Guilloud-Bataille M, Avons P, Patois E, Sempe M. Tracking the development of adiposity from one month of age to adulthood. Ann Hum Biol 1987; 14(2):19–29.

38. Guo SS, Roche AF, Chumlea WC, Gardner JD, Siervogel RM. The predictive value of childhood body mass index values for overweight at age 35 y. Am J Clin Nutr 1994; 59:810–819.

39. Must A, Strauss RS. Risks and consequences of childhood and adolescent obesity. Int J Obes 1999; 23(suppl 2):S2–S11.

40. Braddon FEM, Rodgers B, Wadsworth MEJ, Davies JMC. Onset of obesity in a 36 year birth cohort. BMJ 1986; 293:299–303.

41. Sheldon JH. Maternal obesity. Lancet 1949; 2:869–873.

42. Ohlin A, Rossner S. Maternal body weight development after pregnancy. Int J Obes 1990; 14:159–173.

43. Rossner S. Long term intervention strategies in obesity treatment. Int J Obes 1995; 19:S29–S33.

44. Eriksson KF, Lindgårde E. Prevention of type 2 (non-insulin-dependent) diabetes mellitus by diet and physical exercise: the 6-year Malmö feasibility study. Diabetologia 1991; 34:891–898.

45. Jeffery RW. Community programs for obesity prevention: the Minnesota Heart Health Program. Obes Res 1995; 3:283s–288s.

46. James WPT, Francois P. The choice of cut-off point for distinguishing normal body weight from under-

weight or 'chronic energy deficiency' in adults. Eur J Clin Nutr 1994; 48(S):S179–S184.

47. Kumanyika SK. Minisymposium on obesity: overview and some strategic considerations. Annu Rev Public Health 2001; 22:293–308.

48. Katan MB, Grundy SM, Willett WC. Should a low-fat, high-carbohydrate diet be recommended for everyone? Beyond low-fat diets. N Engl J Med 1997; 337:563–566.

49. Willett WC. Dietary fat and obesity: an unconvincing relation. Am J Clin Nutr 1998; 68(6):1149–1150.

50. Taubes G. Nutrition. The soft science of dietary fat. Science 2001; 291:2536–2545.

51. Frazao E, ed. America's Eating Habits: Changes and Consequences. Washington: USDA Economic Research Services, 1999.

52. Astrup A, Grunwald GK, Melanson EL, Saris WH, Hill JO. The role of low-fat diets in body weight control: a meta-analysis of ad libitum dietary intervention studies. Int J Obes 2000; 24:1545–1552.

53. Bray GA, Popkin BM. Dietary fat intake does affect obesity. Am J Clin Nutr 1998; 68:1157–1173.

54. Astrup A, Toubro S, Raben A, Skov AR. The role of low fats diets and fat substitutes in body weight management: what have we learned from clinical studies? J Am Diet Assoc 1997; 97:82S–87S.

55. Shick SM, Wing RR, Klem ML, McGuire MT, Hill JO, Seagle H. Persons successful at long-term weight loss and maintenance continue to consume a low-energy, low-fat diet. J Am Diet Assoc 1998; 98:408–413.

56. Frost G, Leeds AA, Dore CJ, Madeiros S, Brading S, Dornhorst A. Glycaemic index as a determinant of serum HDL-cholesterol concentration. Lancet 1999; 353: 1045–1048.

57. Liu S, Willett WC, Stampfer MJ, Hu FB, Franz M, Sampson L, Hennekens CH, Manson JE. A prospective study of dietary glycemic load, carbohydrate intake, and risk of coronary heart disease in US women. Am J Clin Nutr 2000; 71(6):1455–1461.

58. Lester IH. Australia's Food and Nutrition Canberra: Australia Government Publishing Service, 1994.

59. Kearney JM, Hulshof KF, Gibney MJ. Eating patterns—temporal distribution, converging and diverging foods, meals eaten inside and outside of the home—implications for developing FBDG. Public Health Nutr 2001; 4(2B):693–698.

60. French SA, Story M, Jeffery RW. Environmental influences on eating and physical activity. Annu Rev Public Health 2001; 22:309–335.

61. Binkley JK, Eales J, Jekanowski M. The relation between dietary change and rising US obesity. Int J Obes 2000; 24:1032–1039.

62. French SA, Harnack L, Jeffery RW. Fast food restaurant use among women in the Pound of Prevention study: dietary, behavioral and demographic correlates. Int J Obes 2000; 24:1353–1359.

63. Young LR, Nestle MS. Portion sizes in dietary assessment: issues and policy implications. Nutr Rev 1995; 53:149–158.

64. Mattes R. Dietary compensation by humans for supplemental energy provided as ethanol or carbohydrate in fluids. Physiol Behav 1996; 59:179–187.

65. De Castro JM. The effects of the spontaneous ingestion of particular foods or beverages on the meal pattern and overall nutrient intake of humans. Physiol Behav 1993; 53:1133–1144.

66. Ludwig DS, Peterson KE, Gortmaker SL. Relation between consumption of sugar-sweetened drinks and childhood obesity: a prospective, observational analysis. Lancet 2001; 357:505–508.

67. Raben A, Møller AC, Vasilaras TH, Astrup A. A randomised 10-week trial of sucrose vs. artificial sweeteners on body weight and blood pressure after 10 weeks. Obes Res 2001; 9(suppl 3):86S.

68. Beverage Marketing Corporation of New York. The Global Multiple Beverage Marketplace. New York: Beverage Marketing Corporation, 2000.

69. James WP. A public health approach to the problem of obesity. Int J Obes 1995; 19(suppl 3):S37–S45.

70. Cox BD. Changes in body measurements. In: Cox BD, Huppert FA, Whitchelow MA, eds. The Health and Lifestyle Survey; Seven Years On. Aldershot: Dartmouth Publishing, 1993:103–117.

71. Prentice AM, Jebb SA. Obesity in Britain: gluttony or sloth? BMJ 1995; 311:437–479.

72. DiPietro L. Physical activity in the prevention of obesity: current evidence and research issues. Med Sci Sports Exerc 1999; 31:S542–S546.

73. Rissanen AM, Heliovaara M, Knekt P, Reunanen A, Aromaa A. Determinants of weight gain and overweight in adult Finns. Eur J Clin Nutr 1991; 45:419–430.

74. Haapanen N, Miilunpalo S, Pasanen M, Oja P, Vuori I. Association between leisure time physical activity and 10-year body mass change among working-aged men and women. Int J Obes 1997; 21:288–296.

75. Williamson DF, Madans J, Anda RF, Kleinman JC, Kahn HS, Byers T. Recreational physical activity and ten-year weight change in a US national cohort. Int J Obes 1993; 17:279–286.

76. Sherwood NE, Jeffery RW, French SA, Hannan PJ, Murray DM. Predictors of weight gain in the Pound of Prevention study. Int J Obes 2000; 24:395–403.

77. Klem ML, Wing RR, McGuire MT, Seagle HM, Hill JO. A descriptive study of individuals successful at long-term maintenance of substantial weight loss. Am J Clin Nutr 1997; 66:239–246.

78. Schoeller DA, Shay K, Kushner RF. How much physical activity is needed to minimize weight gain in previously obese women? Am J Clin Nutr 1997; 66:551–556.

79. Blair SN, Kohl HW, Barlow CE, Paffenbarger RS,

Gibbons LW, Macera CA. Changes in physical fitness and all-cause mortality. A prospective study of healthy and unhealthy men. JAMA 1995; 273:1093–1098.

80. Pate RR, Pratt M, Blair SN, Haskell WL, Macera CA, Bouchard C, Buchner D, Ettinger W, Heath GW, King AC. Physical activity and public health. A recommendation from the Centers for Disease Control and Prevention and the American College of Sports Medicine. JAMA 1995; 273:402–407.

81. Dietz WH, Gortmaker SL. Do we fatten our children at the television set? Obesity and television viewing in children and adolescents. Pediatrics 1985; 75:807–812.

82. Gortmaker SL, Must A, Sobol AM, Peterson K, Colditz GA, Dietz WH. Television viewing as a cause of increasing obesity among children in the United States, 1986–1990. Arch Pediatr Adolesc Med 1996; 150:356–362.

83. Andersen RE, Crespo CJ, Bartlett SJ, Cheskin LJ, Pratt M. Relationship of physical activity and television watching with body weight and level of fatness among children: results from the Third National Health and Nutrition Examination Survey. JAMA 1998; 25:279: 938–942.

84. Robinson TN. Does television cause childhood obesity? JAMA 1998; 279:959–960.

85. Epstein LH, Paluch RA, Gordy CC, Dorn J. Decreasing sedentary behaviors in treating pediatric obesity. Arch Pediatr Adolesc Med 2000; 154:220–226.

86. World Health Organization (WHO). Expert consultation on the optimal duration of exclusive breastfeeding. Conclusions and recommendations. Document A54/INF.DOC./4, Geneva, 28–30 March 2001.

87. Armstrong J, Reilly JJ. Breastfeeding and childhood obesity risk. Obes Res 2001; 9(suppl 3):62S.

88. Gillman MW, Rifas-Shiman SL, Camargo CA, Berkey CS, Frazier AL, Rockett HR, Field AE, Colditz GA. Risk of overweight among adolescents who were breastfed as infants. JAMA 2001; 285:2417–2461.

89. Dietz WH. Breastfeeding may help prevent childhood overweight. JAMA 2001; 285:2506–2567.

90. Von Kries R, Koletzko B, Sauerwald T, Von Mutius E, Barnert D, Grunert V, Von Voss H. Breast feeding and obesity: cross sectional study. BMJ 1999; 319: 147–150.

91. Butte NF. The role of breastfeeding in obesity. Pediatr Clin North Am 2001; 48:189–198.

92. Dutta-Roy AK. Transport mechanisms for long-chain polyunsaturated fatty acids in the human placenta. Am J Clin Nutr 2000; 71(suppl 1):315S–322S.

93. Brown JM, Halvorsen YD, Lea-Currie YR, Geigerman C, McIntosh M. *Trans*-10, *cis*-12, but not *cis*-9, *trans*-11, conjugated linoleic acid attenuates lipogenesis in primary cultures of stromal vascular cells from human adipose tissue. J Nutr 2001; 131(9):2316–2321.

94. Lakin V, Haggarty P, Abramovich DR, Ashton J, Moffat CF, McNeill G, Danielian PJ, Grubb D. Dietary intake and tissue concentration of fatty acids in omnivore, vegetarian and diabetic pregnancy. Prostaglandins Leukot Essent Fatty Acids 1998; 59(3):209–220.

95. Sebire NJ, Jolly M, Harris JP, Wadsworth J, Joffe M, Beard RW, Regan L, Robinson S. Maternal obesity and pregnancy outcome: a study of 287,213 pregnancies in London. Int J Obes 2001; 25:1175–1182.

96. Donath SM, Amir LH. Does maternal obesity adversely affect breastfeeding initiation and duration? J Paediatr Child Health 2000; 36:482–486.

97. Gigante DP, Victora CG, Barros FC. Breast-feeding has a limited long-term effect on anthropometry and body composition of Brazilian mothers. J Nutr 2001; 131:78–84.

98. Janney CA, Zhang D, Sowers M. Lactation and weight retention. Am J Clin Nutr 1997; 66:1116–1124.

99. Barker DJ, Hales CN, Fall CH, Osmond C, Phipps K, Clark PM. Type 2 (non-insulin-dependent) diabetes mellitus, hypertension and hyperlipidaemia (syndrome X): relation to reduced fetal growth. Diabetologia 1993; 36:62–67.

100. Dietz WH, Gortmaker SL. Preventing obesity in children and adolescents. Annu Rev Public Health 2001; 22: 337–353.

101. Gill TP. Key issues in the prevention of obesity. Br Med Bull 1997; 53(2):359–388.

102. Egger G, Swinburn B. An "ecological" approach to the obesity pandemic. BMJ 1997; 315:477–480.

103. Nestle M, Jacobson MF. Halting the obesity epidemic; A public health policy approach. Public Health Rep 2000; 115:12–24.

104. Kumanyika S, Jeffery RW, Morabia A, Ritenbaugh C, Antipatis VJ. Public Health Approaches to the Prevention of Obesity (PHAPO) Working Group of the International Obesity Task Force (IOTF). Obesity prevention: the case for action. Int J Obes Relat Metab Disord 2002; 26:425–436.

105. Parsons TJ, Power C, Logan S, Summerbell CD. Childhood predictors of adult obesity: a systematic review. Int J Obes 1999; 23(suppl 8):S1–S107.

106. Kemper HCG, Post GB, Twisk JWR, Van Mechelen W. Lifestyle and obesity in adolescence and young adulthood: results from the Amsterdam Growth and Health Longitudinal Study (AGHLS). Int J Obes 1999; 23:S34–S40.

107. Campbell K, Waters E, O'Meara S, Summerbell C. Interventions for preventing obesity in children (Cochrane Review). Cochrane Database Syst Rev 2001; 2:CD 001871.

108. Centers for Disease Control and Prevention. Increasing physical activity: a report on recommendations of the Task Force on Community Preventive Services. MMWR 2001; 50:No. RR-18.

109. Luepker RV, Perry CL, McKinlay SM, Nader PR,

Parcel GS, Stone EJ, Webber LS, Elder JP, Feldman HA, Johnson CC. Outcomes of a field trial to improve children's dietary patterns and physical activity. The Child and Adolescent Trial for Cardiovascular Health. CATCH collaborative group. JAMA 1996; 275:768–776.

110. Fardy PS, White RE, Haltiwanger-Schmitz K, Magel JR, McDermott KJ, Clark LT, Hurster MM. Coronary disease risk factor reduction and behavior modification in minority adolescents: the PATH program. J Adolesc Health 1996; 18(4):247–253.

111. Manios Y, Kafatos A. Health and nutrition education in elementary schools: changes in health knowledge, nutrient intakes and physical activity over a six year period. Public Health Nutr 1999; 3:445–448.

111a. Webber LS, Osganian SK, Feldman HA, Wu M, McKenzie TL, Nichaman M, Lytle LA, Edmundson E, Cutler J, Nader PR, Luepker RV (CATCH). Cardiovascular risk factors among children after a $2\frac{1}{2}$-year intervention—The CATCH Study. Prev Med 1996; 25:432–441.

111b. Donnelly JE, Jacobsen DJ, Whatley JE, Hill JO, Swift LL, Cherrington A, Polk B, Tran ZV, Reed G. Nutrition and physical activity program to attenuate obesity and promote physical and metabolic fitness in elementary school children. Obes Res 1996; 4:229–243.

111c. Ewart CK, Young DR, Hagberg JM. Effects of school-based aerobic exercise on blood pressure in adolescent girls at risk for hypertension. Am J Public Health 1998; 88:949–951.

111d. Sallis Jf, McKenzie TL, Alcaraz JE, Kolody B, Faucette N, Hovell MF (SPARK). The effects of a 2-year physical education program (SPARK) on physical activity and fitness in elementary school students. Sports, Play and Active Recreation for Kids. Am J Public Health 1997; 87:1328–1334.

111e. Dwyer T, Coonan WE, Leitch DR, Hetzel BS, Baghurst RA. An investigation of the effects of daily physical activity on the health of primary school students in South Australia. Int J Epidemiol 1983; 12:308–313.

112. Robinson TN. Reducing children's television viewing to prevent obesity: a randomized controlled trial. JAMA 1999; 282:1561–1567.

113. Gortmaker SL, Peterson K, Wiecha J, Sobol AM, Dixit S, Fox MK, Laird N. Reducing obesity via a school-based interdisciplinary intervention among youth: Planet Health. Arch Pediatr Adolesc Med 1999; 153:409–418.

114. Simonetti D'Arca A, Tarsitani G, Cairella M, Siani V, De Filippis S, Mancinelli S, Marazzi MC, Palombi L. Prevention of obesity in elementary and nursery school children. Public Health 1986; 100:166–173.

115. DISC Collaborative Research Group. Efficacy and safe-ty of lowering dietary intake of fat and cholesterol in children with elevated low-density lipoprotein cho-

lesterol. The Dietary Intervention Study in Children (DISC). JAMA 1995; 273:1429–1435.

116. Resnicow K, Robinson TN. School-based cardiovascular disease prevention studies: review and synthesis. Ann Epidemiol 1997; 7:s14–s31.

117. Story M. School based approaches for preventing and treating obesity. Int J Obes 1999; 23:s43–s51.

118. Muller MJ, Asbeck I, Mast M, Langnase K, Grund A. Prevention of obesity—more than an intention. Concept and first results of the Kiel Obesity Prevention Study (KOPS). Int J Obes 2001; 25(suppl 1):S66–S74.

119. Epstein LH, Valoski A, Wing RR, McCurley J. Ten-year outcomes of behavioral family-based treatment for childhood obesity. Health Psychol 1994; 13:373–383.

120. Meyer AJ, Nash JD, McAlister AL, Maccoby N, Farquhar JW. Skills training in a cardiovascular health education campaign. J Consult Clin Psychol 1980; 48:129–142.

121. Wardle J, Rapoport L, Miles A, Afuape T, Duman M. Mass education for obesity prevention: the penetration of the BBC's 'Fighting Fat, Fighting Fit' campaign. Health Educ Res 2001; 16:343–355.

122. Miles A, Rapoport L, Wardle J, Afuape T, Duman M. Using the mass-media to target obesity: an analysis of the characteristics and reported behaviour change of participants in the BBC's 'Fighting Fat, Fighting Fit' campaign. Health Educ Res 2001; 16(3):357–372.

123. Jeffery RW. Minnesota studies on community-based approaches to weight loss and control. Ann Intern Med 1993; 119:719–721.

124. Simmons D, Fleming C, Voyle J, Fou F, Feo S, Gatland B. A pilot urban church-based programme to reduce risk factors for diabetes among Western Samoans in New Zealand. Diabet Med 1998; 15:136–142.

125. Andersen RE, Franckowiak SC, Snyder J, Bartlett SJ, Fontaine KR. Can inexpensive signs encourage the use of stairs? Results from a community intervention. Ann Intern Med 1998; 129:363–369.

126. Brownell KD, Stunkard AJ, Albaum JM. Evaluation and modification of exercise patterns in the natural environment. Am J Psychiatry 1980; 137:1540–1545.

127. Linenger JM, Chesson CV, Nice DS. Physical fitness gains following simple environmental change. Am J Prev Med 1991; 7:298–310.

128. Heirich MA, Foote A, Erfurt JC, Konopka B. Worksite physical fitness programs. Comparing the impact of different program designs on cardiovascular risks. J Occup Med 1993; 35:510–517.

129. Brownson RC, Smith CA, Pratt M, Mack NE, Jackson-Thompson J, Dean CG, Dabney S, Wilkerson JC. Preventing cardiovascular disease through community-based risk reduction: the Bootheel Heart Health Project. Am J Public Health 1996; 86:206–213.

130. Jeffery RW, Wing RR, Thorson C, Burton LR. Use of

personal trainers and financial incentives to increase exercise in a behavioral weight-loss program. J Consult Clin Psychol 1998; 66:777–783.

131. Dunn AL, Marcus BH, Kampert JB, Garcia ME, Kohl HW, Blair SN. Comparison of lifestyle and structured interventions to increase physical activity and cardiorespiratory fitness: a randomized trial. JAMA 1999; 281: 327–334.

132. Mertens IL, Van Gaal LF. Overweight, obesity, and blood pressure: the effects of modest weight reduction. Obes Res 2000; 8(3):270–278.

133. Stamler J, Farinaro E, Mojonnier L, Hall Y, Moss D, Stamler R. Prevention and control of hypertension by nutritional-hygienic means. Long-term experience of the Chicago Coronary Prevention Evaluation Program. JAMA 1980; 243:1819–1823.

134. Torgerson JS, Sjöström L. The Swedish Obese Subjects (SOS) study—rationale and results. Int J Obes 2001; 25(suppl 1):S2–S4.

135. Sacks FM, Svetkey LP, Vollmer WM, Appel LJ, Bray GA, Harsha D, Obarzanek E, Conlin PR, Miller ER, Simons-Morton DG, Karanja N, Lin PH. Effects on blood pressure of reduced dietary sodium and the Dietary Approaches to Stop Hypertension (DASH) diet. DASH–Sodium Collaborative Research Group. N Engl J Med 2001; 344:3–10.

136. Eriksson J, Lindgarde F. Prevention of type 2 (non-insulin-dependent) diabetes mellitus by diet and physical exercise. The 6-year Malmo Feasibility Study. Diabetologia 1991; 34:12891–12898.

137. Pan XR, Li GW, Hu YH, Wang JX, Yang WY, An ZX, Hu ZX, Lin J, Xiao JZ, Cao HB, Liu PA, Jiang XG, Jiang YY, Wang JP, Zheng H, Zhang H, Bennett PH, Howard BV. Effects of diet and exercise in preventing NIDDM in people with impaired glucose tolerance. Diabetes Care 1997; 20:537–544.

138. Tuomilehto J, Lindstrom J, Eriksson JG, Valle TT, Hamalainen H, Ilanne-Parikka P, Keinanen-Kiu-kaanniemi S, Laakso M, Louheranta A, Rastas M, Salminen V, Uusitupa M. Prevention of type 2 diabetes mellitus by changes in lifestyle among subjects with impaired glucose tolerance. N Engl J Med 2001; 344:1343–1350.

139. Diabetes Prevention Program Research Group. Reduction in the incidence of type 2 diabetes with lifestyle intervention or Metformin. N Engl J Med 2002; 346: 393–403.

140. Williamson DF, Pamuk E, Thun M, Flanders D, Byers T, Heath C. Prospective study of intentional weight loss and mortality in never-smoking overweight US white women aged 40–64 years. Am J Epidemiol 1995; 141: 1128–1141.

141. Hankey CR, Wallace AM, Lean ME. Plasma lipids, dehydroepiandosterone sulphate and insulin concentrations in elderly overweight angina patients, and effect of weight loss. Int J Obes 1997; 21:72–77.

142. Dattilo AM, Kris-Etherton PM. Effects of weight reduction on blood lipids and lipoproteins; a meta-analysis. Am J Clin Nutr 1992; 56:320–328.

143. Ornish D, Scherwitz LW, Billings JH, Brown SE, Gould KL, Merritt TA, Sparler S, Armstrong WT, Ports TA, Kirkeeide RL, Hogeboom C, Brand RJ. Intensive lifestyle changes for reversal of coronary heart disease. JAMA 1998; 280:2001–2007.

144. Flechtner-Mors M, Ditschuneit HH, Johnson TD, Suchard MA, Adler G. Metabolic and weight loss effects of long-term dietary intervention in obese patients: four-year results. Obes Res 2000; 8:399–402.

145. Rothacker DQ. Five-year self-management of weight using meal replacements: comparison with matched controls in rural Wisconsin. Nutrition 2000; 16:344–348.

146. Hediger ML, Overpeck MD, Kuczmarski RJ, Ruan WJ. Association between infant breastfeeding and over-weight in young children. JAMA 2001; 285(19):2453–2460.

6

Influence of Obesity-Producing Environments

Boyd Anthony Swinburn and Garry J. Egger

Deakin University, Melbourne, Victoria, Australia

I THE INDIVIDUAL VERSUS THE POPULATION PERSPECTIVE OF OBESITY

A Introduction

Obesity is now at pandemic levels. Its prevalence is increasing in almost all countries—developed and developing (1). To curtail and eventually reverse the rise in obesity prevalence rates, a broad, population-based approach will be needed (1,2). The majority of the current global effort on obesity, however, is centered around establishing biological mechanisms related to energy imbalance and finding appropriate methods of treatment for individuals with obesity. The move to tackling whole populations with obesity requires conceptual shifts at many levels.

B Individual and Population Examples

Consider the following two examples of obesity. The first is Penny who is 45 years old and, apart from a few years around the time of her wedding, has always been quite chubby. Over the last 15 years she has gained a lot more weight and now has a body mass index (BMI) of 34 kg/m^2. Her husband, on the other hand, has a BMI of ~25 kg/m^2, and this has virtually not changed since he left school. The second example is England where the prevalence of obesity (BMI >30 kg/m^2) in 1996 was 17% (3) having increased from 7% in 1980 (4). England's

neighbor just across the English Channel is the Netherlands, where the prevalence of obesity in 1995 was only 8%, up from about 6% in 1981 (5). These two examples illustrate the different perspectives needed for dealing with individuals or populations. The etiologies and management strategies will be quite different for Penny's obesity compared to England's obesity (Table 1).

The etiology of Penny's obesity will tend to be ascribed to genetic, metabolic, hormonal, and behavioral factors, whereas for England it will tend to be environmental, sociocultural, and behavioral. For example, the transport environment in England will stand out as "obesogenic" (obesity promoting) because of its automobile dependence compared to the relatively "leptogenic" (leanness promoting; *leptos* is Greek for thin) transport environment in the Netherlands with its strong emphasis on bicycle and public transport travel.

The management strategies for obesity at the individual and population levels are also quite different (Table 1). The volume of studies and information about weight loss is huge compared to the amount available on population-based prevention. For example, the recent 150-page Report of the British Nutrition Foundation Task Force on Obesity dedicated 51 pages to treatment of individuals and only one page to population prevention strategies (6). This is, in part, because the driving forces for research and action are quite different. For individual treatment, the forces are powerful and immediate; they include the clinical imperative to help people with obesity, the pressure from individuals to lose

Table 1 Differences Between the Individual-Based and Population-Based Approaches to Obesity

	Individual-based approach	Population-based approach
Key measures	Body weight, waist, BMI	Prevalence of overweight and obesity, mean BMI and waist
Key etiology question	Why is this particular person obese (or gaining weight)?	Why does this particular population have a high (or rising) prevalence of obesity?
Main etiological mechanisms	Genetic, metabolic, hormonal, behavioral	Environmental, cultural, behavioral
Key management question	What are the best long-term strategies for reducing the person's body fat?	What are the best long-term strategies for reducing the population's mean BMI?
Main management actions	Patient education, behavioral modification, drugs, surgery	Public education, improving food and physical activity environments, policy, planning
Volume of information on etiology and management	Vast	Minimal
Driving forces for research and action	Immediate and powerful	Distant and weak
Potential for long-term benefit to individuals	Modest	Modest
Potential for long-term benefit to populations	Modest	Significant

weight, and the huge potential profits for pharmaceutical companies from weight loss medications. Contrast this with the relatively weak and distant driving forces for population-based prevention research and action. These are funded largely from government sources, and the lack of political will due to a short-term political focus and limited public pressure for change remain major obstacles. As discussed later, the driving forces for the obesity epidemic are linked to much broader sectors such as transport, the food industry, education, urban planning, building design, and local government, and this adds to the sense of impotence among health authorities about obesity prevention.

As a general rule, individual-directed interventions bring about significant benefits to the individuals but have little impact on the population rates of disease or condition in question and vice versa for population-based interventions, which generally bring little benefit to each individual but have the potential to influence the prevalence or incidence of the condition (7). With obesity, this discrepancy is even more exaggerated (compared to, say, hypertension or hypercholesterolemia) because available individual interventions, apart from surgery, have modest long-term effects for the individuals under treatment (8,9). The efforts on population-based interventions related to obesity are much needed but are still in their infancy (1,10,11).

The potential for populationwide effects is particularly strong for high volume foods or physical activities. For example, a recent survey of fast food outlets in New Zealand showed that the mean fat content of the french fries was 11.5% by weight (12). There was an enormous range across the country, from 5% to 20%, and in many instances the deep-frying practices were very poor. It should be possible to reduce the mean fat content to 9% through a national training program for fast-food outlet operators, which is now under way. If this could be achieved, the consumption of french fries is such that the reduction in fat intake would be ~1/2 kg per capita per year. This is not insubstantial compared to the current increase in weight of the New Zealand adult population of ~1/3 kg per person per year (13).

C   Linking the Individual and Population Approaches

There are synergies to be achieved by bringing the individual and population approaches together. This can be seen most clearly at the general-practice/primary-care level. For example, a general practitioner will have a greater chance of helping Penny to lose weight and keep it off if her obesogenic environments are acknowledged and, where possible, acted upon. Part of Penny's weight gain response to her obesogenic environment may be genetically determined, and recognition of this also helps to remove moral judgments about her obesity and places her individual behaviors into a wider context. The more limited behavior-based perspective can too easily be judged (by her and others) in "sloth-and-gluttony" terms. Penny may even be able to take action to make her own environments more leptogenic such as changing the types of food available at home or on offer at the work cafeteria. She may even decide to remove the batteries from the TV remote control and advocate for bike stands and showers at work.

On the flip side, it makes sense to use the high contact that primary health care has with the public on a regular basis to further the population health goals for obesity. Educating and up-skilling large numbers of patients increases the dissemination of knowledge through the community and promotes advocacy to make healthy choices easier.

II MODELS OF OBESITY INCORPORATING THE INDIVIDUAL AND POPULATION PERSPECTIVES

There are a large number of models in common usage in health promotion and clinical care (14). The value of any particular model is that it helps to explain the problem and to provide a framework for action, and in the obesity area, it should ideally incorporate both treatment and prevention aspects as these should be considered on a continuum. We have found two models of particular value: one is an "ecological model" based on the energy balance equation. The other is the epidemiological triad, which has been successfully applied in other epidemics.

A Ecological Model of Obesity

The energy balance equation is a logical place to start trying to understand obesity at the individual and population level. The most accurate version of the energy balance equation is the "dynamic, physiological" version (15) which incorporates rates of change (16) and an interconversion between energy balance and fat balance (17,18).

Rate of change of energy(fat) stores
= rate of energy(fat) intake
−rate of energy(fat) expenditure

While this equation has served reasonably well as a model for understanding weight gain and obesity at an individual level, it is not helpful in incorporating the broader influences on weight gain and obesity, especially the environmental influences. We have expanded the energy/fat balance equation into an ecological model to help visualize the interplay between the broad influences on energy balance (Fig. 1) (19).

Ecological models help to conceptualize the interdependence of people, their health, and their environments in the broadest sense (20). The model regards an individual's or population's level of obesity at any one time as being at an equilibrium or a "settling point"—the net result of multiple influences on fat mass by acting through the mediators of energy intake (especially through high fat, energy-dense food, and large portion sizes) (21) and/or energy expenditure (especially through the impact of machines on reducing physical activity). The concept of a single, fixed "set point" to explain why people tend to return toward their original body weight following a period of weight loss (22) does not fit with the metabolic evidence (23), and it is an unhelpful term because it is clearly not "set." Most individuals increase their body fat levels over a lifetime, and most populations are getting fatter over time.

The influences are broadly defined as biological, behavioral, and environmental. Biological influences include the effects of genes, hormones, age, gender, ethnicity, and drugs on one or more of the myriad pathways that influence energy balance. The behavioral influences typically attributed to obesity are sloth and gluttony, which imply a willful control over the forces affecting body weight. However, behaviors are the net result of complex factors including habits, knowledge, emotions, cognitions, attitudes, and beliefs. The environmental influences will be expanded upon later.

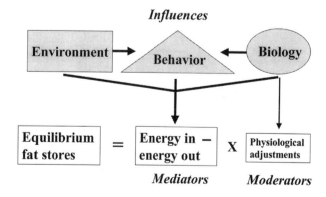

Figure 1 An ecological model of obesity.

Biological differences also explain the heterogeneous physiological adjustments that the body makes in response to weight loss or gain. A period of energy imbalance is moderated by a somewhat exaggerated counterresponse in such things as hunger, metabolic rate, nutrient partitioning, and the energy costs of physical activity (23,24). These all serve to moderate the impact of energy imbalance on changes in fat mass.

B Epidemiological Triad

Another way to visualize these influences is using the classic epidemiological triad (Fig. 2), which has proved to be a robust model with epidemics such as infectious diseases, smoking, coronary heart disease, and injuries (25–27). The Host in Figure 2 encompasses the biological and behavioral influences and the physiological moderators of weight change from the ecological model. The Agent is defined as positive energy balance, and its Vectors are energy-dense food, large portion sizes, time-saving machines (e.g., cars) and time-using machines (e.g., television). These are analogous to the mediators. The Environment is the same in both models. The strategies for intervention are different for each corner of the triad; however, the main lesson learned from other epidemics is that all three corners need to be addressed together. For the host, the intervention strategies encompass both prevention and treatment and range from education (awareness raising to intensive counseling), through behavioral modification, to medical strategies such as drugs and surgery. For the vectors, the strategies are often technology-based such as food technology approaches to reduce the fat content of

food. Unfortunately, many technological advances appear to be the vectors for inactivity (especially cars, television, and computers) with only a few (such as exercise equipment) being the vectors for activity. The underlying drivers for environmental change are often based on profits, policy, or social change (2), with the latter two probably offering more hope for solutions than the first. At a clinical level, the model also is helpful in showing that the individual is part of a wider system including influential environments.

III OBESOGENIC AND LEPTOGENIC ENVIRONMENTS

A central concept to emerge from considering these models is that, while environments are external to the person, they have a powerful influence on the person's behaviors and thus energy balance and obesity. The term *obesogenic environments* can be defined as "the sum of influences that the surroundings, opportunities or conditions of life have on promoting obesity in individuals or populations" (19). By contrast, *leptogenic environments* would promote healthy food choices and encourage regular physical activity. The obesogenic environment is synonymous with other terms which have been coined such as the toxic environment (28) or pathoenvironment (15), but a term for the other end of the spectrum (i.e., the leptogenic environment) may also be of value in defining the direction of desired environmental change.

We have defined environments in a broad sense to include more than just the visible, tangible aspects of the physical environment. They include costs, laws, policies, social and cultural attitudes and values, and indeed any external factors that might affect an individual's behavior. From this perspective, the increasingly obesogenic environments are the fundamental driving forces for the global obesity epidemic (29,30).

IV WHY THE FOCUS ON ENVIRONMENTS?

A broad approach is required for reducing obesity at a population level (10,11). Biological research will continue to map the metabolic and molecular pathways involved in the development of obesity and will therefore help to explain some of the differences in obesity risk among individuals. Identifying key molecules in the pathways may lead to the development of effective drugs to treat obesity, but unless costly, mass medication is undertaken for a large proportion of the pop-

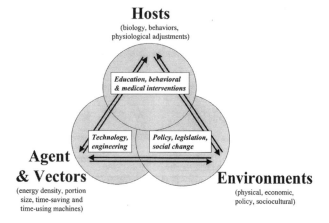

Figure 2 Epidemiological triad as it applies to obesity. The circles refer to the predominant strategies to address each corner of the triad.

ulation, there will be little impact on the population burden of obesity.

One of the primary weight loss interventions aimed at the host is education (including awareness raising, public education, and individual counseling and skills training). The expectation is that new knowledge will be turned into sustained behavior changes. This may be true for some individuals and appears to be a moderately successful approach for obese men (31). However, for most obese people and for population-based prevention, just knowing about what are the healthy choices is a relatively weak force for sustained behavior change (8,32). Education about healthy choices, therefore, appears necessary but not sufficient to reverse obesity.

The key role of environmental change is to "make the healthy choices the easy choices." Unfortunately, the environments in relation to obesity have received little attention to date. Compare the vast human and financial efforts to sequence the human genome with the minor and nascent efforts to sequence the human environment. Yet environmental change can have a major, immediate, and lasting impact on behaviors, especially if it is a "passive" intervention that does not require an active decision by the individual, such as car-free central business districts or lower-fat french fries (see Sec. I.B) or potato chips (below) (33). Table 2 lists some of the key strengths of an environmental/systems-based approach underpinning the obesity prevention efforts.

Obesity, like diabetes and coronary heart disease, has higher prevalence rates among the lower-socioeconomic status (SES) populations in developed countries. Low income and low educational attainment bring reduced options for low-SES groups and a lower uptake of health messages about behavioral changes for a healthy future. One of the key strengths of an environmental focus is its potential impact among lower-SES groups. By influencing the "default" choices in key environments, there is a much greater potential to affect overall diet and physical activity patterns in lower-SES groups than by education strategies alone. Education-based campaigns are complementary to the environmental approach, but the priority needs to be on ensuring that the healthy choices are available first, before embarking upon such campaigns to educate people about taking up those choices.

One of the principles of environmental intervention is to effect small changes in high-volume foods. Take potato chips as an example where, say, 90% of the sales are in the regular, higher-fat chips (35% fat) and 10% of sales are in the lower-fat chips (25%). There are three main options for reducing the population's dietary fat

burden from potato chips by 10%. The first is to reduce the total consumption of chips by 10%, which would probably require a major, sustained public education campaign by health authorities to eat fewer chips, no doubt in the face of stiff opposition from the potato chip manufacturers. The second is to expand the proportion of the sales of lower-fat chips to 44% of the market share. Food companies are already heavily marketing the "healthier" options to the high-income, high-education consumers in an effort to expand that market share. Such healthier options often come at a premium price and are marketed to the healthiest section of the community, making this a relatively ineffective option for reducing the fat intake of low-income people who are at higher risk of obesity. The third option is to reduce the fat content of higher-fat crips from 35% to 31%. This is technologically possible, would not be detectable by the consumer, and impacts on a large section of the community including low-income groups. The barriers to reducing the fat content of the high-volume potato chips are perhaps some increases in cost of production (changing plant and adding fans to blow off the fat after cooking) and the lack of a marketing angle to make it appear worthwhile to the manufacturers.

V DISSECTING OBESOGENIC ENVIRONMENTS: THE ANGELO FRAMEWORK

The development and execution of health promotion programs, including environmental interventions requires the following steps: (1) needs analysis, (2) problem identification, (3) strategy development, (4) intervention, and (5) evaluation (34). Major barriers to progressing through these steps for environmental programs include the lack of suitable paradigms and tools for understanding and measuring the environment (35). We have previously described the development and use of the ANGELO Framework (Analysis Grid for Environments Linked to Obesity) for steps 1 and 2 above (19). This has proved to be a valuable conceptual and practical framework for dissecting the rather nebulous concept of the environment and identifying concrete elements within it which are amenable to measurement and interventions (36–38).

The first step was to dissect eating and physical activity behaviors into the settings in which they occur and then link those settings to the wider sectors that influence them. An example of this analysis is shown in Table 3. The interactions among all these levels can be expanded into a full "causal web" such as the one

Table 2 Strengths of an Environments/Systems-Based Approach to Underpin Obesity Prevention Efforts

Strength	Examples
Addresses underlying causes (i.e., potential for true prevention)	Parental fears for children's safety as the major reason for driving children to school—addressing the substance and perceptions related to the fears is likely to result in more active transport to school.
Becomes structural/systemic	Changing the physical environment for recreation, food laws, local government transport policies, etc., embeds the changes into the system.
Becomes the accepted norm	Regular availability of reduced fat milk, salad options, vegetable-based dishes, etc., makes them normative choices just as legislation quickly made smoke-free indoor environments the norm.
Likely to be sustained	Systemic changes such as safe, attractive cycle networks or healthy school food which are backed by strong policies and traditions are more likely to sustain behaviors over the long term than, say, media campaigns.
Influences the hard-to-reach	Disadvantaged populations such those with low income or low educational attainment tend not to respond to health messages, but they can still benefit from the fast-food outlet that cooks lower-fat french fries.
Less language dependent	Health messages and information are often aimed at a narrow population segment and are often not transmitted in the native tongue of ethnic minorities, but all can take advantage of public transport.
Can address inequities	Environmental interventions can not only reach populations with poor health outcomes but can be differentially targeted to them such as improving bus services, school food programs, and active recreation amenities.
Usually cost-effective	Environmental interventions (especially policy-based initiatives) are relatively inexpensive compared to individual-based approaches and media-based public education campaigns. Even the expensive interventions (e.g., improving public transport) are often cost-effective in the long term.
Changes default behavior	Some food choices are highly influenced by price, labeling, and availability, and changing these factors shifts the default food choices.
Minimizes message distortion	Education messages related to obesity (or foods that might promote weight loss) may be misconstrued or misapplied, and this risk is minimized by a greater emphasis on providing the choices rather than preaching the choices.

developed by the International Obesity Task Force (38). Note that we have included "knowledge" in the analysis because of the important direct influences that environments, particularly the media, have on knowledge of food, nutrition, physical activity, and health.

The ANGELO Framework is a grid composed of two sizes of environment on one axis and four types of environment on the other (Fig. 3) and is used to "scan" the environments in question (19). Individuals interact with the environment in multiple micro (local) environments, or settings, including schools, workplaces, homes, and neighborhoods. Microenvironmental settings, in turn, are influenced by the broader macroenvironments, or sectors (such as the education and health systems, all levels of government, the food industry, and society's attitudes and beliefs), and these tend to be less amenable to the influence of individuals.

Within these settings or sectors there are different types of environment. We have categorized these as physical, economic, policy, or sociocultural. Put in simple terms, one can scan the four types of environment by asking the four respective questions: What is available?

Table 3 Dissection of Some Important Environments That Influence the Mediators of Energy Balance, Energy Intake, and Energy Expenditure

MEDIATOR = ENERGY INTAKE (FAT CONTENT, ENERGY DENSITY, PORTION SIZE)		
Behaviors	Settings	Sectors
Home food	Home	Food industry
Food prepared outside the home	Fast-food outlets	Food industry
	Cafes/restaurants	Food industry
	Institutions	Food industry
	Cafeterias	Food industry
School food	Schools (+ home)	Education sector, food industry
Knowledge	Media	Sectors
Food/nutrition	Curriculum	Education sector
	Health professionals	Health professional training sector
	Popular media	Mass-media sector, food industry
MEDIATOR = ENERGY EXPENDITURE (PHYSICAL ACTIVITY)		
Behaviors	Settings	Sectors
School PE/sports/transport	Schools/transport network	Education sector, local government
Active recreation	Neighborhood (streets, recreation spaces, facilities)	Local government, sports/exercise industry
Passive recreation	Home	Television networks, home entertainment industry
Active transport	Transport network (for walking, cycling, public transport)	Local/central government
Car transport	Transport network (for cars, including parking spaces)	Local/central government
Incidental activity	Home	
	Workplace	Local/central government
Knowledge	Media	Sectors
PA/exercise	Curriculum	Education sector
	Health professionals	Health professional training sector
	Popular media	Mass media sector

Environment size / Environment type	Microenvironment (settings) Food	PA	Macroenvironment (sectors) Food	PA
Physical	What is available?			
Economic	What are the financial factors?			
Policy	What are the rules?			
Sociocultural	What are the attitudes, beliefs, perceptions, and values?			

Figure 3 The ANGELO Framework (Analysis Grid for Environments Linked to Obesity).

What are the financial factors? What are the rules? What are the attitudes, perceptions, values, and beliefs? Both food and physical activity (the two mediators) then become subcategories within these cells and it is either (or both) of these that mediate the effects of the broader environments on body fat levels.

A The Physical Environment

The physical environment ("what is available?") includes not only the visible world (food and physical activity choices) but also less tangible factors such as the availability of educational training opportunities, nutrition and exercise expertise, technological innovations, information, and food labels. Some factors such as the weather or terrain may be important determinants of behavior, but because they are not amenable to influence there is little value in including them in the ANGELO scan, which is selecting factors for potential interventions.

B The Economic Environment

The economic environment ("what are the financial factors?") refers to both the costs related to food and physical activity and the income available to pay for them. These are very important at a household level because of the strong relationship between low incomes and high rates of obesity (40). However, at a macro level, it is the drive to maximize profits of private (and particularly transnational) industries that dominates in a free-market society. In the United States alone, the food industry is the second biggest spender on mass media advertising ($11 billion in 1997) (41). The biggest spenders are companies like Pepsi ($1.2 billion estimated ad spending), MacDonalds ($1 billion), and Coca Cola ($770 million) (42). The budget allocations of local and central governments are tangible indicators of the importance placed on, say, active transport versus car transport or nutrition and physical activity monitoring.

C The Policy Environment

The policy environment ("what are the rules?") refers to laws, regulations, policies (formal or informal), and institutional rules (including in the home) that impact on physical activity and eating behaviors. These "rules" can have profound effects on the behavior of individuals and organizations. Some examples include home rules on television watching (43,44), school food policies (45), regulations (or lack of them) on fast-food advertising on children's television (46), food labeling laws (47), traffic zoning by-laws (48), building codes (limiting stair access), and urban planning regulations (49).

D The Sociocultural Environment

The sociocultural environment ("what are the attitudes, perceptions, values, and beliefs?") establishes the context for what is considered normative behaviors within a particular societal group. At a micro, or setting, level, these sociocultural influences combine to give what is variously described as the culture, ethos, or climate of a school, home, workplace, or neighborhood. In schools, for example, the school ethos is considered a central component of a "health-promoting school" (45). It is influenced by, among other things, the relationships between staff and students, the value a school places on participation in sports and physical education, the degree to which the teachers serve as healthy role models for the students, and how much good nutrition features in the philosophy of the school food service.

Some cultural values or attitudes such as hospitality expectations on hosts to provide and guests to consume large amounts of food could promote overconsumption of food (50). Also, some cultures consider it inappropriate for its members to be physically active, thus promoting inactivity (51). One could therefore consider individuals to be "culturally predisposed to (or protected from) obesity" depending on their cultural affiliations in the same way that they would be considered genetically predisposed or protected according to their genotypes.

At the macroenvironmental level, the mass media are an important sector influencing the sociocultural aspects of food and physical activity (52–54). They directly and indirectly influence society's attitudes, beliefs, and values because they not only reflect and reinforce the "common culture" but also shape it, particularly through the effects of advertising and marketing (55,56).

VI PRIORITIZING ENVIRONMENTAL FACTORS FOR INTERVENTION

Using the ANGELO Framework with a group of stakeholders usually identifies a large number of potential environmental influences that may affect eating and physical activity patterns. The major challenge, then, is to hone them down to a few high-priority areas for further action. The prioritizing criteria should include:

1. Changeability—is the environmental factor amenable to change?
2. Relevance—is the environmental factor a big problem in our area?
3. Impact—what effect will changing the environmental factor have on behavior?

Getting stakeholders to score each element along these criteria quickly sorts out the high priority environmental factors. Action usually takes the form of interventions ("we know enough now to strengthen existing interventions or begin new ones"), research ("we need more hard data before we can proceed to intervention"), or further consultation ("we need more stakeholder consultation before we can prioritize"). We have

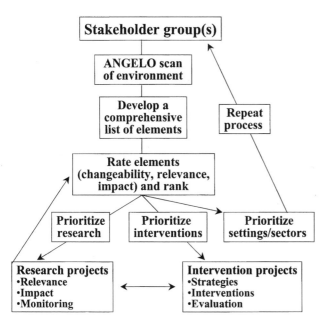

Figure 4 A proposed process for applying the ANGELO Framework to prioritize interventions and research.

found this prioritizing process (as shown in a flow diagram in Fig. 4) to be valuable in a variety of settings (19,36), although in real life such processes rarely proceed along such a linear path.

VII MEASURING ENVIRONMENTAL INDICATORS

Indicators are bits of information that reflect the status of larger systems. They are a way of seeing the big picture by looking at a small piece of it. They tell us which direction the system is going. Indicators are like the gauges and dials of an aircraft's instrument panel. By designing them carefully, watching them closely, and interpreting them wisely, we know the status of our flight and can make good decisions about where to go. Without indicators we're just 'flying by the seat of our pants'. (Sustainable Seattle, 1993. www.scn.org/sustainable/indicat.)

The development of indicators of obesogenic environments (and related behaviors) is a fundamental requirement of an environment or systems-based approach to obesity (57). The indicators are needed primarily to monitor progress over time, but they also allow comparisons among neighborhoods/cities/regions/countries and provide the basis for testing the impact of environmental change and behavior change.

Curtailing and reversing the obesity epidemic will not occur without the underlying environmental driving forces becoming more leptogenic. To positively and systematically influence the environments requires a robust "instrument panel" of indicators. The attributes of an ideal indicator are listed in Table 4, although, as with most measurements in science, all criteria are rarely met. The assessment of the impact of particular environmental factors on a behavior of interest is often problematic. Cross-sectional and ecological studies have inherent limitations in assessing the nature and strength of associations (58), and even intervention studies either are multidimensional or have design weaknesses (such as no control group) that make interpretation difficult (59).

VIII INFLUENCING OBESOGENIC ENVIRONMENTS—GENERAL STRATEGIES

Using the ANGELO Framework with stakeholders across various environments generates dozens, even hundreds, of potential aspects of the environments that might be amenable to leptogenic changes. Several authors have also outlined lists of potential environmental interventions for obesity prevention (19,32,33,39,60–62). The key difficulty in converting good ideas into action is narrowing down the many "could-do" activities into a few "can-do" ones and gaining the community and political commitment to then make them "must-do" actions. This has not been achieved in a coherent way for any population, but based on the experience of other epidemics and the obesity epidemic to date, a few general principles can be extracted.

A Keeping Obesity Prevention Firmly Environment Based

One of the risks to developing a momentum for environment-led obesity prevention is that obesity as an issue gets combined with diabetes and cardiovascular diseases, and then most of the funding and efforts are channeled into clinical interventions and/or mass-media strategies. While the rationale for such clumping is readily defendable and these strategies are important, a primary focus on improving the environments for healthy food and physical activity choices is needed if population-based prevention is to be a priority.

Table 4 Criteria for Ideal Indicators of Obesogenic Environments

Criterion	Comments
Impact	The environmental factor it reflects should have a significant impact on behaviors, e.g., TV advertising on food choices.
Validity	It should faithfully reflect the environmental factor in question, e.g., local government budgets for public transport support and cycleways versus major road works as a true reflection of the public investment in active transport versus car transport.
Responsiveness	It should be able to detect small changes in the environmental factor, e.g., a yes/no question about the presence of a school food policy may not be sensitive enough to detect differences in effectiveness of policies.
Reliability	The intra- and interobserver error and random error should be minimal; e.g., questionnaire-based indicators often need test-retest reliability assessments, whereas the number of cars per household from census data would be considered reliable.
Easy to measure	Ideally it would use data which are already collected for other purposes, e.g., proportion of local government transport funding for active transport versus car transport.
Inexpensive to measure	Questionnaire-based indicators, e.g., sociocultural indicators will be relatively expensive to measure.
Easily understood	Indicators that have complex derivations and are highly adjusted are less likely to be well understood, e.g., access to recreational facilities that is measured using distance-decay formulae and adjusted for attractiveness of the facility and the type of facility.

B Keeping the Interventions Achievable and Sustainable

The vastness of the task of preventing obesity is a classic barrier to action. To build the political and community case for action, the interventions need to be doable. Expanding existing programs that have shown some success (43,63–65), limiting the geographical reach of interventions in the first instance (i.e., establishing demonstration or sentinel sites) or focusing on a small number of settings are all strategies that can overcome the "inertia of enormity." However, a long-term vision (and funding) is needed for the programs to be developed, tested, evaluated, and implemented more widely.

C Priority on Children

Perhaps the strongest case for priority environments to influence are those related to children and adolescents. Nowhere does the ounce of prevention versus the pound of treatment apply more appropriately than with obesity because of the difficulty of losing excess fat once it has been gained. Also the range of achievable environmental interventions for children is greater than for adults (see below).

D Broad-Based Community and Political Commitment

Most of the environments that influence eating and activity patterns lie outside the jurisdiction of health and therefore need the engagement of a range of stakeholders. The strong backing from the community, the setting stakeholders and politicians is vital to securing the momentum and funding for interventions.

E High-Quality Programs

A high-quality program to reduce obesity would have a long duration, be sufficiently well funded to achieve a high dose of the intervention(s) and a wide reach to priority populations, and have robust evaluations. One of the temptations for governments with a low commitment to long-term solutions for obesity is to establish one or two short-term, low-dose, high-profile interventions. Another is to shift the responsibility onto individuals (to make the healthy choices), private industry (to use market forces to create healthy environments), or the health charity sector like heart foundations and cancer societies (to fund the programs). High-dose programs over long periods are needed, and this inevitably means government vision and funding. Evaluation is needed at every step: early formative inquiry, process evaluation (including of the implementation and roll-out phases), outcome analysis, and ongoing monitoring. Highly controlled, one-off interventions provide useful information about efficacy, but what is probably much more valuable is longitudinal evaluation studies (often less well controlled) of the real-world effectiveness of ongoing programs (66).

IX INFLUENCING OBESOGENIC ENVIRONMENTS—PRIORITY SETTINGS

A Schools and Other Educational Settings

1 Rationale and Evidence of Impact

Schools are a natural setting for influencing the food and physical activity environments for several reasons (67): Children are a high-priority population, they are almost all captive in the school environment, they spend a large proportion of their waking hours at school, they eat and do sport and activities at school, there are links to the curriculum, and schools provide some access to the home environment. In a review of environment-based interventions to reduce energy intake or energy density (59), 24 out of the 75 identified studies were school based. There was a wide variety of interventions including changes to the school lunch menus and food choices, award certificates for school canteens, curriculum changes, healthy choice information to students and parents, and changing the price of food items. Overall, the evaluation designs were of mixed quality, but most showed a positive impact on nutrient intake and dietary patterns (63,68,69), nutrition knowledge (70), and food sales (64,71).

Stone et al. (72) reviewed the impact of 14 school-based interventions on physical activity knowledge and behavior. Most of the outcome variables showed significant improvements for the intervention schools or groups. One interdisciplinary intervention program (mainly curriculum based) aimed at influencing the eating patterns, television viewing, and activity levels among 6-to-8-year-old children resulted in a reduction in obesity prevalence among the girls but not the boys (43).

In addition to the areas targeted for intervention in the published studies, there are other areas of growing concern in relation to schools. One is the increasing proportion of children who are being driven to school because of parental fears for the children's safety (from injury from cars) and security (from abduction) (73). In the United Kingdom, the proportion of 7-to-8-year old

children who traveled to school on their own plummeted from 80% in 1971 to only 9% in 1990 (73). Another area of concern is the increasing pressure from soft drink companies on schools to place soft drink vending machines in the schools with contracts for a required volume of sales (32). Also, low participation rates in sports and physical education, particularly among adolescent girls, may set the pattern for activity patterns in adulthood (74).

Despite the crowded curriculum and the pressure on schools and teachers to take on a variety of health programs, there is a strong imperative for schools to be a major setting for obesity prevention. In fact, efforts to prevent obesity could hardly be deemed serious without schools being a central component.

2 Potential Interventions

There are many different models of school food programs depending on the school food services offered (59). Interventions may be in the form of new programs or enhanced existing programs, stand-alone programs, or part of a wider health-promoting schools concept (45). Whatever form they take, they need to be funded to achieve a high enough dose of intervention and achieve a wide enough reach, particularly to schools in disadvantaged areas. The major elements of a school-based programs are: a school food and nutrition policy (including the types of foods and drinks available and promoted at school through the school food service or vending machines); training and resources for teachers and food service staff; guidelines for offering healthy food and drink choices; encouraging healthy options in food brought from home; and curriculum content on food and nutrition.

Increases in sports participation and/or physical education time would need policy-based changes at both the school and education sector levels (75). Similarly, increases in active modes of transport to and from school (walking, cycling, and public transport) will require policy changes at the school and local government levels as well as support from parents and the community. There is a variety of experience in these sorts of programs with some (e.g., supervised road crossings) having a long history and others (e.g., "walking bus," traffic calming around schools, and designated safe walking and cycling routes) are more recent.

3 Indicators of Change

A variety of indicators could be used for the food program such as the proportion of schools with an effective food policy, sales data of indicator foods (such as pies, chips, rolls, and sandwiches), proportion of schools with soft drink vending machines, and proportion of schools involved in various programs. The mode of transport to school and the participation rates in sports and physical education could be important indicators for physical activity.

B   Neighborhoods

1   Rationale and Evidence of Impact

Neighborhoods are a key setting for active recreation. These encompass the walking network (footpaths and walking tracks), the cycling network (roads and cycle paths), informal open recreation spaces such as parks, and formal recreation facilities such as sports grounds or recreation centers. Several studies have found that higher levels of recreational activity correlate with the proximity, density, attractiveness, and safety of recreation facilities or spaces (76–80). Most of these have been cross-sectional or qualitative studies, and it is likely that self-selection bias (individuals motivated to do physical activity choosing to live in areas with good access to recreation facilities) accounts for part of these relationships. Studies that measure the impact of providing and promoting better opportunities for recreational facilities will give a better measure of the strength and direction of the relationship between the recreation environment and physical activity levels (81).

2   Potential Interventions

Enhancing recreational facilities is core business for local governments. While increasing the amount of open recreational space is difficult within an existing environment, protecting the loss of such spaces requires a strong culture within local government of "green preservation" against perpetual commercial pressures. There are, however, a wide variety of enhancements of recreational spaces available to local governments such as extending walking and cycle paths, adding facilities like skateboard ramps, increasing lighting, increasing attractiveness, and reducing crime rates in the area.

3   Indicators of Change

Urban planners have a vast array of classifications, indicators, and standards for recreation amenities (82). They include usage, potential usage, capacity, number of people each facility services, quality measures, and so on. Indicators of access include the density of facilities around a person's house (76) or the number of people living within a given radius of a facility (so-called ped-shed) (83). Ratings of attractiveness or perceived safety

would require questionnaire survey methodology but would also be important to measure. Possibly the fundamental indicator for changes in local government priorities for active recreation environments would be changes in the proportion of their budget that is allocated to parks and recreation facilities.

C   Transport Networks

1   Rationale and Evidence of Impact

Public transport can be included with walking and cycling as active transport because of the regular short walking trips included in the use of public transport. The literature on the impact of land use and transportation systems on physical activity levels is extensive and has been recently reviewed by Frank and Engelke (73). Within the built environment, the land development patterns (i.e., public transport and pedestrian friendly vs. car orientated) and the mode of transport investment (i.e., in public transport, walking and cycling paths vs. highways) are closely interrelated, and between them they have a profound effect on physical activity levels (73). In car-dominated societies, only a minority of trips are walking or cycling (e.g., in the United States it is ~10%), and then most of them are for recreation purposes rather than transportation to a destinaton, whereas in several European countries, walking plus cycling trips equal or exceed car trips (73). This undoubtedly explains part of the differences in obesity prevalence rates between the continents. Single-use, low-density developments necessitate the use of a car.

2   Potential Interventions

Much of the impetus for reducing the dependence on automobile transport relates to reducing emissions, traffic congestion, and transport costs; however, the health benefits are an important additional stimulus for change (84). Because so much of the current built environment is car orientated, interventions will have to "retrofit" existing communities and target emerging communities so that the urban form and transport networks enable or even promote physical activity. Interventions would include promoting higher-density developments, greater mix of land use, a balance between housing and jobs, pedestrian- and cycle-friendly street design, greater investment in public transport, and the designation of streets and areas in the central business districts as car free (48,73). Local governments, nongovernmental organizations, and cycling and walking lobby groups all produce strategy documents replete with ways to promote and support active transport. Governments and communities are grappling with the conversion of the strategies into action. Influencing attitudes toward active transport is also an important part of gaining shifts in modes of transport use because attitudes may be as strongly associated with car transport as land use characteristics (85). If the environment is conducive to active transport, a mass-marketing approach appears to be able to influence long-term behaviors. In a pilot study in Perth, Australia, simple marketing of the active transport options to each household in a suburb resulted in 14% less car travel and increased the use of walking, cycling, and public transport (86). Changes were most marked for short journeys and were sustained over 2 years. Again, modest shifts in transport mode multiplied by the large volumes of short journeys where active transport is an option can result in important increases in physical activity for the population.

3 Indicators of Change

Transport professionals use a vast array of indicators of transport environments and behaviors (87). Many of them are oriented toward measuring car and public transport behaviors, but an expansion of these indicators into measuring how conductive environments are for walking and cycling is clearly achievable. They would need to encompass such factors as perceived safety and security of active transport modes, which are major issues for vulnerable groups like children and the elderly (73).

D Food Industry/Fast-Food Outlets

1 Rationale and Evidence of Impact

Of all the changes in eating patterns coincident with the increase in obesity, the dramatic increase in consumption of food prepared outside the home is probably the most significant. The United States is clearly the world leader in this regard. In 1970, 25% of the food dollar was spent on food prepared outside the home. By 1995, it had climbed to 40% and is projected to rise to 53% by 2010 (32). The settings for eating food prepared outside the home include restaurants, cafeterias, cafes, catered functions, airlines, and the like, but it is the fast-food outlets that are probably the most obesogenic (88). They are more ubiquitous, more heavily advertised, and more highly patronized than other settings, and the drive for fast service places a heavy reliance upon deep-frying cooking methods. Fast foods are one of the most advertised products on television (42), and children are often the targeted market. The fat, sugar, and energy content of foods advertised to children is extremely high com-

pared to their daily needs, and most of the foods advertised fall into the "eat least" or "eat occasionally" sections of the recommended dietary guidelines (46,89,90). Fast food has a higher fat content than the overall diet, and regular consumers of fast food have a higher dietary fat intake and are more likely to gain weight than less regular consumers (reviewed in 32). In addition, portion sizes are increasing, particularly in the United States, as "supersizing" promotions play to the customers' desire for a value-for-money meal or snack (32).

2 Potential Interventions

There are several areas within the fast-food industry sector where feasible intervention strategies could be developed. The New Zealand survey of fast food outlets (outlined in Sec. IB above) found a wide range of fat content of french fries (5–20%) and a high prevalence of practices that could be improved to reduce the fat content of fries (12). For the independent fast-food outlets, the main problem was poor deep-frying techniques due to a lack of training of operators. This led to collaborations among the National Heart Foundation, government health promotion organizations, tertiary technical institutes, and food industry groups to provide training courses around the country. For the chain-based outlets, such as McDonalds and Burger King, where the quality control was good, the reason for the high-fat fries was the use of the 6-to-8-mm shoestring fries rather than the thicker 12- to 14-mm variety. Other strategies (such as consumer education about thin fries being fattier) will be needed to influence this practice.

Nutrition labeling has allowed consumers to make informed choices about processed foods from the supermarket, although it is mainly the more health-conscious and better-educated consumers who use labels to guide food choices (91). It has been suggested that the labeling regulations be extended to include fast-food outlets (nutrition information on menus and/or food wrappers) (32).

A variation on food labeling, "nutrition signposting," might be less complex for consumers and regulators. Nutrition signposting is defined as endorsed signals (e.g., a logo) at point of choice which indicate to the consumer that particular foods, policies, or practices related to food meet certain nutrition standards (92). An example of this is the Pick the Tick program run by the National Heart Foundations of Australia and New Zealand (93). It is widely recognized and used by consumers and has had a significant influence on food formulation of products (92). Applying the Tick to some menu items in fast-food outlets is now being tested in Australia.

In 1990 the American Heart Association halted a proposed endorsement program because of incompatibility with the food regulations. However, nutrition signposting programs continue to operate in various forms in the United States, Singapore, South Africa, Canada, Sweden, and Australia. Evidence of the impact of these programs on food formulation or consumption is simultaneously essential and virtually nonexistent.

The huge television advertising of fast foods to children has been recognized by consumer and health groups as a major and inappropriate force in the shaping of children's diets. Limitations on television advertising to children would give parents a greater chance of moving their children's food choices toward the healthier options. In Sweden, for example, television advertising in children's programs has been banned.

3   Indicators of Change

Potential indicators of change of the obesogenicity of the fast food environment would be sales figures of fast food, the proportion of the food dollar spent on fast food, the average fat content of high volume items such as hot chips, the advertising spend by fast-food chains, and attitudes and beliefs about the role and "status" of fast food in the modern diet.

E   Home Environment

1   Rationale and Evidence of Impact

The home environment is undoubtedly the most important setting in relation to shaping children's eating and physical activity behaviors, but, surprisingly, we know very little about what are those specific home influences (94). As a setting, however, it is difficult to influence because of the sheer numbers and heterogeneity of homes and the limited options for access (with television being the most effective but very expensive access option). Potential areas to target in terms of the home food environment would be the food available and served in the home, the parents as role models for healthy eating, and the "eating ethos" of the household (is a meal simply fuel eaten on the run or in front of television or is it a focus for family communion?). For physical activity/inactivity, the home environment provides rules for television, videotape, Internet, and video game use (95) and establishes the "activity ethos" of the family, again with parents as critical role models. Of all these aspects of the home environment, television viewing has been the most researched (43,96,97). It appears

that gains can be made in obesity prevention through restricting television viewing, although it seems that reduced eating in front of television is at least as important as decreasing inactivity or increasing activity (96).

2   Potential Interventions

Apart from the studies aimed at reducing television viewing, some of which used a locking device on the television (96), there are no major studies to guide potential interventions aimed at influencing the home environment (59,94). The medium for any interventions on the home environment for children and adolescents will have to depend heavily on educating parents. While the use of mass media might achieve the desired reach, it is expensive, and other access points, such as through school or preschool or early childhood health systems, might be more sustainable alternatives.

3   Indicators of Change

Surveys of time spent in front of television, videos, and computer screens are conducted regularly in some countries and are good indicators of inactive recreation. More specific indicators to capture the home environment in terms of the family "rules" or ethos for eating and physical activity would require more extensive household survey questionnaires.

F   Other Potentially Changeable Obesogenic Environments

A variety of other environments warrant consideration for interventions. A few short-term studies have shown that a simple sign on stairs or elevators can increase stair walking (98,99). What is now needed is an implementation program to widely deploy such signs as well as advocacy to influence building codes and architectural designs so that stairs are an attractive easy option for everyday use rather than being hidden and dingy and intended for emergency use only.

The design and development of built environments that are conducive and attractive for physical activity constitute a major challenge. It will be a long process involving urban planners, architects, engineers, government infrastructure departments, and end users, but it is in sympathy with the current drive to make environment and infrastructure decisions more environmentally and socially sound.

Restaurants (59,100), workplaces (59,101,102), supermarkets (59,103), sports venues (104), and whole communities (32,61,105) have been studied as settings for influencing dietary intake and physical activity patterns. The impacts have ranged from none to modest, and many of the interventions have been of relatively short duration. Nevertheless, modest changes adopted by a high proportion of the population are undoubtedly going to be the manner in which the obesity epidemic is to be curtailed. The magnitude of changes seen in individual-based trials cannot expect to be found in population-based interventions.

X CONCLUSIONS

Obesogenic environments are increasingly the predominant driving forces behind the escalating obesity pandemic. It is therefore surprising that little attention has been paid to this area by way of academic analysis, etiological research, and intervention studies. We have proposed a framework for dissecting and analyzing obesogenic environments that we have found to be a useful and robust scanning tool to identify environmental elements worthy of intervention. However, this is only the first stage, and prioritizing the elements or settings to invest in for obesity prevention is difficult in the absence of much evidence to guide decisions. Priorities will vary according to local, regional, and national circumstances, and building intervention efforts onto existing activities will probably be a more successful approach than creating de novo intervention programs. Some of the strategies for reducing obesogenic environments such as banning fast-food advertisements from children's television programs will be met by substantial opposition. One only has to revisit the lessons from the tobacco epidemic to see that the efforts of government, society, and science can overcome such powerful vested interests if they are synergistic and sustained.

We have suggested that the priority population for obesity prevention should be children and adolescents because of the difficulty of reversing obesity in adults once it is established. We have also suggested that the key settings for interventions could be schools and other education settings, neighborhoods, transport networks, fast-food outlets, and home environments. In general, the studies to date have been short to medium term in duration, the study designs have been of mixed quality, and the results have ranged from no effect to modest effect. However, the strength of an environmental approach is that even modest impacts can have positive population benefits if there is a high volume of people exposed to that environment. "Small changes times large volumes" is the nature of both the ascending and descending trajectories of the noncommunicable-disease epidemics.

The challenge ahead of us is to identify obesogenic environments and influence them so that the healthier choices are more available, easier to access, and widely promoted to a large proportion of the community. This will require a paradigm shift within the health sector to see obesogenic environments as the drivers and the nonhealth sectors as essential allies in tackling the obesity epidemic. Similarly, for the nonhealth sectors such as local governments, schools, and the food industry, a paradigm shift is needed for them to see their contributions toward reversing the obesity epidemic.

REFERENCES

1. Obesity: Preventing and Managing the Global Epidemic. Report of a WHO Consultation. WHO Technical Report Series 894. Geneva: World Health Organization, 1998:157–162.
2. Egger G, Swinburn BA. An "ecological" approach to the obesity pandemic. BMJ 1997; 315:477–480.
3. Prescott-Clarke P, Primatesta P. Health Survey for England 1996. London: HMSO, 1998.
4. Knight I. The heights and weights of adults in Great Britain. London: HMSO, 1984.
5. Seidell JC. Time trends in obesity: an epidemiological perspective. Horm Metab Res 1997; 29:155–158.
6. Obesity. The Report of the British Nutrition Foundation Task Force. Oxford: Blackwell Science, 1999.
7. Rose G. The Strategy of Preventive Medicine. London: Oxford University Press, 1993.
8. Swinburn BA, Metcalf PA, Ley SJ. Long term (5 year) effects of a reduced fat diet in individuals with glucose intolerance. Diabetes Care 2001; 24(4):617–624.
9. Brownell K. Relapse and the treatment of obesity. In: Wadden TA, VanItallie TB, eds. Treatment of the Seriously Obese Patient. New York: Guilford Press, 1992: 437–455.
10. Gill T. Key issues in the prevention of obesity. Br Med Bull 1997; 53(2):359–388.
11. James WFT. Epidemiology of obesity. Int J Obes 1992; 16(suppl 2):23–26.
12. Morley John J, Swinburn BA, Metcalf PA, Raza F, Wright H. Fat content of chips, quality of frying fat and deep-frying practices in New Zealand fast food outlets. Aust NZ J Public Health 2002; 26:101–107.
13. Wilson BD, Wilson NC, Russell DG. Obesity and body fat distribution in the New Zealand population. N Z Med J 2001; 114:127–131.
14. Glanz K, Eriksen MP. Individual and community models for dietary behavior change. J Nutr Educ 1993; 25:80–86.
15. Swinburn BA, Ravussin E. Energy and macronutrient metabolism. In: Caterson ID, ed. Baillière's Clinical En-

docrinology and Metabolism: Obesity. Vol. 8. London: Baillière Tindall, 1994:527–548.

16. Alpert S. Growth, thermogenesis, and hyperphagia. Am J Clin Nutr 1990; 48:240–247.

17. Abbott WGH, Howard BV, Christin L, Freymond D, Lillioja S, Boyce VL, Anderson TE, Bogardus C, Ravussin E. Short term energy balance: relationship with protein, carbohydrate, and fat balances. Am J Physiol 1988; 255:E332–E337.

18. Swinburn BA, Ravussin E. Energy balance or fat balance? Am J Clin Nutr 1992; 57(suppl):766S–771S.

19. Swinburn BA, Egger GJ, Raza F. Dissecting obesogenic environments: the development and application of a framework for identifying and prioritising environmental interventions for obesity. Prev Med 1999; 29:563–570.

20. Sallis JF, Owen N. Ecological models. In: Glanz K, Lewis FM, Rimer BK, eds. Health Behavior and Health Education: Theory, Research and Practice. San Francisco: Jossey-Bass, 1996:403–424.

21. Prentice A. Manipulation of dietary fat and energy density and subsequent effects on substrate flux and food intake. Am J Clin Nutr 1998; 67(suppl):535S–541S.

22. Keesey RE. The body weight set-point. What can you tell your patients? Postgrad Med 1988; 83:114–127.

23. Ravussin E, Swinburn BA. Metabolic predictors of obesity: cross-sectional versus longitudinal data. Int J Obes 1994; 17(suppl 3):S28–S31.

24. Leibel RL, Rosenbaum M, Hirsch J. Changes in energy expenditure from altered body weight. N Engl J Med 1995; 332:621–628.

25. Teris M. Epidemiology and the public health movement. J Publ Health Policy 1987; 8(3):315–329.

26. Haddon W. Advances in the epidemiology of injuries as a basis for public policy. Public Health Rep 1980; 95(5):411–420.

27. Chapman S. Unwrapping gossamer with boxing gloves. BMJ 1993; 307:429–432.

28. Battle EK, Brownell KD. Confrontng the risng tide of eating disorders and obesity: treatment versus prevention and policy. Addict Behav 1996; 21:755–765.

29. Salbe AD, Ravussin E. The determinants of obesity. In: Bouchard C, ed. Physical Activity and Obesity. Champagne, IL: Human Kinetics, 2000:69–102.

30. Hill JO, Peters JC. Environmental contributions to the obesity epidemic. Science 1998; 280:1371–1374.

31. Egger G, Bolton A, O'Neill M, Freeman D. Effectiveness of an abdominal obesity reduction programme in men: the GutBusters 'waist loss' programme. Int J Obes 1996; 20:227–231.

32. French SA, Story M, Jeffrey RW. Environmental influences on eating and physical activity. Ann Rev Public Health 2001; 22:309–335.

33. King AC. Community and public health approaches to the promotion of physical activity. Med Sci Sports Exerc 1994; 26:1405–1412.

34. Egger G, Spark R, Donovan R. Health Promotion: Strategies and Methods. 2d ed. Sydney: McGraw-Hill, 1999:113–122.

35. Nutbeam D. Creating health-promoting environments: overcoming barriers to action. Aust N Z J Public Health 1997; 21(4):355–359.

36. Egger G, Fisher G, Piers S, Bedford K, Morseau G, Sabasio S, Taipim B, Bam G, Assan M, Mills P. Abdominal obesity reduction in indigenous men. Int J Obes 1999; 23:564–569.

37. Acting on Australia's Weight. National Medical and Health Research Council. Canberra: Commonwealth of Australia, 1997.

38. Balancing Policies for Healthy Weight: Preparing an Action Plan for the Prevention and Management of Overweight and Obesity. London: International Obesity Task Force, 2000:32–36.

39. Kumanyika SK. Mini symposium on obesity: overview and some strategic considerations. Annu Rev Public Health 2001; 22:293–308.

40. Aguirre P. Socioanthropological aspects of obesity in poverty. In: Pena M, Bacallo J, eds. Obesity and Poverty. A New Public Health Challenge. Scientific publication No. 576. Washington: Pan-American Health Organization, 2000.

41. Gallo AE. Food advertising in the United States. In: Frazao E, ed. America's Eating Habits: Changes and Consequences Washington: USDA/Econ Res Serv, 1999:173–180.

42. Advertising Age. 1999. Leading National Advertisers. http://www.adage.com.

43. Gortmaker SL, Peterson K, Wiecha J, Sobol AM, Dixit S, Fox MK, Laird N. Reducing obesity via a school-based interdisciplinary intervention among youth: Planet Health. Arch Pediatr Adolesc Med 1999; 153:409–418.

44. Epstein LH, Valoski A, Wing RR, Mc Curley J. Ten-year outcomes of behavioural family-based treatment for childhood obesity. Health Psychol 1994; 13:373–383.

45. Booth ML, Samdal O. Health-promoting schools in Australia: models and measurements. Aust N Z J Public Health 1997; 21(4):365–370.

46. Dibb S, Castwell A. Easy to swallow, hard to stomach: the results of a survey of food advertising on television. London: National Food Alliance, 1995.

47. Glanz K, Mullis RM. Environmental interventions to promote healthy eating: a review of models, programs, and evidence. Health Ed Q 1988; 15:395–415.

48. Crawford JH. Carfree Cities. Utrecht: International Books, 2000.

49. Cervero R, Gorham R. Commuting in transit versus automobile neighborhoods. J Am Plan Assoc 1995; 61:210–225.

50. Packard DP, McWilliams M. Cultural foods heritage of Middle Eastern immigrants. Nutr Today 1993; 28:6–13.

51. Stahl T, Rutten A, Nutbeam D, Bauman A, Kannas L, Abel T, Luschen G, Rodriguez DJA, Vinck J, Van der Zee J. The importance of the social environment for physically active lifestyle—results from an international study. Soc Sci Med 2001; 52:1–10.

52. MacLaren T. Messages for the masses: food and nurition issues on television. J Am Diet Assoc 1997; 97(7):733–738.

53. Hertzler AA, Grun I. Potential nutrition messages in magazines read by college students. Adolescence 1990; 25(99):717–723.

54. Strasburger VC. Adolescent and the Media: Medical and Psychological Impact. California: Sage, 1995.

55. Billington R, Strawbridge S, Greensides L, Fitzsimmons A. Culture and Society. London: Macmillan Education, 1991:156–171.

56. Serwer AE. McDonalds conquers the world. Fortune 1994; 130(8):103–107.

57. Cheadle A, Kristal A, Wagner E, Patrick D, Koespell T. Environmental indicators: a tool for evaluating community-based health promotion programs. Am J Prev Med 1992; 8:345–350.

58. Beaglehole R, Bonita R, Kjellstrom T. Basic Epidemiology. Geneva: World Health Organization, 1993: 31–53.

59. Hider P. Environmental interventions to reduce energy intake or density. A critical appraisal of the literature. NZHTA Report 2001 4(2). Christchurch: New Zealand Health Technology Assessment, 2001.

60. Nestle M, Jacobson MF. Halting the obesity epidemic: a public health policy approach. Public Health Rep 2000; 115:1–13.

61. Sallis JF, Bauman A, Pratt M. Environmental and policy interventions to promote physical activity. Am J Prev Med 1998; 15:379–397.

62. King AC, Jeffrey RW, Fridinger F, Dusenbury L, Provence S, Hedlund SA, Spangler K. Environmental and policy approaches to cardiovascular disease prevention through physical activity: issues and opportunities. Health Educ Q 1995; 22(4):499–511.

63. Luepker RV, Perry CL, McKinlay SM, Nader PR, Parcel GS, Stone EJ, Webber LS, Elder JP, Feldman HA, Johnson CC, Kelder SH, Wu M. Outcomes of a field trial to improve children's dietary patterns and physical activity. The Child and Adolescent Trial for Cardiovascular Health (CATCH). JAMA 1996; 275: 768–776.

64. Carter MA, Swinburn B. Measuring the impact of a school food programme on food sales. Health Prom Int 1999; 14:307–316.

65. Linenger JM, Chesson CV, Nice DS. Physical fitness gains following simple environmental change. Am J Prev Med 1991; 7:298–310.

66. Truswell AS. Levels and kinds of evidence for public-health nutrition. Lancet 2001; 357:1061–1062.

67. Resnicow K, Robinson TN. School-based cardiovas-cular disease prevention studies: review and synthesis. Ann Epidemiol 1997; S7:S14–S31.

68. Synder P, Anliker J, Cunningham-Sabo L, Dixon L, Altaha J, Chamberlain A, Davis S, Evans M, Hurley J, Weber JL. The Pathways Study: a model for lowering the fat in school menus. Am J Clin Nutr 1999; 69(suppl 4):810S–815S.

69. Snyder P, Story M, Trenkner L. Reducing fat and sodium in school lunch programs: the Lunchpower intervention study. J Am Diet Assoc 1992; 92:1087–1091.

70. Dollahite J, Hosig K, White K, Rodibaugh R, Holmes T. Impact of a school-based community intervention program on nutrition knowledge and food choices in elementary school children in the rural Arkansas Delta. J Nutr Ed 1998; 30:289–301.

71. Meiselman H, Hedderley D, Staddon S, Pierson B, Symonds C. Effect of effort on meal selection and acceptability in a student cafeteria. Appetite 1994; 23:43–55.

72. Stone EJ, McKenzie TL, Welk GJ, Booth ML. Effects of physical activity interventions in youth. A review and synthesis. Am J Prev Med 1998; 15:298–315.

73. Frank LD, Engelke P. How Land Use and Transportation Systems Impact Public Health: A literature review of the relationship between physical activity and the built form. Report to the Centers for Disease Control and Prevention. Atlanta: Georgia Institute of Technology, 2001. http://www.cdc.nccdphp/dnpa/pdf/aces-workingpaper1.pdf.

74. Booth M, Maskill P, McClelland L, Phongsavan P, Okley T, Patterson J, Wright J, Bauman A, Baur L. NSW Schools Fitness and Physical Activity Survey. Sydney: NSW Department of School Education, 1997.

75. Dwyer T, Coonan WE, Leitch DR, Hetzel BS, Baghurst KA. An investigation of the effects of daily physical activity on the health of primary school students in South Australia. Int J Epidemiol 1983; 12(3):308–313.

76. Sallis JF, Hovell MF, Hofstetter CR, Edler JP, Hackley M, Caspersen CJ, Powell KE. Distance between homes and exercise facilities related to frequency of exercise in San Diego residents. Public Health Rep 1990; 105(2): 179–185.

77. Bauman A, Smith B, Stoker L, Bellew B, Booth M. Geographical influences upon physical activity participation: evidence of a 'coastal effect'. Aust N Z J Public Health 1999; 23(3):322–324.

78. Wright C, MacDougall C, Atkinson R, Booth B. Exercise in Daily Life: Supportive Environments. National Heart Foundation of Australia report Adelaide: Commonwealth of Australia, 1996.

79. Rutten A, Abel T, Kannas L, Von Lengerke T, Luschen G, Diaz JA, Vinck J, Van der Zee J. Self reported physical activity, public health and perceived environment: results from a comparative European study. J Epidemiol Community Health 2001; 55(2):139–146.

80. Corti B, Donovan RJ, D'Arcy C, Holman J. Factors influencing the use of physical activity facilities: results

from qualitative research. Health Prom J Aust 1996; 6(1):16–21.

81. Housmann RA, Brown DR, Jackson-Thompson J, King AC, Balone BR, Sallis JF. Promoting physical activity in rural counties—walking trails access, use and effects. Am J Prev Med 2000; 18:235–241.

82. Lancaster RA, ed. Recreation, Park and Open Space Standards and Guidelines. Virginia: National Recreation and Park Association, 1983.

83. Llewelyn-Davies. Sustainable Residential Quality—New Approaches to Urban Living. London: London Planning Advisory Committee, 1997.

84. Dora C. A different route to health: implications of transport policies. BMJ 1999; 318:1686–1689.

85. Kitamura R, Mokhtarian PL, Laidet L. A micro-analysis of land use and travel in five neighborhoods in the San Francisco Bay area. Transportation 1997; 24:125–158.

86. TravelSmart (Transport). www.travelsmart.transport.wa.gov.au.

87. Bachels M, Newman P, Kenworthy J. Indicators of Urban Transport Efficiency in New Zealand's Main Cities: An International City Comparison of Transport, Land Use and Economic Indicators. Perth: Institute for Science and Technology Policy, Murdoch University, 1999.

88. Jeffrey RW, French SA. Epidemic obesity in the United States: are fast foods and television viewing contributing? Am J Publ Health 1998; 88:277–280.

89. Wilson N, Quigley R, Mansoor O. Food advertisements on TV: a health hazard for children. Aust N Z J Public Health 1999; 23(6):647–650.

90. Hill JM, Radimer KL. A content analysis of food advertisements in television for Australian children. Aust N Z J Public Health 1997; 54(4):174–181.

91. Guthrie JF, Kox JJ, Cleveland LE, Welsh S. Who uses nutrition labeling and what effects does label use have on diet quality? J Nutr Educ 1995; 27:163–172.

92. Young L, Swinburn B. The impact of the Pick the Tick food information program on salt content of food in New Zealand. Health Prom Int 2002; 17:13–19.

93. Noakes M, Crawford D. The National Heart Foundations 'Pick the Tick' Program: consumer awareness,

attitudes and interpretation. Food Aust 1991; 43:262–266.

94. Campbell K, Crawford D. Family food environments as determinants of preschool-aged children's eating behaviours: implications for obesity prevention policy. A review. Aust J Nutr Diet 2001; 58(1):19–25.

95. American Academy of Pediatrics Committee on Communications. Children, adolescents and television. Pediatrics 1995; 96(4):786–787.

96. Robinson TN. Reducing children's television viewing to prevent obesity. A randomized controlled trial. JAMA 1999; 282(16):1561–1567.

97. Dietz WH, Gortmaker SL. Preventing obesity in children and adolescents. Annu Rev Public Health 2001; 22:337–353.

98. Russell WD, Dzewaltowski DA, Ryan GJ. The effectiveness of a point-of-decision prompt in deterring sedentary behavior. Am J Health Prom 1999; 13(5): 257–259.

99. Brownell KD, Stunkard AJ, Albaum JM. Evaluation and modification of exercise patterns in the natural environment. Am J Psychiatry 1980; 137:1540–1545.

100. Colby J, Elder J, Peterson G, Knisley P, Carleton R. Promoting the selection of health food through menu item description in a family style restaurant. Am J Prev Med 1987; 3:171–177.

101. Chu C, Driscoll T, Dwyer S. The health-promoting workplace: an integrative perspective. Aust N Z J Public Health 1997; 21(4):377–384.

102. Schmitz M, Fielding J. Point-of-choice nutrition labeling—evaluation in a worksite cafeteria. J Nutr Educ 1986; 18(suppl 1):S65–S68.

103. Winett R, Wagner J, Moore J, Walker W, Hite L. An experimental evaluation of a prototype public access nutrition information system for supermarkets. Health Psychol 1991; 10:75–78.

104. Corti B, Holman CDJ. Warning: attending a sport, racing or arts venue may be beneficial to your health. Aust N Z J Public Health 1997; 21(4):371–376.

105. Bell AC, Swinburn BA, Amosa H, Scragg RK. A nutrition and exercise intervention program for controlling weight in Samoan communities in New Zealand. Int J Obes 2001; 25:920–927.

7

Prevention and Management of Dyslipidemia and the Metabolic Syndrome in Obese Patients

Scott M. Grundy

University of Texas Southwestern Medical Center at Dallas, Dallas, Texas, U.S.A.

I INTRODUCTION

The increasing prevalence of obesity in the United States and worldwide is a cause of great concern both for the health of individuals and for national health care systems. The underlying causes of the obesity epidemic are largely the product of what might be called "progress" in human civilization. These include increased availability of inexpensive food, urbanization, and technological advances that promote sedentary lifestyles. The combination of increased availability of food and lessened demand for physical activity combine to produce the progressive increase in body weight of individuals throughout the world. The public health consequences of these changes are enormous and pose a challenge to health policy at every level. A fundamental question has emerged: *How do we approach the emerging epidemic of obesity?*

The medical and psychological complications to which obesity can contribute are far-reaching. Obesity can adversely affect many body systems as well as behavior. Immediate effects can be a decrease in self-respect, lack of social acceptance, and loss of a feeling of well-being. In the long term, obesity contributes to several chronic diseases that can shorten life. Among these are coronary heart disease (CHD), stroke, and adult-onset (type 2) diabetes. This last, type 2 diabetes, carries a myriad of secondary complications including heart failure, kidney failure, loss of limbs, and infec-

tions. Obesity also predisposes to gallstones, sleep apnea, osteoarthritis, and various gynecological problems. Thus, among risk factors for chronc disease, obesity is near the top of the list.

II PREVENTION OF OBESITY: THE ULTIMATE GOAL

A high priority for health care in our society is to prevent the development of mass population obesity. Prevention strategy is directed first to factors leading to obesity in childhood, adolescence, and young adulthood. Nonetheless, prevention must extend into middle age and the later years, where changes in body composition accentuate the adverse effects of excess body fat. Once obesity becomes established, attention must turn to reducing excess both weight as well as to preventing further weight gain. At this time too, medical intervention must aim to prevent the complications of obesity, particularly cardiovascular disease and type 2 diabetes. This chapter will briefly address prevention of obesity in the general population and will then focus on the clinical management of overweight/obese patients with particular attention to preventing medical complications.

In the approach to the problem of obesity a clear distinction cannot be drawn between "prevention" and "treatment." Except when severe obesity is present, obesity per se does not cause physical limitation. Instead, associated medical problems usually develop insidiously over a period of many years. Once obesity is established, aims of management are twofold: (a) prevention of the medical complications, and (b) elimination of excess body fat. Unfortunately, clinical weight-reduction therapy has met with only limited success. Certainly with therapy some obese patients will effectively lose weight, others will lose small amounts, and some will be able to prevent further weight gain; but still others will continue to gain weight. Efforts to achieve weight reduction are warranted, but in view of the limited success of weight reduction programs, parallel intervention to prevent the complications of obesity must come into play.

III COMPLICATIONS OF OBESITY AND THE METABOLIC SYNDROME

The complications of obesity—psychological, functional, and metabolic—are listed in Tables 1 and 2. In many social circles, obesity is not acceptable. Its presence, although common, still leads to social discrimination, followed by feelings of psychological inadequacy and guilt. If obesity is severe, it can impair mobility and musculoskeletal functions. But the major health consequences of obesity lie in the metabolic sphere. The metabolic abnormalities induced by obesity frequently contribute to cardiovascular disease, type 2 diabetes, fatty liver, gallstones, and polycystic ovary syndrome, among others (1,2).

Table 1 ATP III Classification of LDL, Total, and HDL Cholesterol (mg/dL)

LDL cholesterol—primary target of therapy	
<100	Optimal
100–129	Near optimal/ above optimal
130–159	Borderline high
160–189	High
≥190	Very high
Total cholesterol	
<200	Desirable
200–239	Borderline high
≥240	High
HDL cholesterol	
<40	Low
≥60	High

Table 2 Classification of Major Nonlipid Risk Factors

Cigarette smoking (any smoking in past year)
Hypertension (BP ≥ 140/90 mmHg or on antihypertensive medication)
Low HDL cholesterol (<40 mg/dL)[a]
Family history of premature CHD (CHD in male first-degree relative <55 years; CHD in female first-degree relative <65 years)
Age (men ≥ years; women ≥ 55 years)

[a] HDL cholesterol ≥ 60 mg/dL counts as a "negative" risk factor: its presence removes one risk factor from the total count.

Of particular importance for cardiovascular risk, obesity is almost always present in persons who manifest an aggregation of cardiovascular risk factors called the metabolic syndrome (3–6). In the United States, this syndrom is emerging as a major contributor to cardiovascular disease. In addition, it commonly precedes the development of type 2 diabetes (7). The metabolic syndrome typically consists of two underlying risk factors and five metabolic risk factors (8). Various combinations of these risk factors can occur in one individual to enhance cardiovascular risk. The essential features of the metabolic syndrome are the following:

Underlying risk factors
    Obesity (especially abdominal obesity)
    Physical inactivity
Metabolic risk factors
    Atherogenic dyslipidemia
    Raised blood pressure
    Insulin resistance ± elevated plasma glucose
    Pro-thrombotic state
    Pro-inflammatory state

The metabolic syndrome received increased emphasis as a major, multifaceted cardiovascular risk factor in the National Cholesterol Education Program's Adult Treatment Panel (ATP III) report (8). ATP III chooses the term "metabolic syndrome" over others that have been used. Some of these other terms are:

Insulin resistance syndrome
Syndrome X (or metabolic syndrome X)
Multiple metabolic syndrome or dysmetabolic syndrome
Deadly quartet

ATP III favored "metabolic syndrome" because it is the most widely used and seems to apply most directly to clinical practice. "Multiple metabolic syndrome" and "dysmetabolic syndrome" are employed less frequently.

Syndrome X offers some confusion with the cardiac syndrome X ("microvascular angina"); also, it does not point to a metabolic origin. Endocrinologists and diabetologists often prefer the "insulin resistance syndrome," which focuses on the common association between multiple risk factors and the presence of insulin resistance. On the other hand, that insulin resistance directly causes this syndrome has not been documented.

The causes of the metabolic syndrome have not been fully elucidated. Nonetheless, obesity and lack of physical activity are important underlying causes (3). The syndrome appears to arise in large part out of an overloading of tissues, particularly the liver and muscle, with lipid. With obesity, nonesterified fatty acids (NEFAs) are elevated; this excess NEFA provides more energy substrate than is needed for normal metabolism. The accumulation of lipid in both liver and muscle contribute importantly to both insulin resistance and the metabolic syndrome. Beyond obesity and physical inactivity, however, genetic factors also are involved. The role of genetics is demonstrated by the variable expression of the metabolic syndrome in the presence of obesity and physical inactivity. Severity of the several risk factors of the syndrome varies widely among individuals and populations. The high prevalence of the metabolic syndrome, coronary heart disease, and type 2 diabetes in people of South Asian origin provides strong evidence that genetic factors play a role (9). Reasons for the increased CHD risk in persons with the metabolic syndrome remain to be fully understood. The specific role of each risk factor has been difficult to determine. Even so, most of the risk factors associated with this syndrome appear to have atherogenic potential. Thus, the increased risk for CHD in patients with the metabolic syndrome almost certainly derives from multiple factors.

IV PUBLIC HEALTH APPROACHES TO PRIMARY PREVENTION OF OBESITY

A Prevention of Childhood and Adolescent Obesity

Obesity in childhood and adolescence is increasing at an alarming rate (10). This increase appears to be largely due to societal changes. Nowadays children generally do not to walk to school. Compared to the past, less time is devoted to physical activity in school. After school, children have fewer opportunities for playing outside. Many go straight home and lock themselves in, waiting for parents to come home from work. At home, they settle down into chairs and watch television. Snacking while watching TV is common at this time.

Surfing the Internet and playing video games commonly takes time away from outside activities (11). The availability of cheap food enhances caloric intake. When busy parents return home at night, they often prefer eating out to preparing healthy meals at home. A trip for hamburgers or pizza typically provides both diversion and unneeded calories. All of these factors combine to promote weight gain in children and adolescents.

To reverse these trends, it will be necessary to bring about major changes in the behavior of society as well as individuals (12). New recreational facilities are needed to promote physical activity. Safe havens for physical play are required. Schools need to spend more time in teaching healthy life habits. Parents must be made aware of how to improve the household to reduce the tendency for weight gain in the family. School lunches should be modified to be less calorically dense as well as healthier. These social issues and will require a concerted effort at local, state, and national levels.

The medical model for treatment of obesity in childhood so far had only limited success. Reports of success in achieving weight loss through professional intervention for individual obese children have not been encouraging. Thus, to deal with the problem of population childhood obesity, the social changes described above undoubtedly will be required.

B Prevention of Obesity in Adults

Many people make it through adolescence without developing obesity. In fact, in our society, a great deal of weight gain typically occurs between ages 20 and 50 years. This gain is the result of several factors: decreasing physical activity, "stress" eating at both home and work, and for women, weight gain with pregnancy (13–15). The increase of body weight during young adulthood lays the foundation for the medical consequences of obesity.

Prevention of adult-onset obesity again must focus on social factors. Here, public education and enhanced awareness of the dangers of weight gain are needed. Many young adults are not yet tuned into the health drawbacks of obesity, and they fail to take precautions to avoid it at this stage. Consequently, a more intensive educational effort for this age range is required. Adults must restructure their lives to allow more time for exercise, to minimize use of "labor-saving devices," and to limit portion sizes of their food choices. Whether large-scale social changes beyond education can be brought into play to prevent obesity in adults is uncertain.

After age 50, many people do not gain further weight. Although weight gain can occur, overweight and obesity assume a new dimension in the later stages of life. Even when absolute weight does not increase, changes in body composition begin to accelerate. Foremost is a decline in muscle mass (16,17). As a result, the ratio of adipose tissue to muscle mass usually is higher in older people than in middle age. This change shifts the metabolic balance in ways that favor the development of insulin resistance and the metabolic syndrome [18–20]. Loss of muscle mass is brought about in part by an increasingly sedentary lifestyle. In addition, metabolic changes accompanying aging, which are not well understood, probably play a role. In any case, loss of muscle mass makes older people more susceptible to health consequences of obesity.

V CLINICAL MANAGEMENT OF ADULTS WITH ESTABLISHED OBESITY

Clinical treatment of obesity in childhood and adolescence is beyond the scope of this chapter. The Obesity Education Initiative (OEI) of the National Institutes of Health provides a reasonable approach to the management of adults with established obesity (1,2). Similar guidelines are available from other sources (2). The OEI report focuses primarily on weight reduction strategies; although it indicated the need to evaluate coexisting risk factors, it did not directly recommend their management before instituting weight reduction. The ATP III report, on the other hand, placed priority on initiating therapies for risk factors before dealing with the problem of obesity. ATP III contends that risk factors typically impart a more immediate risk to patients than does obesity itself; thus, risk factor control takes precedence in clinical management. The present chapter will attempt to integrate OEI and ATP III reports so as to facilitate both weight reduction and treatment of metabolic risk factors. Both OEI and ATP III base recommendations on available scientific evidence. They contain a large number of references and evidence tables. They are both available on the National Heart Lung and Blood Institute website (www.nhlbi.nih.gov). The current chapter summarizes key features of these guidelines but does not detail the literature available in the reports. They can be obtained from the website or corresponding publications of the reports.

VI CLINICAL ASSESSMENT IN PERSONS WHO ARE OVERWEIGHT OR OBESE

Clinical management of overweight/obese patients includes identification of risk factors, among which

are several body weight parameters and detection of comorbidities accompanying excess body weight.

A Assessment of Risk Factors

Overall, the greatest danger of overweight/obesity is the development of cardiovascular disease. Moreover, in the long term obesity predisposes to type 2 diabetes, which is itself a risk factor for cardiovascular disease. ATP III provides useful classifications for lipid and nonlipid risk factors. These classifications are shown in Tables 1 and 2, respectively. In ATP III, estimates are made of a person's absolute risk using Framingham risk scoring, which is available through the NHLBI (http://www.nhlbi.nih.gov/guidelines/cholesterol/profmats.htm). This scoring estimates the 10-year risk for developing myocardial infarction or coronary death. It is based on absolute levels of the following risk factors: total cholesterol, HDL cholesterol, blood pressure, smoking history, and age. Framingham scoring can be carried out either by manual scoring or with a simple computer program, both of which are available on the NHLBI website. In addition, ATP III defines the metabolic syndrome for clinical practice according to five clinical features (Table 3). According to ATP III, three of five of these clinical features constitute a clinical diagnosis of the metabolic syndrome. In addition, however,

Table 3 Clinical Identification of the Metabolic Syndrome—Any Three of the Following

Risk factor	Defining level
Abdominal obesity[a]	Waist circumference[b]
Men	>102 cm (>40 in)
Women	>88 cm (>35 in)
Triglycerides	≥150 mg/dL
HDL cholesterol	
Men	<40 mg/dL
Women	<50 mg/dL
Blood pressure	≥130/≥85 mmHg
Fasting glucose	≥110 mg/dL

[a] Overweight and obesity are associated with insulin resistance and the metabolic syndrome. However, the presence of abdominal obesity is more highly correlated with the metabolic risk factors than is an elevated BMI. Therefore, the simple measure of waist circumference is recommended to identify the body weight component of the metabolic syndrome.
[b] Some male patients can develop multiple metabolic risk factors when the waist circumference is only marginally increased, e.g., 94–102 cm (37–39 in). Such patients may have a strong genetic contribution to insulin resistance. They should benefit from changes in life habits, similarly to men with categorical increases in waist circumference.

it was recognized that there are other "hidden" metabolic risk factors. These are risk factors that are not routinely detected in clinical practice, but could be identified with special testing. They include the following:

Insulin resistance (with elevated plasma insulin)
Prothrombotic state (with elevated plasma fibrinogen and PAI-1)
Proinflammatory state [with elevated high-sensitivity C-reactive protein (hs-CRP)]
Fatty liver

B   Assessment for Underlying Risk Factors

1   Overweight/Obesity

a.   Body Mass Index

According to the OEI report (1,2), overweight is defined as a body mass index (BMI) of 25–29.9 kg/m^2 and obesity by a BMI of 30 kg/m^2. Several methods can be used to calculate total body fat: total body water, total body potassium, bioelectrical impedance, and dual-energy x-ray absorptiometry. However, in the clinical setting, BMI is the best indicator of body fat, importantly, the BMI provides a more accurate measure of total body fat than does weight alone. Nonetheless, simply measuring body weight is a practical approach to follow weight changes. The BMI is calculated as follows:

$$BMI = weight\ (kg)/height\ squared\ (m^2)$$

To estimate BMI from pounds and inches use:

$$[weight\ (pounds)/height\ (inches)^2] \times 703(1 lb$$
$$= 0.4536\ kg)(1\ in = 2.54\ cm = 0.0254\ m)$$

A patient should be weighed with shoes off and clad only in a light robe or undergarments.

The relation between BMI and disease risk varies among individuals and among different populations. Highly muscular individuals often have a BMI placing them in an overweight category when body fat content is not high. Also, in very short persons (under 5 feet), high BMIs may not reflect a high body fat. In addition, susceptibility to risk factors at a given BMI varies among individuals. Some individuals may have risk factors in the absence of a high BMI; in these persons, genetic causes of risk factors may be predominant.

Clinical judgment must be used in interpreting BMI in situations in which it may not be an accurate indicator of total body at, e.g., the presence of edema, high muscularity, muscle wasting, or for very short people.

The relationship between BMI and body fat content varies with age, sex, and possibly ethnicity because of differences in factors such as composition of lean tissue, sitting height, and hydration state. For example, older persons often have less muscle mass and more fat for a given BMI than younger persons, women usually have more fat for a given BMI than men, and clinical edema gives erroneously high BMIs.

b.   Waist Circumference

Excess fat in the abdomen independently predicts risk factors and morbidity. Research has shown that the waist circumference correlates with the amount of fat in the abdomen, and thus is an indicator of the severity of abdominal obesity (Table 4). In ATP III (8), increased waist circumference was identified as a strong obesity-associated clinical correlate of the metabolic syndrome. "Waist" circumference (1,2) is used instead of "abdominal" circumference because it more accurately describes the anatomical site of measurement. Abdominal fat has three compartments: visceral, retroperitoneal, and subcutaneous. Some studies suggest that visceral fat is the most strongly correlated with risk factors, whereas others indicate that the subcutaneous component is the most highly correlated with insulin resistance. Regardless, the presence of increased total abdominal fat is to be an independent risk predictor even when the BMI is not markedly increased. Therefore, waist or abdominal circumference, as well as BMI, should be measured.

Although waist circumference and BMI are interrelated, waist circumference carries extra prediction of risk beyond that of BMI (1,2). Waist circumference measurement is particularly useful in patients who are categorized as normal or overweight on the BMI scale. At BMIs >35, waist circumference has little added predictive power of disease risk beyond BMI.

A high waist circumference carries increased risk for type 2 diabetes, dyslipidemia, hypertension, and CVD when a BMI ranges between 25 and 34.9 kg/m^2. The clinician should keep in mild that ethnic and age-related differences in body fat distribution can that modify the predictive power of waist circumference. In general, and particularly in some populations (e.g., Asians), waist

Table 4   Definition of Abdominal Obesity

Gender	Waist circumference
Men	>102 cm (>40 in)
Women	>88 cm (35 in)

circumference is a better indicator of relative disease risk than is BMI. Waist circumference in particular assumes greater value than BMI for estimating risk for obesity-related disease at older ages.

2 Physical Inactivity

Sedentary life habits are a major underlying risk factor for both cardiovascular disease and type 2 diabetes (22). The detection of physical inactivity can be assessed in two ways: (1) by history, and (2) by detection of cardiovascular fitness. Since the recommendation for physical activity calls for 30 min of moderately intense activity daily, lesser amounts of activity constitute varying degrees of physical inactivity. Some investigators contend that quantitative measures of cardiovascular fitness through exercise testing provide a more reliable indication of physical activity status with respect to future cardiovascular risk; this advantage, however, has not been proven with certainty (23).

C Detection of Comorbidities

Patients who are overweight/obese should be questioned for the presence of existing comorbidities (Table 5). When suspected, further diagnostic testing may be required. Diseases that are commonly present in overweight/obese persons are coronary heart disease, type 2 diabetes, gallstones, osteoarthritis, and sleep apnea. Patients with severe obesity may also exhibit pulmonary disease and/or dysmobility. These condi-

Table 5 Complications of Obesity

Development of risk factors
  Hypertension
  Dyslipidemia
  Insulin resistance
  Impaired fasting glucose
Risk factor–related chronic diseases
  Coronary heart disease
  Stroke
  Type 2 diabetes
Comorbidities
  Osteoarthritis
  Some types of cancer (endometrial, prostate, colon)
  Sleep apnea and other respiratory disorders
  Gallstones
  Menstrual irregularities and polycystic ovary syndrome
  Complications of pregnancy
  Stress incontinence
  Psychological disorders (e.g., depression)
  Fatty liver (rarely cirrhosis)
  Impaired mobility (severe obesity)

tions may require clinical intervention independent of risk factor management and weight reduction.

VII MANAGEMENT OF RISK FACTORS IN OVERWEIGHT/OBESE PERSONS

In patients who are overweight/obese, clinical focus should be directed first to the risk factors associated with obesity. Most of these risk factors relate to cardiovascular disease, but some may indicate an increased susceptibility to type 2 diabetes. Management of the metabolic risk factors that are characteristic of the metabolic syndrome will be discussed. However, consideration will be given first to management of elevated low-density lipoprotein (LDL) cholesterol, which is the prime risk factor for development of atherosclerotic coronary heart disease.

A Elevated LDL Cholesterol

Serum LDL cholesterol is the primary target of cholesterol-lowering therapy. Overweight and obesity contribute to elevations of LDL cholesterol. Moreover, at any given level of LDL cholesterol, the presence of obesity-induced metabolic syndrome raises the risk for CHD. For this reason, particular attention should be given reducing LDL cholesterol levels in overweight/obese patients who are identified as having the metabolic syndrome. In this section, the key recommendations of ATP III for management of elevated LDL cholesterol levels will be summarized (8). These recommendations apply particularly to patients who are overweight or obese. The primary sequence of therapy in ATP III is to direct attention first toward elevated LDL cholesterol; the metabolic syndrome is a secondary target of therapy. In other words, the goals for LDL therapy are first achieved before turning to the risk factors of the metabolic syndrome. Of course, if cigarette smoking or categorical hypertension is present, intervention on these risk factors will be needed from the outset. After intervention on the major risk factors is established, attention can turn to control of the metabolic risk factors. The latter features weight reduction and increased exercise.

Therapeutic modalities for LDL cholesterol lowering include both nondrug and drug therapies. The former are designated *therapeutic lifestyle changes (TLC)*. The components of TLC specifically directed toward LDL lowering are:

Reduced intakes of saturated fats (<7% of total calories) and cholesterol (<200 mg/d)

> Therapeutic options for enhancing LDL lowering, such as plant stanols/sterols (2 g/d) and increased viscous (soluble) fiber (10–25 g/d)
>
> Weight reduction

As the first step of TLC, intakes of saturated fats and cholesterol are reduced first to lower LDL cholesterol. To improve overall health, ATP III's therapeutic diet generally corresponds to the recommendations embodied in the Dietary Guidelines for Americans 2000. One exception is that in ATP III total fat is allowed to range from 25% to 35% of total calories provided saturated fats and trans fatty acids are kept low. A higher intake of total fat, mostly in the form of unsaturated fat, can help to reduce triglycerides and raise HDL cholesterol in persons with the metabolic syndrome. In accordance with the Dietary Guidelines, moderate physical activity is encouraged. After 6 weeks of reducing saturated fats and cholesterol, the LDL response is determined; if the LDL cholesterol goal has not been achieved, other therapeutic options for LDL lowering such as plant stanol/sterols and viscous fiber can be added. After maximum reduction of LDL cholesterol with dietary therapy, emphasis shifts to management of the metabolic syndrome and associated lipid risk factors (see below).

Several drugs are available for lipid lowering (Table 6). The major drugs available for LDL lowering are bile acid sequestrants and HMG CoA reductase inhibitors (statins). Other drugs—nicotoinic acid and fibrate—moderately lower LDL levels, but they primarily reduce triglycerides and raise HDL levels.

Table 7 defines LDL cholesterol goals and cut points for initiation of TLC and for consideration of drug therapy for persons with four categories of risk: (1) *high-risk patients* (CHD and CHD risk equivalents); (2) *moderately high risk* persons with *multiple (2 +) risk factors (10-year risk 10–20%)*; (3) *moderate-risk* persons with *multiple (2 +) risk factors (10-year risk < 10%)*; and (3) *lower-risk* persons with 0–1 risk factor. The management of each group will be considered briefly.

1 High-Risk Patients: CHD and CHD Risk Equivalents

The high-risk category includes patients with established CHD and CHD risk equivalents. Established CHD includes a history of myocardial infarction, unstable angina, stable angina, and coronary artery procedures (coronary angioplasty, coronary bypass operation). CHD risk equivalents are present in (1) patients with clinical forms of noncoronary atherosclerotic disease (peripheral arterial disease, abdominal aortic aneurysm, and symptomatic carotid artery disease (carotid transient ischemic attacks and carotid strokes); (2) patients with diabetes; and (3) persons whose 10-year risk for CHD is estimated to be >20% by Framingham risk scoring. For high-risk patients with CHD and CHD risk equivalents, LDL-lowering therapy greatly reduces risk for major coronary events and stroke and yields highly favorable cost-effectiveness ratios. *If baseline LDL cholesterol is ≥130 mg/dL*, intensive lifestyle therapy and maximal control of other risk factors should be started. Moreover, for most patients, an LDL-lowering drug will be required to achieve an LDL cholesterol <100 mg/dL; thus, an LDL cholesterol lowering drug can be started simultaneously with TLC to attain the goal of therapy. *If baseline (or on-treatment) LDL cholesterol levels are <130 mg/dL*, either at baseline or on LDL-lowering therapy, several therapeutic approaches are available:

1. Initiate or intensify lifestyle and/or drug therapies specifically to achieve the goals for LDL lowering therapy.

2. Emphasize weight reduction and increased physical activity in persons with the metabolic syndrome.

3. Delay use of LDL-lowering therapies and institute treatment of other lipid or nonlipid risk factors; consider use of other lipid-modifying drugs (e.g., nicotinic acid or fibric acid) if the patient has elevated triglyceride or low HDL cholesterol.

2 Moderately High Risk Patients: Multiple (2 +) Risk Factors and a 10-Year Risk of 10–20%

In this category, the goal for LDL cholesterol is <130 mg/dL. The therapeutic aim is to reduce short-term risk as well as long-term risk for CHD. If baseline LDL cholesterol is ≥130 mg/dL, TLC is initiated and maintained for 3 months. If LDL remains ≥130 mg/dL after 3 months of TLC, consideration can be given to starting an LDL-lowering drug to achieve the LDL goal of <130 mg/dL. Use of LDL-lowering drugs at this risk level reduces CHD risk and is cost-effective. If the LDL falls to <130 mg/dL on TLC alone, TLC can be continued without adding drugs. In older persons (≥65 years), clinical judgment is required for how intensively to apply these guidelines; a variety of factors, including concomitant illnesses, general health status, and social issues may influence treatment decisions and may suggest a more conservative approach.

Table 6 Drugs Affecting Lipoprotein Metabolism

Drug class, agents and daily doses	Lipid/lipoprotein effects			Side effects	Contraindications	Clinical trial results
Bile acid sequestrants[a]	LDL C	↓15–30%		Gastrointestinal distress	Absolute: dysbetalipoproteinemia TG >400 mg/dL	Reduced major coronary events and CHD deaths
	HDL C	↑ 3–5%		Constipation	Relative: TG >200 mg/dL	
	TG	No change or increase		Decreased absorption of other drugs		
HMG CoA reductase inhibitors (statins)[b]	LDL C	↓18–55%		Myopathy	Absolute: Active or chronic liver disease	Reduced major coronary events, CHD deaths, need for coronary procedures, stroke, and total mortality
	HDL C	↑ 5–15%		Increased liver enzymes	Relative: Concomitant use of certain drugs[c]	
	TG	↓ 7–30%				
Nicotinic acid[d]	LDL C	↓ 5–25%		Flushing	Absolute: Chronic liver disease Severe gout	Reduced major coronary events, and possibly, total mortality
	HDL C	↑15–35%		Hyperglycemia	Relative: Diabetes	
	TG	↓20–50%		Hyperuricemia (or gout)	Hyperuricemia	
				Upper-GI distress; hepatotoxicity	Peptic ulcer disease	
Fibric acids[e]	LDL C	↓ 5–20% (may be increased in patients with high TG)		Dyspepsia	Absolute:	Reduced major coronary events.
	HDL C	↑10–20%		Gallstones	Severe renal disease	Increased non-CHD mortality (in 2/5 clinical trials)
	TG	↓10–50%		Myopathy	Severe hepatic disease	

TG, triglyceride.

[a] Cholestyramine (4–16 g), colestipol (5–20 g), colesevelam (2.6–3.8 g).

[b] Lovastatin (20–80 mg), pravastatin (20–40 mg), simvastatin (20–80 mg), fluvastatin (20–80 mg), atorvastatin (10–80 mg); standard starting doses of statins are lovastatin (40 mg), pravastatin (40 mg), simvastatin (20 mg), fluvastatin (40 mg), and atorvastatin (10 mg).

[c] Cyclosporine, gemfibrozil (or niacin), macrolide antibiotics, various antifungal agents, and cytochrome P-450 inhibitors.

[d] Immediate release (crystaline) nicotinic acid (1.5–3 g), extended release nicotinic acid (Niaspan) (1–2 g), sustained release nicotinic acid (1–2 g).

[e] Gemfibrozil (600 mg BID), fenofibrate (200 mg), clofibrate (1000 mg BID).

Table 7 LDL Cholesterol Goals and Cutpoints for Therapeutic Lifestyle Changes and Drug Therapy in Different Risk Categories

Risk category	LDL goal	LDL level at which to initiate therapeutic lifestyle changes	LDL level at which to consider drug therapy
High risk (10-year risk >20%)[a]	<100 mg/dL	≥100 mg/dL	≥130 mg/dL (100–129 mg/dL: drug optional)
Moderately high risk (2+ risk factors and 10-year risk 10–20% or metabolic syndrome)	<130 mg/dL	≥130 mg/dL	≥130 mg/dL (after dietary therapy)
Moderate risk (2+ risk factors; 10-year risk <10%)	<130 mg/dL	≥130 mg/dL	≥160 mg/dL (after dietary therapy)
Lower risk (0–1 risk factor)	<160 mg/dL	≥160 mg/dL	≥190 mg/dL (160–189 mg/dL: LDL-lowering drug optional)

[a] The high risk category includes patients with established CHD and CHD risk equivalents. Established CHD includes a history of myocardial infarction, unstable angina, stable angina, and coronary artery procedures (coronary angioplasty, coronary bypass operation). CHD risk equivalents are present in patients with clinical forms of noncoronary atherosclerotic disease (peripheral arterial disease, abdominal aortic aneurysm, and symptomatic carotid artery disease (carotid transient ischemic attacks and carotid strokes), patients with diabetes, and persons whose 10-year risk for CHD is estimated to be >20% by Framingham risk scoring.

3 Moderate-Risk Patients: Multiple (2+) Risk Factors and a 10-Year Risk of <10%

Here the goal for LDL cholesterol also is <130 mg/dL. The therapeutic aim, however, is primarily to reduce longer-term risk. If baseline LDL cholesterol is ≥130 mg/dL, the TLC diet is initiated to reduce LDL cholesterol. If LDL is <160 mg/dL on TLC alone, it should be continued. LDL-lowering drugs generally are not recommended because the patient is not at high short-term risk. On the other hand, if LDL cholesterol is ≥160 mg/dL, drug therapy can be considered to achieve an LDL cholesterol <130 mg/dL; the primary aim is to reduce long-term risk. Cost-effectiveness is marginal, but drug therapy can be justified to slow development of coronary atherosclerosis and to reduce long-term risk for CHD.

4 Lower-Risk Patients: 0–1 Risk Factor

Most persons with 0–1 risk factor have a 10-year risk <10%. They are managed according to Table 4. The goal for LDL cholesterol in this risk category is <160 mg/dL. The primary aim of therapy is to reduce long-term risk. First-line therapy is TLC. If after 3 months of TLC the LDL cholesterol is <160 mg/dL, TLC is continued. However, if LDL cholesterol is 160–189 mg/dL after an adequate trial of TLC, drug therapy is optional depending on clinical judgment. Factors favoring use of drugs include: (1) a severe single risk factor (heavy cigarette smoking, poorly controlled hypertension, strong family history of premature CHD, or very low HDL cholesterol); (2) multiple life-habit risk factors and emerging risk factors (if measured); (3) 10-year risk approaching 10% (if measured). If LDL cholesterol is ≥190 mg/dL despite TLC, drug therapy should be considered to achieve the LDL goal of <160 mg/dL. The purpose of using LDL-lowering drugs in persons with 0–1 risk factor and elevated LDL cholesterol (≥160 mg/dL) is to slow the development of coronary atherosclerosis, which will reduce long-term risk. This aim may conflict with cost-effectiveness considerations; thus, clinical judgment is required in selection of persons for drug therapy, although a strong case can be made for using drugs when LDL cholesterol remains ≥190 mg/dL after TLC. For persons whose LDL cholesterol levels are already below goal levels upon first encounter, instructions for appropriate changes in life habits, periodic follow-up, and control of other risk factors are needed.

B Metabolic Risk Factors (Metabolic Syndrome)

1 Atherogenic Dyslipidemia

Elevations of triglycerides and low levels of high-density lipoprotein (HDL) are common in overweight/obese patients. They are especially common when patients have other risk factors of the metabolic syndrome (4–6). ATP III classification of serum triglycerides is shown in Table 8. In patients with atherogenic dyslipidemia [(triglyceride ≥150 mg/dL, small LDL particles, and low HDL cholesterol (<40 mg/dL)], a three-part ther-

Table 8 ATP III Classification of Serum Triglycerides (mg/dL)

<150	Normal
150–199	Borderline high
200–499	High
≥500	Very high

apeutic strategy is required. First, the LDL cholesterol goal should be achieved (Table 6). Second, underlying risk factors—overweight/obesity and physical inactivity—should be treated as described later in this chapter. And third, consideration can be given to treatment of atherogenic dyslipidemia with drug therapy, particularly if lipid levels remain abnormal after an effort to achieve significant weight reduction. For patients who have high triglycerides (200–499 mg/dL), a secondary goal of cholesterol-lowering therapy is non-HDL cholesterol (total cholesterol minus HDL cholesterol). Non-HDL cholesterol consists of LDL + VLDL cholesterol. When patients have a triglyceride level in the range of 200–499 mg/dL, the secondary goal of therapy is a non-HDL cholesterol level of 30 mg/dL above the LDL goal (Table 9). In some patients, the non-HDL cholesterol goal can be achieved by statin therapy, because statins lower both LDL cholesterol and VLDL cholesterol. Alternatively, a statin can be combined with either a fibrate or nicotinic acid. The use of combined drug therapy is particularly attractive when the HDL cholesterol level is low. Finally, it should be noted that when triglyceride levels are >500 mg/dL, the primary goal becomes to lower triglycerides to prevent the development of acute pancreatitis. The favored drug in this case is a fibrate (gemfibrozil or fenofibrate). Once the triglycerides are reduced to <500 mg/dL, consideration can then be given to adding an LDL-lowering drug. For patients with triglyceride >500 mg/dL, statin therapy is not indicated as the first drug; it will not effectively lower triglyceride levels.

2   Raised Blood Pressure

The National High Blood Pressure Education Program (NHBPEP) also recommends that lifestyle changes should be first-line therapy for elevated blood pressure. Recommendations for blood pressure are described in the JNC VI report (24). These recommendations have been amplified recently by reports on the efficacy of the DASH diet for reducing blood pressure (25). This diet resembles that for cholesterol control, but places special emphasis on increased intakes of fruits and vegetables,

higher potassium consumption, low sodium intakes, and alcohol restriction. Lifestyle therapies for blood pressure control also emphasize weight reduction and increased physical activity. All of these dietary recommendations apply equally well to patients with diabetes. Although the first-line approach to controlling elevated blood pressure is through lifestyle changes, many patients with high blood pressure will also require blood pressure–lowering drugs. Fortunately, a large number of safe and effective drugs are available for treatment of elevated blood pressure. It has been estimated that about 60 million Americans have high blood pressure, and a large fraction of these are overweight and have the metabolic syndrome. The magnitude of this problem thus is evident. Effective treatment of high blood pressure is required to reduce risk for stroke as well as heart attack.

3   Insulin Resistance, Impaired Fasting Glucose, and Type 2 Diabetes

Insulin resistance is present in most persons with the metabolic syndrome. Some investigators believe that insulin resistance is the underlying cause of the metabolic syndrome (26,27). In the final analysis, however, the causes of insulin resistance are also the causes of the metabolic syndrome (3). These include genetic predisposition, overweight/obesity, and physical inactivity. A genetic predisposition to insulin resistance appears to reside in abnormalities in the insulin-signaling pathway. Overweight/obesity and physical inactivity further impair insulin signaling. Treatment of the underlying causes of the metabolic syndrome thus is synonymous with "treatment of insulin resistance." Primary clinical therapy includes weight reduction and increased physical activity. Both have been shown to reduce insulin resistance and to mitigate the risk factors of the metabolic syndrome. In addition, there is a growing interest in the use of drugs to modify insulin resistance and to

Table 9 Comparison of LDL Cholesterol and Non-HDL Cholesterol Goals for Three Risk Categories

Risk category	LDL goal (mg/dL)	Non-HDL goal (mg/dL)
CHD and CHD risk equivalent (10-year risk for CHD >20%)	<100	<130
Multiple (2+) risk factors and 10-year risk ≤20%	<130	<160
0–1 Risk factor	<160	<190

reduce risk accompanying the metabolic syndrome. One class of drugs includes the glitazones, which are peroxisome proliferator–activated receptor-gamma (PPAR-γ) agonists. These drugs may have several actions including suppression of release of nonesterified fatty acids (NEFAs) by adipose tissue (28). Although these agents are promising, they are associated with some side effects that at present limit their use to treatment of patients with clinical type 2 diabetes. They may, however, be a prototype for newer agents that are both more effective and safer and can be used to reduce insulin resistance in patients with the metabolic syndrome and who do not have frank diabetes. Metformin is another drug that reduces insulin resistance, and some workers contend that it may be useful in some forms of insulin resistance, e.g., polycystic ovary syndrome (29,30).

A borderline-high glucose [impaired fasting glucose (110–126 mg/dL)] is commonly associated with insulin resistance and the metabolic syndrome. Patients with borderline elevations of glucose are at increased risk for both cardiovascular disease and type 2 diabetes. The goal in management of overweight or obese patients with impaired fasting glucose is twofold: to reduce risk for cardiovascular disease, and to delay the onset of diabetes. Therapeutic approaches to reduce insulin resistance may help to mitigate *all* of the risk factors of the metabolic syndrome and thus reduce the risk for cardiovascular disease. First-line therapies are weight reduction and increased physical activity. Therefore, all overweight/obese persons with impaired fasting glucose should be encouraged to lose weight and exercise more. One of the most important aims in the medical management of obese persons is to prevent the onset of adult-onset (type 2) diabetes.

A recent study carried out and completed by the National Institute of Diabetes and Digestive and Kidney Diseases (NIDDK) examined whether dietary or drug therapy can prevent the conversion of impaired fasting glucose (IFG) into type 2 diabetes. The trial was the Diabetes Prevention Program (DPP), a major clinical trial comparing diet and exercise to treatment with metformin in 3234 people with impaired glucose tolerance, a condition that often precedes diabetes (31,32). The results of this study have recently been summarized online, although they have not been published (http://www.hhs.gov/news/press/2001pres/20010808a.html). Participants randomly assigned to intensive lifestyle intervention reduced their risk of getting type 2 diabetes by 58%. On average, this group maintained their physical activity at 30 min/d, usually with walking or other moderate intensity exercise, and lost 5–7% of

their body weight. Participants randomized to treatment with metformin reduced their risk of getting type 2 diabetes by 31%. Of the 3234 participants enrolled in the DPP, 45% are from minority groups that suffer disproportionately from type 2 diabetes: African-American, Hispanic-Americans, Asian-Americans, Pacific Islanders, and American Indians. The trial also recruited other groups known to be at higher risk for type 2 diabetes, including individuals age 60 and older, women with a history of gestational diabetes, and people with a first-degree relative with type 2 diabetes.

The use of drugs that reduce insulin resistance is particularly attractive for patients with borderline elevations of plasma glucose. It is possible that such drugs will forestall the development of type 2 diabetes. In fact, the same NIH study mentioned above indicated that one such drug, metformin, will reduce the number of overweight persons who actually become diabetic. This study also started off with another drug, troglitazone, but hepatotoxicity led to discontinuation of this arm of the study. Other "glitazones" that are not hepatotoxic might be employed as an alternative to troglitazone for prevention of type 2 diabetes in patients with borderline-high glucose. These drugs are currently being used to treat the high blood glucose of some patients with established diabetes, but at present they are not approved for prevention of diabetes.

When the fasting plasma glucose exceeds 126 mg/dL on multiple measurements, a diagnosis of type 2 diabetes can be made. At this stage risk for cardiovascular disease, particularly CHD, is markedly increased. ATP III defined diabetes, especially type 2 diabetes, as a CHD risk equivalent. In patients with diabetes, the LDL cholesterol goal is a level < 100 mg/dL. The goal for blood pressure control is a level < 130/85 mm Hg. The American Diabetes Association provides recommendations for control of plasma glucose (33). If possible, the hemoglobin A1c level should be kept < 7%. One important approach to control of plasma glucose is to initiate weight reduction and increased physical activity. Thus, therapeutic lifestyle changes, as outlined in this chapter, should be employed in all patients with type 2 diabetes.

4 Prothrombotic State

A tendency to form blood clots, which can result in coronary thrombosis (heart attack), is characteristic of the metabolic syndrome. Obese people are also more likely to have deep-vein thrombosis. The physician must decide whether to start chronic and low-dose aspirin therapy in patients with the metabolic syndrome. If patients are properly selected, they can achieve a significant reduction in risk for heart attack and stroke (34).

5 Proinflammatory State

Obese persons also have a tendency to chronic inflammation in the arteries, causing plaque buildup and heart attack. There are no proven ways to reduce this chronic inflammation. However, recent research strongly suggests that high intakes of vitamin E will reduce inflammation (35). Because of this result, it may be advisable to prescribe vitamin E for obese persons with the metabolic syndrome; however, benefit has yet to be proven through large, controlled clinical trials.

VIII UNDERLYING RISK FACTORS: OVERWEIGHT/OBESITY AND PHYSICAL INACTIVITY

These risk factors will be considered together because they are closely intertwined. In particular, management of physical inactivity is one therapy for obesity. Approaches to management of overweight/obesity including the following:

    Energy-restricted diets
    Increased physical activity
    Behavior modification
    Pharmacotherapy
    Surgical therapy

The first three are standard therapies. Pharmacotherapy and surgical therapy are reserved for special cases. They are used mainly for more severe forms of obesity, particularly to control comorbidities. Theoretically, they could be considered for patients with type 2 diabetes, although they have not been thoroughly evaluated in such patients. The following approach to weight loss in overweight/obese persons at risk for cardiovascular disease or type 2 diabetes is taken in large part from recommendations of the OEI report (1,2).

A Energy-Restricted Diets

A decrease in energy intake is the most important dietary component of weight loss and maintenance. Low-calorie diets often reduce total body weight by an average of 8% over a period of 6 months. Included in this average are individuals who did not lose weight; thus a 10% loss is feasible. A decrease of 500–1000

kcal/d will produce a weight loss 1–2 lbs/week, and a decrease of 300–500 kcal/d, 1/2–1 lb/wk.

The weight loss component of dietary therapy consists mainly in instructing patients on how to consume fewer calories The key is a moderate reduction in caloric intake. This will achieve a slow but progressive weight loss. Caloric intake need be reduced only enough to maintain the desired weight. At this caloric intake, excess weight will gradually vanish. In practice, somewhat greater caloric deficits are generally used during active weight loss. Recommended dietary therapy for weight loss in overweight patients is a low-calorie diet (1000–1800 kcal/d). The low-calorie diet should be distinguished from a very low calorie diet (250–800 kcal/d); Very low calorie diets have generally failed to achieve and maintain weight loss over the long term. In fact, clinical trials reveal that low-calorie diets are as effective as very low calorie diets for producing weight loss after 1 year. Although more weight is initially lost with very low calorie diets, more is usually regained. Importantly, rapid weight reduction fails to allow for gradual acquisition of new eating behavior. Slower weight loss allows more time to adjust eating habits.

Follow-up of very low calorie diets reveal that patients are at increased risk of cholesterol gallstones. Low-calorie diets are more likely to be successful if a patient's food preferences are included. Certainly all of the recommended dietary allowances should be met, even if a dietary supplement is needed. During low-calorie diet therapy, educational efforts should focus on the following topics: energy value of different foods; food composition—fats, carbohydrates (including dietary fiber), and proteins; reading nutrition labels to determine caloric content and food composition; new habits of purchasing (preference to low-calorie) foods; food preparation and avoiding adding high-calorie ingredients during cooking (e.g., fats and oils); avoiding overconsumption of high-calorie foods (both high-fat and high-carbohydrate foods); maintain adequate water intake; reducing portion sizes; and limiting alcohol consumption.

The rate of weight loss generally diminishes after 6 months. Behavior therapy is helpful in addition to low-calorie diets. Frequent clinical visits during initial weight reduction will facilitate reaching the goals of therapy. During active weight loss, visits of once per month or more often with a health professional helps to promote weight reduction. Weekly group meetings are low cost, and can contribute to favorable behavior changes. Adequate time must be made available to convey information, to reinforce behavioral and dietary messages, and to monitor the patient's response.

B Increased Physical Activity

An increase in physical activity promotes weight loss through increased expenditure of energy and possibly through inhibition of food intake. Physical activity also helps to maintain a desirable weight and to reduce CHD risk beyond that produced by weight reduction alone. Several experts contend that a decrease in the amount of energy expended for work, transportation, and personal chores is a major cause of obesity in the United States. They note that total caloric intake has not increased over the last few decades; instead, the caloric imbalance leading to overweight and obesity is the result of a substantial decrease in physical activity and, consequently, a decrease in daily energy expenditure. This hypothesis is intriguing but not proven. Regardless, increased regular physical activity is the way to achieve this goal of augmenting daily energy expenditure.

Increased physical activity improves cardiorespiratory fitness, with or without weight loss. The latter improves the quality of life in overweight patients by improving mood, self-esteem, and physical function in daily activities. Physical activity reduces elevated levels of CVD risk factors, including blood pressure and triglycerides, increases HDL cholesterol, and improves glucose tolerance with or without weight loss. Furthermore, the more active an individual is, the lower the risk for CVD morbidity and mortality, and diabetes. Physical activity apparently has a favorable effect on distribution of body fat. Several studies showed an inverse association between energy expenditure through physical activity and several indicators of body fat distribution. Only a few randomized controlled trials that have tested the effect of physical activity on weight loss measured waist circumference. In some (but not all) studies, physical activity was found to produce only modest weight loss and decreased waist circumference.

Many people live sedentary lives, have little training or skills in physical activity, and are difficult to motivate toward increasing their activity. For these reasons, starting a physical activity regimen may require supervision for many people. The need to avoid injury during physical activity is high. Extremely obese persons may need to start with simple exercises that can gradually be intensified. A decision must be made whether exercise testing for cardiopulmonary disease is needed before starting physical activity regimen. This decision should be based on a patient's age, symptoms, and concomitant risk factors.

For most obese persons, physical activity should be initiated slowly. Initial activities may be walking or swimming at a slow pace. Gradually, the patient may engage in more strenuous activities, such as fitness walking, cycling, rowing, cross-country skiing, aerobic dancing, and rope jumping. Jogging provides a high-intensity aerobic exercise. If jogging is recommended, the patient's ability to do this must first be assessed because it can cause orthopedic injuries. Competitive sports, such as tennis and volleyball, can motivate people to exercise, but care must be taken to avoid injury, especially in older people. Because amounts of activity are functions of duration, intensity, and frequency, the same amounts of activity can be obtained in longer sessions of moderately intense activities (such as brisk walking) as in shorter sessions of more strenuous activities (such as running). Daily walking is one good form of exercise, particularly those who are overweight or obese. Its helpful to start by walking 10 min 3 days a week, and can build to 30–45 min of more intense walking at least 5 days a week. With this exercise, an additional 100–200 calories per day of physical activity can be used. Although other forms of physical activity are acceptable, walking is particularly attractive because of its safety and accessibility.

Reducing sedentary time is another approach to increasing activity. Patients also should be encouraged to build physical activities into their lives. They should consider leaving public transportation one stop before the usual one, parking farther than usual from work or shopping, walking up stairs instead of taking elevators or escalators, gardening, and walking a dog every day. Of course, attention should be given to exercising in safe areas, e.g., community parks, gyms, pools, health clubs, an area of the home perhaps outfitted with a stationary bicycle or a treadmill. Helpful hints are planning exercise in advance, budgeting necessary time, and documenting duration and intensity of exercise.

C Behavior Therapy

Behavioral strategies help to reinforce changes in diet and physical activity. Without new habits, long-term weight reduction is unlikely to succeed. Most people unfortunately return to baseline weights without continued behavior modification. Learning how to include behavior modification in weight reduction therapy is essential. Behavior therapy is designed to permanently alter eating and activity habits.

Behavior therapy is based on the following principles: (1) by changing eating and physical activity habits, it is possible to change body weight; (2) patterns of eating and physical activity are learned behaviors that can be modified; and (3) to change these patterns over the long term, the environment must be changed. Behavior therapies are designed to promote compliance with dietary therapy and/or increased physical activity; they are important components of weight loss therapy.

Various strategies of behavioral therapy can be employed. Therapies can be applied either on an individual basis or in groups. Group therapy is less expensive. Included in behavorial therapy are self-monitoring of eating and exercise, and objectifying one's own behavior through observation and recording. Patients should learn to record amounts and types of food consumed, the caloric values, and nutrient composition. Record keeping will add insight to personal behavior. Patients should record time, place, and feelings related to eating and physical activity. The following lists several components of behavioral therapy.

1. *Stress management*. Stress can trigger overeating that can be countered by stress management. Stress control employs coping strategies, meditation, and relaxation techniques.

2. *Stimulus control*. High-risk situations that promote incidental eating should be identified. Obese patients can learn to shop carefully for healthy foods, keep high-calorie foods out of the house, limit the times and places of eating, and consciously avoid situations in which overeating occurs.

3. *Problem solving*. Self-correction of problems includes identifying weight-related problems, generating possible solutions and choosing one, planning and implementing the healthier alternative, and evaluating the outcome of possible behavioral changes. Patients should reevaluate setbacks in behavior and learn from them.

4. *Contingency management*. Rewards for specific actions can help to change behavior. These rewards can either be verbal, social, or tangible (e.g., monetary). And they can come from the professional team or from the patients themselves.

5. *Cognitive restructuring*. Unrealistic goals, inaccurate beliefs, and self-defeating thoughts and feelings often stand in the way of successful weight reduction.

6. *Social support*. A strong system of social support is an important component of weight loss therapy. Professionals should recruit family members, friends, or colleagues for assistance. Weight reduction support groups also can be used. A restructuring of family eating habits can also assist in therapy directed toward individuals. (Often, more than one family member is overweight, and thus several persons in the family may benefit from a modification of family eating habits.)

D   Weight Reduction Pharmacotherapy

The purpose of weight loss and weight maintenance is to reduce health risks. If weight is regained, health risks increase once more. The majority of persons who lose weight regain it, so the challenge to the patient and the practitioner is to maintain the weight loss. Because of the tendency to regain weight after weight loss, the use of long-term medication to aid in the treatment of obesity may be indicated in some carefully selected patients.

One weight loss drug is sibutramine. It has norepinephrine and serotonin effects. Another new agent, orlistat, has a different mechanism of action, the blockage of fat absorption. Very few trials longer than 6 months have been done with any drug. These drugs are effective but modest in their ability to produce weight loss. Net weight loss attributable to drugs generally has been reported to be in the range of 2–10 kg (4.4–22 lb), although some patients lose significantly more weight. It is not possible to predict how much weight an individual may lose. Most of the weight loss usually occurs in the first 6 months of therapy.

With sibutramine there is a tendency for increased blood pressure and pulse rate. People with a history of high blood pressure, CHD, congestive heart failure, arrhythmias, or stroke should not take sibutramine, and all patients taking the medication should have their blood pressure monitored on a regular basis. With orlistat, there is a possible decrease in the absorption of fat-soluble vitamins; overcoming this may require vitamin supplementation.

Given that adverse events may occur with drug therapy, it seems wise, until further safety data are available, to use weight loss drugs cautiously. Furthermore, drugs should be used only as part of a comprehensive program that includes behavior therapy, diet, and physical activity. Appropriate monitoring for side effects must be continued while drugs are part of the regimen. Patients will need to return for follow-up in 2–4 weeks, then monthly for 3 months, and then every 3 months for the first year after starting the medication. Drugs should be used only in the context of a long-term treatment strategy.

E   Weight Loss Surgery

Surgery is one option for weight reduction for some patients with severe and resistant obesity. The aim of surgery is to reduce net food intake. Generally weight loss surgery should be reserved for patients with severe obesity, in whom other therapies have failed, and who are suffering from the complications of obesity. Surgical interventions commonly used include gastroplasty, gastric partitioning, and gastric bypass. Treatment of clinically severe obesity involves an effort to create a caloric deficit sufficient to result in weight loss and reduction of weight-associated risk factors or comorbidities. Surgical approaches can result in substantial weight loss, i.e., from 50 kg (110 lb) to as much as 100 kg (220 lb) over a period of 6 months to 1 year. Compared to other interventions available, surgery has produced the longest period of sustained weight loss. Assessing both perioperative risk and long-term complications is important and requires assessing the risk/benefit ratio in each case. Patients whose BMI is ≥40 kg/m^2 are potential candidates for surgery because obesity severely impairs the quality of their lives. Less severely obese patients (BMIs between 35 and 39.9 kg/m^2) may also be considered for surgery if they have comorbid conditions (e.g., sleep apnea, uncontrolled type 2 diabetes). In one study, patients with diabetes undergoing the surgical procedure had a decrease in mortality rate for each year of follow-up compared to nonsurgery patients. The major limitation of gastric surgery for obesity is the occurrence of side effects which are various and occur either in the perioperative period or long term.

IX SUMMARY

Obesity is emerging as one of the most serious health problems both in the United States and worldwide. It is the major reason why cardiovascular disease will become the No. 1 killer of the 21st century and why the prevalence of diabetes threatens to triple over the next 30 years. Obesity is thus a health problem of the first magnitude and deserves increased attention in both public health and medical fields. Except for patients with severe obesity in whom excess body fat directly interferes with bodily functions (e.g., mobility or breathing), overweight/obesity should be viewed as an underlying risk factor for chronic diseases. Foremost among these are cardiovascular disease and diabetes. Thus the clinical approach to overweight/obese patients requires that excess body weight be considered in the context of all risk factors. The intensity of clinical management of patients thus depends on the total risk profiles. This maxim holds for management of overweight/obesity as well as for other risk factors. Nonetheless, early intervention on underlying risk factors (overweight/obesity and physical inactivity) may forestall the development of other risk factors later in life.

REFERENCES

1. Executive summary of the clinical guidelines on the identification, evaluation, and treatment of overweight and obesity in adults. Arch Intern Med 1998; 158(17):1855–1867.
2. Clinical guidelines on the identification, evaluation, and treatment of overweight and obesity in adults—the evidence report. National Institutes of Health. Obes Res 1998; 6(suppl 2):51S–209S.
3. Grundy SM. Metabolic complications of obesity. Endocrine 2000; 13(2):155–165.
4. Grundy SM. Hypertriglyceridemia, insulin resistance, and the metabolic syndrome. Am J Cardiol 1999; 83(9B):25F–29F.
5. Grundy SM. Hypertriglyceridemia, atherogenic dyslipidemia, and the metabolic syndrome. Am J Cardiol 1998; 81(4A):18B–25B.
6. Grundy SM. Small LDL. atherogenic dyslipidemia, and the metabolic syndrome. Circulation 1997; 95(1):1–4.
7. Haffner SM, Stern MP, Hazuda HP, Mitchell BD, Patterson JK. Cardiovascular risk factors in confirmed prediabetic individuals. Does the clock for coronary heart disease start ticking before the onset of clinical diabetes? JAMA 1990; 263(21):2893–2898.
8. Executive Summary of the Third Report of the National Cholesterol Education Program (NCEP) Expert Panel on Detection, Evaluation, and Treatment of High Blood Cholesterol in Adults (Adult Treatment Panel III). JAMA 2001; 285(19):2486–2497.
9. Cappuccio FP. Ethnicity and cardiovascular risk: variations in people of African ancestry and South Asian origin. J Hum Hypertens 1997; 11(9):571–576.
10. Styne DM. Childhood an adolescent obesity. Prevalence and significance. Pediatr Clin North Am 2001; 48(4):823–854.
11. Robinson TN. Television viewing and childhood obesity. Pediatr Clin North Am 2001; 48:1017–1025.
12. Dietz WH, Gortmaker SL. Preventing obesity in children and adolescents. Annu Rev Public Health 2001; 22:337–353.
13. DiPietro L. Physical activity in the prevention of obesity: current evidence and research issues. Med Sci Sports Exerc 1999; 31(11 suppl):S542–S546.
14. Schoeller DA. Balancing energy expenditure and body weight. Am J Clin Nutr 1998; 68(4):956S–961S.
15. Seidell JC. Obesity in Europe: scaling an epidemic. Int J Obes Relat Metab Disord 1995; 19(suppl 3):S1–S4.
16. Westerterp KR. Daily physical activity, aging and body composition. J Nutr Health Aging 2000; 4(4):239–242.
17. Seidell JC, Visscher TL. Body weight and weight change and their health implications for the elderly. Eur J Clin Nutr 2000; 54(suppl 3):S33–S39.
18. Ryan AS. Insulin resistance with aging: effects of diet and exercise. Sports Med 2000; 30(5):327–346.

19. Barzilai N, Gupta G. Interaction between aging and syndrome X: new insights on the pathophysiology of fat distribution. Ann NY Acad Sci 1999; 892:58–72.

20. Paolisso G, Tagliamonte MR, Rizzo MR, Giugliano D. Advancing age and insulin resistance: new facts about an ancient history. Eur J Clin Invest 1999; 29(9):758–769.

21. Nawaz H, Katz DL. American College of Preventive Medicine Practice Policy statement. Weight management counseling of overweight adults. Am J Prev Med 2001; 21(1):73–78.

22. Epstein S, Sivarajan Froelicher ES, Froelicher VF, Pina IL, Pollock ML. Statement on exercise: benefits and recommendations for physical activity programs for all Americans. Circulation 1996; 94:857–862.

23. Blair SN, Cheng Y, Holder JS. Is physical activity or physical fitness more important in defining health benefits? Med Sci Sports Exerc 2001; 33(6 suppl):S379–S399.

24. The sixth report of the Joint National Committee on prevention, detection, evaluation, and treatment of high blood pressure. Arch Intern Med 1997; 157(21):2413–2446.

25. Sacks FM, Svetkey LP, Vollmer WM, Appel LJ, Bray GA, Harsha D, Obarzanek E, Conlin PR, Miller ERIII, Simons-Morton DG, Karanja N, Lin PH. Effects on blood pressure of reduced dietary sodium and the Dietary Approaches to Stop Hypertension (DASH) diet. DASH-Sodium Collaborative Research Group. N Engl J Med 2001; 344(1):3–10.

26. Reaven GM. Insulin resistance: a chicken that has come to roost. Ann NY Acad Sci 1999; 892:45–57.

27. DeFronzo RA. Insulin resistance: a multifaceted syndrome responsible for NIDDM, obesity, hypertension, dyslipidaemia and atherosclerosis. Neth J Med 1997; 50(5):191–197.

28. Lebovitz HE, Banerji MA. Insulin resistance and its treatment by thiazolidinediones. Recent Prog Horm Res 2001; 56:265–294.

29. Norman RJ, Kidson WJ, Cuneo RC, Zacharin MR. Metformin and intervention in polycystic ovary syndrome. Endocrine Society of Australia, the Australian Diabetes Society and the Australian Paediatric Endocrine Group. Med J Aust 2001; 174(11):580–583.

30. Kowalska I, Kinalski M, Straczkowski M, Wolczyski S, Kinalska I. Insulin, leptin, IGF-I and insulin-dependent protein concentrations after insulin-sensitizing therapy in obese women with polycystic ovary syndrome. Eur J Endocrinol 2001; 144(5):509–515.

31. Diabetes Prevention Program. Design and methods for a clinical trial in the prevention of type 2 diabetes. Diabetes Care 1999; 22(4):623–634.

32. Diabetes Prevention Program. Baseline charcteristics of the randomized cohort. Diabetes Care 2000; 23(11):1619–1629.

33. American Diabetes Association. The Diabetes Desk Professional Edition: How to Control and Manage Diabetes Mellitus, 2001.

34. American Diabetes Association. Aspirin therapy in diabetes. Diabetes Care 1997; 20(11):1772–1773.

35. Devaraj S, Jialal I. Alpha tocopherol supplementation decreases serum C-reactive protein and monocyte interleukin-6 levels in normal volunteers and type 2 diabetic patients. Free Radic Biol Med 2000; 29(8):790–792.

8

Obesity and Eating Disorders

Susan Z. Yanovski

National Institute of Diabetes and Digestive and Kidney Diseases, National Institutes of Health, Bethesda, Maryland, U.S.A.

Albert J. Stunkard

University of Pennsylvania School of Medicine, Philadelphia, Pennsylvania, U.S.A.

I INTRODUCTION

Eating disorders are psychophysiological disturbances characterized by abnormalities in affects, cognitions, and behaviors regarding food intake and body image. While predominantly affecting adolescent and young adult women, these illnesses affect individuals of both sexes and a wide range of ages. Eating disorders are also found across the spectrum of weights, from the emaciated individual with anorexia nervosa to the severely obese patient with binge eating disorder. Left untreated, eating disorders can result in severe functional disability, or even death, in individuals at an otherwise healthy time of life.

Disordered eating may manifest itself through dietary restriction, binge eating, or both. Other inappropriate compensatory behaviors used to control weight include vomiting, abuse of diuretics, laxatives, anorexiant medications, or thyroid hormones, and excessive exercise.

Binge eating is defined as eating, in a discrete period of time (e.g., within any 2-hr period), an amount of food that is definitely larger than most people would eat in a similar period of time *plus* a sense of lack of control over eaing during the episode (e.g., a feeling that one cannot stop eating or control what or how much one is eating (1). Note that both consumption of an objectively large

amount of food and a sense of loss of control are necessary for the definition of a binge episode. Loss of control in the absence of consumption of a large amount of food (e.g., a self-described "binge" consisting of two cookies) is considered a "subjective" bulimic episode. Conversely, an objectively large amount of food consumed without a concomitant feeling of loss of control is considered an "objective" overeating episode (2).

II DIAGNOSTIC CHARACTERISTICS

Anorexia nervosa is characterized by refusal to maintain a normal body weight, along with a fear of gaining weight. Diagnostic criteria for anorexia nervosa are shown in Table 1. The Diagnostic and Statistical Manual of Mental Disorders, 4th Edition (DSM-IV) (1) criteria divide anorexia into the restricting and binge-eating/purging subtypes. Approximately 50% of patients with anorexia nervosa experience binge eating and/or purging at some point in their illness (3).

Bulimia nervosa is characterized by frequent episodes of binge eating accompanied by emotional distress, plus the presence of frequent compensatory behaviors to avoid weight gain (Table 1) (1). The DSM-IV further classifies patients as belonging to the purging or nonpurging subtypes. Purging is common in bulimia nervosa, and

Table 1 Diagnostic Criteria for Eating Disorders

Anorexia nervosa
  A. Refusal to maintain body weight at or above a minimally normal weight for age and height
  B. Intense fear of gaining weight or becoming fat, even though underweight
  C. Disturbance in the way in which one's body or shape is experienced
  D. In postmenarchal females, amenorrhea
  E. Type:
      Restricting type
      Binge-eating/purging type
Bulimia nervosa
  A. Recurrent episodes of binge eating
  B. Recurrent inappropriate compensatory behaviors to prevent weight gain
  C. The binge eating and inappropriate compensatory behaviors both occur, on average, at least twice a week for 3 months
  D. Self-evaluation is unduly influenced by body weight and shape
  E. Type:
      Purging type
      Nonpurging type
Binge eating disorder[a]
  A. Recurrent episodes of binge eating
  B. The binge eating episodes are associated with at least three behavioral indicators of loss of control
  C. Marked distress regarding binge eating
  D. The binge eating occurs, on average, at least 2 days a week for 6 months
  E. The binge eating is not associated with the regular use of inappropriate compensatory behaviors and does not occur
     exclusively during the course of anorexia nervosa or bulimia nervosa
Night eating syndrome[b]
  A. Morning anorexia, even if the subject eats breakfast
  B. Evening hyperphagia; at least 50% of the daily caloric intake is consumed in snacks after the last evening meal
  C. Awakenings at least three nights a week
  D. Frequent consumption of snacks during the awakenings
  E. The pattern occurs for a period of at least 3 months

---

[a] Diagnostic criteria for binge eating disorder are listed in the Appendix of the DSM-IV as an example of eating disorder, not otherwise specified.
[b] Criteria proposed by Birketvedt et al. (7).
Source: Ref. 1.

includes vomiting (80–90%) and laxative use (38–75%) (4,5). Less common forms of purging include diuretic abuse, abuse of thyroid hormone or anorexiant medications, induction of vomiting through use of ipecac, and use of enemas. Diabetics have been known to withhold insulin to avoid weight gain (6).

Binge eating disorder is an eating disorder characterized by frequent episodes of binge eating accompanied by emotional distress, but without the regular use of compensatory behaviors (Table 1). Binge eating disorder is listed in the DSM-IV in an appendix as an example of an Eating Disorder Not Otherwise Specified (EDNOS). A diagnosis of EDNOS is also used for disordered eating that does not meet criteria for one of the established eating disorders (e.g., purging only once weekly, weight loss without amenorrhea, etc.).

Night Eating Syndrome is characterized by morning anorexia, evening and nighttime overeating, sleep onset and sleep maintenance insomnia, and the consumption of high carbohydrate snacks during many of the awakenings. It was described recently in detail by Birketvedt et al. (7). Diagnostic criteria for this syndrome are evolving, and it is not included as a diagnostic category in the DSM-IV. Proposed clinical criteria are shown in Table 1.

III EPIDEMIOLOGY

Anorexia nervosa, as categorized by the DSM-IV, is relatively uncommon, affecting 0.5–1% of adolescent and young adult women (8,9), although a much larger percentage experience subthreshold symptoms. Approximately 10% of patients with anorexia nervosa are male (9). There is some evidence that the incidence of anorexia nervosa is increasing among adolescents, but not among adults (10,11). Although most individuals with anorexia nervosa are adolescents or young adults, onset has been reported in prepubertal children and postmenopausal women (12). It is more common in industrialized societies where food is plentiful and thinness is valued, but anorexia nervosa is found in individuals from all cultures and social strata (13,14).

The prevalence of bulimia nervosa has been estimated at 1–3% of high school and college-age women (8,9), although a much greater percentage engage in bulimic behaviors, such as binge eating and/or purging, that are not of sufficient frequency or duration to meet criteria for the disorder. Five percent to 15% of patients with bulimia nervosa are male (15–17), and it is more frequent in homosexual men (18 and athletes who must "make weight" for competition, such as wrestlers (19). Bulimia nervosa is found in all racial, ethnic, and socioeconomic groups (15,16). A substantial subset of patients with bulimia nervosa have previously met criteria for anorexia nervosa (20).

Binge eating disorder (BED) is the most common eating disorder, affecting < 3% of the general population (21). The prevalence among overweight persons is higher, with increasing prevalence as degree of obesity and intensity of treatment increases. Although initial reports suggested a prevalence of up to 30% of obese individuals seeking specialized treatment, such as very low calorie diet programs (22,23), diagnosis made by clinical interview shows a much lower prevalence, even in clinical populations, in whom the prevalence is generally 10–15% (21). The prevalence of binge eating disorder among severely obese individuals undergoing bariatric surgery, however, is high even when made by clinical interview, and may exceed 50% (9,24,25). Unlike anorexia nervosa and bulimia nervosa, a large proportion of individuals with BED are men, estimated at 40% in the original field studies (22,23). The age at diagnosis of BED is older than that seen in anorexia nervosa or bulimia nervosa, averaging in the mid-to late thirties; however, age of onset of significant binge eating is often a decade or more earlier. An age-matched study of patients with bulimia nervosa and binge eating disorder showed a younger age of onset of binge eating behavior among those with BED (14.3 vs. 19.8 years), although both groups reported first dieting at similar ages (15.0 vs. 16.2 years) (26). In addition, among those with BED, the age of onset of binge eating as well as age at which symptoms met criteria for BED was significantly lower in those whom reported that age of binge eating preceded age of first diet (27).

The night eating syndrome has been reported in 1.5% of the general population (28), and is more common among obese persons than the nonobese. It may also increase with increasing adiposity. Studies have found a prevalence of 8.9% in an obesity clinic (29), 12% of obese patients in a nutrition clinic (30), and 27% among candidates for obesity surgery (28).

IV PATHOPHYSIOLOGY

A Individual and Familial Factors

A number of psychological factors have been described in patients with eating disorders, including difficulties in self-esteem and self-regulation, along with a sense of ineffectiveness and helplessness. Eating disorders, in this view, represent the attempt of the patient to gain control in the arena of eating and weight. Girls who are conflicted about maturation and sexuality are felt to be particularly prone to the development of anorexia nervosa. There are limitations in determining the premorbid psychological factors that may predispose to the development of eating disorders, primary among which is that this information has generally been obtained retrospectively, after the eating disorder has developed. A community-based study found that nonspecific risk factors such as adverse childhood experiences, negative comments about weight and shape, parental depression, and a predisposition towards obesity increased the likelihood of developing BED (31).

B Sociocultural Factors

It has been proposed that "dieting disorders" is a more proper term than "eating disorder" because the underlying essential feature of anorexia nervosa, bulimia nervosa, and associated conditions is the "inappropriate and excessive pursuit of thinness" (32). For individuals with either anorexia nervosa or bulimia nervosa, attempts at weight loss and dietary restriction (often severe) almost invariably precede the development of the significant symptoms of disordered eating. The current cultural milieu, in which thinness, fitness, and body shapes that are impossible for most women to obtain are prized, no doubt contributes to the dissatisfaction with body size and shape that is normative among women. While most women have tried to lose weight, relatively few develop eating disorders, leading some investigators to suggest that dieting may be a "necessary, but insufficient" condition for the development of eating disorders (33). The relationship between dietary restraint and binge eating is complex, and many factors, including the type and degree of dietary restraint, individual psychological and biological predispositions, and the sociocultural milieu, may contribute to binge eating in the susceptible individual.

The link between dieting and the development of disordered eating is even less in binge eating disorder than in anorexia or bulimia nervosa. A recent review of the literature by the National Task Force on the Prevention and Treatment of Obesity concluded that "moderate caloric restriction, in combination with behavioral weight loss treatment does not seem to cause clinically significant binge eating in adults pre-existing binge eating problems and might ameliorate binge eating, and least in the short term, in those reporting recurrent binge eating before treatment" (34). Studies to date have indicated that binge eating precedes or occurs at approximately the same time as first attempts of weight loss in about half of all subjects (22,27,35); however, these studies have the disadvantage of being retrospective. Berkowitz et al. (36) have evaluated obese adolescent girls, many of whom had not previously attempted weight loss, and found a significant percentage who nonetheless reported serious difficulties with binge eating. Some studies suggest that, rather than being "restrained" eaters obese binge eaters exhibit high levels of disinhibition, or loss of control due to affective, pharmacological, or cognitive stimuli (32, 33,35,37–39). Marcus et al. (40) have found that, when compared to bulimia nervosa patients, obese binge eaters report less dietary restraint, but score similarly on other measures of eating disorders psychopathology regarding weight and shape (40). This finding has implications for the modification of treatments developed for bulimia nervosa to address the special needs of non-purging obese binge eaters.

The evidence that dieting plays a causal role in the night eating syndrome is even weaker than in binge eating disorder. Although stress appears to play a role in precipitation night eating, dieting does not appear to contribute to this stress (41).

C Affective Disorders

Affective disorders are common among patients with eating disorders, leading some researchers to postulate that eating disorders are a variant of affective disorders. Comorbid major depression is frequent among patients with eating disorders (42,43), occurring in over half of all patients in some series. In addition, family history of affective disorders is often more frequent among patients than controls. The response of symptoms to antidepressant treatment, in both bulimia nervosa and binge eating disorder, has been proposed as further evidence of this link. However, it is unknown if the

depression seen in bulimia nervosa and binge eating disorder is primary, secondary to the eating disorder, or due to an underlying common pathogenesis. Dysfunction of the serotonergic pathways, which could affect both appetite and mood, has been postulated as one such possible mechanism (44). While depression is common in patients with anorexia nervosa, at least some of these symptoms may be secondary to the accompanying starvation, as similar affective symptoms have been produced in normal volunteers undergoing long-term semistarvation (45). Therefore, the relationship between eating disorders and affective disorders remains unclear. Depression is a prominent feature of the night eating syndrome, and it follows a diurnal course, unlike that of the usual depressive episode. Thus, dysphoria is lowest in the morning and becomes more severe during the afternoon, reaching its peak during the evening hours (7).

D Other Comorbid Psychiatric Conditions

Obsessive-compulsive disorder is reportedly more frequent in both anorexia nervosa and bulimia nervosa (46,47), and some researchers have speculated that disturbances in neurally active substances, such as 5HIAA, brought about by starvation, binge eating, or purging, may contribute to the perpetuation of compulsive behaviors in patients with these disorders (46–49). Among individuals with binge eating disorder, no increase in either obsessive-compulsive disorder or obsessive-compulsive personality disorder has been noted (50). Other anxiety and related disorders, such as generalized anxiety disorder and phobias, are also common in eating disorders (51,52).

Personality disorders involving impulsivity (including borderline personality disorder) are found more frequently in those with eating disorders involving binge eating than among controls, across the weight spectrum. For example, one study found that obese individuals with binge eating disorder have a 14% prevalence of borderline personality disorder versus only 1% of obese individuals without binge eating disorder (50). Avoidant personality disorder has also been reported to be more prevalent among these subjects with than without binge eating disorder (50,53).

Binge eating is also associated with a higher likelihood of substance abuse than is seen in control populations, in the binge eating subtype of anorexia nervosa (54), bulimia nervosa (55), and binge eating disorder (22). Among obese individuals, a family history of substance abuse is more likely among individuals with than without binge eating disorder (54). Similarly, studies of patients with bulimia nervosa and the purging subtype of anorexia nervosa have found increased rates of substance abuse in among relatives of patients compared with controls (56).

To summarize, psychiatric comorbidity is common in patients with eating disorders. Among obese individuals, the presence of binge eating disorder may explain the increased levels of psychopathology previously attributed to the presence of obesity per se (50,52,57).

E   Biological Predisposition

Family and twin data suggest that there may heritable factors that predispose to susceptibility for developing eating disorders (58,59). While there appear to be familial factors involved in the development of anorexia and bulimia nervosa, further study is necessary to sort out the magnitude of additive genetic factors with those of shared environment (60). Studies are currently in progress to identify genetic factors contributing to the pathogenesis of anorexia and bulimia nervosa (61).

Although abnormalities in numerous neuroendocrine and metabolic systems have been described in eating disorders, it is often difficult to sort out the effects of semistarvation or purging behaviors from disturbances that might be primary (62). While many of the metabolic abnormalities seen with eating disorders normalize after recovery, suggesting a state, rather than trait, component (63), some researchers have found persistent abnormalities after recovery from anorexia or bulimia nervosa (46,64,65). Few data are available to support preexisting neuroendocrine or other physiological differences among those who will later develop eating disorders, but the possibility exists that a biological vulnerability to eating disorders interacts with environmental factors to increase the likelihood of their development.

F   Sexual Abuse

The contribution of sexual abuse to the development of eating disorders remains controversial. While some authors have cited sexual abuse as a major causal factor in eating disorders (66), others have found that the prevalence of sexual abuse is no greater in eating disordered patients than in patients being treated for other psychiatric disorders (67). It has been suggested that some types of sexual abuse, such as earlier and more persistent abuse, may predispose to eating disorders (68), and that it is binge eating, rather than dietary restriction, that is associated with sexual abuse (69,70). Although sexual abuse may play a direct role in the

development of eating disorders for some patients, it appears to be a risk factor for psychiatric disorders in general, rather than specific for eating disorders (68).

G   Addiction

Addiction has been postulated to play a role in disordered eating, with some individuals addicted to certain foods or combinations of foods. Although substance abuse and other impulse control disorders are associated with binge eating in some studies, there is no evidence that "addiction" to foods such as refined flour, simple sugars, or carbohydrates occurs or triggers binge episodes (71). An interesting finding, however, is that both lean and obese female binge eaters, women with binge eating disorder, who prefer to binge on foods that are both sweet and high in fat, may decrease their intake of these foods selectively when given naloxone (72). The role of β-endorphins and other endogenous opioids in the development or maintenance of binge eating, while unknown, is intriguing.

V   SIGNS AND SYMPTOMS

Eating disorders are often "hidden disorders" and will not be recognized without gentle probing by the clinician. Both anorexia nervosa and bulimia nervosa, however, are associated with a host of medical complications, affecting virtually every organ system.

A   Anorexia Nervosa

In patients with anorexia nervosa, emaciation will be obvious. Often, the patient is brought to the clinician's attention by the family, who are concerned about weight loss. The patient frequently tries to minimize concerns about her intake and low body weight, and may resort to subterfuge, such as wearing heavy clothing while being weighed.

Although physical complaints are remarkably few given the degree of emaciation (73), patients present with a variety of signs and symptoms referable to low body weight, including constipation, abdominal pain, cold intolerance, hypothermia, hypotension, bradycardia, edema, lanugo, and dry skin (74).

Amenorrhea, as one of the necessary criteria for diagnosis, is present in all anorexic women, but anorexic men also show evidence of a hypogonadal state. Laboratory abnormalities, particularly in patients who purge, are frequent, and include electrolyte abnormalities, elevation of liver enzymes, elevated blood urea

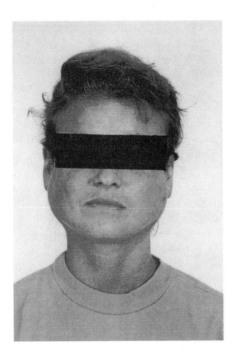

Figure 1 Bilateral parotid gland swelling associated with bulimia nervosa. (From Ref. 151a.)

the most frequent reason for presentation to a general practitioner of the bulimic patient was to request a weight loss diet (82). Other common presenting complaints include gastrointestinal symptoms, such as bloating or constipation, and amenorrhea or irregular cycles (83). Rarely, patients may present with palpitations or cardiac arrhythmias secondary to electrolyte imbalance. Pathognomonic signs in bulimia nervosa include a "chipmunk" cheek appearance, due to non-inflammatory stimulation of the salivary glands, particularly the parotids (84) (Fig. 1). Erosions of the lingual surface of the teeth and multiple dental caries are seen, due to the exposure to acid from repeated vomiting (85). Russell's sign (86) (scarring and abrasions on the dorsum of the hands during self-induced vomiting) can also be seen (Fig. 2). Laboratory abnormalities, which may be frequent in purging patients, include metabolic alkalosis and hypokalemia (87).

Hyperamylasemia is seen in about one-third of actively binge eating/purging patients and is due to elevation of the salivary isoenzyme, secondary to vomiting (73,88). Rare but serious complications of bulimia nervosa include Mallory-Weiss tears of the esophagus due to forceful vomiting, and cardiomyopathy secondary to ipecac abuse.

nitrogen, leukopenia, thrombocytopenia, and normochromic normocytic anemia (73–75). Leptin levels are decreased in patients in anorexia nervosa, consistent with their low fat mass (76).

Anorexia nervosa, with its resultant hypoestrogenemic and hypercotisolemic state, predisposes patients to osteoporosis, which may be severe. The best predictors of bone loss are low body weight, early onset, and long duration of amenorrhea (77,78). The role of estrogen replacement in anorexia nervosa in order to prevent osteoporosis is controversial, with studies yielding mixed results (79,80). The role of bisphosphonates in treating the osteopenia of anorexia nervosa has not been established. Calcium and vitamin D supplementation are recommended (75). Bone density does improve with weight recovery and resumption of menses, although it usually remains significantly below control levels many years later (77,81). Periodic assessment of bone mineral density by dual-energy x-ray absorptiometry is can be helpful in following the patient's fracture risk (75).

B Bulimia Nervosa

Patients with bulimia nervosa frequently show no abnormalities on physical examination. In one study,

C Binge Eating Disorder

Patients with binge eating disorder are frequently obese and may present with obesity-associated disorders. Patients with binge eating disorder are also more likely

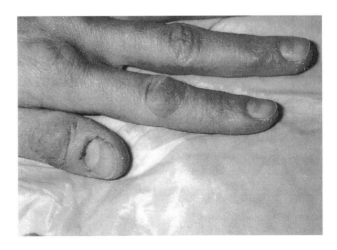

Figure 2 Scarring on the dorsum of the hand due to self-induced vomiting.

than obese nonbinge eaters to present with signs of gastrointestinal disturbance, such as nausea, vomiting, abdominal pain, and bloating (89).

D Night Eating Syndrome

A characteristic circadian neuroendocrine pattern has been observed in a study of the night eating syndrome (7). The presence of elevated 24-hr levels of cortisol provides a biological marker of the stress under which patients are laboring. Blunting of the expected nighttime rise in melatonin and leptin was also found, in intriguing association with the impaired sleep and nighttime snacking of the night eating syndrome.

VI TREATMENT

A Anorexia Nervosa

Anorexia nervosa is treated through a combination of nutritional rehabilitation and psychotherapy, with the goals of weight restoration, development of healthy eating habits, improvement in moods/behaviors, reduction in obsessions with thinness, and amelioration of concomitant physical and psychiatric symptoms (8).

1 Nutritional Rehabilitation

Nutritional rehabilitation is crucial and should be accomplished either prior to or concomitant with psychotherapy. The involvement of a dietician for meal planning is helpful. Refeeding should be slow and cautious, to prevent edema and cardiac failure (90). Use of enteral or parenteral feeding is generally unnecessary, unless life-threatening inanition is present and the patient refuses oral feeding (8). Behavioral modification, in which privileges are tied to specified weight gain, may be useful in the initial stages for promoting increased intake.

2 Psychotherapy

Psychotherapy may be provided individually or in groups. In younger patients with anorexia nervosa, who frequently live with their family of origin, family therapy is also used. Individual psychological therapies include cognitive behavioral psychotherapy, in which faulty cognition regarding eating and weight is examined, and psychodynamic or interpersonal psychotherapy, in which the patient's current interpersonal relationships with others are explored. Cognitive behavioral psychotherapy is described in more detail below.

In patients undergoing inpatient or partial hospitalization, the therapeutic milieu is also an integral part of treatment.

In the current climate of managed care, inpatient treatment is increasingly being replaced by less expensive and less intensive therapies, including outpatient care and partial hospitalization (91). One randomized study has shown good outcomes in anorexic patients assigned to outpatient treatment (92). However, many experts believe that inpatient treatment is preferable for all but the most mild forms of anorexia nervosa (8). While anorexia nervosa is the diagnosis most likely to require hospitalization, there are indications for hospitalization in patients with any of the eating disorders (Table 2).

3 Medications

Medications are less often used in the treatment of anorexia nervosa than in bulimia nervosa. Few medications have proven effective in long-term studies. There has been a recent resurgence of interest in the use of antipsychotic medications in the treatment of anorexia nervosa, particularly the atypical neuroleptics, which often promote weight gain (93,94). However, at this time data on their safety and effectiveness in this population are preliminary. Although antidepressant medications can be useful in patients with concomitant depression, it is generally preferable to reassess mood after nutritional rehabilitation, as semistarvation can produce both cognitive and affective changes. There are some data, however, that fluoxetine may be useful in preventing relapse after weight restoration (95).

To summarize, the role of medication in the treatment of anorexia nervosa is limited at present. While some reports suggest the potential for modest improve-

Table 2 Indications for Hospitalization in Eating Disorders

Medical
  Extreme emaciation (e.g., <70% of ideal body weight)
  Dangerous medical complications (e.g., renal failure,
    hypokalemia, arrhythmias)
  Intercurrent infection
  Suicidal tendencies or attempts
Psychosocial
  Marked family disturbance inaccessible to treatment
  Inability to function at work or school
Psychotherapeutic
  Previous treatment failures
  Nonavailability of specialized treatment in the community
  Failure to respond to optimal outpatient care

ments in selected subgroups of patients with certain medications, more research is needed to further characterize the optimal use of these agents.

B Bulimia Nervosa

Bulimia nervosa is generally treated in an outpatient setting. Both psychotherapy and medication have been shown to be efficacious in the treatment of bulimia nervosa.

1 Cognitive-Behavioral Psychotherapy (CBT)

CBT is the most well-studied psychological treatment for bulimia nervosa and is generally considered first-line treatment for this disorder (96,97). Originally adapted for use in eating disorders by Fairburn, CBT is based on the premise that central to the disorder are maladaptive cognitions regarding the fundamental importance of weight and shape. In this model, the extremes of dietary restraint that are used to control weight lead to compensatory binge eating. Thus, the modification of these abnormal attitudes and behaviors of weight and shape may be expected to ameliorate the consequent dietary restriction, binge eating, and purging. While modifications of the technique are frequent, the original program consisted of time-limited, individual treatment given over 20 weeks (98).

Studies of treatment efficacy show very good short-term outcomes for CBT. Reviews have shown mean reductions in binge eating and purging of from 40% to 97%, with about half of patients, on average, "abstinent" from binge eating or purging at the end of treatment (97). CBT has also been show to produce more rapid improvement in symptoms than nonspecific supportive psychotherapy (99).

2 Interpersonal Psychotherapy (IPT)

IPT has also been shown to improve symptoms in bulimia nervosa. This type of psychotherapy, originally developed for the treatment of depression, has been adapted for the treatment of eating disorders. In contrast to CBT, which focuses on the elimination of dietary restriction and distorted cognitions about weight and shape, IPT focuses on improving negative moods and low self-esteem that may trigger binge eating, through the mastery of social and interpersonal relationships (100). Research suggests that CBT is superior to IPT at 1 year in some measures of treatment effectiveness, including percentage recovered or remitted, or with improved eating attitudes and behaviors (101,102). At longer-term follow-up, however, IPT and CBT appear to have similar effectiveness (102–104).

3 Antidepressant Medications

Antidepressants, including tricyclics, monoamine oxidase (MAO) inhibitors, atypical antidepressants, and selective serotonin reuptake inhibitors (SSRIs), are frequently used in the treatment of bulimia nervosa and have been proven effective in numerous studies (97). MAO inhibitors have the disadvantage of requiring restriction of certain foods, which may be difficult for some bulimic patients. SSRIs, such as fluoxetine, have fewer adverse effects than tricyclics and MAO inhibitors. While some SSRIs, such as fluoxetine and sertraline, don't cause weight gain, and may even cause weight loss, over the short term, weight generally returns to baseline with longer-term (i.e., > 6 months) treatment (105). Fluoxetine is currently FDA approved for the treatment of bulimia nervosa. Bupropion is contraindicated in patients with anorexia or bulimia nervosa because of an increased incidence of seizures (106). While trials with a variety of antidepressant agents of different classes have shown short-term efficacy in reduction of binge eating, there are a number of limitations to these studies. Most were conducted using fixed dosages over relatively short periods of time and involved populations of normal-weight, purging women. Thus, the optimal dose ranges, duration of treatment, and treatment response in the nonpurging bulimic patient are not clear. In a dose response study of fluoxetine for bulimia nervosa, the most effective dose was 60 mg/d, significantly higher than that usually used for depression (107). Both patients with and without a history of depression appear to show similar improvement in bulimic symptoms with antidepressant treatment (97,108).

Antidepressant treatment, while more effective than placebo, is not a "magic bullet." Although antidepressant medications reduce frequency of binge eating in bulimic patients, only ~25% respond with complete abstinence from binge eating/purging (109). In addition, many patients who show initial improvement later relapse, despite continued use of the drug (108,109). Most experts do not recommend medication alone in the treatment of bulimia nervosa (97,108). There is some support for switching antidepressant medications if a patient fails to respond to one drug (109,110).

4 Other Pharmacotherapeutic Agents

Other pharmacotherapeutic agents that have been evaluated for bulimia nervosa include anticonvulsants, lithium carbonate, L-tryptophan, and naltrexone. However, none of these agents has been consistently shown to be useful for treatment of this disorder (97,108). One trial evaluating the efficacy of fenfluramine versus desipramine in 22 patients with bulimia nervosa found decreases in binge eating and improvement in depression over the 15-week trial period with both agents (111). Although both drugs reduced binge eating and vomiting, only fenfluramine produced a small weight loss. However, a larger placebo-controlled study of dexfenfluramine in 42 patients found no antidepressant effect for dexfenfluramine and a slight weight gain (112). In addition, patients who experienced the most symptomatic improvement in binge eating/purging showed a paradoxical tendency to drop out of the study. Another controlled trial of dexfenfluramine versus placebo found no advantage over brief psychotherapy alone in the treatment of bulimia nervosa (113). A recent double-blind placebo-controlled trial found that short-term treatment with the serotonin receptor antagonist ondansetron significantly reduced binge eating/purging in patients with bulimia nervosa (114).

5 Combined Medication and Psychotherapy

Medications and psychotherapy are often used in combination. Studies have found that CBT added to medication is more efficacious than medication alone (108, 115). While one study found that medication added to CBT provided little additional benefit (102,116) to study patients who received state-of the-art CBT in an intensive outpatient setting, the results may not be applicable to patients receiving less intensive psychotherapeutic treatment. Another study did find a small additional benefit to adding antidepressant medication to CBT (115). In addition, fluoxetine was shown in one study to be helpful in patients who had either not responded to, or had relapsed after, a course of CBT or IPT (117). It is reasonable to add an antidepressant medication (such as an SSRI or tricyclic) to psychotherapy if a patient does not have an adequate response to psychotherapy.

6 Support/Self-Help Groups

Support/self-help groups are commonly used in bulimia nervosa. These may be led by professionals or laypersons. Twelve-step programs, such as Overeaters Anonymous, are helpful for some patients, although controlled studies of their efficacy are not available. There is increasing interest in developing and evaluating stepped-care approaches, in which guided or unguided self-help manuals are used initially, supplemented by medication if needed, within the primary care setting

(108). Referral for more intensive psychotherapy would be reserved for those who failed to respond to initial interventions. A supervised cognitive-behavioral self-help approach, using a manual, has been shown to reduce bulimic symptoms in carefully selected patients (118,119).

C Binge Eating Disorder

Binge eating disorder is generally treated with similar therapies to bulimia nervosa, including cognitive behavioral and interpersonal psychotherapy and antidepressant medications. Any consideration of the treatment of binge eating disorder must begin with recognition of the unusual instability of the disorder. As Fairburn et al. (120) have noted, "unlike bulimia nervosa, binge eating disorder is an unstable state with a strong tendency toward spontaneous remission." In one study, a 4-week placebo run-in revealed a decrease in the frequency of binge eating of 70% (from 6.0 to 1.8 binge episodes per week) (121). Alger et al. (122) showed a similar 68% placebo response. Even in a wait-list control, binge eating decreased by 38% during a 3-month period.

1 Psychotherapy and Weight Loss Treatment

Both CBT (100,123) and IPT (100) have been shown to promote reductions in binge eating for up to 12 months following treatment. Treatment is generally similar to that used for bulimia nervosa, with some modifications. It has been hoped that, as these psychotherapies may work through differing mechanisms, patients failing to improve with one form of psychotherapy might respond favorably to another. However, a study using IPT as "salvage" therapy for patients who failed to respond to CBT found no additional benefit of IPT in this group (124). Another form of psychotherapy, dialectical behavior therapy (DBT), has recently been adapted for use in binge eating disorder (125). DBT is an empirically validated treatment for individuals with borderline personality disorder, which conceptualizes pathologic behaviors as faulty attempts at affect regulation (126). The treatment attempts to teach clients more functional methods of dealing with negative emotions.

Because many patients with BED are obese, and because eating disorder treatment alone does not lead to weight loss, researchers have sought to determine whether those with BED can lose weight with traditional weight loss treatments. Perhaps because of the instability of the diagnosis of BED, most studies find that, in the short term, binge eaters can lose weight well in standard weight loss treatment programs that don't address binge eating (127–130), although some studies have found a greater risk of dropping out of treatment or earlier regain of lost weight (130–132). One study, however, has found less frequent treatment attrition among obese women with binge eating disorder than among those without the disorder (133), while another has found episodic overeaters, who do not experience feelings of loss of control, to be at risk for attrition (134).

A frequent concern in using calorie-restricted diets in obese patients is that such dietary restriction will trigger the onset of binge eating in those who have not previously experienced this problem and will worsen binge eating in those already affected. Although one study found that a third of nonbinge eaters reported episodes they labeled as "binges" after a very low calorie diet program (135), others have found that weight loss treatment actually improves binge eating and associated psychopathology over the short term (37,38,127) and does not induce binge eating in obese subjects who previously reported no difficulties in this area (38). A recent review of the literature concluded that weight loss treatment does not have an adverse affect on binge eating in patients with binge eating disorder (34).

Sequencing of treatment for the eating disorder and obesity has been proposed an one possible means of improving outcome in patients with both binge eating disorder and obesity. One study that treated 93 obese women diagnosed with BED with a sequence of CBT followed by behavioral weight loss treatment found that, on average, weight lost during the weight loss treatment phase was not maintained. However, those who stopped binge eating during the CBT phase were able to maintain a weight loss of 4.0 kg over the follow-up period, suggesting that successful elimination of binge eating may improve long-term weight maintenance (136).

2 Medication

Antidepressant medication is frequently used in the treatment of binge eating disorder, although few studies of its efficacy have been published (107). Agras et al. (127) found that adding desipramine to a combination of CBT and behavioral weight loss treatment did not provide any additional benefit in reduction of binge eating. However, those on medication did maintain a significantly larger weight loss at 3-month posttreatment follow-up, as well as favorable reductions in disinhibition.

Fluoxetine has been evaluated as a weight loss agent in a group of obese individuals that included binge and nonbinge eaters (137). That study demonstrated significant weight loss in both groups while medication was continued, but no differential advantage was found for binge eaters. The effects of fluoxetine on binge eating frequency or severity were not measured. A small open-label trial using a combination of phentermine and fluoxetine as an adjunct to a 20-week CBT program showed significant reductions in binge frequency and distress, along with significant weight loss, at the end of the active treatment period. Medication duration was variable (1–25 months), and only 25% of patients continued taking medication throughout the study and follow-up periods. However, most of the weight was regained by 18-month follow-up, and the authors concluded that addition of phentermine/fluoxetine to CBT had little long-term benefit (138).

A report of an 8-week, double-blind, placebo-controlled trial using dexfenfluramine in obese individuals with binge eating disorder found significant decreases in binge frequency in the active treatment group compared with placebo, although neither group lost weight during the treatment period (121). Another open-label trial using the fenfluramine/phentermine combination found that after 24 weeks of treatment, binge eaters improved eating patterns and depression scores, and achieved similar weight loss to nonbinge eaters (139). Although fenfluramine and dexfenfluramine were withdrawn from the market due to their implication in the development of valvular heart disease, currently available weight loss medications are being studied in populations with binge eating disorder.

A few preliminary studies have suggested that opiate antagonists such as naltrexone (122,139,140) or naloxone (72) may eventually play a role in the treatment of binge eating disorder, but such approaches are still experimental.

3 Self Help

A cognitive behavioral self-help program for binge eating, either used alone or with guidance, has been found to be useful. The frequency of binge eating during a 12-week study fell by 53% in the pure self-help condition, significantly more than the 38% fall in the wait-list control group ($P < .05$) (141). Use of a self-help manual for binge eating has also been shown to improve eating behavior, reduce shape and weight concerns, and improve general psychological functioning in obese women with binge eating disorder (142).

D Night Eating Syndrome

The first trials of treatment of the night eating syndrome are just getting under way, and there are no guidelines for treatment. Anecdotal reports and the blunted night-time rise in melatonin seen in pilot studies suggest that this agent might prove helpful. However, at this time data are not available on its safety or efficacy for this condition, or on the optimal dosage and timing.

VII PROGNOSIS

A Anorexia Nervosa

Anorexia nervosa is a condition with severe morbidity and a high mortality, estimated at up to 20% over 20 years, although most studies show considerably lower rates, closer to 5% (143–145). The major reasons for death include starvation, suicide, and cardiac arrhythmias due to fluid and electrolyte imbalance (144, 145). A 10-year follow-up study of 76 severely ill anorexics found high rates of chronicity, with 41% experiencing bulimic episodes 10 years after initial treatment, and a 13-fold increase in mortality (146). Less than one-quarter of patients in that series were considered fully recovered. In a review of 14 outcome studies, Herzog et al. (144) report that 22–70% of patients were within the normal weight range at follow-up, while 15–43% were considered underweight. Overweight is not common among patients with a history of anorexia nervosa. Even when overweight is defined as 10% above "standard" weight, studies report a prevalence of only 2–10% (144). The same review reported that abnormal eating behaviors remain common over the long term in anorexia nervosa, with 23–67% reporting continued dieting, and up to half reporting binge eating and/or purging. A long-term study of patients with anorexia nervosa found that 10% met criteria for bulimia nervosa, purging subtype, at 6-year follow-up (143). Thus, while about half of all patients report normal weight over the long term, reproductive function, psychological well-being, and attitudes toward food and weight remain abnormal for the majority of patients with anorexia nervosa. While these studies are often of patients hospitalized at tertiary referral centers and may reflect the "worst-case scenario," it is clear that for many patients anorexia nervosa remains a chronic and persistent disorder.

Predictors of poor outcome in anorexia nervosa include long duration of illness, comorbid personality disorder, low body weight, and the presence of bulimic symptoms (143,144).

B Bulimia Nervosa

Mortality due to bulimia nervosa appears to be uncommon, although few studies have been published. Crude mortality rates for bulimia nervosa have been estimated at < 1% (147). A long-term study of 246 women with eating disorders studied for up to 11 years recorded seven deaths, all in patients with a history of anorexia nervosa, purging type. No deaths occurred in the 110 patients with bulimia nervosa who did not have a history of anorexia. (145).

While psychotherapy and pharmacotherapy lead to significant reductions in binge eating and purging behaviors, success, defined as complete "abstinence" from symptomatic behaviors, is much more variable.

A review of 88 studies that followed bulimic subjects for at least 6 months found that 5–10 years after presentation, ~50% of women had entirely recovered from the disorder, while almost 20% continued to meet DSM-IV criteria for bulimia nervosa. The course appeared to be remitting and relapsing for many, with ~30% experiencing relapse (147). There are few consistent prognostic indicators, although some studies have found personality disorders involving impulsivity, history of substance abuse, and longer duration of illness at time of presentation to be predict more negative treatment outcomes (147,148). No relationship has been found between pretreatment levels of binge eating or vomiting and treatment response.

A 5-year natural history study in a community-based cohort of women who met criteria for bulimia nervosa at baseline found that while there was a tendency for gradual improvement, between half and two-thirds of the sample met criteria for some sort of eating disorder at each 15-month assessment period, but most did not continue to meet DSM-IV criteria for bulimia nervosa. A relapsing and remitting course was common (120).

Most studies do not find a link between depression at presentation and treatment outcome (97), although improvement in bulimic symptoms leads to a reduction in depressive symptoms (149).

C Binge Eating Disorder

There appears to be a strong tendency toward spontaneous remission in binge eating disorder. Fichter et al. (150) reported that an 82% decrease in binge eating frequency during treatment was maintained at a 3-year follow-up. In a community-based natural history study, Fairburn and colleagues found that there was a tendency for improvement over time, with only 18% of the binge eating disorder cohort meeting DSM-IV diagnostic criteria at 5-year follow-up. However, there was a tendency toward continued weight gain, and the prevalence of obesity (BMI >30) increased from 21% to 39% during the 5-year period (120).

D   Night Eating Syndrome

Information about prognosis in the night eating syndrome is limited to retrospective reports, which suggest that it follows a chronic course, exacerbated by stressful situations (41). The syndrome appears to be of prognostic significance in its own right. Obese persons suffering from night eating syndrome have great difficulty in lowing weight and may pay a high price in emotional disturbance if they try (151).

REFERENCES

1. American Psychiatric Association. Diagnostic and Statistical Manual of Mental Disorders, 4th ed. Washington: American Psychiatric Association, 1994.
2. Fairburn CG, Cooper Z. The eating disorder examination. 12th ed. In: Fairburn CG, Wilson GT, eds. Binge Eating: Nature, Assessment, and Treatment. New York: Guilford Press, 1993:317–360.
3. Casper RC, Eckert ED, Halmi KA, Goldberg SC, Davis JM. Bulimia: its incidence and clinical importance in patients with anorexia nervosa. Arch Gen Psychiatry 1980; 37:1030–1035.
4. Gwirtsman HE. Laxative and emetic abuse in bulimia nervosa. In: Yager J, Gwirtsman H, Edelstein CK, eds. Special Problems in the Management of Eating Disorders. Washington: American Psychiatric Press, 1991.
5. Pryor T, Wiederman MW, McGilley B. Laxative abuse among women with eating disorders: an indication of psychopathology? Int J Eat Disord 1996; 20:13–18.
6. Jones JM, Lawson ML, Daneman D, Olmsted MP, Rodin G. Eating disorders in adolescent females with and without type 1 diabetes: cross sectional study. BMJ 2000; 320:1563–1566.
7. Birketvedt GS, Florholmen J, Sundsfjord J, Osterud B, Dinges D, Bilker W. Behavioral and neuroendocrine characteristics of the night-eating syndrome [see comments]. JAMA 1999; 282:657–663.
8. American Psychiatric Association. Practice guideline for eating disorders. Am J Psychiatry 1993; 150:212–228.
9. Hsu LK. Epidemiology of the eating disorders. Psychiatr Clin North Am 1996; 19:681–700.
10. Lucas AR, Crowson CS, O'Fallon WM, Melton LJ III. The ups and downs of anorexia nervosa. Int J Eat Disord 1999; 26:397–405.
11. Lucas AR, Beard CM, O'Fallon WM, Kurland LT. 50-year trends in the incidence of anorexia nervosa in Rochester, Minn.: a population-based study. Am J Psychiatry 1991; 148:917–922.
12. Garner DM. Pathogenesis of anorexia nervosa. Lancet 1993; 341:1631–1635.
13. Rastam M, Gillberg C. The family background in anorexia nervosa: a population-based study [see comments]. J Am Acad Child Adolesc Psychiatry 1991; 30:283–289.
14. Pate JE, Pumariega AJ, Hester C, Garner DM. Cross-cultural patterns in eating disorders: a review [see comments]. J Am Acad Child Adolesc Psychiatry 1992; 31:802–809.
15. Pemberton AR, Vernon SW, Lee ES. Prevalence and correlates of bulimia nervosa and bulimic behaviors in a racially diverse sample of undergraduate students in two universities in southeast Texas. Am J Epidemiol 1996; 144:450–455.
16. Warheit GJ, Langer LM, Zimmerman RS, Biafora FA. Prevalence of bulimic behaviors and bulimia among a sample of the general population. Am J Epidemiol 1993; 137:569–576.
17. Carlat DJ, Camargo CA Jr. Review of bulimia nervosa in males. Am J Psychiatry 1991; 148:831–843.
18. Carlat DJ, Camargo CA Jr, Herzog DB. Eating disorders in males: a report on 135 patients. Am J Psychiatry 1997; 154:1127–1132.
19. Oppliger RA, Landry GL, Foster SW, Lambrecht AC. Bulimic behaviors among interscholastic wrestlers: a statewide survey. Pediatrics 1993; 91:826–831.
20. White JH. Symptom development in bulimia nervosa: a comparison of women with and without a history of anorexia nervosa. Arch Psychiatr Nurs 2000; 14:81–92.
21. Yanovski SZ. Diagnosis and prevalence of eating disorders in obesity. In: Ailhaud G, Guy-Grand B, eds. Progress in Obesity Research. London: John Libby, 1999:229–236.
22. Spitzer RL, Yanovski S, Wadden T, Wing R, Marcus MD, Stunkard A, et al. Binge eating disorder: its further validation in a multisite study. Int J Eat Disord 1993; 13:137–153.
23. Spitzer RL, Devlin M, Walsh BT, Hasin D, Wing R, Marcus M, et al. Binge eating disorder: a multisite field trial of the diagnostic criteria. Int J Eat Disord 1992; 11:191–203.
24. Adami GF, Gandolfo P, Bauer B, Scopinaro N. Binge eating in massively obese patients undergoing bariatric surgery. Int J Eat Disord 1995; 17:45–50.
25. Hsu LK, Betancourt S, Sullivan SP. Eating disturbances before and after vertical banded gastroplasty: a pilot study. Int J Eat Disord 1996; 19:23–34.
26. Raymond NC, Mussell MP, Mitchell JE, De Zwaan M, Crosby RD. An age-matched comparison of subjects with binge eating disorder and bulimia nervosa. Int J Eat Disord 1995; 18:135–143.
27. Spurrell EB, Wilfley DE, Tanofsky MB, Brownell KD. Age of onset for binge eating: are there different pathways to binge eating? Int J Eat Disord 1997; 21:55–65.
28. Rand CS, Macgregor AM, Stunkard AJ. The night

eating syndrome in the general population and among postoperative obesity surgery patients. Int J Eat Disord 1997; 22:65–69.

29. Stunkard A, Berkowitz R, Wadden T, Tanrikut C, Reiss E, Young L. Binge eating disorder and the night-eating syndrome. Int J Obes Relat Metab Disord 1996; 20:1–6.

30. Stunkard AJ. Eating patterns and obesity. Psychol Bull 1959; 33:284–294.

31. Fairburn CG, Doll HA, Welch SL, Hay PJ, Davies BA, O'Connor ME. Risk factors for binge eating disorder: a community-based, case-control study. Arch Gen Psychiatry 1998; 55:425–432.

32. Beumont PJ, Garner DM, Touyz SW. Diagnoses of eating or dieting disorders: what may we learn from past mistakes? Int J Eat Disord 1994; 16:349–362.

33. Wilson GT. Relation of dieting and voluntary weight loss to psychological functioning and binge eating. Ann Intern Med 1993; 119:727–730.

34. National Task Force on the Prevention and Treatment of Obesity. Dieting and the development of eating disorders in overweight and obese adults. Arch Intern Med 2000; 160:2581–2589.

35. Wilson GT, Nonas CA, Rosenblum GD. Assessment of binge eating in obese patients. Int J Eat Disord 1993; 13:25–33.

36. Berkowitz R, Stunkard AJ, Stallings VA. Binge-eating disorder in obese adolescent girls. Ann NY Acad Sci 1993; 699:200–206.

37. Marcus MD, Wing RR, Fairburn CG. Cognitive treatment of binge eating v. behavioral weight control in the treatment of binge eating disorder [abstr]. Ann Behav Med 1995; 17:S090.

38. Yanovski SZ, Sebring NG. Recorded food intake of obese women with binge eating disorder before and after weight loss. Int J Eat Disord 1994; 15:135–150.

39. Yanovski SZ. The chicken or the egg: binge eating disorder and dietary restraint. Appetite 1995; 24:258.

40. Marcus MD, Smith D, Santelli R, Kaye W. Characterization of eating disordered behavior in obese binge eaters. Int J Eat Disord 1993; 12:249–256.

41. Stunkard AJ, Grace WJ, Wolfe HG. The night-eating syndrome: a pattern of food intake among certain obese patients. Am J Med 1955; 10:78–86.

42. Casper RC. Depression and eating disorders. Depress Anxiety 1998; 8(suppl 1):96–104.

43. Mussell MP, Peterson CB, Weller CL, Crosby RD, De Zwaan M, Mitchell JE. Differences in body image and depression among obese women with and without binge eating disorder. Obes Res 1996; 4:431–439.

44. Weltzin TE, Fernstrom MH, Kaye WH. Serotonin and bulimia nervosa. Nutr Rev 1994; 52:399–408.

45. Keys A, Brozek J, Henschel A, et al. The Biology of Human Starvation. Minneapolis: University of Minnesota Press, 1950.

46. Von Ranson KM, Kaye WH, Weltzin TE, Rao R,

Matsunaga H. Obsessive-compulsive disorder symptoms before and after recovery from bulimia nervosa. Am J Psychiatry 1999; 156:1703–1708.

47. Hsu LK, Kaye W, Weltzin T. Are the eating disorders related to obsessive compulsive disorder? Int J Eat Disord 1993; 14:305–318.

48. Kaye W, Strober M, Stein D, Gendall K. New directions in treatment research of anorexia and bulimia nervosa. Biol Psychiatry 1999; 45:1285–1292.

49. Marcus MD. Binge eating in obesity. In: Fairburn CG, Wilson GT, eds. Binge Eating: Nature, Assessment and Treatment. New York: Guilford Press, 1999:77–96.

50. Yanovski SZ, Nelson JE, Dubbert BK, Spitzer RL. Association of binge eating disorder and psychiatric comorbidity in obese subjects [published erratum appears in Am J Psychiatry 1993; 150(12):1910]. Am J Psychiatry 1993; 150:1472–1479.

51. Godart NT, Flament MF, Lecrubier Y, Jeammet P. Anxiety disorders in anorexia nervosa and bulimia nervosa: co-morbidity and chronology of appearance. Eur Psychiatry 2000; 15:38–45.

52. Antony MM, Johnson WG, Carr-Nangle RE, Abel JL. Psychopathology correlates of binge eating and binge eating disorder. Compr Psychiatry 1994; 35:386–392.

53. Specker S, De Zwaan M, Raymond N, Mitchell J. Psychopathology in subgroups of obese women with and without binge eating disorder. Compr Psychiatry 1994; 35:185–190.

54. Garner DM. Binge eating in anorexia nervosa. In: Fairburn CG, Wilson GT, eds. Binge Eating: Nature, Assessment, and Treatment New York: Guilford Press, 1993:50–76.

55. Wiederman MW, Pryor T. Substance use among women with eating disorders. Int J Eat Disord 1996; 20:163–168.

56. Hudson JI, Pope HG Jr, Jonas JM, Yurgelun-Todd D, Frankenburg FR. A controlled family history study of bulimia. Psychol Med 1987; 17:883–890.

57. Telch CF, Stice E. Psychiatric comorbidity in women with binge eating disorder: prevalence rates from a non-treatment-seeking sample. J Consult Clin Psychol 1998; 66:768–776.

58. Wade TD, Bulik CM, Neale M, Kendler KS. Anorexia nervosa and major depression: shared genetic and environmental risk factors. Am J Psychiatry 2000; 157: 469–471.

59. Strober M, Freeman R, Lampert C, Diamond J, Kaye W. Controlled family study of anorexia nervosa and bulimia nervosa: evidence of shared liability and transmission of partial syndromes. Am J Psychiatry 2000; 157:393–401.

60. Bulik CM, Sullivan PF, Wade TD, Kendler KS. Twin studies of eating disorders: a review. Int J Eat Disord 2000; 27:1–20.

61. Kaye WH, Lilenfeld LR, Berrettini WH, Strober M, Devlin B, Klump KL. A search for susceptibility loci for anorexia nervosa: methods and sample description. Biol Psychiatry 2000; 47:794–803.

62. Yanovski SZ. Biological correlates of binge eating. Addict Behav 1995; 20:705–712.

63. Wolfe BE, Metzger ED, Levine JM, Finkelstein DM, Cooper TB, Jimerson DC. Serotonin function following remission from bulimia nervosa. Neuropsychopharmacology 2000; 22:257–263.

64. Frank GK, Kaye WH, Altemus M, Greeno CG. CSF oxytocin and vasopressin levels after recovery from bulimia nervosa and anorexia nervosa, bulimic subtype. Biol Psychiatry 2000; 48:315–318.

65. Kaye WH, Gendall K, Kye C. The role of the central nervous system in the psychoneuroendocrine disturbances of anorexia and bulimia nervosa. Psychiatr Clin North Am 1998; 21:381–396.

66. Hall RC, Tice L, Beresford TP, Wooley B, Hall AK. Sexual abuse in patients with anorexia nervosa and bulimia. Psychosomatics 1989; 30:73–79.

67. Connors ME, Morse W. Sexual abuse and eating disorders: a review. Int J Eat Disord 1993; 13:1–11.

68. Welch SL, Fairburn CG. Childhood sexual and physical abuse as risk factors for the development of bulimia nervosa: a community-based case control study [see comments]. Child Abuse Negl 1996; 20:633–642.

69. Wonderlich SA, Brewerton TD, Jocic Z, Dansky BS, Abbott DW. Relationship of childhood sexual abuse and eating disorders. J Am Acad Child Adolesc Psychiatry 1997; 36:1107–1115.

70. Moyer DM, DiPietro L, Berkowitz RI, Stunkard AJ. Childhood sexual abuse and precursors of binge eating in an adolescent female population. Int J Eat Disord 1997; 21:23–30.

71. Wilson GT. Binge eating and addictive disorders. In: Fairburn CG, Wilson GT, eds. Binge Eating: Nature Assessment and Treatment. New York: Guilford Press, 1993:97–120.

72. Drewnowski A, Krahn DD, Demitrack MA, Nairn K, Gosnell BA. Naloxone, an opiate blocker, reduces the consumption of sweet high-fat foods in obese and lean female binge eaters. Am J Clin Nutr 1995; 61:1206–1212.

73. Mitchell JE. Medical complications of anorexia nervosa and bulimia. Psychiatr Med 1983; 1:229–255.

74. Brown JM, Mehler PS, Harris RH. Medical complications occurring in adolescents with anorexia nervosa [see comments]. West J Med 2000; 172:189–193.

75. Becker AE, Grinspoon SK, Klibanski A, Herzog DB. Eating disorders [see comments]. N Engl J Med 1999; 340:1092–1098.

76. Grinspoon S, Gulick T, Askari H, Landt M, Lee K, Anderson E. Serum leptin levels in women with anorexia nervosa. J Clin Endocrinol Metab 1996; 81:3861–3863.

77. Lucas AR, Melton LJ III, Crowson CS, O'Fallon WM. Long-term fracture risk among women with anorexia nervosa: a population-based cohort study. Mayo Clin Proc 1999; 74:972–977.

78. Soyka LA, Grinspoon S, Levitsky LL, Herzog DB, Klibanski A. The effects of anorexia nervosa on bone metabolism in female adolescents. J Clin Endocrinol Metab 1999; 84:4489–4496.

79. Grinspoon S, Herzog D, Klibanski A. Mechanisms and treatment options for bone loss in anorexia nervosa. Psychopharmacol Bull 1997; 33:399–404.

80. Klibanski A, Biller BM, Schoenfeld DA, Herzog DB, Saxe VC. The effects of estrogen administration on trabecular bone loss in young women with anorexia nervosa. J Clin Endocrinol Metab 1995; 80:898–904.

81. Hartman D, Crisp A, Rooney B, Rackow C, Atkinson R, Patel S. Bone density of women who have recovered from anorexia nervosa. Int J Eat Disord 2000; 28:107–112.

82. King MB. Eating disorders in a general practice population. Prevalence, characteristics and follow-up at 12 to 18 months. Psychol Med Monogr Suppl 1989; 14:1–34.

83. McClain CJ, Humphries LL, Hill KK, Nickl NJ. Gastrointestinal and nutritional aspects of eating disorders. J Am Coll Nutr 1993; 12:466–474.

84. Levin PA, Falko JM, Dixon K, Gallup EM, Saunders W. Benign parotid enlargement in bulimia. Ann Intern Med 1980; 93:827–829.

85. Roberts MW, Li SH. Oral findings in anorexia nervosa and bulimia nervosa: a study of 47 cases. J Am Dent Assoc 1987; 115:407–410.

86. Russell G. Bulimia nervosa: an ominous variant of anorexia nervosa. Psychol Med 1979; 9:429–448.

87. Mitchell JE, Specker SM, De Zwaan M. Comorbidity and medical complications of bulimia nervosa. J Clin Psychiatry 1991; 52(suppl):13–20.

88. Gwirtsman HE, Kaye WH, George DT, Carosella NW, Greene RC, Jimerson DC. Hyperamylasemia and its relationship to binge-purge episodes: development of a clinically relevant laboratory test [see comments]. J Clin Psychiatry 1989; 50:196–204.

89. Crowell MD, Cheskin LJ, Musial F. Prevalence of gastrointestinal symptoms in obese and normal weight binge eaters. Am J Gastroenterol 1994; 89:387–391.

90. Solomon SM, Kirby DF. The refeeding syndrome: a review [see comments]. J Parenter Enteral Nutr 1990; 14:90–97.

91. Kaye WH, Kaplan AS, Zucker ML. Treating eating-disorder patients in a managed care environment. Contemporary American issues and Canadian response. Psychiatr Clin North Am 1996; 19:793–810.

92. Gowers S, Norton K, Halek C, Crisp AH. Outcome of outpatient psychotherapy in a random allocation treatment study of anorexia nervosa. Int J Eat Disord 1994; 15:165–177.

93. Jensen VS, Mejlhede A. Anorexia nervosa: treatment with olanzapine [letter]. Br J Psychiatry 2000; 177:87.

94. Newman-Toker J. Risperidone in anorexia nervosa [letter]. J Am Acad Child Adolesc Psychiatry 2000; 39:941–942.

95. Kaye WH, Klump KL, Frank GK, Strober M. Anorexia and bulimia nervosa. Annu Rev Med 2000; 51:299–313.

96. Wilson GT. Cognitive behavior therapy for eating disorders: progress and problems. Behav Res Ther 1999; 37(suppl 1):S79–S95.

97. Peterson CB, Mitchell JE. Psychosocial and pharmacological treatment of eating disorders: a review of research findings. J Clin Psychol 1999; 55:685–697.

98. Wilson GT, Fairburn CG. Cognitive treatments for eating disorders. J Consult Clin Psychol 1993; 61:261–269.

99. Wilson GT, Loeb KL, Walsh BT, Labouvie E, Petkova E, Liu X. Psychological versus pharmacological treatments of bulimia nervosa: predictors and processes of change. J Consult Clin Psychol 1999; 67:451–459.

100. Wilfley DE, Agras WS, Telch CF, Rossiter EM, Schneider JA, Cole AG. Group cognitive-behavioral therapy and group interpersonal psychotherapy for the nonpurging bulimic individual: a controlled comparison. J Consult Clin Psychol 1993; 61:296–305.

101. Fairburn CG, Jones R, Peveler RC, Carr SJ, Solomon RA, O'Connor ME. Three psychological treatments for bulimia nervosa. A comparative trial. Arch Gen Psychiatry 1991; 48:463–469.

102. Agras WS, Walsh T, Fairburn CG, Wilson GT, Kraemer HC. A multicenter comparison of cognitive-behavioral therapy and interpersonal psychotherapy for bulimia nervosa. Arch Gen Psychiatry 2000; 57: 459–466.

103. Fairburn CG, Jones R, Peveler RC, Hope RA, O'Connor M. Psychotherapy and bulimia nervosa. Longer-term effects of interpersonal psychotherapy, behavior therapy, and cognitive behavior therapy. Arch Gen Psychiatry 1993; 50:419–428.

104. Fairburn CG, Norman PA, Welch SL, O'Connor ME, Doll HA, Peveler RC. A prospective study of outcome in bulimia nervosa and the long-term effects of three psychological treatments. Arch Gen Psychiatry 1995; 52:304–312.

105. National Task Force on the Prevention and Treatment of Obesity. Long-term pharmacotherapy in the management of obesity. JAMA 1996; 276:1907–1915.

106. Horne RL, Ferguson JM, Pope HG, Hudson JI, Lineberry CG, Ascher J. Treatment of bulimia with bupropion: a multicenter controlled trial. J Clin Psychiatry 1988; 49:262–266.

107. Goldstein DJ, Wilson MG, Thompson VL, Potvin JH, Rampey AH. Long-term fluoxetine treatment of bulimia nervosa. Fluoxetine Bulimia Nervosa Research Group. Br J Psychiatry 1995; 166:660–666.

108. Walsh BT, Devlin MJ. Pharmacotherapy of bulimia nervosa and binge eating disorder. Addict Behav 1995; 20:757–764.

109. Agras WS. Pharmacotherapy of bulimia nervosa and binge eating disorder: longer-term outcomes. Psychopharmacol Bull 1997; 33:433–436.

110. Mitchell JE, Pyle RL, Eckert ED, Hatsukami D, Pomeroy C, Zimmerman R. Response to alternative antidepressants in imipramine nonresponders with bulimia nervosa. J Clin Psychopharmacol 1989; 9: 291–293.

111. Blouin AG, Blouin JH, Perez EL, Bushnik T, Zuro C, Mulder E. Treatment of bulimia with fenfluramine and desipramine. J Clin Psychopharmacol 1988; 8:261–269.

112. Russell GF, Checkley SA, Feldman J, Eisler I. A controlled trial of d-fenfluramine in bulimia nervosa. Clin Neuropharmacol 1988; 11(suppl 1):S146–S159.

113. Fahy TA, Eisler I, Russell GF. A placebo-controlled trial of d-fenfluramine in bulimia nervosa. Br J Psychiatry 1993; 162:597–603.

114. Faris PL, Kim SW, Meller WH, Goodale RL, Oakman SA, Hofbauer RD. Effect of decreasing afferent vagal activity with ondansetron on symptoms of bulimia nervosa: a randomised, double-blind trial [see comments]. Lancet 2000; 355:792–797.

115. Walsh BT, Wilson GT, Loeb KL, Devlin MJ, Pike KM, Roose SP. Medication and psychotherapy in the treatment of bulimia nervosa. Am J Psychiatry 1997; 154: 523–531.

116. Mitchell JE, Pyle RL, Eckert ED, Hatsukami D, Pomeroy C, Zimmerman R. A comparison study of antidepressants and structured intensive group psychotherapy in the treatment of bulimia nervosa. Arch Gen Psychiatry 1990; 47:149–157.

117. Walsh BT, Agras WS, Devlin MJ, Fairburn CG, Wilson GT, Kahn C. Fluoxetine for bulimia nervosa following poor response to psychotherapy. Am J Psychiatry 2000; 157:1332–1334.

118. Cooper PJ, Coker S, Fleming C. An evaluation of the efficacy of supervised cognitive behavioral self-help bulimia nervosa. J Psychosom Res 1996; 40:281–287.

119. Thiels C, Schmidt U, Treasure J, Garthe R, Troop N. Guided self-change for bulimia nervosa incorporating use of a self-care manual. Am J Psychiatry 1998; 155: 947–953.

120. Fairburn CG, Cooper Z, Doll HA, Norman P, O'Connor M. The natural course of bulimia nervosa and binge eating disorder in young women. Arch Gen Psychiatry 2000; 57:659–665.

121. Stunkard A, Berkowitz R, Tanrikut C, Reiss E, Young L. d-Fenfluramine treatment of binge eating disorder. Am J Psychiatry 1996; 153:1455–1459.

122. Alger SA, Schwalberg MD, Bigaouette JM, Michalek AV, Howard LJ. Effect of a tricyclic antidepressant and opiate antagonist on binge-eating behavior in normoweight bulimic and obese, binge-eating subjects. Am J Clin Nutr 1991; 53:865–871.

123. Telch CF, Agras WS, Rossiter EM, Wilfley D,

Kenardy J. Group cognitive-behavioral treatment for the nonpurging bulimic: an initial evaluation. J Consult Clin Psychol 1990; 58:629–635.

124. Agras WS, Telch CF, Arnow B, Eldredge K, Detzer MJ, Henderson J. Does interpersonal therapy help patients with binge eating disorder who fail to respond to cognitive-behavioral therapy? J Consult Clin Psychol 1995; 63:356–360.

125. Wiser S, Telch CF. Dialectical behavior therapy for binge-eating disorder. J Clin Psychol 1999; 55:755–768.

126. Linehan MM. Dialectical behavior therapy for borderline personality disorder. Theory and method. Bull Menninger Clin 1987; 51:261–276.

127. Agras WS, Telch CF, Arnow BA, Eldredge KL, Wilfley D, Raeburn SD. Weight loss, cognitive-behavioral, and desipramine treatments in binge eating disorder. An additive design. Behav Ther 1994; 25:225–238.

128. Gladis MM, Wadden TA, Vogt R, Foster G, Kuehnel RH, Bartlett SJ. Behavioral treatment of obese binge eaters: do they need different care? J Psychosom Res 1998; 44:375–384.

129. Wadden TA, Foster GD, Letizia KA. Response of obese binge eaters to treatment by behavior therapy combined with very low calorie diet. J Consult Clin Psychol 1992; 60:808–811.

130. Yanovski SZ, Gormally JF, Lesser MS, Gwirtsman HE, Yanovski JA. Binge eating disorder affects outcome of comprehensive very-low-calorie diet treatment. Obes Res 1994; 2:205–212.

131. Marcus MD, Wing RR, Hopkins J. Obese binge eaters: affect, cognitions, and response to behavioral weight control. J Consult Clin Psychol 1988; 56:433–439.

132. Loro AD, Orleans CS. Binge eating in obesity: preliminary findings and guidelines for behavioral analysis and treatment. Addict Behav 1981; 6:155–166.

133. Ho KS, Nichaman MZ, Taylor WC, Lee ES, Foreyt JP. Binge eating disorder, retention, and dropout in an adult obesity program. Int J Eat Disord 1995; 18:291–294.

134. Wadden TA, Foster GD, Letizia KA. Response of obese binge eaters to treatment by behavior therapy combined with very low calorie diet. J Consult Clin Psychol 1992; 60:808–811.

135. Telch CF, Agras WS. The effects of a very-low-calorie diet on binge eating. Behav Ther 1993; 24:177–193.

136. Agras WS, Telch CF, Arnow B, Eldredge K, Marnell M. One-year follow-up of cognitive-behavioral therapy for obese individuals with binge eating disorder. J Consult Clin Psychol 1997; 65:343–347.

137. Marcus MD, Wing RR, Ewing L, Kern E, McDermott M, Gooding W. A double-blind, placebo-controlled trial of fluoxetine plus behavior modification in the treatment of obese binge-eaters and non-binge-eaters. Am J Psychiatry 1990; 147:876–881.

138. Devlin MJ, Goldfein JA, Carino JS, Wolk SL. Open treatment of overweight binge eaters with phentermine and fluoxetine as an adjunct to cognitive-behavioral therapy. Int J Eat Disord 2000; 28:325–332.

139. Alger SA, Malone M, Cerulli J, Fein S, Howard L. Beneficial effects of pharmacotherapy on weight loss, depressive symptoms, and eating patterns in obese binge eaters and non-binge eaters. Obes Res 1999; 7:469–476.

140. Marrazzi MA, Markham KM, Kinzie J, Luby ED. Binge eating disorder: response to naltrexone. Int J Obes Relat Metab Disord 1995; 19:143–145.

141. Carter JC, Fairburn CG. Cognitive-behavioral self-help for binge eating disorder: a controlled effectiveness study. J Consult Clin Psychol 1998; 66:616–623.

142. Loeb KL, Wilson GT, Gilbert JS, Labouvie E. Guided and unguided self-help for binge eating. Behav Res Ther 2000; 38:259–272.

143. Fichter MM, Quadflieg N. Six-year course and outcome of anorexia nervosa. Int J Eat Disord 1999; 26:359–385.

144. Herzog DB, Keller MB, Lavori PW. Outcome in anorexia nervosa and bulimia nervosa. A review of the literature. J Nerv Ment Dis 1988; 176:131–143.

145. Herzog DB, Greenwood DN, Dorer DJ, Flores AT, Ekeblad ER, Richards A. Mortality in eating disorders: a descriptive study. Int J Eat Disord 2000; 28:20–26.

146. Eckert ED, Halmi KA, Marchi P, Grove W, Crosby R. Ten-year follow-up of anorexia nervosa: clinical course and outcome. Psychol Med 1995; 25:143–156.

147. Keel PK, Mitchell JE. Outcome in bulimia nervosa [see comments]. Am J Psychiatry 1997; 154:313–321.

148. Herzog DB, Dorer DJ, Keel PK, Selwyn SE, Ekeblad ER, Flores AT. Recovery and relapse in anorexia and bulimia nervosa: a 7.5-year follow-up study. J Am Acad Child Adolesc Psychiatry 1999; 38:829–837.

149. Wilson GT, Rossiter E, Kleifield EI, Lindholm L. Cognitive-behavioral treatment of bulimia nervosa: a controlled evaluation. Behav Res Ther 1986; 24:277–288.

150. Fichter MM, Quadflieg N, Gnutzmann A. Binge eating disorder: treatment outcome over a 6-year course. J Psychosom Res 1998; 44:385–405.

151. Stunkard AJ. Night eating. In: Stunkard, AJ, ed. The Pain of Obesity. Palo Alto: Bull Publishing, 1976:41–63.

151a. Yanovski SZ. Bulimia nervosa: the role of the family physician. Am Fam Physician 1991; 44:1234.

9

Behavioral Approaches to the Treatment of Obesity

Rena R. Wing

Brown Medical School, Providence, Rhode Island, U.S.A.

I THE BEHAVIORAL APPROACH TO OBESITY: A THEORETICAL OVERVIEW

The behavioral approach to obesity grew out of Learning Theory (1,2) and was first applied to the treatment of obesity between 1960 and 1970 (3,4). The primary assumptions of the behavioral approach are that (1) eating and exercise behaviors affect body weight; by changing eating and exercise behaviors it is possible to change body weight; (2) eating and exercise patterns are learned behaviors and, like other learned behaviors, can be modified; and (3) to modify these behaviors long term, it is necessary to change the environment that influences them.

The behavioral approach does not deny that an individual's genetic background may have a strong influence on their body weight. However, despite a predisposition to be a certain weight, changes in energy balance (i.e., decreases in energy intake and/or increases in energy expenditure) will produce weight loss.

Likewise, the behavioral approach recognizes the importance of an individual's past history. The individual's family and cultural background influence body weight by determining food preferences, food choices, and the preferred level of physical activity. However, while accepting the importance of historical antecedents, the focus of a behavioral approach is on current behaviors and the environmental factors controlling these current behaviors.

The essence of the behavioral approach to obesity is the functional analysis of behavior, delineating the association between eating and exercise behaviors and environmental events such as time of day, presence of other people, mood, and other activities (5,6). Patients are asked to monitor their eating and exercise behaviors to determine specific problem areas that should be targeted in treatment. The environment controlling these behaviors is then restructured to modify these problem behaviors.

A key technique in behavioral approaches is self-monitoring (7), which involves writing down exactly what is eaten and what type of physical activity is performed. This record allows the patient and therapist to identify problem behaviors that might be changed. For example, the self-monitoring record may reveal that a large percentage of an individual's calories is consumed in the form of desserts, that between-meal eating constitutes a major problem, or that an individual's portion sizes are unusually large. Alternatively, the individual may consume relatively few calories but lead a very sedentary lifestyle. These different behavior patterns would lead to different targets for the behavior change intervention.

Often in changing overall behavior, it is necessary to break the target behavior into several components, and then to work on each part in turn (i.e., "shape" the behavior). For example, to lower calorie intake in an overweight individual, a therapist might work first on

147

A   →   B   ←   C
Antecedents   **Behavior**   **Consequences**

Figure 1 A-B-C model of the behavioral approach to the treatment of obesity.

reducing calories consumed at breakfast, and later move to lunch and dinner, or focus initially on decreasing the quantity of food consumed (i.e., portion sizes) and later work on changing the quality of the diet.

After defining the behavior to be changed, the next step is to change the environment that controls the behavior. The behavioral approach assumes that behavior is controlled by *antecedents*, or cues in the environment that set the stage for the behavior, and by *consequences*, or reinforcers, that come after the behavior and lead to its recurrence (8). This A-B-C model is shown schematically in Figure 1. For example, the sight of food on a buffet table may lead a person to overeat, or the cue of seeing someone else eating may arouse feelings of hunger. Likewise, the positive consequences that come from the good taste of food or from reduction in feelings of hunger may lead to continued selection of these food items.

In the behavioral approach to weight control, patients are taught to restructure their home environment so that it will elicit the desired behaviors. These techniques are called stimulus control strategies (3,4). For example, patients are encouraged to refrain from purchasing high-calorie desserts, and to store all high-calorie foods in difficult-to-reach places; simultaneously they are taught to buy more fruits and vegetables and to keep them readily accessible. Patients are also taught strategies for changing thoughts and emotions, which can serve as powerful cues for overeating, and strategies for dealing with social cues and social pressure to overeat.

Patients in weight control programs often observe that they don't have the necessary "willpower" to avoid unhealthy foods. The behavioral approach is designed to restructure the environment to minimize the need for willpower. For example, if a patient opens the refrigerator and finds only low-calorie food items available, the chances are good that the patient will select a low-calorie item (even if the person lacks willpower). Likewise, if the patient plans ahead to meet a friend at the park for a walk after work, the chances are increased that the patient will actually take a walk. By planning ahead and developing a structure at a point in time when will power isn't required, patients can increase the likelihood that the desirable behavior will occur.

Finally, since environmental consequences are believed to play an important role in influencing behavior, behavioral programs attempt to develop new reinforcement contingencies. Behavior therapists use reinforcers, such as praise and positive feedback, to encourage patients to adopt new healthier eating and exercise behaviors and teach patients to reinforce themselves for appropriate behavior change. Some behavioral programs also include more formal reinforcement systems, such as contingency procedures where patients deposit money with the therapist and earn back portions of their money contingent on behavior change (9,10).

II HISTORY OF BEHAVIORAL APPROACHES TO OBESITY

A Development of Treatments from 1970 to 1990

The earliest report of a behavioral treatment program for obesity was by Stuart, who successfully treated eight overweight women (4). These women experienced an average weight loss of 17 kg over a 12-month period, ranging from a weight loss of 12–21 kg. It should be noted that Stuart (an eminent behavior therapist) conducted the treatment program himself, selecting each patient individually and tailoring the program to fit the needs of the individual patient. At the start of therapy, the treatment sessions were scheduled frequently (several times per week), and then gradually less frequently. Eating and exercise behaviors were targeted, and patients weighed themselves four times each day. The program included cognitive interventions, as patients were taught to deal with their weight-related fears, and the patients were helped to develop new hobbies as alternative sources of reinforcement.

Stuart's successful report led to a flood of behavioral research studies. These studies in the early 1970s typically involved 10 weeks of group treatment with mildly overweight subjects, and were often conducted as part of a student's doctoral dissertation (5,11). Thus, in many ways these studies represented an abrupt departure from Stuart's landmark treatment. The emphasis in these programs was on changing eating patterns (where and when foods were eaten), but the nutritional aspects of the diet (number of calories, macronutrient distribution) were ignored, in part to distinguish behavioral treatment from traditional dieting interventions. These early studies showed that behavior modification was more effective than nutrition education (12) or psychotherapy (13). On average, participants lost 3.8 kg over an 8.4-week treatment interval (5). When followed up an average of 15.5 weeks later, participants had maintained a weight loss of 4.0 kg.

The evolution of behavioral treatments from 1974 to 1990 is shown clearly in Table 1. As seen in this table, behavioral treatments gradually evolved over this period (1974–1990) to include heavier participants (from 73 to 92 kg at entry), longer treatment intervals (from 8.4 to 21.3 weeks in length), and longer follow-up durations (increasing to a yearlong follow-up). The program itself changed as well, placing far greater emphasis on nutrition (14). Patients in behavioral programs were now given calorie goals (usually 1200–1500 kcal/d) and self-monitored not only the events surrounding eating but also exactly what they ate (8,15). Calorie goals for exercise were also prescribed. Cognitive behavioral strategies were given greater emphasis (2), and financial incentives were often utilized. Thus, behavioral programs evolved from teaching strictly behavioral strategies to focusing equally on diet, exercise, and behavior modification. With this longer, more inclusive, intervention, average weight losses increased from 3.8 kg in 1974 to 8.5 kg in 1990. At 1-year follow-up, subjects maintained an average weight loss of 5.6 kg (66% of their initial weight loss).

B Refining Treatments—1990–2000

Research during the period of 1990–2000 has been designed to evaluate new strategies that might increase the magnitude of weight loss achieved in behavioral programs. Interestingly, years 1990–1995 focused mainly on diet, whereas 1996–2000 stressed physical activity. Each of these areas will be described in detail in later sections of this chapter.

Estimating the magnitude of weight loss that can be achieved with current behavioral weight loss programs is difficult, because a variety of different approaches have often been tried within one study. Therefore, rather than tabulating results of all treatment studies and all intervention groups, Table 2 presents a highly selected listing of 12 of the largest, longest studies. Two of these 12 studies compared very low calorie diets with low-calorie diets (16,17); results from the low-calorie conditions are included in the table to provide a more accurate appraisal of the usual outcome in behavioral programs. Similarly, treatment conditions which include diet plus exercise were selected (aerobic exercise was selected if several types of exercise), since this is the recommended approach to behavioral treatment. Finally, if a study included several treatment groups that were prescribed diet plus exercise, results from the most effective intervention were used to determine what can be achieved in current intervention studies.

Table 3 averages across the treatment groups listed in Table 2. Comparing Table 3 with Table 1, it appears that there has continued to be improvement in treatment outcomes over this decade. Whereas in 1988–1990, the average patient lost 8.5 kg over 21 weeks, currently the average patient loses 10.4 kg over 5 months. Some of this improvement may be due to the fact that not all treatment groups are tabulated for 1990–2000; as noted above, the most effective low-calorie diet plus exercise intervention in each trial has been selected. However, much of the improvement appears to be the result of stronger behavioral techniques. These stronger behavioral techniques will be discussed in subsequent sections of this chapter.

Follow-up also appears to be improving. When re-examined at ~18 months (i.e., 1 year later), patients in

Table 1 Summary Analysis of Selected Studies from 1974 to 1990 Providing Treatment by Behavior Therapy and Conventional Reducing Diet

	1974	1978	1984	1985–1987	1988–1990
No. of studies included	15	17	15	13	5
Sample size	53.1	54.0	71.3	71.6	21.2
Initial weight (kg)	73.4	87.3	88.7	87.2	91.9
Initial % overweight	49.4	48.6	48.1	56.2	59.8
Length of treatment (weeks)	8.4	10.5	13.2	15.6	21.3
Weight loss (kg)	3.8	4.2	6.9	8.4	8.5
Loss per week (kg)	0.5	0.4	0.5	0.5	0.4
Attrition (%)	11.4	12.9	10.6	13.8	21.8
Length of follow-up (weeks)	15.5	30.3	58.4	48.3	53
Loss at follow-up	4.0	4.1	4.4	5.3	5.6

Source: Ref. 14.

Table 2 Results of Selected Behavioral Weight Loss Trials, 1990–2000

First author	Treatment format	Initial weight (kg)	Weight loss (kg)			
			Month 6	Month 12	Month 18	Month 24
Wadden (16)	Weekly for 12 mo, biweekly mo 12–18, low-calorie diet	106	11.9	14.4	12.2	
Wing (17)	Weekly for 12 mo, no Tx after 12 mo, low-calorie diet	106	13.5	10.5		5.7
Viegener (18)	Weekly for 6 mo, biweekly 6–12 mo, low-calorie diet	96	10.2	9.0		
Jeffery (19)	Weekly for 6 mo, monthly, 6–18 mo, SBT + food provision	90	10.0	9.1	6.4	
Wing (20)	Weekly for 6 mo, varied for next 12 mo, SBT + food provision or menus	86	12.0		6.9	
Wadden (21)	Weekly for 6 mo, biweekly 6–12 mo, aerobic exercise 2–3/wk	96	16.2	13.7		8.5
Jeffery (22)	Weekly BT for 6 mo, monthly 6–18 mo, exercise on own	86	8.3		7.6	
Jakicic (23)	Weekly for 6 mo, biweekly 7–12 mo, monthly 12–18 mo, long-bout exercise	90	~7.5		5.8	
Perri (24)	Weekly for 6 mo, biweekly 6–12 mo, lifestyle exercise	88	10.6	12.4	11.9[a]	
Andersen (25)	Weekly 4 mo, lifestyle exercise	89	7.9[b]		7.1[c]	
Leermakers (26)	Weekly 6 mo, biweekly 6–12 mo, weight-focused maintenance	85	8.7	8.5	7.9	
Foreyt (27)	Weekly for 3 mo, biweekly/monthly for 3–12 mo, diet + exercise	97	6.9[d]	8.1		

BT, behavioral treatment; SBT, standard behavioral treatment.
[a] = 15 months.
[b] = 4 months.
[c] = 16 months.
[d] = 3 months.

studies conducted from 1900–2000 maintained a weight loss of 8.1 kg, or 82% of their initial weight loss. Again, this compares very favorably with the 5.6-kg loss at follow-up reported in 1988–1990.

Figure 2 presents the data from the 1990–2000 studies in graphical form showing the pattern of weight changes over time and the consistency of results across the 12 studies. There is a tight clustering of results at 6 months, suggesting that initial weight losses are produced quite consistently across different studies, different investigators, and different treatment populations (the only two outliers are the two studies that had 3- and 4-month treatments). Weight losses at 12 months (mean = 10.35 kg) are comparable to those seen at 6 months (mean = 10.37 kg). Studies with 18-month data (N = 7 studies) show an average weight loss of 8.2 kg at this time. Thus weight regain appears to occur during the 12-to-18-month window.

Only two studies provided 24-month data. In these studies the average weight loss was 7.1 kg at 24 months, quite comparable to the results for studies with 18-month data. Since the two studies with 24-month follow-up included a full 12 months of treatment, the 24-month point actually reflects results 1 year after the end of weekly treatment, perhaps explaining the similarity between the 18-month and 24-month results. No studies were found that included 30-month, 36-month, or longer follow-up.

Table 3 Summary of Results of Selected Behavioral Weight Loss Trials, 1990–2000

Number of treatment trials	12
Initial treatment	
Duration	5.6 months
Weight loss	10.4 kg
Final follow-up	
Duration	17.6 months
Weight loss	8.1 kg
% of Weight loss retained	82%

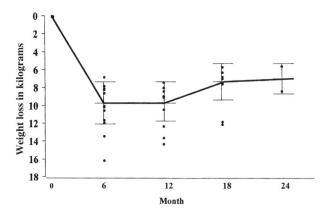

Figure 2 Weight loss outcome in behavioral treatments from 1990 to 2000.

Thus, results of behavioral programs appear to be continuing to improve—albeit only slightly. The strongest behavioral programs now produce weight losses of 10.4 kg, with maintenance of an 8.1-kg weight loss 1 year later.

III DESCRIPTION OF CURRENT BEHAVIORAL TREATMENT PROGRAMS

Over time, behavioral programs have become fairly standardized. Therefore it is possible to describe a "typical" program. These current programs differ quite markedly from both Stuart's early intervention and from the theoretical description of a behavioral program provided at the start of this chapter.

Currently almost all behavioral programs are delivered in groups of 10–20 patients (8,14). With this many patients in a group, it is difficult to conduct an individualized functional analysis of behavior. The program is offered as a series of lessons, and the entire group of participants receives lesson 1 on week 1, lesson 2 on week 2, etc. There is no assessment of whether the lessons relate to the individual participant's problem areas or whether the participant has mastered the skill before moving on to the next skill. However, individualization of treatment occurs through lessons on problem solving, allowing participants the opportunity to focus on their specific problem areas. Therapists for behavioral programs are likewise quite different. Some programs use one therapist throughout, but many use a team of therapists (including a behavior therapist, an exercise physiologist, and a nutritionist) and rotate therapists by topic. Treatment usually involves weekly meetings for

16–24 weeks (with some programs now using yearlong programs) and then less frequent contact.

Key strategies in current behavioral program include the following:

A Self-Monitoring

Patients in behavioral programs are taught to write down everything they eat and the calories in these foods. Recently, many program have begun to teach patients to also self-monitor the grams of fat in each food. After a few weeks in the program, self-monitoring of physical activity is added (with activity monitored either in minutes or in calories expended). Self-monitoring is prescribed daily throughout the initial 20- to 24-week program and periodically (or daily) during maintenance. Self-monitoring is often considered the sine qua non of behavioral programs, and continued adherence to self-monitoring predicts long-term maintenance of weight loss (28,29).

B Goal Setting

The goal in behavioral programs is to achieve a weight loss of 1–2 lb/week (0.5–1 kg). To accomplish this, patients are given goals for total calories (usually 1000–1500 kcal/d), for grams of fat (usually given in grams of fat per day and set at a level to achieve a 20–30% fat diet), and for physical activity (gradually increased from 250 kcal/week to 1000 kcal/week). Patients may also set specific behavioral goals to achieve during various weeks of the project. Short-term goals the participant can reasonably be expected to achieve are emphasized (30).

C Nutrition

The nutritional aspects of weight loss are now given far more attention in behavioral weight loss programs (8,15). Virtually all programs ask participants to record what they are eating and the calorie and/or fat content of those foods. Lessons on healthy eating, which emphasize increasing intake of complex carbohydrates and fiber and decreasing dietary fat, are usually included. Moreover, the specific skills required to be able to consume a low-fat diet are taught during the course of the program, with lessons on topics such as recipe modification, label reading, restaurant eating, and demonstrations of special cooking skills such as stir-fry cooking. Thus, nutrition is taught both through educational classes designed to increase knowledge of what should be consumed, and through demonstrations of how to accomplish the complex task of going from a high-calorie, high-fat diet to a lower-calorie, lower-fat regimen.

D Exercise

Exercise is given a great deal of attention in behavioral weight loss programs because exercise is the single best predictor of long-term weight maintenance (31). Correlational studies comparing successful and unsuccessful weight losers consistently show that successful weight losers are best distinguished by their self-reported exercise behavior (32–34). The association between exercise and long-term weight loss has been observed in men, women, children, and adolescents, and is seen in programs involving low-calorie diets and very low calorie diets (31). In addition, randomized controlled trials, in which diet alone, exercise alone, and diet plus exercise are compared, consistently show that the combination of diet plus exercise produces the best long-term results (35–37).

To increase exercise, participants in behavioral programs are given goals for exercise, and these goals are gradually increased over time to "shape" an exercise routine. Most programs encourage patients to gradually work up to 1000 calories/week of exercise, which can be accomplished by walking 10 miles a week (2 miles on 5 days each week).

Behavioral treatment programs often distinguish between *lifestyle exercise*, such as using stairs instead of elevators or parking farther from the store, and *programmed exercise*, in which a specific time is set aside for the purpose of exercise. Both types of exercise are strongly encouraged in behavioral treatment programs. Moreover, based on Epstein et al.'s recent findings that decreasing sedentary activities such as TV watching is very effective in promoting weight loss (38), many programs now include lessons on this topic as well.

Again, as in discussing nutrition, behavioral programs help patients learn the specific skills required to become more active, such as learning to monitor their heart rate to determine the intensity of exercise, learning how to dress for exercise in cold or hot weather, and learning how to deal with barriers that make exercise difficult. Some behavioral programs include supervised exercise sessions to model these skills and help provide participants with social support for exercise (39).

E Stimulus Control

Stimulus control techniques remain the hallmark of behavioral treatment programs (3,4). Based on the assumption that behaviors are controlled by environmental antecedents, participants in weight control programs are taught to change the environment they live in, so that there are an increased number of cues for appropriate diet and exercise behaviors and fewer cues for inappropriate behaviors. Specifically, participants in behavioral weight control programs are taught to increase their purchase of fruits and vegetables, to wash and prepare these foods for easy eating, and to place these foods prominently in the refrigerator. In contrast, high-fat/high-calorie products are to be decreased. If it is necessary to purchase these foods at all, they are to be stored in opaque containers or high cupboards, since "out-of-sight, out-of-mind." Some programs also encourage participants to select a designated eating place and to restrict all eating to that place, and to separate eating from other activities (such as watching television or reading). In this way, behavioral programs seek to limit the cues associated with eating.

F Problem Solving

The problem-solving approach of D'Zurilla and Goldfried (40) is taught to participants in weight control programs. Participants learn to identify situations that pose a problem for their eating and exercise behaviors, to use brainstorming to generate possible solutions to the problem, to select one solution to try, and then to evaluate the success of their attempt. Through training in problem solving, behavioral programs are able to individualize the group-based weight control program and to teach patients strategies for dealing with their own personal problem areas.

G Cognitive Restructuring

The cues for overeating and underexercising include not only physical cues such as the sight and smell of food, but also cognitive cues. A person's thoughts, such as the thought "I've had a bad day. I deserve a treat. I'll go for some ice cream" can lead to inappropriate behavior. Dividing the world into good and bad foods, developing excuses or rationalizations for inappropriate behavior, and making comparisons with others can all serve as negative thoughts. Behavioral programs teach participants to recognize that they are having these negative thoughts, to understand the function these thoughts serve for the participant, and then to counter these negative thoughts with more positive self-statements (41,42).

H Relapse Prevention

Based on Marlatt and Gordon's theory of the relapse process (43,44), behavioral weight control programs now emphasize that lapses (or slips) are a natural part of the weight loss process. Patients are taught to anticipate the types of situations that might cause them to lapse and to plan strategies for coping with these situations. The goal is to keep lapses from becoming relapses.

IV RECENT EFFORTS TO IMPROVE TREATMENT OUTCOME

In an effort to improve treatment outcome, behavioral research from 1990 to 2000 focused on strengthening the dietary component of the weight loss program, strengthening the exercise component, and/or strengthening the manner in which the behavioral strategies are implemented. Each of these areas of research will be discussed in turn.

A Strengthening the Dietary Component

1 Combining Behavior Modification and Very Low Calorie Diet

One approach to improving weight loss in behavioral treatment programs is to improve initial weight loss by using stricter dietary approaches, such as very low calorie diets (VLCDs). VLCDs are diets of < 800 kcal/d, usually consumed as liquid formula or as lean meat, fish, and fowl (45). These diets have been shown to produce excellent weight losses (9 kg in 12 weeks) (45, 46) and appear to be safe when used with carefully selected patients and appropriate medical monitoring (45). By using VLCDs to produce large initial weight losses and behavioral training to improve maintenance, it was hoped that a more successful treatment approach could be developed.

In one of the earliest studies of the combination of behavior modification and a VLCD (Table 4), Wadden and colleagues (47) randomly assigned 59 overweight subjects to one of three conditions: an 8-week VLCD administered in a physician's office with no behavioral counseling (VLCD alone); a 20-week group behavioral weight loss program that used a balanced low-calorie diet throughout (BT + LCD); or a 20-week group behavioral program that included an 8-week period of VLCD (BT + VLCD). Subjects in the VLCD alone group lost 14.1 kg during the 8-week diet, but then rapidly regained their weight, maintaining a weight loss of 4.1 kg at 1-year follow-up (i.e., maintaining only 29% of their initial weight loss). Better results were obtained in the BT + VLCD condition which lost 19.3 kg initially and maintained a weight loss of 12.9 kg at 1 year. However, while the initial weight losses in the BT + VLCD condition were better than those in the BT + LCD (19.3 vs. 14.3 kg, respectively), at 1 year follow-up weight losses were no longer significantly different (12.9 vs. 9.5 kg in BT + VLCD vs. BT + LCD conditions, respectively). Thus, the greater initial weight losses in the VLCD were not successful in producing significantly better long-term results.

A similar finding occurred in the Wing et al. (48) study with a sample of 36 obese patients with NIDDM. At the end of a 20-week behavioral program which included an 8-week period of VLCD, weight losses averaged 18.6 kg and were significantly greater than those obtained when a 1000- to 1500-kcal LCD was used throughout (10.1 kg). At 1-year follow-up, subjects in the BT + VLCD condition had regained 54% of their initial weight loss, compared to only 33% in the BT + LCD group; consequently, the overall weight losses (8.6 for BT + VLCD vs. 6.8 kg for BT + LCD) no longer differed significantly between the two treatment groups.

These studies of VLCDs were indeed successful in improving initial weight loss, as researchers had anticipated; however, increasing initial weight loss did not improve long-term outcome. Rather, it simply increased the magnitude of weight regained. To try to better maintain these larger initial weight losses, several inves-

Table 4 Weight Loss in Long-Term Studies of Behavioral Interventions with VLCD Versus LCD

	Short-term results			Long-term results		
		Weight loss			Weight loss	
Trial	Duration	LCD	VLCD	Duration	LCD	VLCD
Wadden (47)	20 wk	14.3 kg	19.3 kg*	52 wk	9.5 kg	12.9 kg
Wing (48)	20 wk	10.1 kg	18.6 kg*	72 wk	6.8 kg	8.6 kg
Wadden (16)	52 wk	14.4 kg	17.3 kg	78 wk	12.2 kg	10.9 kg
Wing (17)	50 wk	10.5 kg	14.2 kg*	102 wk	5.7 kg	7.2 kg

* Difference in weight loss between LCD and VLCD significant at $P < .05$.

tigators have recently used VLCDs in combination with yearlong behavioral programs. Wadden and colleagues (16) randomly assigned 49 overweight women to a behavioral treatment program which involved 52 weekly meetings and either used a balanced low-calorie diet throughout (1200 kcal/d) or included 16 weeks of VLCD. All subjects were then seen biweekly from week 52 to week 72. The BT + VLCD condition achieved their maximum weight loss at 6 months (21.1 kg) and then gradually regained (17.3 kg at 12 months and 10.9 kg at 18 months). The BT + LCD group lost significantly less weight initially (11.86 kg at 26 weeks), but then continued to lose weight between 26 and 52 weeks (14.4 kg at 52 weeks). Consequently by week 52, differences between the VLCD and LCD condition were no longer significant. After week 52, subjects in the BT + LCD group regained weight despite continued contact, achieving a final weight loss of 12.2 kg at 18 months. Subjects in the LCD condition regained much less than the VLCD subjects, so that at the end of the study, overall weight loss in the BT + LCD condition exceeded but did not differ significantly from that of the BT + VLCD condition (12.2 kg vs. 10.9 kg).

Wing and colleagues (17) also examined the possibility of using the VLCD in the context of a yearlong behavioral treatment program. These investigators studied 93 patients with NIDDM and randomly assigned them to either a balanced low-calorie diet (1000–1200 kcal/d) throughout the 52 weeks or to a program that included two 12-week periods of VLCD. Subjects in the BT + VLCD condition consumed 400 kcal/d for weeks 1–12 and 24–36 and then gradually increased their intake after these periods until they were eating 1000–1200 kcal/d. After 24 weeks of treatment, subjects in the BT + VLCD condition had lost 16.4 kg, while those in the BT + LCD condition had lost only 12.3 kg. Despite continued weekly contact and the use of a second 12-week interval of the VLCD, both groups regained approximately 2 kg over the next 6 months. At the end of the yearlong program, the BT + VLCD group had lost 14.2 kg versus 10.5 kg in the BT + LCD conditions. This difference approached statistical significance ($P = .057$), but is of questionable clinical significance. Treatment was then terminated, and subjects were recontacted 1 year later. At that time, the VLCD group maintained a weight loss of 7.2 kg versus 5.7 kg in the LCD group.

Very low calorie diets pose an interesting dilemma for behavior therapists. These regimens have been successful in accomplishing what they are designed to accomplish, namely, increasing the magnitude of initial weight loss. The diets are well tolerated by patients, and

most patients find them easier to follow than balanced low-calorie diets. They have also improved glycemic control (49). Moreover, it appears that VLCDs of 800 kcal/d are just as effective for weight loss as those with 400–600 kcal, and reduce the risks and the need for medical monitoring (50). However, to date it has not been possible to develop approaches that are effective in maintaining the large initial weight losses obtained with VLCDs. Creative approaches to using VLCDs that allow these regimens to be used over longer intervals may be helpful. For example, Williams et al. (51) recently tested the efficacy of using intermittent VLCDs for individuals with type 2 diabetes. These investigators suggested that periodic VLCDs might improve both weight loss and glycemic control in patients with diabetes. One group of participants received a standard 20-week behavioral program with a 1500- to 1800-kcal diet throughout. A second group used a VLCD 1 day each week, and a third group used the VLCD for 5 consecutive days every 5 weeks. Weight loss for the standard group averaged 5.4 kg over 20 weeks, compared to 9.6 kg in the 1 day/week group and 10.4 kg in the 5 day/week group. The 5 day/week regimen also increased the percent of participants losing more than 5 kg (93% vs. 50–69%) and the percent who normalized glycemic control (47% vs. 8% in SBT). It remains unclear whether this intermittent regimen also improves long-term weight loss. Further research with novel approaches to using VLCDs is clearly warranted.

2 Low-Fat Diets

Another approach to improving weight loss in behavioral treatment programs has been to emphasize decreasing dietary fat intake, instead of or in addition to decreasing total calories. This approach is based on studies suggesting that subjects who are allowed to consume as much low-fat, high-carbohydrate food as they desire will decrease their calorie intake and lose weight (52,53).

There have been several recent behavioral studies addressing the effects of restricting fat intake (Table 5). Jeffery and colleagues (54) compared the effectiveness of the usual behavioral approach of restricting calorie intake, with a program based on restricting only the intake of dietary fat. Moderately overweight women (N = 122) were recruited; half of the women were given a fat goal (20 g fat/d), but no calorie goal; the other half were given a calorie goal (1000–1200 kcal/d), but no dietary fat goal. Both groups were seen weekly for 6 weeks, biweekly for 20 weeks and then monthly through 18 months. Weight losses at the end of 6 months were

Table 5 Weight Loss in Long-Term Studies of Behavioral Interventions with Low-Fat Versus Low-Calorie Diets

| | Short-term results | | | | Long-term results | | | |
| | | Weight loss | | | | | Weight loss | | |
Trial	Duration	Low cal	Low fat	Low cal/low fat	Duration	Low cal	Low fat	Low cal/low fat
Jeffery (54)	24 wk	3.7 kg	4.6 kg	—	78 wk	+ 1.8 kg	+ .4 kg	—
Schlundt (55)	20 wk	—	4.6 kg	8.8 kg*	36–52 wk	—	2.6 kg	5.5 kg*
Pascale (56)								
NIDDM	16 wk	4.6 kg	—	7.7 kg*	52 wk	1.0 kg	—	5.2 kg*
FH+	16 wk	6.9 kg	—	7.5 kg	52 wk	3.2 kg	—	3.1 kg
Viegener (18)	24 wk	8.9 kg	10.2 kg	—	52 wk	9.0 kg	9.0 kg	—

*Difference in weight loss between groups significant at $P < .05$.

comparable in the two conditions: 4.6 kg for fat restriction and 3.7 kg for calorie restriction. Likewise, no differences between conditions were seen at 12 or 18 months. By 18 months, both treatment groups had returned to their baseline levels. The weight losses of the calorie restriction condition are modest compared to most recent behavioral weight control studies, which is not readily explained but may have been due to the fact that only six weekly meetings were held before turning to biweekly sessions.

Another group of investigators compared a low-fat, unrestricted-carbohydrate diet to the combination of calorie plus fat restriction. Schlundt et al. (55) randomly assigned 60 overweight subjects to a low fat dietary intervention (20 g fat) with either ad libitum carbohydrate intake or with calories restricted to 1200 kcal/d for women and 1500 for men. Forty-nine of the 60 subjects completed the 20-week treatment program. At the end of the 20 weeks, subjects in the low-fat, ad libitum carbohydrate condition had lost less weight than those who had both calorie and fat restriction (4.6 kg vs. 8.8 kg). Follow-up occurred after 9–12 months but included only 58% of the initial cohort. In these participants, follow-up weight losses averaged 2.6 kg for the ad libitum carbohydrate diet and 5.5 kg for the calorie-restricted subjects.

A calorie plus fat restriction condition similar to that used by Schlundt et al. (55) was also used by Pascale and colleagues (56), but compared in this study to the standard behavior approach of calorie restriction. Ninety subjects were studied, half with type 2 diabetes and half with a family history of diabetes. Subjects in the calorie restriction condition were instructed to consume 1000–1500 kcal/d, depending on initial body weight, and monitored the calories in each food they consumed. Those in the calorie plus fat restriction group were given a similar calorie goal, but in addition were also given a

fat gram goal corresponding to a fat intake of ≤20% of calories. These individuals recorded the calories and the grams of fat in each food they consumed. In the sample of NIDDMs, significant differences were seen between the two diet interventions, with greater weight loss in the calorie plus fat restriction condition both at the end of the 16-week treatment program (7.7 kg vs. 4.6 kg) and at 1 year follow-up (5.2 kg vs. 1.0 kg). There were no significant differences between the diet groups in the cohort of individuals at risk for diabetes. Weight losses in the calorie restriction alone condition in the diabetic patients were poorer than would be expected based on other similar studies.

The best overall results in a dietary comparison study were reported by Viegener et al. (18). Eighty-five obese women were randomly assigned to either follow a 1200-kcal/d diet throughout or to alternate between an 800-kcal/d low-fat diet used 4 days per week and the 1200-kcal regimen. In this alternating condition, subjects were taught to restrict their fat intake to <25% of total calories on the 1200-kcal days and to <15% on the 800-kcal days. The goal of achieving "fat-free" days was also introduced during this program, and subjects were gradually encouraged to develop 4 fat-free days per week.

The dropout rate from this study was quite high (26%), but in the subjects who completed the 6-month behavioral program there was a tendency toward greater weight losses in the alternating low-fat diet condition at months 1–4 of the program. At the end of the 6-month treatment, weight losses were comparable (8.9 kg in standard low-calorie and 10.2 kg in alternating low-fat). Subjects were then offered a chance to participate in a maintenance program with meetings held every 2 weeks for 6 months. Weight losses at the end of this 6-month maintenance program remained excellent in both groups (9.0 kg in both standard and alternating low-fat).

Thus, taken as a whole, these studies suggest some potential benefit to a low-calorie low-fat regimen, versus the traditional calorie focused approach. However the differences are not very substantial. Moreover, the fact that several of the studies had a significant dropout rate makes conclusions from these studies more difficult. Additional evidence suggesting the importance of reducing dietary fat in behavioral weight control studies comes from a correlational analysis by Harris and colleagues (57) of predictors of weight loss over an 18-month program in 82 men and 75 women. Changes in BMI were more strongly associated with changes in dietary fat intake than with changes in total calories. Moreover, decreases in consumption of certain specific foods—beef, hot dogs, and sweets—were associated with weight losses, as were increases in consumption of vegetables and increases in physical activity.

3   Providing More Structure Regarding Dietary Intake

As noted in the overview of the behavioral approach to obesity, teaching patients to rearrange their home environment is a key behavioral treatment strategy. Typically, participants in behavioral weight control programs are encouraged to remove the high-calorie, high-fat foods from their home and to replace these items with healthier alternatives. Jeffery and colleagues (19) argued that better weight losses might be obtained if therapists intervened more directly on the home environment, by actually providing patients with the food they should eat in appropriate portion sizes. To test this hypothesis, these investigators recruited 202 overweight patients (half at the University of Minnesota and half at the University of Pittsburgh) and randomly assigned these participants to one of five groups. Group 1 was a no treatment control group that received no weight control intervention and was simply followed over time. Group 2 received a standard behavioral treatment program (SBT) with weekly meetings for 20 weeks and then monthly meetings and weekly weigh-ins through an 18-month treatment program. These participants were given a daily calorie goal of 1000 or 1500 kcal (depending on their initial weight) and encouraged to restrict their intake of dietary fat. In group 3, the standard behavioral program was supplemented by actual food provision. The calorie goals remained at 1000–1500 kcal/d, but subjects in group 3 were given a box of food each week that contained exactly what should be eaten for five breakfasts and five dinners each week. Patients selected their own lunches and all three meals on the other two days each week.

Group 4 was designed to test their hypothesis that more direct reinforcement for weight loss might improve treatment outcome. The subjects in this group received the SBT, and in addition could earn up to $25 each week for losing weight and maintaining their weight loss. Group 5 included SBT, food provision, and payment for weight loss.

The main finding in this study (Fig. 3) was that food provision significantly increased weight loss. Weight losses with SBT averaged 7.7, 4.5, and 4.1 kg at 6, 12, and 18 months, compared to 10.1, 9.1, and 6.4 with addition of food. Provision of incentives had no effect on weight loss.

After the 18-month program, all intervention was terminated and subjects were recontacted at 30 months to assess weight maintenance (58). Unfortunately, subjects in all four of the active treatment groups maintained weight losses of only 1.4–2.2 kg. These weight losses at 30 months were better than in the no-treatment control group, but did not differ among the four active treatment groups.

Since the use of food provision improved weight losses during the initial treatment program, actually doubling the results at month 12, a subsequent study was designed to determine which component of food provision was responsible for its success (20). Food provision includes actual food, which is provided free to subjects, and a meal plan specifying which foods should be eaten at which times. To determine which of

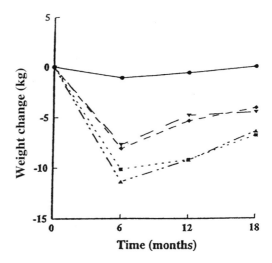

Figure 3   Weight change at 6, 12, and 18 months by treatment group. ●, Control; ▼, SBT; ◆, SBT + incentives; ■, SBT + food; ▲, SBT + food + incentives. SBT, standard behavioral treatment. (From Ref. 19.)

these components is necessary, 163 overweight women were recruited, and the women were randomly assigned to either a standard behavioral program (SBT), SBT plus meal plans and grocery lists, SBT plus meal plans plus food provided on a cost-sharing basis, or SBT plus meal plans plus food provided free. Results at the end of the 6-month study showed that subjects in the SBT condition had lost 8.0 kg. Weight loss as in the other three conditions, which were given meal plans or meal plans plus food, were all significantly better than those achieved by the SBT condition, and did not differ from each other (12.0, 11.7, and 11.4 kg, for groups 2–4 respectively). From these results, it appears that the most important component of food provision is the provision of structured meal plans and grocery lists; no further benefit was seen by actually giving food to the patients.

The meal plan and grocery lists appear to improve weight loss by changing the foods available in the home and creating a more regular meal pattern. Interestingly, the meal plans and grocery lists exerted as much of an effect on these variables as actual food provision. Subjects in the treatment groups that were given either meal plans or actual food reported an increase in the number of days per week that they ate breakfast, an increase in the number of days that they ate lunch, and a decrease in the frequency of snacks. Likewise, when asked to survey their homes and to indicate what foods were currently stored in their home, subjects given meal plans and those who were given the food reported greater increases than subjects in the SBT condition in the number of fruits/vegetables, low-fat meats, medium-fat meats, breads/cereals, and low-calorie frozen entrees. Subjects in these conditions also reported less difficulty having appropriate foods available, estimating portion sizes, finding time to plan meals, and controlling eating when not hungry. On all these measures, the patients who were given the meal plans and grocery lists reported changes that were comparable to those in subjects who were actually given the food.

Several other studies have achieved excellent weight losses using portion-controlled diets, in which some or all of the participants' food is provided to them. These diets often involve a combination of liquid formula and regular food, and are designed for calorie levels of ~1000 kcal/d. Wadden and colleagues (21) used a 900–925 kcal/d diet that included four servings of liquid formula diet (at 150 kcal/serving) and a prepackaged entree plus salad for dinner. After 18 weeks on this regimen, conventional foods were gradually reintroduced and calories increased to 1500 kcal/d. Average weight loss was 16.5 kg at 24 weeks. Participants continued to attend treatment meeting for a full year, and at week 48 had maintained a weight loss of 15.1 kg.

A portion-controlled diet using Slim-Fast has also been shown to improve short and long-term weight losses (59). Participants (n = 100) were asked to consume a 1200–1500 kcal/d diet, but were randomly assigned to use either a self-selected diet of conventional foods or a daily regimen of 2 Slim-Fast meal replacements and 2 Slim-Fast snack bars plus a healthy dinner. At the end of 3 months, the conventional diet group had lost 1.3 kg, versus 7.1 kg in the Slim-Fast group. Subsequently, both groups of participants were instructed to consume one Slim-Fast meal and one Slim-Fast snack bar each day for the next 24 months. At months 27, mean weight losses were 7.7 kg for the conventional-food group and 10.4 kg for the Slim-Fast group. Four-year follow-up data (60) were available for 75% of the original 100 participants (Fig. 4). Those in the Slim-Fast group maintained a weight loss of 9.5 kg at 4 years, whereas the conventional groups weight loss was 4.1 kg. The excellent results from these portion-controlled diets suggest that it is the structure, rather than the calorie levels of VLCDs that makes these regimens effective. By using diets of 1000–1500 kcal/d rather than 400–800 kcal VCLDs, and having patients continue to consume regular food in addition to liquid formula, it appears possible to achieve large weight losses without the subsequent marked weight regain.

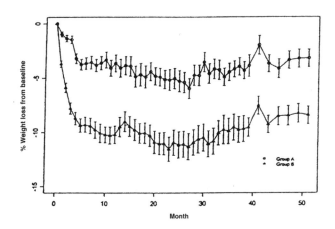

Figure 4 Mean (± SEM) percentage change from initial body weight in patients during 51 months of treatment with an energy-restricted diet (1200–1500 kcal/d). Data were analyzed on an available case basis. Patients received either a conventional energy-restricted diet (control group A, O) or a diet with two meals and snack replacements (group B, △) for 3 months. During the remaining 4 years, all patients received one meal and snack replacement daily. (From Ref. 60.)

B Strengthening the Exercise Component

As noted above, exercise is a key component of behavioral weight loss program, and has been strongly associated with the long-term maintenance of weight loss. Previous to 1990, there were a number of behavioral treatment studies showing that the combination of diet plus exercise was more effective for long-term weight control than diet or exercise alone (35,36,61). Foreyt and colleagues (27) recently replicated this finding in a study of 165 mildly overweight adults who were randomly assigned to exercise only, diet only, diet plus exercise, or a waiting list control. Each group attended 12 weekly meetings, followed by three biweekly meetings and eight monthly meetings. The goal for the exercise groups was to complete three to five aerobic exercise sessions per week, each session lasting 45 mins. The diet program focused on reducing fat to <30% of calories and utilized the Help Your Heart Eating Plan. At the end of 12 weeks, the two diet groups had lost significantly more weight (7.1 kg for diet only and 6.9 kg for diet plus exercise) than the exercise-alone condition (0.32 kg) or the waiting list control (0.98 kg). Approximately 75% of participants completed the 1-year study. At that time, the diet plus exercise group maintained a weight loss of 8.1 kg, which was significantly greater than the exercise-alone condition (2.7 kg), but not different from diet alone (6.3 kg).

Leermakers et al. (26) examined the effect of focusing on exercise during the maintenance phase. All participants (N = 67) received the same initial 6-month weight loss program and were then randomly assigned to an exercise-focused maintenance program or a weight-focused maintenance program. Both maintenance programs involved 6 months of biweekly treatment contact. The exercise-focused program included supervised walking sessions, contingencies for exercise, and relapse prevention strategies focused on maintaining physical activity. The weight-focused program involved general problem solving of weight-related problems. At month 12, the weight-focused group maintained a weight loss of 7.9 kg, versus 5.2 kg (P < .05) in the exercise-focused intervention. Perhaps with the extensive focus on exercise, participants neglected to maintain their dietary change.

Rather than simply addressing the issue of whether exercise is important to include in the behavioral treatment or maintenance component of obesity programs, investigators have begun to ask what type of exercise is best to prescribe (i.e., what type of exercise will produce the greatest adherence and best long-term weight loss) and how best to prescribe exercise to promote adherence.

1 Home-Based Versus Supervised Exercise

Physical activity researchers have shown that it is possible to increase fitness using either supervised exercise or home-based physical activity (62). In weight loss programs, however, home-based programs appear to produce better maintenance of weight loss (Table 6). Andersen and colleagues (25) randomly assigned overweight participants to weight loss programs that involved either three supervised sessions of aerobic dance each week for 16 weeks or home-based activity (goal of 30 min of moderate to vigorous activity most days in the week). Weight losses in the two groups were similar at week 16 (8.3 kg for aerobics and 7.9 kg for lifestyle), but the aerobic dance group regained 1.6 kg from week 16 to 1-year follow-up whereas the lifestyle group regained .08 kg (P = .06). Perri and colleagues (24) also found evidence of similar initial weight losses in home-based and supervised programs, but better maintenance of weight loss in the home-based program. Forty-nine obese women participated in a yearlong behavioral weight loss program. All participants were instructed to complete a moderate intensity walking program (30 min/d on 5 days per week), but half completed this activity on their own, at home, whereas the other half attended three supervised group exercise

Table 6 Effects of Supervised Versus Home-Based Exercise Programs for Long-Term Weight Loss

| | Short-term results | | | Long-term results | | |
| | | Weight loss | | | Weight loss | |
Trial	Duration	Supervised	Home-based	Duration	Supervised	Home-based
Andersen (25)	16 wk	8.3 kg	7.9 kg	68 wk	6.7 kg	7.8 kg*
Perri (24)	26 wk	9.3 kg	10.4 kg	64 wk	7.0 kg	11.6 kg*

* P < .5 for difference in weight regain.

sessions per week for 26 weeks and then two supervised groups exercise sessions per week. Weight losses at 6 months were 10.4 kg for home-based and 9.3 kg for supervised groups. At month 15, the home-based program had an average weight loss of 11.6 kg, versus 7.0 kg in the supervised program. Thus, home-based exercise appears most effective for long-term weight loss maintenance.

2 Short Bouts Versus Long Bouts

Home-based and supervised exercise prescriptions differ in many ways, including the location used for exercise (and the convenience of access to this location), whether the activity is done alone or with others, and the flexibility regarding when the exercise is performed. Since lack of time is the most commonly reported barrier to physical activity, another important difference may be in the duration of each episode of activity. In supervised exercise programs, participants typically complete an hour of exercise three times a week. In home-based programs, the emphasis is on accumulating activity, with a goal of being active for 30 min each day. Jakicic et al. (23,63) have conducted two weight loss studies examining the effect of prescribing exercise in long bouts (40-min sessions) versus several shorter bouts (four 10-min sessions). In the first study (63), the use of short bouts led to better exercise adherence and somewhat greater weight losses at 6 months. The second study, which involved a larger number of participants (N = 148) and continued for 18 months, suggested that long and short bouts can be equally effective for exercise adherence, weight loss, and long-term changes in fitness (23). At 18 months weight losses averaged −5.8 kg for the long-bout group and −3.7 kg for the short-bout group, a nonsignificant difference. Thus, short bouts of exercise may be helpful as participants are beginning to increase their physical activity and represent a useful option for long-term participation in activity.

3 Providing Home Exercise Equipment

Another way to maximize adherence to physical activity may be to provide participants with home exercise equipment. Jakicic and colleagues observed a significant correlation between number of pieces of exercise equipment in one's home and activity level (64). Although the direction of causation cannot be determined from these correlational data, it is possible that providing home equipment to participants would increase physical activity since the equipment may serve as a cue for activity and reduce some of the barriers to exercise. The benefit of providing home exercise equipment was

examined in the study of long and short bouts of exercise described above (23). Participants were randomly assigned to long exercise bouts (40-min bouts 5 d/wk), short bouts (four 10-min bouts 5 d/wk), or short bouts with provision of a home treadmill. The group given the treadmill had higher physical activity levels from 13 to 18 months and better maintenance of weight loss over the 18-month study (Fig. 5). At month 18, the group given the treadmill had an average weight loss of 7.4 kg, compared to 3.7 kg in the short-bout group without treadmills.

4 Personal Trainers and Financial Incentives

As described above, the behavioral approach suggests that by changing antecedents and consequences, it is possible to change behavior. Jeffery and colleagues (22) applied this model to increasing physical activity in participants in a weight loss program. They recruited 193 participants and randomly assigned them to one of five conditions. Group 1 received a standard behavioral program, with home-based exercise and a goal of

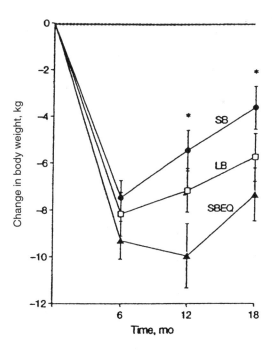

Figure 5 Changes in weight loss among treatment groups across 18 months of treatment (mean [SEM]). Asterisk indicates that data for the short-bout exercise (SB) group and multiple short-bout exercises plus home exercise equipment (SBEQ) group were significantly different ($P < .05$) at the same time period. LB indicates long-bout exercise. Error bars indicate standard error of the mean. (From Ref. 23.)

expending 1000 kcal/wk in physical activity. Group 2 received the same behavioral program and same exercise goal, but these participants were asked to attend three supervised exercise sessions (walking at a track) each week for 18 months. Group 3 had the same interventions as group 2, except that they were provided a personal trainer/coach who called them regularly to encourage them to exercise and met them at the exercise facility and walked with them. This strategy was designed to increase the cues for exercise. Group 4 had the same intervention as group 2, but they could earn small financial incentives for attending the supervised exercise sessions ($1–3/session), thus increasing the positive consequence of exercising. Group 5 had the combination of the personal trainers/coaches and incentives.

The personal coaches and the incentives both significantly increased the number of supervised activity sessions attended by participants (Table 7). Group 2 attended 35 scheduled exercise sessions on average; the use of coaches increased this to an average of 80 walks and the use of incentives increased this to 66 walks (each approach thus approximately doubled attendance at exercise sessions). When the two approaches were combined (group 5), there was an additive effect, and participants attended an average of 103 sessions. However, increased attendance at exercise sessions did not result in increased overall physical activity (all groups exceeded the 1000 kcal/wk goal) or improved weight loss. Group 1, which had home-based exercise, actually maintained the largest weight loss (7.6 kg), confirming findings from the Perri (24) and Andersen (25) studies described above. Average weight losses at 18 months were 3.8, 2.9, 4.5, and 5.1 kg for groups 2–5, respectively. Hence, the cues and incentives increased the targeted behavior (attendance at exercise sessions), but this behavior did not increase overall physical activity (participants appeared to substitute the supervised

activity for other approaches to activity) or long-term weight losses.

5   Resistance Versus Aerobic Exercise

Behavioral weight loss programs typically stress aerobic exercise, such as walking or bicycling. Since resistance exercises may increase lean muscle mass, such changes may offset the decrease in metabolic rate that occurs with weight reduction. However, studies comparing aerobic and resistance exercise have typically reported no differences in long-term weight loss (65). For example, Wadden and colleagues (21) randomly assigned 128 obese women to diet alone, diet plus aerobic training, diet plus strength training, or diet plus the combination of aerobic plus strength training. All participants received the same 48-week behavioral program and were prescribed the same portion-controlled diet (discussed above). Those in the exercise conditions attended supervised sessions three times per week for the first 28 weeks of the program and then two times per week through week 48. There were no significant differences in weight loss for the four conditions at week 24 or week 48 (14.4, 13.7, 17.2, and 15.2 kg for the four conditions at week 48, respectively). Participants in all four conditions regained 35–55% of their weight loss over the subsequent year of follow-up; at week 100, there was again no significant difference among conditions (overall weight loss of 13.7–17.2 kg). The excellent weight loss in all four conditions support the use of the portion-controlled diet, but there is no evidence from this study of any differences due to the type of exercise prescribed.

6   Increasing Physical Activity Versus Decreasing Sedentary Behavior

Epstein and colleagues (38) recently reported the results of a treatment program for overweight children that

Table 7   Effects of Supervised Walks, Exercise Coaches, and Financial Incentives on Attendance, Activity Level, and Weight Loss

Group	No. of walks attended[a]	Self-reported activity at 18 months	Weight loss at 18 months
SBT[b]	—	1119 kcal/wk	7.6 kg*
SBT + supervised walks	35	1063 kcal/wk	3.8 kg
SBT + walks + coach	80*	1294 kcal/wk	2.9 kg
SBT + walks + $	66*	1426 kcal/wk	4.5 kg
SBT + walks + coach + $	103*	1272 kcal/wk	5.1 kg

[a] Out of 222 total possible.
[b] SBT = standard behavioral treatment.
* Difference between conditions is significant at $P < .05$.
Source: Ref. 22.

focused on increasing physical activity versus a program that focused on decreasing sedentary activities or the combination. In the decreasing sedentary activity condition, the amount of time that the children could spend watching television or playing computer games was gradually reduced. At 1-year follow-up, the group that was taught to decrease sedentary activities had greater decreases in percent overweight than the group that was taught to increase aerobic exercise or the combination group. All groups increased in fitness, suggesting that the decrease sedentary activity group had used their extra time for more physical activities. In addition, children in the decreasing sedentary activity group increased their liking of high-intensity physical activities more than the exercise conditions. These results suggest an interesting new approach that could be used to change activity level in overweight adults.

7 Increasing the Amount of Physical Activity That Is Prescribed

Behavioral weight loss programs traditionally prescribe gradual increases in activity to a goal of 1000 kcal/wk. The rationale for selecting this goal is unclear, and recent studies suggest that higher levels of activity may be associated with better weight loss maintenance. For example, in the National Weight Control Registry (66), successful weight loss maintainers are asked to complete the Paffenbarger Activity Questionnaire, indicating their current level of activity. Table 8 shows on average these individuals report expending 2800 kcal/wk. Similar levels of physical activity were reported by the highest quartile of exercisers in the Jeffery et al. study (22), described above, who also had the best long-term weight loss. Jakicic et al. (23) found that participants who reported at least 200 min of activity per week had better weight losses at 18 months than those reporting 150 min or less. Unpublished data from these participants who exercised ≥200 min showed exercise levels of approximately 2500 kcal/wk.

There are several clinical trials currently underway testing higher dose of exercise. Key questions being examined are whether it is possible to achieve such high levels of exercise in a randomly selected group of overweight patients, whether higher levels of exercise are associated with injury, and finally whether higher levels of exercise produce better maintenance of weight loss.

C Strengthening the Behavioral Component

The studies by Jeffery (19), Wing (20), and Jakicic (23) described above are designed to strengthen the behavioral component of weight loss programs by more directly modifying the home environment. Other recent approaches to improving behavioral programs have included lengthening the program, increasing social support and motivation for weight loss, and increasing the target audience. Each of these approaches will be discussed below.

1 Lengthening Treatment

Over the period of 1970–1990, behavioral weight loss programs gradually succeeded in producing larger initial weight losses. Part of this improvement appeared to be due to lengthening of the treatment program. Whereas in 1974 the average treatment lasted 8 weeks and weight loss averaged 3.8 kg (0.5 kg weight loss per week), by 1990, the program had been increased to 21 weeks, and the weight loss had increased to 8.5 kg (0.4 kg weight loss per week).

To more systematically investigate the effect of treatment length on outcome, Perri and colleagues compared a standard 20-week program to a 40-week program (67). The material presented was identical in the two conditions, but the 40-week program covered the lessons more gradually. At week 20, weight losses were comparable (8.9 kg in standard 20-week program and 10.1 kg in extended program). However, when treatment was terminated, subjects in the 20-week program began to

Table 8 Exercise Habits (kcal/wk) Reported by Successful Weight Loss Maintainers

	Energy expenditure (kcal/wk) of successful weight maintainers in NWCR (66)	Subjects in top quartile of energy expenditure in TRIM study (22)
Walking	1093	1125
Stair climbing	188	259
Sports		
Light	211	167
Medium	526	390
Heavy	798	608
Total	2829	2559

regain weight, whereas those in extended treatment (who continued to participate in weekly therapy) increased their weight loss, thus producing significant differences between conditions at week 40 (6.4 kg in standard program vs. 13.6 kg in extended). Between weeks 40 and 72, both groups regained weight, but at week 72, the extended condition maintained a significantly greater weight loss (9.8 kg vs. 4.6 kg).

While these data clearly show that lengthening treatment improves weight loss, it has been suggested that such continued contact merely delays the point at which weight regain occurs. The standard condition regained 28% of their initial weight loss in the 20 weeks following cessation of therapy; the extended condition regained the identical percent of their weight loss in the 32 weeks following the end of their treatment. Although it would thus appear that extended treatment is not helping participants learn the behavioral skills to a greater extent, that relapse can be delayed is an important step forward—especially if by continuing to lengthen programs, relapse can be pushed further and further back in time.

Based on these findings, several recent treatment studies have evaluated yearlong behavioral programs (16,17,68). Subjects in the Wadden et al. study (16) continued to lose weight over time, with weight losses averaging 11.9 kg at 26 weeks and 14.4 kg at 1 year. Wing et al. (17) found that the weight losses were best at 6 months (12.3 kg) and then subjects regained weight, maintaining a weight loss of 10.5 kg at 1 year. The changes between weeks 24 and 48 varied by treatment condition in the Andersen et al. study (68). From these results, it would appear that lengthening treatments to 1 year may be warranted. However, as noted by several of these investigators, attendance declines tremendously over time, and the cost:benefit of extending treatment from 24 weeks to 52 is questionable.

Continuing to have regular contact with patients after the initial treatment program has also been shown to be beneficial for long-term maintenance of weight loss. Perri and colleagues (69) treated 123 women in a standard 20-week behavioral weight loss program, followed by different types of maintenance interventions over the subsequent year. One group of women received no further treatment contact over the year of follow-up; the others received 26 biweekly treatment contacts focusing on problem solving, problem solving plus aerobic exercise, problem solving plus social support, or problem solving plus aerobic exercise and social support. All four of the groups that received continued contact maintained their weight losses better than the no-contact condition, with no significant differences

among the four conditions. Other studies have shown benefit of phone contact during the maintenance period (70,71). Thus, providing some form of ongoing contact with participants appears to improve long-term outcome.

2 Increasing Social Support and Motivation for Weight Loss

Another approach to providing ongoing support for the participant is to involve significant others in the treatment program. For example, spouses have been involved in a variety of behavioral weight loss programs; a meta-analysis of this literature found a small positive effect on weight loss through 2–3 months of follow-up but not thereafter (72). Wing and colleagues (73) examined the effect of natural and experimentally created social support. Participants enrolled in a weight loss program either alone or with three friends or family members (thus, this aspect of the study was not randomized). These individuals or small groups were then randomly assigned to a standard behavioral program or to a program with enhanced social support strategies (intragroup cooperation and intergroup competition activities). Participants recruited with friends had better weight losses at the end of the 4-month treatment and at 10-month follow-up than participants recruited alone. Both recruitment strategy and the social support intervention affected maintenance of weight loss from month 4 to month 10. Among participants recruited alone and given the standard behavioral treatment (representing the typical approach to recruitment and intervention), only 24% maintained their weight loss in full from month 4 to month 10. In contrast, 66% of those recruited with friends and given the social support intervention maintained their weight loss in full.

Attention should also be given to a recent report evaluating the Trevose behavior modification program (74). This program is lay led and charges no fees. Standard behavioral strategies are presented at each weekly group meeting. There are two unique aspects of this program: first, it is indefinite in length, and second, attendance and achieving weight loss goals are strictly enforced for continued participation. At entry participants set a weight loss goal that must be within the normal weight range and represents a weight loss of 9–45 kg. During the first 5 weeks (an initial trial period), attendance is required and participants must achieve a weight loss of 15% of their weight loss goal. Subsequently, absences may be excused but failure to attend or meet the cumulative weight loss goals (22% of the total goal at 2 months, 30% at 3 months, and so forth until 90% of the goal is achieved) results in dismissal from the program. Attendance requirements are gradually decreased after achieving the weight loss goal.

Latner et al. (74) described the outcome of all applicants to the Trevose program from 1992 to 1993. Of the 329 who applied, 286 were invited to join, 202 entered week 1 of the program, and 171 (52%) completed the 5-week trial. Thereafter, 105 of these 171 entrants completed year 1, 54 completed year 3, and 37 completed year 5. The 37 who completed year 5 maintained a weight loss of 15.7 kg at 5 years. While this represents only 11% of the original applicant pool, it is still unusual to obtain a 15.7-kg weight loss at 5 years for even 10% of the patient population. Moreover, 5-year weight loss data were collected by self-report from 77 of the 171 participants who completed the 5-week trial period but were no longer in the program. Their average weight loss was 11.44 kg. Thus, the approach used in this program clearly deserves further empirical investigation. By requiring attendance and success at achieving realistic weight loss goals, this approach may help identify those participants who are most motivated to succeed.

3 Increasing the Audience

In an effort to increase the audience served by behavioral weight loss programs, investigators have studied various media-based interventions. Although these programs have not achieved weight losses comparable to face-to-face programs, they may prove useful in reducing the cost of delivering treatments, expanding the number of individuals who are willing to participate, and providing a way to maintain long-term contact with participants.

Telephone calls have been used primarily as a way to maintain contact with participants during the maintenance phase of treatment. Wing and colleagues (75) suggested that an important effect of such calls would be to prompt participants to continue to self-monitor their diet, exercise, and body weight. Consequently, after successful completion of a 6-month weight loss program (weight loss of > 4 kg), participants were randomly assigned to either no contact control or to receive weekly calls from a research assistant who collected data from the participant's self-monitoring record. Call completion and self-reported adherence to self-monitoring were significantly related to weight regain over the yearlong intervention, but average weight regain in the phone maintenance condition did not differ significantly from the control condition (3.9 kg. vs. 5.6 kg.). Similarly use of telephone calls as the

primary mode of intervention (after two initial group meetings) did not increase weight loss relative to a no-contact condition (76).

Several studies here suggested that television might be a useful way to provide weight loss programming. In one study, an 8-week cable TV weight loss program produced weight losses equivalent to a face-to-face program (77). Harvey-Berino (78) used an interactive television technology, where participants can see and hear the therapists and the other participants. Weight losses were again comparable for those assigned to receive the 12-week program via interactive TV (−7.6 kg.) and those who participated in a face-to-face program (−7.9 kg.).

Computer technology has also been applied to weight loss, with most studies investigating the effects of hand-held computers for self-monitoring and reinforcement (79,80). More recently, Tate and colleagues (81) used the Internet and e-mail to deliver a more complete behavioral program. Ninety-one participants were randomly assigned to a 6-month weight loss program of either Internet education or Internet behavior therapy. The Internet education condition was given access to a website which provided an organized directory of Internet weight loss resources related to self-monitoring, diet/nutrition, and physical activity. The Internet behavior therapy program included in addition 24 weekly behavioral lessons sent via e-mail, weekly online submission of self-monitoring diaries, individualized therapist feedback via e-mail, and an online bulletin board. The Internet behavior therapy group lost significantly more weight than the education group over the 6-month program (4.1 kg vs 1.6 kg), and more participants achieved the 5% weight loss goal (45% vs. 22%). Login frequency was significantly correlated with weight loss. As the number of households with computers and Internet access is increasing rapidly, further research using this technology to provide behavioral treatment of obesity is clearly warranted.

V CONCLUSIONS

Behavioral treatment programs focus on teaching participants to change their diet (calories and percent of fat consumed) and their exercise behaviors. It appears that there has been a fair amount of standardization in the way in which participants are helped to make these lifestyle changes. Currently, strong behavioral programs produce weight losses of 10.4 kg at the end of 6 months. When followed up ~1 year later, participants maintain a weight loss of 8.1 kg. Thus, there appears to have been a gradual improvement in treatment outcome results over the past 10 years.

Recent efforts to improve weight loss results have focused on strengthening the diet and exercise components in weight loss programs. Very low calorie diets have been shown to improve initial weight losses, but it has been difficult to maintain these weight losses long term. Better long-term results are seen with dietary approaches such as food provision, structured meal plans and grocery lists, or meal replacement products that provide a high degree of structure for patients but use calorie intake goals of 1000–1500 kcal.

Research in the area of physical activity has shown benefits to home-based rather than supervised exercise. Related to this emphasis on lifestyle activity, there have been several studies indicating that exercise can be effective when divided into multiple short bouts and that providing home exercise equipment to participants increases their long-term adherence. Although participants in behavioral weight control programs are encouraged to gradually increase their physical activity to 1000 kcal/wk, there is increasing evidence that successful long-term weight losers may expend approximately 2500 kcal/wk in physical activity.

Behavioral researchers have also examined several other approaches to improving outcome, including lengthening the intervention program, and increasing social support and motivation. Telephone calls have been shown to be a useful approach to extending treatment contact. Most recently, the Internet has been used to deliver a behavioral weight loss program. Further research using the Internet to increase the audience for behavioral weight loss programs is clearly warranted.

ACKNOWLEDGMENTS

Preparation of this chapter was supported by NIH grants HL41330 and DK57413.

REFERENCES

1. Skinner BF. The Behavior of Organisms: An Experimental Analysis. New York: Appleton-Century-Crofts, 1938.
2. Bandura A. Social Learning Theory. Eaglewood Cliffs, NJ: Prentice-Hall, 1977.
3. Ferster CB, Nurnberger JI, Levitt EB. The control of eating. J Mathetics 1962; 1:87–109.
4. Stuart RB. Behavioral control of overeating. Behav Res Ther 1967; 5:357–365.
5. Brownell KD, Wadden TA. Behavior therapy for obesity: modern approaches and better results. In: Brownell KD, Foreyt JP, eds. Handbook of Eating Disorders: Physiology, Psychology, and Treatment of Obesity, Anorexia and Bulimia. New York: Basic Books, 1986:180–198.
6. Wadden TA, Bell ST. Obesity. In: Bellack AS, Hersen M, Kazdin A, eds. International Handbook of Behavior Modification and Therapy. Vol II. New York: Plenum Press, 1990:449–472.
7. Kazdin AE. Self-monitoring and behavior change. In: Mahoney MJ, Thoresen CF, eds. Self-Control: Power to the Person. Monterey, CA: Brooks/Cole, 1974.
8. Wing RR. Behavioral strategies for weight reduction in obese type II diabetic patients. Diabetes Care 1989; 12:139–144.
9. Jeffery RW, Thompson PD, Wing RR. Effects on weight reduction of strong monetary contracts for calorie restriction or weight loss. Behav Res Ther 1978; 16:363–369.
10. Jeffery RW, Gerber WM, Rosenthal BS, Lindquist RA. Monetary contracts in weight control: effectiveness of group and individual contracts of varying size. J Consult Clin Psychol 1983; 51(2):242–248.
11. Jeffery RW, Wing RR, Stunkard AJ. Behavioral treatment of obesity: the state of the art. Behav Ther 1978; 9:189–199.
12. McReynolds WT, Lutz RN, Paulsen BK, Kohrs MB. Weight loss resulting from two behavior modification procedures with nutritionists as therapists. Behav Ther 1976; 7:283–291.
13. Penick Sb, Filion R, Fox S, Stunkard AJ. Behavior modification in the treament of obesity. Psychosom Med 1971; 33:49–55.
14. Wadden TA. The treatment of obesity: an overview. In: Stunkard AJ, Wadden TA, eds. Obesity Theory and Therapy. New York: Raven Press, 1993:197–218.
15. Brownell KD. The LEARN Program for Weight Control. Dallas: American Health, 1991.
16. Wadden TA, Foster GD, Letizia KA. One-year behavioral treatment of obesity: comparison of moderate and severe caloric restriction and the effects of weight maintenance therapy. J Consult Clin Psychol 1994; 62:165–171.
17. Wing RR, Blair E, Marcus M, Epstein LH, Harvey J. Year-long weight loss treatment for obese patients with type II diabetes: does inclusion of an intermittent very low calorie diet improve outcome? Am J Med 1994; 97:354–362.
18. Viegener BJ, Perri MG, Nezu AM, Renjilian DA, McKelvey WF, Schein RL. Effects of an intermittent, low-fat, low-calorie diet in the behavioral treatment of obesity. Behav Ther 1990; 21:499–509.
19. Jeffery RW, Wing RR, Thorson C, Burton LR, Raether C, Harvey J, Mullen M. Strengthening behavioral interventions for weight loss: a randomized trial of food

provision and monetary incentives. J Consult Clin Psychol 1993; 61:1038–1045.

20. Wing RR, Jeffery RW, Burton LR, Thorson C, Sperber Nissinoff K, Baxter JE. Food provision vs. structured meal plans in the behavioral treatment of obesity. Int J Obes 1996; 20:56–62.

21. Wadden TA, Vogt RA, Andersen RE, Bartlett SJ, Foster GD, Kuehnel RH, Wilk J, Weinstock R, Buckenmeyer P, Berkowitz RI, Steen SN. Exercise in the treatment of obesity: effects of four interventions on body composition, resting energy expenditure, appetite, and mood. J Consult Clin Psychol 1997; 65:269–277.

22. Jeffery RW, Wing RR, Thorson C, Burton LC. Use of personal trainers and financial incentives to increase exercise in a behavioral weight-loss program. J Consult Clin Psychol 1998; 66:777–783.

23. Jakicic J, Wing R, Winters C. Effects of intermittent exercise and use of home exercise equipment on adherence, weight loss, and fitness in overweight women. JAMA 1999; 282:1554–1560.

24. Perri MG, Martin AD, Leermakers EA, Sears SF, Notelovitz M. Effects of group-versus home-based exercise in the treatment of obesity. J Consult Clin Psychol 1997; 65:278–285.

25. Andersen R, Frankowiak S, Snyder J, Bartlett S, Fontaine K. Effects of lifestyle activity vs. structured aerobic exercise in obese women: a randomized trial. JAMA 1998; 281:335–340.

26. Leermakers EA, Perri MG, Shigaki CL, Fuller PR. Effects of exercise-focussed versus weight focussed maintenance programs on the management of obesity. Addict Behav 1999; 24:219–227.

27. Foreyt JP, Goodrick GK, Reeves RS, Raynaud AS, Darnell L, Brown AH, Gotto AM. Response of free-living adults to behavioral treatment of obesity: attrition and compliance to exercise. Behav Ther 1993; 24:659–669.

28. Wadden TA, Letizia KA. Predictors of attrition and weight loss in patients treated by moderate and severe caloric restriction. In: Wadden TA, Van Itallie TB, eds. Treatment of the Seriously Obese Patient. New York: Guilford Press, 1992:383–410.

29. Guare JC, Wing RR, Marcus MD, Epstein LH, Burton LR, Gooding WE. Analysis of changes in eating behavior and weight loss in type II diabetic patients. Diabetes Care 1989; 12:500–503.

30. Bandura A, Simon KM. The role of proximal intentions in self-regulation of refractory behavior. Cognit Ther Res 1977; 1:177–193.

31. Pronk NP, Wing RR. Physical activity and long-term maintenance of weight loss. Obes Res 1994; 2:587–599.

32. Kayman S, Bruvold W, Stern JS. Maintenance and relapse after weight loss in women: behavioral aspects. Am J Clin Nutr 1990; 52:800–807.

33. Jeffery RW, Bjornson-Benson WM, Rosenthal BS, Lindquist RA, Kurth CL, Johnson SL. Correlates of weight loss and its maintenance over two years of follow-up among middle-aged men. Prev Med 1984; 13:155–168.

34. Colvin RH, Olson SB. Winners revisited: an 18-month follow-up of our successful weight losers. Addict Behav 1984; 9:305–306.

35. Dahlkoetter J, Callahan EJ, Linton J. Obesity and the unbalanced energy equation: exercise versus eating habit change. J Consult Clin Psychol 1979; 47:898–905.

36. Stalonas PM, Johnson WG, Christ M. Behavior modification for obesity: the evaluation of exercise, contingency management, and program adherence. J Consult Clin Psychol 1978; 46:463–469.

37. Wing RR, Epstein LH, Paternostro-Bayles M, Kriska A, Nowalk MP, Gooding W. Exercise in a behavioural weight control programme for obese patients with type 2 (non-insulin-dependent) diabetes. Diabetologia 1988; 31:902–909.

38. Epstein LH, Valoski AM, Vara LS, McCurley J, Wisniewski L, Kalarchian MA, Klein KR, Shrager LR. Effects of decreasing sedentary behavior and increasing activity on weight change in obese children. Health Psychol 1995; 14:109–115.

39. Craighead LW, Blum MD. Supervised exercise in behavioral treatment for moderate obesity. Behav Ther 1989; 20:49–59.

40. D'Zurilla TJ, Goldfried MR. Problem solving and behavior modification. J Abnorm Psychol 1971; 78:107–126.

41. Beck AT. Cognitive Therapy and the Emotional Disorders. New York: International Universities Press, 1976.

42. Mahoney MJ, Mahoney K. Permanent Weight Control: A Total Solution to the Dieter's Dilemma. New York: W. W. Norton, 1976.

43. Marlatt GA, Gordon JR. Determinants of relapse: Implications for the maintenance of behavior change. In: Davidson PO, Davidson SM, eds. Behavioral Medicine: Changing Health Lifestyles. New York: Brunner/Mazel, 1979:410–452.

44. Marlatt GA, Gordon JR. Relapse Prevention: Maintenance Strategies in Addictive Behavior Change. New York: Guilford, 1985.

45. National Task Force on the prevention and treatment of obesity. Very low-calorie diets. JAMA 1993; 270(8):967–974.

46. Wadden TA, Stunkard AJ, Brownell KD. Very low calorie diets: their efficacy, safety, and future. Ann Intern Med 1983; 99:675–684.

47. Wadden TA, Stunkard AJ. Controlled trial of very low calorie diet, behavior therapy, and their combination in the treatment of obesity. J Consult Clin Psychol 1986; 54:482–488.

48. Wing RR, Marcus MD, Salata R, Epstein LH, Miaskiewicz S, Blair EH. Effects of a very-low-calorie diet on long-term glycemic control in obese type 2 diabetic subjects. Arch Intern Med 1991; 151:1334–1340.

49. Wing RR, Blair EH, Bononi P, Marcus MD, Watanabe R, Bergman RN. Caloric restriction per se is a significant factor in improvements in glycemic control and insulin sensitivity during weight loss in obese NIDDM patients. Diabetes Care 1994; 17:30–36.

50. Foster GD, Wadden TA, Peterson FJ, Letizia KA, Bartlett SJ, Conill AM. A controlled comparison of three very-low-calorie diets; effects on weight, body composition, and symptoms. Am J Clin Nutr 1992; 55:811–817.

51. Williams KV, Mullen ML, Kelley DE, Wing RR. The effect of short periods of caloric restriction on weight loss and glycemic control in type 2 diabetes. Diabetes Care 1998; 21:2–8.

52. Insull W, Henderson MM, Prentice RL, Thompson DJ, Clifford C, Goldman S, Gorbach S, Moskowitz M, Thompson R, Woods M. Results of a randomized feasibility study of a low-fat diet. Arch Intern Med 1990; 150:421–427.

53. Kendall A, Levitsky DA, Strupp BJ, Lissner L. Weight loss on a low-fat diet: consequence of the imprecision of the control of food intake in humans. Am J Clin Nutr 1991; 53:1124–1129.

54. Jeffery RW, Hellerstedt WL, French SA, Baxter JE. A randomized trial of counseling for fat restriction versus calorie restriction in the treatment of obesity. Int J Obes 1995; 19:132–137.

55. Schlundt DG, Hill JO, Pope-Cordle J, Arnold D, Virts KL, Katahn M. Randomized evaluation of a low fat ad libitum carbohydrate diet for weight reduction. Int J Obes 1993; 17:623–629.

56. Pascale RW, Wing RR, Butler BA, Mullen M, Bononi P. Effects of a behavioral weight loss program stressing calorie restriction versus calorie plus fat restriction in obese individuals with NIDDM or a family history of diabetes. Diabetes Care 1995; 18(9):1241–1248.

57. Harris JK, French SA, Jeffery RW, McGovern PG, Wing RR. Dietary and physical activity correlates of long-term weight loss. Obes Res 1994; 2(4):307–313.

58. Jeffery RW, Wing RR. Long-term effects of interventions for weight loss using food provision and monetary incentives. J Consult Clin Psychol 1995; 63:793–796.

59. Ditschuneit HH, Flechtner-Mors M, Johnson TD, Adler G. Metabolic and weight-loss effects of a long-term dietary intervention in obese patients. Am J Clin Nutr 1999; 69:198–204.

60. Flechtner-Mors M, Ditschuneit HH, Johnson TD, Suchard MA, Adler G. Metabolic and weight loss effects of long-term dietary intervention in obese patients: four-year results. Obes Res 2000; 8:399–402.

61. Pavlou KN, Krey S, Steffee WP. Exercise as an adjunct to weight loss and maintenance in moderately obese subjects. Am J Clin Nutr 1989; 49:1115–1123.

62. Dunn AL, Marcus BH, Kampert JB, Garcia ME, Kohl HW, Blair SN. Comparison of lifestyle and structured interventions to increase physical activity and cardio-respiratory fitness: a randomized trial. JAMA 1999; 281:327–334.

63. Jakicic JM, Wing RR, Butler BA, Robertson RJ. Prescribing exercise in multiple short bouts versus one continuous bout: effects on adherence, cardiorespiratory fitness, and weight loss in overweight women. Int J Obes 1995; 19:893–901.

64. Jakicic JM, Wing RR, Butler BA, Jeffery RW. The relationship between presence of exercise equipment in the home and physical activity level. Am J Health Promot 1997; 11:363–365.

65. Wing R. Physical activity in the treatment of the adulthood overweight and obesity: current evidence and research issues. Med Sci Sports Exerc 1999; 31:S547–S552.

66. Klem ML, Wing RR, McGuire MT, Seagle HM, Hill JO. A descriptive study of individuals successful at long-term maintenance of substantial weight loss. Am J Clin Nutr 1997; 66:239–246.

67. Perri MG, Nezu AM, Patti ET, McCann KL. Effect of length of treatment on weight loss. J Consult Clin Psychol 1989; 57(3):450–452.

68. Andersen RE, Wadden TA, Bartlett SJ, Vogt RA, Weinstock RS. Relation of weight loss to changes in serum lipids and lipoproteins in obese women. Am J Clin Nutr 1995; 62:350–357.

69. Perri MG, McAllister DA, Gange JJ, Jordan RC, McAdoo WG, Nezu AM. Effects of four maintenance programs on the long-term management of obesity. J Consult Clin Psychol 1988; 56:529–534.

70. Perri MG, Shapiro RM, Ludwig WW, Twentyman CT, McAdoo WG. Maintenance strategies for the treatment of obesity: an evaluation of relapse prevention training and posttreatment contact by mail and telephone. J Consult Clin Psychol 1984; 52:404–413.

71. King AC, Frey-Hewitt B, Dreon DM, Wood PD. The effects of minimal intervention strategies on long-term outcomes in men. Arch Intern Med 1989; 149:2741–2746.

72. Black DR, Gleser LJ, Kooyers KJ. A meta-analytic evaluation of couples weight-loss programs. Health Psychol 1990; 9:330–347.

73. Wing RR, Jeffery RW. Benefits of recruiting participants with friends and increasing social support for weight loss maintenance. J Consult Clin Psychol 1999; 67:132–138.

74. Latner JS, Wison GT, Jackson ML, Labouvie E. Effective long-term treatment of obesity: a continuing care model. Int J Obes 2000; 24:893–898.

75. Wing RR, Jeffery RW, Hellerstedt WL, Burton LR. Effect of frequent phone contacts and optional food provision on maintenance of weight loss. Ann Behav Med 1996; 8:172–176.

76. Hellerstedt W, Jeffery R. The effects of a telephone-based intervention on weight loss. Am J Health Promot 1997; 11:177–182.

77. Meyers A, Graves T, Whelan J, Barclay D. An eval-

uation of a television-delivered behavioral weight loss program: are the ratings acceptable? J Consult Clin Psychol 1996; 64:172–178.

78. Harvey-Berino J. Changing health behavior via tele-communications technology: using interactive television to treat obesity. Behav Ther 1998; 29:505–519.

79. Burnett KF, Taylor CB, Agras WS. Ambulatory computer-assisted therapy for obesity: a new frontier for behavior therapy. J Consul Clin Psychol 1985; 53: 698–703.

80. Taylor CB, Agras WS, Losch M, Plante TG, Burnett K. Improving the effectiveness of computer-assisted weight loss. Behav Ther 1991; 22:229–236.

81. Tate DF, Wing RR, Winett RA. Using internet technology to deliver a behavioral weight loss program. JAMA 2000; 285:1172–1177.

10

Exercise as a Treatment for Obesity

Wayne C. Miller

The George Washington University, Washington, D.C., U.S.A.

Thomas A. Wadden

University of Pennsylvania School of Medicine, Philadelphia, Pennsylvania, U.S.A.

I INTRODUCTION

Ask a group of obese individuals what they should do to lose weight, and virtually all will note the need to exercise more. They are equally likely to volunteer that they do not enjoy exercising or do not have time for it. This is a central challenge for obese patients and their practitioners. Given findings that regular physical activity is the most reliable correlate of long-term weight control, how can practitioners help overweight and obese individuals develop and maintain a program of regular physical activity?

This chapter discusses the effects of exercise on body composition, metabolism, and health, as well as the role of exercise in inducing and maintaining weight loss. We also review components of an exercise prescription and examine the benefits of increasing lifestyle activity, combined with efforts to decrease sedentary behavior. These latter two targets underscore the objective of increasing physical activity, not simply exercise. Physical activity has been defined as "any bodily movement produced by skeletal muscles ... which results in energy expenditure" (1). Exercise is a subset of physical activity and may be viewed as "planned, structured, and repetitive bodily movement done to improve or maintain one or more components of physical fitness" (1). From this perspective, watching 2 fewer hours a day of television would not constitute exercising more but it could, by

decreasing sedentary time, increase spontaneous physical activity.

II PHYSIOLOGICAL ASPECTS OF EXERCISE TRAINING FOR WEIGHT LOSS

A Exercise and Metabolism

1 Energy Cost of Physical Activity

The 24-h energy expenditure can be broken down into several components, including resting metabolic rate (RMR), the thermic effect of feeding, and the energy cost of physical activity. Less than 20% of the RMR is attributed to skeletal muscle (1). Nonetheless, the factor that can cause the most dramatic effect on metabolic rate is strenuous exercise. During strenuous exercise, the total energy expenditure of the body may increase 15–25 times above resting levels (1). This enormous elevation in the body's metabolic rate is the result of a 200-fold increase in the energy requirement of exercising muscles (1). In terms of measurement, the resting energy expenditure of a 70-kg human is approximately 1.2 kcal/min (5.0 kJ), whereas the energy cost during strenuous exercise can be 18–30 kcal/min (75–125 kJ) (1). At first glance, these numbers look promising for weight loss; in that the energy cost of a 60-min exercise bout would be from 1080 to 1800 kcal (4518–7531 kJ). This translates into an exercise-induced weight loss of about one-third to one-half pound a day.

However, theoretical estimates of energy expenditure during exercise, such as those previously described, are not realistic for the overweight or obese individual for several reasons. For example, an intense exercise bout lasting 60 min is beyond the reach of most overweight people (2), since the functional capacity of the overweight person is generally much less than that of the normal-weight individual. Overweight people who have a history of inactivity generally can only increase their total energy expenditure by about eightfold during maximal exercise exertion (2,3), and most of these people find it very difficult to sustain an exercise intensity of 75% maximal effort for 20 min (2). Therefore, the best initial expectation for the overweight person would be to exercise for 20 min at an intensity that is six times the RMR (6 METS, or 6 metabolic equivalents). Under these conditions (20 min at 6 METS), the predicted energy expenditure of the exercise session would only be ~150 kcal (628 kJ).

As we have shown above, some of the failure for exercise programs to produce expected outcomes in the obese may be attributed to the inappropriate application of data derived from normal weight or athletic populations to the obese (3). Accordingly, practitioners are cautioned against using prediction equations and metabolic estimates for obese individuals until the predictors have been validated for the obese (2,3). (More on the use of prediction equations for energy expenditure in the obese is given later in this chapter; see Sec. II.C.)

Although it may seem that the absolute contribution of the energy cost of activity to offset the daily energy balance during weight loss treatment is small, the relative contribution of exercise to the 24-h energy expenditure is important. Even the 20-min exercise bout described above may account for 10% or more of the daily energy expenditure for an obese person. Furthermore, exercise may have a metabolic effect beyond that which is accounted for during the actual exercise session itself.

2   Exercise and Resting Metabolic Rate

The RMR accounts for ~60–75% of the total energy expenditure. Therefore, anything that alters the RMR has the potential to significantly impact body weight. The association between obesity and an impaired RMR has received considerable attention, as have how diet and exercise affect RMR (4,5). It is well known that caloric restriction produces a rapid reduction in RMR

of up to 20%. This reduction in RMR may account for some of the plateau in weight loss observed even when energy intake is held at a reduced level. On the contrary, it is also well known that exercise increases the RMR, but the magnitude and duration of the increase post exercise are not well understood. Furthermore, it is not clear how the exercise prescription can be optimized to enhance RMR and offset any metabolic decline produced by restrictive dieting.

Early work revealed that daily aerobic exercise at 60% of VO₂max, initiated 2 weeks after a very low calorie diet (500 kcal/d, 2092 kJ/d), normalized the diet-induced depression in RMR and attenuated the diet-induced loss in lean body mass (4). A later study found that when aerobic exercise was initiated simultaneously with a severely restricted diet, RMR was maintained, but the diet-induced loss in lean tissue was not safeguarded (5). Other studies, in which diet and exercise were initiated simultaneously, have shown that exercise neither minimized the loss of lean tissue nor maintained RMR (6,7). Although the data are not consistently clear, the American College of Sports Medicine attests that exercise helps maintain the RMR and slows the rate of fat-free tissue loss that occurs when a person loses weight by severe caloric restriction (1). Whether exercise completely offsets the diet-induced reduction or only partially offsets the diet-induced reduction in RMR may depend on the severity and duration of the diet restrictions; type, duration, and intensity of exercise; and the magnitude of changes in body composition.

The most extensive review of the effect of exercise on RMR was performed several years ago by Ballor and Poehlman (8). This meta-analytical review pooled together data from 33 reports, which included 60 group means from weight loss studies using either diet only or diet plus aerobic exercise interventions. The analysis revealed that there were no significant exercise or gender effects on RMR during weight loss. When diet-induced reductions in RMR were corrected for changes in body weight, RMR was reduced by less than 2% ($P < .05$). These meta-analytical data indicate that exercise training does not differentially affect RMR during weight loss, or enhance RMR during weight loss, and that reductions in RMR normally seen during weight loss are proportional to the loss of the metabolically active tissue (8). More recent investigations infer that aerobic exercise training does not automatically increase RMR significantly. For example, Wilmore et al. (9) showed that RMR remained unchanged following 20 weeks of aerobic exercise training in men and women of all ages, in spite of a large increase of 18% in VO₂max. However, subjects in this study were not necessarily overweight, nor were they attempting to lose weight during the exercise intervention.

Nonetheless, aerobic exercise may prevent the common age-related decline in RMR (10). Endurance-trained, middle-aged and older women presented a 10% higher RMR than sedentary women, when RMR was adjusted for body composition. Although descriptive in nature, these data suggest that exercise may help prevent the age-related weight gain seen in sedentary women, and that the protective mechanism may be an altered RMR.

Since it is well accepted that strength training can increase muscle mass, and that muscle mass is very active metabolically, Byrne and Wilmore (11) have recently examined how strength training may differentially affect RMR in comparison to aerobic exercise training. This cross-sectional study found that there was no significant difference in RMR among strength-trained, aerobically trained, and untrained women. In a randomized controlled clinical trial, moderately obese men and women were assigned to one of three groups; diet plus strength training, diet plus aerobic training, or diet only (12). The exercise protocols were designed to be isoenergetic. The mean weight loss among groups did not differ significantly after 8 weeks, but the strength-trained group lost less lean tissue mass than the other two groups. The RMR declined significantly in each group, with no difference among groups. These data indicate that neither strength training nor aerobic exercise training prevents the decline in RMR caused by restrictive dieting (12).

The relationship among diet, exercise, and metabolism is complex. Diet and exercise do affect metabolic rate, but for how long and by how much remains unclear. Severely restrictive diets generally result in a transient decrease in metabolic rate, but whether this decrease is sustained has not been clearly shown. It may be that the variability in the metabolic response to diet restriction and exercise among individuals is influenced by the type of obesity (gluteal-femoral or abdominal), the cellular expression of obesity (hypertrophic or hyperplastic), and/or the genotype of obesity (8). Some of the variation in the literature with respect to the effects of exercise training on RMR may also be related to the length of time between the last exercise training session and measurement of RMR. Herring et al. (13) reported that RMR was elevated immediately following an exercise session, but that within 39 hr of the cessation of exercise the RMR had dropped 8%. It may be that in order to demonstrate a true exercise-induced elevation in RMR, which would enhance weight control success, the exercise stimulus must be repeated daily or several times per week. Accordingly, the incremental effects of the energy cost of exercise itself combined with the incremental effects of the temporary postexercise elevations in metabolic rate may act synergistically to enhance weight loss success and long-term reduced weight maintenance.

3 Excess Postexercise Oxygen Consumption

It is well established that metabolic rate (measured as oxygen consumption) remains elevated for some period of time following exercise (14–20). This phenomenon has been termed excess postexercise oxygen consumption (EPOC). Studies have shown that the magnitude of EPOC is linearly related to the duration and intensity of exercise (14,15,17,19), and that EPOC following a moderate intensity exercise bout (70% VO_2max) accounts for ~15% of the total energy cost of the exercise (15). The time for metabolism to return to baseline following an acute exercise session can vary from as little as 20 min to 12 hr, depending on both the duration and intensity of exercise (15,16,18,19). Thus, one can see that over a period of months or more, increments of EPOC may play a contributing role in weight loss or reduced weight maintenance for the person struggling with body weight.

Gaesser and Brooks have identified several factors as contributing to EPOC (20). Intermediary substrates, such as lactate and free fatty acids, continue to be oxidized at an elevated rate following an exercise bout. The cost of replenishing glycogen stores also adds to the EPOC. Circulatory levels of catecholamines and other hormones, which stimulate metabolism, remain elevated post exercise. Increased respiration and elevated heart rate also add to the metabolic rate following exercise. Body temperature can remain elevated for as long as 2 hr after exercise, and this thermic response will raise energy expenditure slightly.

Although several studies have examined the possibility of a metabolic defect in RMR, 24-hr energy expenditure, or the thermic effect of food for obese compared to lean people, only a few studies have evaluated EPOC in the obese. Broeder et al. (21) examined five borderline obese men (23.5 ± 1.3% body fat) and five lean men (<15% body fat) for their metabolic response to exercise. Each group performed two exercise bouts, one at 30% of VO_2max and another exercise bout at 60% of VO_2max. Energy expenditure during each exercise session was 720 kcal (3.1 MJ), while oxygen consumption was measured for 180 minutes post exercise. The low-intensity exercise session did not elicit any EPOC compared to preexercise RMR for either group, but the moderate-intensity exercise elicited an EPOC that was 13.5% above RMR, for each group. The authors attributed the failure to show significant differences in EPOC between lean and borderline obese groups to a small sample number.

Although Segal et al. (22) did not study EPOC directly, they did study the postprandial thermogenesis in the obese compared to the lean at rest, during exercise, and postexercise. Eight lean men ($10 \pm 1\%$ body fat) and eight obese men ($30 \pm 2\%$ body fat) exercised for 30 min on a cycle ergometer at their ventilatory threshold (borderline anaerobiosis). Results showed that the 3-hr thermic effect of food was significantly higher for the lean than the obese men during rest (44 ± 7 vs. 28 ± 4 kcal, 184 ± 29 vs. 117 ± 17 kJ), during exercise (19 ± 3 vs. 6 ± 3 kcal, 79 ± 13 vs. 25 ± 12 kJ), and postexercise (44 ± 7 vs. 16 ± 5 kcal, 184 ± 29 vs. 67 ± 21 kJ). Even though the EPOC measurements in this study were confounded with diet-induced thermogenesis, the data showed obese men to have lower metabolic rates postexercise than the lean men.

In another study, 10 lean women (BMI <25) and 10 obese women (BMI 30–45) performed exercise at 60–65% of VO_2max on a cycle ergometer for 13 min (23). EPOC effects lasted for 30 min postexercise for both groups, but there was no significant difference in EPOC or postexercise respiratory exchange ratio between groups.

Although the data on EPOC in overweight people are sparse, findings seem to indicate that the EPOC effect for lean and overweight individuals is similar. Therefore, one would not expect that a defect in EPOC would hinder weight control efforts for the obese. Furthermore, the beneficial effects of EPOC in the overall energy expenditure for the obese should encourage the use of exercise as a tool in weight management.

4 Exercise and Substrate Use

Exercise professionals often prescribe different exercise protocols for the obese person compared to the normal weight individual based on two assumptions: (1) that the obese person is less fit than the normal weight individual, so the metabolic substrate response during exercise is different from the normal weight person; and (2) that low- to moderate-intensity aerobic exercise will allow the body to use more fat as an energy source, thus hastening the loss of body fat in the obese individual (24–26). Despite several research efforts, no significant relationship between body fatness and substrate utilization in response to the same relative exercise intensity (% VO_2max) has been found

(2,27). Therefore, if substrate utilization is a concern in exercise programming for previously sedentary individuals, exercise protocols need not be differentiated on the basis of the severity of obesity (2).

The second assumption is supported by data demonstrating that fat oxidation during exercise at 65% VO_2max is greater than at 85% VO_2max (28), while fat oxidation at 33% VO_2max is even greater than at 65% VO_2max (29). Furthermore, even with a higher total energy expenditure during a 15-min exercise bout at 75% VO_2max, more total fat-derived energy was expended during 15 min of exercise at 50% VO_2max (2). The assumption is also supported by data showing that peripheral lipolysis is maximally stimulated at low exercise intensities (28).

Most obese individuals find it difficult to sustain an exercise session for 15 min when the intensity is >70% of VO_2max (2). Thus, it may be unrealistic to expect obese men and women in weight loss treatment to exercise at a high intensity for 20–60 min. The most feasible application of the data would be an exercise prescription calling for low to moderate intensity.

B Health Benefits of Exercise Training with or Without Substantial Weight Loss

Normalization of body weight or body fat content through exercise is not necessary to improve health of obese individuals with metabolic disorders that are thought to be weight related. For example, Lamarche and associates (30) have shown that a 6-month exercise program consisting of four to five weekly 90-min exercise sessions at 55% of VO_2max improved metabolic profile of obese women in spite of the fact that these women gained 2.3 kg body weight and 2.8 kg body fat during the same time period. Brown et al. (31) have shown that only seven days of aerobic exercise improved insulin sensitivity and glucose-stimulated plasma insulin levels in obese women. Furthermore, some studies have shown that fitness, rather than fatness, is the determinant for disease and mortality (32–34). Although it is not well understood how fitness and fatness interplay as determinants of health and disease, it is well established in the literature that regular exercise participation will improve the health of all people, regardless of size (1,30,31,35,36). For some of these people, improvement in health will correlate well with weight loss, and for other people the correlation may be low because the improvement in health precedes or supercedes weight loss.

Diabetes or poor glucose control, cardiovascular disease, and hypertension are the three commonest comorbidities for obesity. The risks and symptoms for each of these can be prevented, ameliorated, or eliminated with regular physical activity. Table 1 enumerates the benefits of regular exercise participation for people of all sizes, irrespective of the amount of weight they might lose during the program. Accordingly, exercise should be part of any obesity intervention, regardless of whether the primary outcome measures for success are weight related or health related.

C The Exercise Prescription

Physical fitness is evaluated in terms of body composition (% body fat), cardiovascular capacity (VO_2 max), muscular strength and endurance, and flexibility. The ideal would be for all persons to participate in an exercise training program to improve or maintain fitness in each of these categories. However, the majority of Americans do not participate in any type of regular

Table 1 Health Benefits of Exercise

1. Maintenance of reduced body weight and body fat content
2. Prevention of weight/fat regain
3. Reduced systolic and diastolic blood pressure, control of hypertension
4. Decreased resting heart rate, increased stroke volume, increased cardiac output
5. Reduced blood lipids: LDL cholesterol, VLDL cholesterol, triglycerides, free fatty acids
6. Increased blood high-density lipoproteins
7. Reduced cardiovascular disease risk
8. Increased blood glucose control, reduction in oral hypoglycemic medications, reduction in insulin dosage, increased insulin sensitivity
9. Decreased cancer risk: colon, breast, prostrate, lung
10. Decreased bone and joint problems
11. Increased aerobic capacity
12. Increased functional capacity
13. Increased muscular function
14. Increased psychological profile: decreased stress, decreased depression, increased self-esteem, decreased body image disparagement, decreased eating pathology
15. Decreased mortality risk
16. Increased immunity
17. Increased pulmonary function
18. Increased or maintenance of bone mineral density
19. Decreased risk of stroke
20. Maintenance or increase in lean body mass
21. Augmentation in RMR and/or 24-hr energy expenditure (dependent upon changes in body composition, exercise protocol, and accompanying diet)

exercise program. To promote the message of increased activity for all Americans, the American College of Sports Medicine (ACSM) and the Centers for Disease Control (CDC) have recommended that every adult should accumulate 30 min or more of moderate-intensity physical activity on most, preferably all, days of the week (35). Moderate activity in this recommendation is defined as activity that elicits an energy expenditure of three to six times resting metabolic rate (3–6 METS). In layman's terms, this means simple activities such as walking, gardening, playing golf, walking the dog; as well as incorporating more activity into one's lifestyle, like using the stairs instead of the elevator, parking the car at the far end of the lot, etc. Those who follow these recommendations for activity will experience many of the health-related benefits of physical activity (Table 1), but they may not improve their fitness level (35).

Physical fitness, however, is not a dichotomy, but a continuum. Once physical activity becomes a part of one's lifestyle, higher levels of fitness can be achieved by participating in a more structured exercise program. Since it is beyond the scope of this chapter to detail how to prescribe exercise for cardiovascular fitness, muscular strength and endurance, and flexibility, the reader is referred elsewhere (1,35,36). The remainder of this section, however, will give some specifics for cardiovascular exercise training, in that this component of fitness is most closely related to health improvement for the obese. The term "cardiovascular exercise training" is synonymous with the more familiar term, aerobic exercise training.

Improvements in cardiovascular fitness, or aerobic capacity, are directly related to two principles of exercise training—overload and specificity. The overload principle states that an organ, tissue, or system will improve its functional capacity only if it is exposed to a load to which it is not normally accustomed. Repeated exposure to this overload, or exercise stress, causes an adaptation, which improves functional capacity. The principle of specificity states that the training effects derived from an exercise program are specific to the organ, tissue, or system being overloaded. The application of these two principles means that specific muscles, tissues, or energy systems will improve their functional capacity only if the exercise prescription is structured to overload those very same muscles, tissues, or energy systems. The achievement of the desired training effect is therefore accomplished through an exercise prescription that specifies the proper type, frequency, duration, and intensity of exercise required to overload the muscles, tissues, and/or energy system wherein the specific training adaptation is desired.

The overall objective of exercise participation for the overweight person is to bring about a physiological change that will improve the health status of the individual, as well as prevent future disease. As mentioned earlier in this chapter, most people must overcome several obstacles or barriers to exercise, before exercise participation becomes part of their lifestyle. Thus, the art of exercise prescription is the successful integration of exercise science with behavioral techniques that result in long-term program adherence and attainment of the individual's goals (36).

1 Type or Mode of Exercise

The overload principle can be applied to the cardiovascular system in two ways, pressure overload and volume overload. Pressure overload is found when peripheral resistance in the circulatory system is increased, and the heart has to beat harder to overcome this resistance. This condition is called hypertension or high blood pressure, and is an unhealthy and dangerous way to overload the cardiovascular system. The healthy way to overload the system is through volume overload. In volume overloading, the cardiac muscle is overloaded by pumping a larger volume of blood than that to which it is accustomed. Volume overloading is achieved best when the exercise uses large muscle groups over prolonged periods of time in activities that are rhythmic and continuous. Thus, the type of exercise necessary for improving cardiovascular function or aerobic fitness is one that is continuous and rhythmic and that uses the large muscle groups. Examples of good "aerobic exercises" are walking, jogging, cycling, dancing, or endurance games.

2 Frequency of Exercise

The exercise stimulus must be applied repeatedly in order to achieve and maintain the desired adaptation in the cardiovascular system. The minimal frequency of activity is three times a week. However, for weight loss, daily exercise is recommended (1,36).

3 Duration of Exercise

The duration of each exercise bout should be 20–60 min of continuous or intermittent (10 min minimum) bouts of exercise accumulated throughout the day (36). The duration of the exercise bout depends on exercise intensity (see below). Low- to moderate-intensity exercises can be maintained for a longer period of time than high-intensity exercise. As discussed previously (see Sec.

II.A.4), the best exercise for the overweight person attempting weight loss is an exercise of low to moderate intensity and long duration.

4 Intensity of Exercise

The final criterion to meet for overloading the cardiovascular system during exercise training relates to the intensity of the exercise bout. In order to achieve the benefits of an aerobic training, one needs to exercise at an intensity of 40–80% of maximal aerobic capacity (VO_2max). Individuals who are severely obese and unconditioned should exercise at the lower end of the intensity range (40–60% of VO_2max), while those persons who are accustomed to exercise can exercise at the higher intensity of the range (60–80% VO_2max). The best indicator available outside the laboratory for estimating aerobic intensity during exercise is heart rate. The relationship between heart rate and aerobic metabolism is valid only if the exercise is prolonged and aerobic in nature—meaning that the type of exercise is continuous and rhythmic and uses the large muscle groups. The formula for calculating the proper intensity for the exercise session is as follows (36):

$$E.H.R. = (D.I. \times H.R.R.) + R.H.R.$$

where E.H.R. = exercise heart rate in beats per minute; D.I. = desired exercise intensity or desired percentage of VO_2max expressed as a decimal (e.g., 40% = 0.40); H.R.R. = heart rate range or maximal heart rate minus resting heart rate; and R.H.R. = resting heart rate. Maximal heart rate for the obese can be estimated (3) by the formula:

$$200 - (0.5 \times age)$$

Adjustments in the exercise prescription should be made according to individual needs and any existing comorbidities or relative contraindications (1,36). If vigorous activity is planned, the exercise session should be preceded by a warm-up period and followed by a cool-down period, each consisting of several minutes of aerobic activity (e.g., walking). Medical parameters such as heart rate, blood pressure, and blood glucose may need to be monitored for patients with existing comorbidities.

5 Dose-Response Considerations for Predicting Weight Loss Through Exercise

The most extensive review of the dose-response relationship between exercise and weight loss was recently performed by Ross and Janssen (37). Nine randomized control trials (RTC) and 22 nonrandomized trials, which used exercise only to induce weight loss, were retrieved from the literature for the years 1966 through 2000. Differences in effect were clearly seen when the studies were dichotomized according to length of treatment. The short-term (<16-wk) RTC were characterized by a relatively high energy expenditure (~2200 kcal/wk, 9.2 MJ) that corresponded to an average weight loss of 0.26 kg/wk. In contrast, the long-term (≥26-wk) RTC were characterized by energy expenditures of ~1100 kcal/wk (4.6 MJ), which corresponded to an average weight loss of only 0.06 kg/wk. For the nonrandomized trials, the short-term (≤16-wk) studies also reported greater reductions in body weight (0.18 kg/wk) than the long-term (≥20-wk) studies (0.06 kg/wk). When data from the short-term RCT were combined with the short-term nonrandomized trials, weight loss was positively related to energy expenditure or volume of exercise (37). However, for the long-term studies no dose-response relationship was found (37). Weight loss achieved in the short-term studies reached 85% of that predicted, but reached only 30% of that predicted for the long-term studies.

The reason weight loss was not as tightly coupled with exercise volume in the long-term studies as in the short-term studies is not clear. The authors suggest that one source of error could be found in the estimates of exercise-induced energy expenditure (37). Another possibility is that exercise adherence decreased over the time of treatment, which would have a more dramatic effect for the long-term studies than for the short-term studies.

Nonetheless, the authors suggest that if the goal is to use exercise alone as a strategy for weight reduction, practitioners prescribe exercise programs wherein the predicted energy expenditure approximates 3000–3500 kcal/wk (12.5–14.6 MJ) (37). This means that the exercise prescription would require 45–60 min of aerobic exercise at an intensity of 60% VO_2max on most days of the week (38). A program of this nature is consistent with recommendations for exercise needed for improvements in cardiovascular fitness, but much more rigorous than that which is suggested for improvements in health (35,36). Thus, it is suggested that the initial goal of the exercise prescription be to increase the energy expenditure of daily activity by 300–400 kcal/wk (1255–1673 kJ); with the ultimate goal of progressively increasing the volume of exercise by adjusting its duration and intensity so that the target of 3000—3500 kcal/wk (12.5–14.6 MJ) can be achieved safely for the patient.

Table 2 Equations for Predicting the Energy Cost of Walking and Running over Level Ground[a]

| Walking | kcal/min = 0.343 × S × T |
| Jogging/running | kcal/min = 0.686 × S × T |

[a] Where 1 kcal = 4.184 kJ; S = speed in m/min; 1 mile/hr = 26.8 m/min; T = time in minutes.

An estimate of the net energy cost for walking or jogging/running can be obtained by the use of the formulas (1,36) shown in Table 2. It must be remembered that these equations will only provide estimates, and that the accuracy of the estimates may vary for extremely large persons or persons with a very high percentage of body fat. The most accurate measure of the energy cost of activity can be obtained through direct metabolic measures.

III EXERCISE AND WEIGHT LOSS

A Exercise Alone for Inducing Weight Loss

Weight loss can be induced by increasing energy expenditure (i.e., exercising more), by decreasing energy intake (i.e., eating less), or by combining the two. Expert panels have recommended combining exercise with diet, in part, because exercise alone produces only marginal weight loss (39–41). Studies of this issue were recently reviewed by a panel convened by the National Heart, Lung and Blood Institute (NHLBI) (41). The panel found that in 10 of 12 investigations, exercise produced larger weight losses than no-exercise control conditions; however, the mean difference in weight loss was only 2.4 kg (41). A meta-analysis by Garrow and Summerbell (42) found that obese men treated by exercise alone lost an average of only 3.0 kg and women and average of 1.6 kg. Two additional meta-analyses reported a loss of 0.1 kg per week achieved with exercise alone (43,44), comparable to the rate reported by Garrow and Summerbell (42). Wing's (45) review of this literature reached the same conclusion; exercise alone produced small weight losses that were significantly, but only modestly, greater than those observed in no-treatment control groups.

Reasons for these relatively small losses are easy to understand. In most studies, the exercise regimen consisted of walking three or four times week for 20–40 min per bout. Participants, thus, were expected to expend anywhere from 300 to 900 kcal (1255–3765 kJ) above the RMR each week, which would result in a loss of ~0.1 kg per week.

More aggressive exercise interventions may induce larger weight losses. Sopko and colleagues (46), for example, randomly assigned obese men to one of four groups: (1) no-treatment control; (2) diet-induced weight loss; (3) exercise-induced weight loss; and (4) exercise without weight loss (as a result of caloric compensation). The energy deficit in the diet and exercise conditions designed for weight loss (i.e., groups 2 and 3) was ~3500 kcal (14.6 MJ) per week (i.e., the equivalent of walking 30–35 miles per week). After 12 weeks, both groups reduced body weight by 6 kg. Other well-controlled studies have reported similar findings (47). Thus, a high-frequency/high-intensity exercise program potentially could be used to induce losses of 5% or more of initial weight. Most obese individuals, however, are unlikely to tolerate such a program. Many are deconditioned as a result of months or years of inactivity, and others have joint and other problems that preclude vigorous activity. Adherence to exercise regimens also declines over time, as discussed later.

1   Achieving a 5–10% Weight Loss

A growing body of evidence indicates that small weight losses, as little as 5–10% of initial weight, are sufficient to improve many of the health complications of obesity including essential hypertension, type 2 diabetes, and dyslipidemia (39–41). The data reviewed above, however, suggest that exercise alone will not help the majority of overweight and obese individuals reach this weight loss goal. That is a principal reason that expert panels have recommended that exercise be combined with diet. As discussed in the next sections, the combination of diet and exercise is likely to produce a more satisfactory outcome than either approach used alone.

B   Exercise Plus Caloric Restriction for Inducing Weight Loss

Caloric restriction (i.e., dieting) remains the cornerstone of most weight loss interventions, principally because overweight and obese individuals find it easier to achieve negative energy balance by reducing their energy intake than by increasing their energy expenditure (48). In behavioral weight loss programs, women typically are instructed to consume a 1200-to-1500-kcal/d (5.0–6.3 MJ) diet composed of conventional foods and men a similar diet of 1500–1800 kcal/d (6.3–7.5 MJ). This intervention, combined with weekly group treatment sessions, produces an average loss of 8–10% of initial weight in 16–26 weeks (48). Mean losses may be increased to 15–25% of initial weight by the use (for several months) of a very low calorie diet (VLCD), proving 400–800 kcal/d (1675–3350 kJ) (49).

1   Effects of Adding Exercise

Numerous studies have examined the effects on weight loss of adding exercise to caloric restriction. Perri and colleagues (50), for example, compared the combination of diet plus group behavior modification with the same intervention combined with a walking program designed to expend 800 kcal (3350 kJ) a week. After 20 weeks, participants in the first group lost 8.2 kg, compared with a loss of 10.6 kg for those in the exercise group. Perri's findings are typical of those reviewed by the NHLBI expert panel (41); 12 of 15 studies found greater weight loss in the diet-plus-exercise group than in the diet-alone group, with a mean difference of 1.9 kg. Wing (45), in reviewing most of the same studies, noted that while the weight losses were greater in diet-plus-exercise conditions, only two of 12 studies showed statistically significant differences between diet-alone and diet-plus-exercise groups.

These modest benefits of exercise may be masked in studies of VLCDs in which the marked restriction of calories and carbohydrates results in large losses not only of fat but also of water and lean body mass (49). Wadden and colleagues (51), for example, examined weight loss of patients who consumed a 925 kcal/d (3870 kJ) diet for 16 of the first 24 weeks and were randomly assigned to one of four conditions: no exercise; aerobic exercise; strength training; or aerobic plus strength training. Participants in the three exercise conditions attended three supervised sessions a week. At the end of 24 weeks, participants in the four conditions lost 18.6%, 16.4%, 18.1%, and 19.9% of initial weight, respectively. Thus, supervised exercise training appeared to have no effect on weight loss in the short term. Donnelly and colleagues (52) reached the same conclusions with a VLCD that provided 520 kcal/d (2176 kJ), as did Hammer and colleagues (53) with a diet providing 800 kcal/d (3350 kJ).

2   Inducing Versus Maintaining Weight Loss

It is possible, as noted previously, that larger weight losses could be induced with exercise plus diet by using more aggressive exercise interventions. Patients might, however, compensate for more vigorous exercise by either decreasing their spontaneous physical activity (during the remainder of the day) and/or by increasing their energy intake.

As discussed in later sections of this chapter, exercise's greatest benefit appears to be in facilitating the maintenance of weight loss (and improving cardiovascular health) rather than in inducing larger weight losses. We have found that overweight and obese individuals frequently become discouraged when they have exercised several times during the week only to find at the weekly weigh-in that they have not lost weight. At such times some participants conclude that increasing their physical activity is a waste of time, particularly if they do not enjoy it. For this reason, we now encourage patients to increase their physical activity for the sake of improving their cardiovascular health and quality of life. We explicitly discourage them from linking exercise to losing weight. Regular exercise is critical for maintaining weight loss but not for inducing it.

C   Role of Exercise in Maintaining Weight Loss

Improving the maintenance of weight loss remains a central goal of obesity research. A new generation of weight loss medications holds promise of facilitating this goal (54), but, for now, exercise appears to be the best bet for long-term weight control. This conclusion is based on case studies, correlational investigations, and randomized controlled trials.

1   Case Studies

Several studies have identified groups of individuals who by their own reports, or as documented by medical records, lost substantial amounts of weight and kept it off (55–59). Almost invariably, such individuals reported that they exercised frequently and regularly. Kayman and colleagues (56), for example, examined weight maintainers (i.e., women who had lost 20% of initial weight and maintained it for at least 2 years), weight regainers (i.e., those who had lost 20% but regained it), and normal-weight controls (i.e., women who had always been average weight). Exercise was the principal variable that distinguished weight maintainers from regainers; 90% of maintainers and 82% of controls reported that they exercised on a regular basis (i.e., >3 days per week for ≥30 min), whereas only 34% of regainers reported doing so.

Similar findings have been reported from the National Weight Control Registry, which includes a total of 784 males and females who have maintained an average weight loss of 30 kg for an average of 5.6 years (57). Participants in the National Registry reported expending ~ 2830 kcal per week (11.8 MJ), or the equivalent of walking about 28 miles per week (or more than 1 hr a day, every day).

2   Correlational Studies

A second set of studies followed patients prospectively, after they finished participating in randomized weight loss trials, and examined correlates of long-term weight change (60,61). Participants who maintained larger weight losses at subsequent evaluations reported higher levels of physical activity during the follow-up period.

While suggestive, such data cannot prove definitively that exercise improves the maintenance of weight loss. It is impossible to determine whether exercise promoted weight loss or, instead, was merely a marker for other behaviors, such as keeping food records or eating a low-calorie diet, that were related to weight control. It is also unclear whether participants maintained their weight loss because they continued to exercise, or continued to exercise because they maintained their weight. We have observed that some patients regain weight, despite their reporting high levels of physical activity. They became discouraged and stopped exercising, thus giving the mistaken impression that lack of exercise was responsible for their weight gain.

3   Randomized Control Trials

Randomized controlled trials (RCTs) ultimately are needed to demonstrate a causal relationship between exercise and the maintenance of weight loss. These studies typically have compared diet alone, exercise alone, and the combination of diet plus exercise, and have included follow-up evaluations of 1 year or more. In these studies, patients participated in a supervised exercise program for 16–52 weeks, after which contact was limited to periodic follow-up evaluations. Participants in the exercise conditions were instructed to maintain their physical activity during follow-up.

Surprisingly, RCTs have provided only limited evidence of the benefits of a supervised exercise program for facilitating the maintenance of weight loss. As reviewed by Wing (45), only two of six studies found a significantly greater weight loss at follow-up in patients originally treated by diet plus exercise, compared to diet alone. Similarly, a meta-analysis by Miller and colleagues (62) found no differences in weight loss, or percent of weight loss retained, between diet-plus-exercise and diet-alone groups at 1 year. While the NHLBI review (41) reported greater weight loss in combined diet-plus-exercise conditions (1.5–3 kg greater), this assessment was limited to only three studies. Taken together, these studies suggest that an initial supervised exercise intervention only modestly improves the long-term maintenance of weight loss (and not sufficiently to reach statistical significance) (45).

This finding does not necessarily contradict the correlational data reviewed earlier that showed a strong relationship between exercise and weight loss maintenance. The most likely explanation for the absence of effects in RCTs is that exercise adherence declined over time, particularly during follow-up, but even during the initial period of supervised exercise training. Perri and colleagues (63), for example, found that obese women attended 90% of possible supervised exercise sessions during the first month of treatment, but only 30% of sessions during the 12th (and last) month. Wadden and colleagues (64) similarly found that obese women attended 90% of possible exercise sessions during the first 8 weeks but only 57% of sessions from week 25 to 40. Not surprisingly, only 50% of participants reported exercising regularly in the 4 months preceding a 1-year follow-up evaluation, at which time there were no significant differences in weight loss among patients who originally had been treated by diet combined with no exercise, aerobic exercise, strength training, or combined training (51). Clearly, several initial months of supervised exercise instruction will not improve the maintenance of weight loss if patients fail to continue to exercise. Despite the lack of significant differences among treatment groups in the study by Wadden and colleagues (51), the more times per week patients reported exercising during the follow-up period, the greater was their weight loss at the 1-year follow-up ($r = .48$) and the less weight they regained at this time ($r = -.44$).

4 Volume of Exercise

A consistent finding from both these correlational studies and randomized trial is "the more exercise, the better the maintenance of weight loss." Patients who expended 1500–2500 kcal (6.3–10.5 MJ) a week (or more) were more likely to maintain their full end-of-treatment weight loss (60,65,66). This amount of exercise is double or more the goal targeted in earlier studies.

D Overcoming Barriers to Exercise Adherence

Recent research on exercise and weight control has explored methods of increasing patients' long-term adherence to physical activity. Understanding the causes of inactivity may help in this regard. Common barriers to physical activity include inclement weather, dislike of vigorous exercise, disruption of routine, and lack time (67). Of these, time constraints are probably noted most frequently by the patient.

1 Short-Bout Activity

Investigators have addressed this problem by examining the effects of daily multiple short bouts (e.g., 10 min) of activity, compared with the effects of one long bout (e.g., 30–60 min). The rationale is that it may be easier to find 10 min to exercise on several occasions during the day (e.g., before breakfast, at lunchtime, etc.) than to schedule one 30-to-60-min block. Two studies of average weight volunteers found that three daily brief bouts of jogging (at 65–80% of maximum heart rate) were sufficient to significantly improve fitness, as assessed by maximal oxygen consumption (68,69). Jakicic and colleagues (70) extended this approach to obese women in a weight loss program and showed that daily multiple short bouts of physical activity significantly improved exercise adherence, compared with single long bouts. Participants in the short-bout condition reported exercising on significantly more days of the program (87 days vs. 70 days, respectively). Their superior exercise adherence was associated with a trend ($P < .07$) toward greater weight losses (-8.9 kg vs. -6.4 kg, respectively). In addition, there were equivalent improvements in the two conditions in cardiorespiratory fitness.

In a longer-term follow-up study, Jakicic and colleagues (65) compared the effects of multiple short-bout exercise (10-min bouts), multiple short-bout exercise with home exercise equipment (i.e., a treadmill), and longer-bout exercise (40 min). After 18 month, short- and long-bout groups had similar weight losses and improvements in cardiorespiratory fitness, again suggesting at least comparable benefits of short- and long-bout exercise. Participants with the home exercise equipment maintained a higher level of exercise than participants in the short- and long-bout groups who were not provided treadmills.

2 Home-Based Versus On-Site Exercise

Additional studies have shown the potential benefits of exercising at home rather than at a health club or gym. In a 1-year study of nonobese, older adults, King and colleagues (71) found that patients who participated in a home-based program of high intensity walking (i.e., 73–

88% of maximum heart rate) reported completing significantly more exercise bouts than individuals who were required to walk on site in a group (79% vs. 53% adherence, respectively). Differences in adherence between conditions were maintained at 1-year follow-up. Perri and colleagues (63) compared these same approaches in obese women, all of whom received a comprehensive, 1-year behavioral weight loss program. During the last 6 months, participants who were assigned to walk at home reported completing significantly more exercise bouts than those assigned to an on-site, group walking program (72% vs. 54% adherence, respectively). This superior exercise adherence was associated with significantly better maintenance of weight loss (from month 6 to month 15) in the at-home exercisers.

3 Lifestyle Activity: An Alternative to Exercise

The above studies improved adherence by incorporating short bouts of activity and by having participants exercise at home. Nevertheless, these investigations all required participants to exercise at a relatively high intensity (i.e., ~60–80% of maximum heart rate). Lifestyle activity, by contrast, involves increasing physical activity throughout the day, without concern for the intensity of the activity. As Epstein (72) has noted, "Lifestyle exercise involves a less structured exercise program that does not emphasize intensity. If the goal of the exercise is to produce weight loss, then the energy expenditure, and not the exercise intensity, is the important factor" (p 166). From this perspective, small daily increases in physical activity (such as walking rather than riding, taking stairs rather than elevators, or throwing out remote control devices) could improve weight control without obese individuals ever having to break a sweat.

Lifestyle activity has numerous potential advantages over structured exercise including reducing patients' negative attitudes and improving their self-efficacy concerning physical activity (73,74). Obese individuals, in particular, report negative attitudes toward exercise because they believe it is associated with exhaustion, pain, or other physical discomfort, as well as potential shame and embarrassment. Many report a history of weight-related teasing (75). Beliefs that exercise bouts must be both strenuous and long are likely to contribute to obese individuals' low exercise self-efficacy (i.e., their belief that they do not have the skills or ability to exercise). Lifestyle activity could markedly decrease these barriers.

Several studies now support the benefits of increased lifestyle activity for weight control. Epstein and colleagues (76) showed that obese children who were assigned to diet plus lifestyle activity or diet plus structured aerobic exercise achieved comparable reductions in percent overweight during the first 2 months. At 6 and 17 months, however, the lifestyle participants displayed significantly better maintenance of weight loss, a finding attributed to their superior activity adherence. These findings were replicated in a subsequent study (77). More recently, Andersen and colleagues (78) demonstrated the benefits of lifestyle activity in obese women. Forty women were treated by a group behavior weight loss program that included a 1200–1500 kcal/d (5.0–6.3 MJ) diet. Participants prescribed either lifestyle activity or structured on-site exercise (three times a week for 45 min at 7–8.5 METS) both lost ~8.5 kg at the end of treatment. One year later, the lifestyle participants had maintained their full end-of-treatment weight loss, compared with a gain of 1.6 kg for women in the structured exercise program ($P < .06$). Comparable improvements in cardiovascular risk factors were observed in the two groups, as they were in a 2-year study of non-obese adults (79). Taken together, these findings suggest that lifestyle activity may be the treatment of choice for overweight and obese individuals who report that they hate to exercise. Further studies are needed to confirm this view.

4 Decreasing Sedentary Behavior

Efforts to control body weight may be aided not only by increasing programmed or lifestyle behavior but also by targeting reductions in sedentary behavior. American children, for example, watch an average of 24 hr of television a week, during which time they expend minimal energy and may increase energy intake because of exposure to food advertising. Efforts to decrease inactivity, such as by imposing television or video game blackouts for part of the day, could increase spontaneous physical activity and thus contribute to weight control. This is precisely what Epstein and colleagues (80) found in a treatment study of obese children. Patients who were reinforced for decreasing their physical inactivity achieved better maintenance of weight loss than those who were reinforced to increase their physical activity (79). Robinson (81) similarly showed that a program designed to reduce the number of hours children watched television and played video games resulted in a relative reduction in body weight. Studies are now needed that target the reduction in sedentary behaviors in overweight and obese adults.

IV CONCLUSIONS

Exercise can be a valuable tool in the treatment of obesity. Exercise increases energy expenditure and may slow the rate of lean tissue loss that occurs with severe dieting. The effects of exercise training on RMR may vary among individuals, but the effects seem to be related primarily to dietary intake and body composition. Severe restrictions in energy intake may reduce the RMR by up to 20%, but this effect may be offset somewhat if the individual exercises during the dieting period. Any changes in RMR seen with diet and exercise are probably related more to changes in lean tissue mass rather than a relative change in RMR (energy expenditure per kg lean tissue). The summation of the effects of repeated bouts of exercise on EPOC will assist in weight loss by contributing to a negative energy balance over time. The health benefits of exercise training can be obtained with or without large reductions in body weight. The safest, most effective exercise program for the overweight person would be a program of aerobic exercise, performed 5–7 days per week, accumulating 40–60 min of exercise per day, at an intensity of 40–60% of VO_2max (60–80% for those already acclimated to exercise training). Clearly, this is a goal toward which obese individuals should progress gradually.

The amount of weight loss attributed to exercise, with or without accompanying dietary restrictions, is minimal (0.1–0.2 kg/wk). However, when exercise is combined with a weight-reducing diet, 10–25% of initial body weight can be lost. Exercise is a common component in all studies demonstrating sustained reduced weight maintenance. Hence, continued exercise is currently the best guarantee for maintaining weight loss. The most critical component of the exercise prescription is the volume of exercise, meaning the total energy expenditure achieved through exercise is more important than the intensity or duration of the exercise bout. However, individual barriers to exercise and activity must be factored into the exercise prescription so that the exercise behaviors are sustained. Increasing activities of daily living, while reducing sedentary behavior may initially upset the energy balance enough for some individuals to lose weight.

Exercise should be part of all weight loss and weight maintenance programs. The components of the exercise prescription should be planned so that the maximum amount of energy is expended in a safe exercise bout that is within the framework of the patient's lifestyle. As exercise becomes a sustained behavior, the intensity and/or duration of exercise can be increased in order to gain more pronounced fitness benefits.

REFERENCES

1. American College of Sports Medicine. ACSM's Resource Manual for Guidelines for Exercise Testing and Prescription. 4th ed. Philadelphia: Lippincott Williams & Wilkins, 2001:17, 277–307, 499–512.
2. Granat-Steffan H, Elliott W, Miller WC, Fernhall B. Substrate utilization during submaximal exercise in obese and normal-weight women. Eur J Appl Physiol 1999; 80:233–239.
3. Miller WC, Wallace JP, Eggert KE. Predicting max HR and the HR-VO₂max relationship for exercise in obesity. Med Sci Sports Exerc 1993; 25:1077–1081.
4. Mole PA, Stern JS, Schulze CL, Bernauer EM, Holcomb BJ. Exercise reverses depressed metabolic rate produced by severe caloric restriction. Med Sci Sports Exerc 1989; 21:29–33.
5. Mole PA. Daily exercise enhances fat utilization and maintains metabolic rate during severe energy restriction in humans. Sports Med Training Rehab 1996; 7:39–48.
6. Phinney SD, LaGrange BM, O'Connel M, Danforth E Jr. Effects of aerobic exercise on energy expenditure and nitrogen balance during very low calorie dieting. Metabolism 1988; 37:758–764.
7. Van Dale D, Saris WHM, Schoffelen PFM, Hoor F. Does exercise give an additional effect in weight reduction regimens? Int J Obes 1987; 11:367–375.
8. Ballor DL, Poehlman ET. A meta-analysis of the effects of exercise and/or dietary restriction on resting metabolic rate. Eur J Appl Physiol 1995; 71:535–542.
9. Wilmore JH, Stanforth PR, Hudspeth LA, Gagnon J, Daw EW, Leon AS, Rao DC, Skinner JS, Bouchard C. Alterations in resting metabolic rate as a consequence of 20 wk of endurance training: the HERITAGE Family Study. Am J Clin Nutr 1998; 68:66–71.
10. Van Pelt RE, Jones PP, Davy KP, Desouza CA, Tanaka H, Davy BM, Seals DR. Regular exercise and the age-related decline in resting metabolic rate in women. J Clin Endocrinol Metab 1997; 10:3208–3212.
11. Byrne HK, Wilmore JH. The relationship of mode and intensity of training on resting metabolic rate in women. Int J Sport Nutr Exerc Metab 2001; 11:1–14.
12. Geliebter A, Maher MM, Gerace L, Bernard G, Heymsfield SB, Hashim SA. Effects of strength or aerobic training on body composition, resting metabolic rate, and peak oxygen consumption in obese dieting subjects. Am J Clin Nutr 1997; 66:557–563.
13. Herring JL, Mole PA, Meredith CN, Stern JS. Effect of

suspending exercise training on resting metabolic rate in women. Med Sci Sports Exerc 1992; 24:59–65.

14. Bahr R, Sejersted OM. Effect of intensity of exercise on postexercise O_2 consumption. Metabolism 1991; 40:836–841.

15. Bahr R, Hansson P, Sejersted OM. Effect of duration of exercise on excess postexercise O_2 consumption. J Appl Physiol 1987; 62:485–490.

16. Bielinski R, Schutz Y, Jaquier E. Energy metabolism during the postexercise recovery in man. Am J Clin Nutr 1985; 42:69–82.

17. Brehm B, Gutin B. Recovery energy expenditure for steady state exercise in runners and nonexercisers. Med Sci Sports Exerc 1986; 18:205–210.

18. Freedman-Akabas S, Colt E, Kissileff HR, Pi-Sunyer FX. Lack of sustained increase in VO_2max following exercise in fit and unfit subjects. Am J Clin Nutr 1985; 41:545–549.

19. Sedlock DA, Fissinger JA, Melby CL. Effect of exercise intensity and duration on postexercise energy expenditure. Med Sci Sports Exerc 1989; 21:662–666.

20. Gaesser G, Brooks GA. Metabolic basis of excess postexercise oxygen consumption: a review. Med Sci Sports Exerc 1984; 16:29–43.

21. Broeder CE, Brenner M, Hofman Z, Paijmans IJM, Thomas EL, Wilmore JH. The metabolic consequences of low and moderate intensity exercise with or without feeding in lean and borderline obese males. Int J Obes 1991; 15:95–104.

22. Segal RK, Gutin B, Nyman AM, Pi-Sunyer FX. Thermic effect of food at rest, during exercise, and after exercise in lean and obese men of similar body weight. J Clin Invest 1985; 76:1107–1112.

23. Cormmett AD. Excess post-exercise oxygen consumption following acute aerobic and resistance exercise in lean and obese women. J Am Coll Med 2001; 33(suppl 5):515.

24. Gaterade Sports Science Institute. Commonly asked questions regarding nutrition and exercise: what does the scientific literature suggest? (A roundtable with James O. Hill, William D. McArdle, Jean T. Snook, and Jack Wilmore.) Sports Sci Roundtable 1992; 9:1–4.

25. La Forge R, Kosich D. Fat burning: just the facts. Idea Today 1995; January;65–70.

26. Wilmore JH, Costill DL. Physiology of Sport and Exercise. Champaign, IL: Human Kinetics, 1994:500–504.

27. Geerling BJ, Alles MS, Murgatroyd PR, Goldberg GR, Harding M, Prentice AM. Fatness in relation to substrate oxidation during exercise. Int J Obes 1994; 18:453–459.

28. Romijn JA, Coyle EF, Sidossis LS, Gastaldelli A, Horowitz JF, Endert E, Wolfe RR. Regulation of endogenous fat and carbohydrate metabolism in relation to exercise intensity and duration. Am J Physiol 1993; 265: E380–E391.

29. Thompson DL, Townsend KM, Boughey R, Patterson K, Bassett DR Jr. Substrate use during and following moderate- and low-intensity exercise: implications for weight control. Eur J Appl Physiol 1998; 78:43–49.

30. Lamarche B, Despres J-P, Pouliot M-C, Moorjani S, Lupien P-L, Theriault G, Tremblay A, Nadeau A, Bouchard C. Is body fat loss a determinant factor in the improvement of carbohydrate and lipid metabolism following aerobic exercise training in obese women? Metabolism 1992; 41:1249–1256.

31. Brown MD, Moore GE, Korytkowski MT, McCole SD, Hagberg JM. Improvement in insulin sensitivity by short-term exercise training in hypertensive African-American women. Hypertension 1997; 30:1549–1553.

32. Barlow CE, Kohl HWIII, Gibbons LW, Blair SN. Physical fitness, mortality and obesity. Int J Obes 1995; 19(suppl 4):S41–S44.

33. Blair SN, Kampert JB, Kohl III HW, Barlow CE, Macera CA, Paffenbarger RS Jr, Gibbons LW. Influences of cardiorespiratory fitness and other precursors on cardiovascular disease and all-cause mortality in men and women. JAMA 1996; 276:205–210.

34. Blair SN, Kohl III HW, Barlow CE. Physical activity, physical fitness, and all-cause mortality in women: do women need to be active? Am Coll Nutr 1993; 12:368–371.

35. Pate RR, Pratt M, Blair SN, Haskell WL, Macera CA, Bouchard C, Buchner D, Ettinger W, Heath GW, King AC, Kriska A, Leon AS, Marcus BH, Morris J, Paffenbarger RS, Patrick K, Pollock ML, Rippe JM, Sallis J, Wilmore JH. A recommendation from the Centers for Disease Control and Prevention and the American College of Sports Medicine. JAMA 1995; 273:402–407.

36. American College of Sports Medicine. ACSM's Guidelines for Exercise Testing and Prescription. 6th ed. Philadelphia: Lippincott Williams & Wilkins, 2000:137–164, 302–303.

37. Ross R, Janssen I. Physical activity, total regional obesity: dose-response considerations. Med Sci Sports Exerc 2001; 33(suppl):S521–S527.

38. Ross R, Dagnone D, Jones PHJ, Smith H, , Paddags A, Hudson R, Janssen I. Reduction in obesity and related cormobid conditions after diet-induced weight loss or exercise-induced weight loss in men: a randomized controlled trial. Ann Intern Med 2000; 133:92–103.

39. Institute of Medicine. Weighing the Options: Criteria for Evaluating Weight Management Programs. Washington: Government Printing Office, 1995.

40. World Health Organization. Obesity: Preventing and Managing the Global Epidemic Geneva: World Health Organization, 1998.

41. NHLBI. Clinical guidelines on the identification, evaluation, and treatment of overweight and obesity in adults: the evidence report. Obes Res 1998; 6:51S–210S.

42. Garrow JS, Summerbell CD. Meta-analysis: Effect of exercise, with or without dieting, on the body composi-

tion of overweight subjects. Eur J Clin Nutr 1995; 49:1–10.

43. Epstein LH, Wing RR. Aerobic exercise and weight. Addict Behav 1980; 5:371–388.

44. Ballor DL, Keesey RE. A meta-analysis of the factors affecting exercise induced changes in body mass, fat mass, and fat-free mass in males and females. Int J Obes 1991; 15:717–726.

45. Wing RR. Physical activity in the treatment of the adulthood overweight and obesity: current evidence and research issues. Med Sci Sports Exerc 1999; 31:S547–S552.

46. Sopko G, Leon AS, Jacobs DR Jr, Foster N, Moy J, Kuba K, Anderson JT, Casal D, McNally C, Frantz I. The effects of exercise and weight loss on plasma lipids in young obese men. Metabolism 1985; 34:227–236.

47. Bouchard C, Tremblay A, Nadeau A, Dussault J, Depres JP, Theriault G, Lupien PJ, Serresse O, Boulay MR, Fournier G. Long-term exercise training with constant energy intake: effect on body composition and selected metabolic variables. Int J Obes 1990; 14:57–73.

48. Wadden TA, Foster GD. Behavioral treatment of obesity. Med Clin North Am 2000; 84:441–461.

49. National Task Force on the Prevention and Treatment of Obesity. Very low calorie diets. JAMA 1993; 270:967–974.

50. Perri MG, McAdoo WG, McAllister DA, Laurer JB, Yancey DZ. Enhancing the efficacy of behavior therapy for obesity: effects of aerobic exercise and a multi component maintenance program. J Consult Clin Psychol 1986; 54:670–675.

51. Wadden TA, Vogt RA, Foster GD, Anderson DA. Exercise and the maintenance of weight loss: one-year follow-up of a controlled clinical trial. J Consult Clin Psychol 1998; 66:429–433.

52. Donnelly JE, Pronk NP, Jacobson MS, Jakicic JM. Effects of very low calorie diets and physical training regimens on body composition and resting energy expenditure in obese females. Am J Clin Nutr 1991; 54:56–61.

53. Hammer RL, Barrier CA, Roundy ES, Bradford JM, Fisher AG. Calorie-restricted low-fat diet and exercise in obese women. Am J Clin Nutr 1989; 49:77–85.

54. Bray GA, Greenway FL. Current and potential drugs for treatment of obesity. Endocr Rev 2000; 20:805–875.

55. Colvin RH, Ohlson SB. A descriptive analysis of men and women who have lost significant weight and are highly successful at maintaining the weight loss. Addict Behav 1983; 8:281–295.

56. Kayman S, Bruvold W, Stern JS. Maintenance and relapse after weight loss in women: behavioral aspects. Am J Clin Nutr 1990; 52:800–807.

57. Klem ML, Wing RR, McGuire MT, Seagle HM, Hill JO. A descriptive study of individuals successful at long-term maintenance of substantial weight loss. Am J Clin Nutr 1997; 66:239–246.

58. Pronk NP, Wing RR. Physical activity and long-term maintenance of weight loss. Obes Res 1994; 2:587–599.

59. Marston AR, Criss J. Maintenance of successful weight loss: incidence and prediction. Int J Obes 1984; 8:587–599.

60. Hartmann WM, Stroud M, Sweet DM, Saxton J. Long-term maintenance of weight loss following supplemented fasting. Int J Eating Disord 1993; 14:87–93.

61. Jeffrey RW, Bjornson-Benson WM, Rosenthal BS, Lindquist RA, Kurth CL, Johnson SL. Correlates of weight loss and its maintenance over two years of follow-up among middle-aged men. Prev Med 1984; 13:155–168.

62. Miller WC, Koceja DM, Hamilton EJ. A meta-analysis of the past 25 years of weight loss research using diet, exercise, or diet plus exercise intervention. Int J Obes 1997; 21:941–947.

63. Perri MG, Martin AD, Leermakers EA, Sears SF. Effects of group- versus home-based exercise training in healthy older men and women. J Consult Clin Psychol 1997; 65:278–285.

64. Wadden TA, Vogt RA, Anderson RE, Bartlett SJ, Foster GD, Kuehnel RH, Wilk JE, Weinstock RS, Buckenmeyer P, Berkowitz RA, Steen SN. Exercise in the treatment of obesity: effects of four interventions on body composition, resting energy expenditure, appetite and mood. J Consult Clin Psychol 1997; 65:269–277.

65. Jakicic J, Wing R, Winters C. Effects of intermittent exercise and use of home exercise equipment on adherence, weight loss, and fitness in overweight women. JAMA 1999; 282:1554–1560.

66. Jeffrey RW, Wing RR, Thorson C, Burton LR. Use of personal trainers and financial incentives to increase exercise in a behavioral weight loss program. J Consult Clin Psychol 1998; 66:777–783.

67. Dishman RK, Sallis JF. Determinants and interventions for physical activity and exercise. In: Bouchard C, Shephard RJ, Stephens T, eds. Physical Activity, Fitness, and Health. Champaign, IL: Human Kinetics, 1994:214–238.

68. DeBusk RF, Stenestrand U, Sheehan M, Haskell W. Training effects of long versus short bouts of exercise in healthy subject. Am J Cardiol 1990; 65:1010–1013.

69. Ebisu T. Splitting the distance of endurance running: on cardiovascular endurance and blood lipids. Jpn J Phys Educ 1985; 30:37–43.

70. Jakicic JM, Wing RR, Butler BA, Robertson RJ. Prescribing exercise in multiple short bouts versus one continuous bout: effects on adherence, cardiorespiratory fitness, and weight loss in overweight women. Int J Obes 1995; 19:893–901.

71. King AC, Haskell WL, Taylor CB, Kramer HC, DeBusk RF. Group- vs. home-based exercise training in healthy older men and women. JAMA 1991; 266:1535–1542.

72. Epstein LH. Treatment of childhood obesity. In: Foreyt JP, Brownell KD, eds. Handbook of Eating Disorders:

Physiology, Psychology, and Treatment of Obesity, Anorexia, and Bulimia. New York: Basic Books, 1986:159–
179.

73. Brownell KD, Stunkard AJ. Physical activity in the
development and control of obesity. In: Stunkard AJ, ed.
Obesity. Philadelphia: Saunders, 1980:300–324.

74. Dunn AL, Anderson RE, Jakicic JM. Lifestyle physical
activity interventions: history, short- and long-term
effects, and recommendations. Am J Prev Med 1998;
15:398–412.

75. Grilo CM, Wilfley D, Brownell KD, Rodin J. Teasing,
body image, and self-esteem in a clinical sample of obese
women. Addict Behav 1994; 19:443–450.

76. Epstein LH, Wing RR, Koeske R, Ossip DJ, Beck S. A
comparison of lifestyle change and programmed aerobic
exercise on weight and fitness changes in obese children.
Behav Ther 1982; 13:651–665.

77. Epstein LH, Wing RR, Koeske R, Valoski A. A comparison of lifestyle exercise, aerobic exercise, and calis-
thenics on weight loss in obese children. Behav Ther
1982; 16:345–356.

78. Andersen RE, Wadden TA, Bartlett SJ, Zemel BS, Verde
TJ, Franckowiak SC. Effects of lifestyle activity vs. structured aerobic exercise in obese women: a randomized
trial. JAMA 1999; 281:335–340.

79. Dunn AL, Marcus BH, Kampert JB, Garcia ME, Kohl
HW, Blair SN. Comparison of lifestyle and structured
interventions to increase physical activity and cardiorespiratory fitness. JAMA 1999; 281:327–334.

80. Epstein LH, Valoski A, Vara L, McCurley J, Wisniewski
L, Kalarchian MA, Klein KR, Shrager LR. Effects of
decreasing sedentary behavior and increasing activity on
weight change in obese children. Health Psychol 1995;
14:109–115.

81. Robinson TN. Television viewing and childhood obesity. Pediatr Clin North Am 2001; 48:1017–1025.

11

Preventing Weight Regain After Weight Loss

Michael G. Perri

University of Florida, Gainesville, Florida, U.S.A.

John P. Foreyt

Baylor College of Medicine, Houston, Texas, U.S.A.

I OVERVIEW

For most dieters, a regaining of lost weight is an all too common experience. Indeed, virtually all interventions for weight loss show limited or even poor long-term effectiveness. This sobering reality was reflected in a comprehensive review of nonsurgical treatments of obesity conducted by the Institute of Medicine (IOM). In its report, the IOM concluded: "those who complete weight-loss programs lose approximately 10 percent of their body weight, only to regain two thirds of it back within one year and almost all of it back within 5 years" (1).

In this chapter, we address the question of whether it is possible to prevent the regaining of weight that invariably seems to follow treatment-induced weight loss. We begin by reviewing the long-term outcomes of lifestyle interventions and by describing some of the physiological, environmental, and psychological factors that contribute to weight regain following weight loss. Next, we examine methods designed specifically to prevent regaining of lost weight including strategies such as extended treatment, skills training, portion-controlled diets, monetary incentives, social support, physical activity, and pharmacotherapy. We conclude the chapter by discussing future directions for the prevention of weight regain in the management of obesity.

II LONG-TERM EFFECTS OF OBESITY TREATMENT

Numerous reviews have documented the effects of lifestyle interventions (2–5). Randomized trials conducted in the past decade show that lifestyle interventions, delivered in weekly group sessions over the course of 4–6 months, typically produce mean posttreatment weight reductions of ~8.5 kg. Weight losses of this magnitude usually result in beneficial changes in blood pressure, blood glucose, lipid profiles, and psychological well-being (3,6). However, the clinical significance of 5–10% reductions in body weight is ultimately determined by long-term rather than short-term outcomes. If the weight reduction is not maintained, it is unlikely that the health benefits derived from that weight loss will be achieved or sustained.

Table 1 summarizes the results of 10 behavioral weight loss intervention studies with follow-ups of 2 or more years (7–17). The initial weight changes in these studies ranged from 4.5 to 14.3 kg with a mean loss of 9.0 kg (unadjusted for study n). The magnitude of initial losses appears to reflect the pretreatment weight of the samples, the length of initial treatment, and the degree of caloric restriction. Studies with heavier subjects, longer initial treatments, or daily energy intakes <1000 kcal showed larger initial losses. Final follow-up evaluations,

Table 1 Behavioral Weight Loss Interventions with Follow-ups of 2 or More Years

Study (Ref.)	(n)	Treatment length (wk)	Pre-tx wt (kg)	Initial loss (kg)	Follow-up (yr)	Net loss (kg) at follow-up	Initial loss maintained
Bjorvell and Rossner (8)	49	6 (inpt)[a]	125	12.6	10–12	10.6	89%
Flechtner-Mors et al. (9)	75	12[b]	93	4.2	4.0	6.8	122%
Gotestam (10)	11	16	87	9.4	3.0	2.1	22%
Graham et al. (11)	60	NA	NA	4.5	4.5	3.3	74%
Kramer et al. (12)	152	15	97	11.5	4–5	2.7	23%
Murphy et al. (13)	33	10	88	7.4	3.0	0.5	7%
Stalonas et al. (14)	36	10	82	4.8	5.0	+0.7	None
Stunkard and Penick (15)	26	12	NA	8.0	5.0	4.4	55%
Wadden et al. (16)	16	26	122	14.3	3.0	4.8	33%
Wadden et al. (17)	22	26	106	13.0	5.0	+2.7	None

[a] Included initial 6-week inpatient stay with a 600 kcal/day diet followed by a 4-year follow-up program.
[b] Included the use of meal replacements (1 meal and 1 snack per day) over 4 years of follow-up.

conducted 2–12 years after initial treatment, showed mean weight changes that ranged from a gain of 2.7 kg to a net loss of 10.6 kg. There was a mean net loss of 3.2 kg (unadjusted for sample n) across all studies.

If we consider long-term maintenance of a 5-kg loss or a 5% reduction in body weight as reflecting a clinically significant outcome (1), then only two of the 10 interventions showed successful long-term results. The two exceptions were studies conducted in Europe (7–9), each of which included an intensive, 4-year maintenance program that incorporated ongoing therapist contacts and either the use of meal replacements (9) or occasional periods of very low calorie diets for patients who relapsed (7,8). Omitting these two studies from consideration owing to the intensive nature of their maintenance regimens, the follow-up data in Table 1 show a reliable pattern of weight regain following behavioral treatment. Approximately 4 years after initial treatment, participants have regained 76% of their initial losses and have managed to maintain a mean net loss from baseline of 1.8 kg.

In evaluating the significance of a 1.8-kg loss four years after behavioral treatment, we must consider what might have happened if the obese individual had never entered treatment (18). Secular trend data suggest that the natural course of obesity in untreated adults entails steady weight gain (19) with obese individuals gaining ~0.6 kg per year (20). Accordingly, a long-term finding of the maintenance of a small amount of weight loss may represent a relatively favorable outcome. Furthermore, simply examining mean weight changes may obscure the fact that some subsets of treatment participants achieve clinically significant long-term outcomes (i.e., maintenance of losses of 5 kg or 5% of body weight). For example, in the Kramer et al. (12) study,

the mean net weight loss at 4.5-year follow-up was 2.7 kg; however, ~20% of the participants maintained losses ≥5 kg for 4 or more years. In contrast, a recent community-based study showed that among adults who lost 5% or more of their baseline BMIs, fewer than 5% successfully maintained their reductions for 2 years (21). Collectively, such findings suggest a significant percentage of participants in lifestyle treatments achieve successful long-term outcomes.

III CONCEPTUALIZATION OF THE PROBLEM OF WEIGHT REGAIN

A complex interaction of physiological, environmental, and psychological factors makes the maintenance of lost weight difficult to achieve. Following a period of restrictive dieting, people often experience a heightened sensitivity to palatable food (22). Consequently, exposure to an environment rich in tasty high-fat, high-calorie foods virtually guarantees occasional lapses in dietary control (23,24). Moreover, increased caloric intake during the postdieting period may easily translate into weight regain. During the postdieting period, a variety of physiological processes, including reduced metabolic rate (25–28), changes in catecholamine excretion and thyroid function (29), and increased lipoprotein lipase activity (30,31), may facilitate the regaining of lost weight. Thus, even minor periods of positive energy balance may readily result in weight gain.

As a consequence of this unfriendly combination of factors, most individuals experience some regaining of weight during the postdieting period. Moreover, the weight gain often occurs at a time when there is less contact with a health care provider and fewer reinforcers to maintain adherence to changes in diet and activity. In addition, the most satisfying aspect of treatment, namely, weight loss, usually ceases with the completion of treatment. Consequently, the dieter sees a high behavioral "cost" of continued dietary control and little "benefit" in terms of weight loss. Without professional assistance, a sense of hopelessness may ensue, and a small weight regain may lead to attributions of personal ineffectiveness, negative emotions, and an abandonment of the weight control endeavor (32,33).

This problem is further compounded by unrealistic weight loss expectations, a minimization of the importance of "modest" weight losses, and a failure to achieve personal goals. Virtually all obese clients begin weight loss therapy with unrealistically high expectations about the amount of weight loss they can achieve. For example, Foster et al. (34) found that obese persons commonly expect to lose 25–32% of their body weight—reductions of a magnitude that can only be reliably accomplished through surgery. Such unreasonable expectations may lead obese patients to discount the beneficial impact of modest weight losses such as the 5–10% reductions that are typically accomplished with lifestyle interventions. This mismatch between expected and actual weight changes may lead to demoralization and poor maintenance of the behavioral changes needed to sustain weight loss. Moreover, many obese persons expect that losing weight will help them to realize other personal goals such as improving their physical attractiveness and gaining greater approval and affection from others (35). When these personal goals go unfulfilled, disappointment follows and the motivation to continue with weight management evaporates.

IV MAINTENANCE STRATEGIES

Long-term outcome in weight management may be improved by implementing strategies specifically designed to maintain the behavioral changes accomplished in initial treatment. The various maintenance methods that have been evaluated include extended treatments, skills training, provision of portion-controlled foods, social support, exercise/physical activity, monetary incentives for weight loss and exercise, multicomponent programs, and pharmacotherapy. In this section, we summarize the effectiveness of these strategies.

A Extended Treatment/Professional Contact

Over the past two decades, the magnitude of weight reductions accomplished with behavioral lifestyle treatments has doubled. The increase in weight loss appears to be the result of increases in the length of treatment (i.e., from 10–12 weekly sessions in the 1980s up to current standard of 20–24 weekly sessions). The longer obese patients are in treatment, the longer they adhere to prescribed changes in eating and exercise behaviors. The effects of length of treatment on continued adherence and weight loss have been demonstrated experimentally. Perri and colleagues (36) investigated whether extending treatment would improve adherence and weight loss by comparing a standard 20-week program with an extended 40-week program. The results indicated that the extended treatment significantly improved outcome compared to the standard program. From week 20 to week 40, participants in extended treatment increased their weight losses by 35% while those in the standard length program regained a small amount of weight. Furthermore, the weight loss and adherence data showed that the longer participants were in treatment the longer they adhered to the behaviors necessary for weight loss. Thus, extending the length of treatment may help patients to sustain the behavioral changes required to maintain lost weight.

Table 2 presents the results of 14 studies in which behavioral treatment was extended beyond 6 months through the use of weekly or biweekly treatment sessions (36–49). On average, treatment in the extended-intervention groups in these 14 studies included 42.5 sessions over the course of 54.3 weeks. Approximately 1 year after the initiation of treatment, those groups that received extended treatment maintained 95% of their initial weight losses. The inclusion of a control group (i.e., behavioral treatment without extended contact) in four of the studies allows a rough comparison of behavioral treatment with and without extended contact. The groups *without* extended contact maintained ~61.5% of their initial weight reductions. Evaluating the impact of extended contact by comparison with the standard-length treatment suggests a beneficial impact for extended treatment (i.e., 95% vs. 61.5% maintenance of initial weight loss). Furthermore, the results of additional follow-ups conducted on average 22 months after the initiation of treatment showed that the extended treatment groups maintained 65.8% of their initial reductions. In contrast, the groups without extended contact maintained only 38.3% of their initial reductions.

Collectively, these findings suggest that extended treatment improves long-term outcome. However, following the conclusion of the extended contact periods, participants gradually begin to regain weight. Such findings may be interpreted as reflecting the futility of lifestyle interventions (50,51) or the necessity of taking a continuous care approach to the management of obesity (52).

Table 2 Behavioral/Lifestyle Interventions with Professional Contact Extended Beyond 6 Months Through Weekly or Biweekly Sessions

Study (Ref.)	(n)	Initial treatment length (wk)	Mean initial weight loss (kg)	Type and number of extended contact sessions	Length of extended contact period (wk)	Net loss after extended contact (kg)	Percent of initial loss maintained	Additional follow-up without contact (wk)	Net loss at follow-up (kg)	Percent of initial loss maintained
Jakicic et al. (37)	148	26 Lb	8.2	13 bw	26	7.0	85%	26	5.8	71%
		26 Sb	7.5	13 bw	26	5.7	76%	26	3.7[a]	49%
		26 SbE	9.3	13 bw	26	10.0	108%	26	7.4[b]	80%
Leermakers et al. (38)	28	26	9.6	EF 13 bw	26	7.9	82%	26	5.2	54%[a]
	20	26	8.7	WF 13 bw	26	8.5	98%	26	7.9	91%[b]
Perri et al. (39)	16	20	10.3	None		7.8[a]	76%	48	3.1[a]	30%
	27	20	10.7	15 bw	30	11.5[b]	107%	48	6.4[b]	60%
Perri et al. (40)	16	20	10.8	None		5.7[a]	53%	26	3.6[a]	33%
	19	20	13.2	26 bw	52	12.9[b]	98%	26	11.4[b]	86%
Perri et al.	16	20	8.9	None		6.4[a]	71%	32	4.6[a]	52%
	16	20	10.1	20 wk	20	13.6[b]	135%	32	9.9[b]	98%
Perri et al. (36)	24	26 H	10.4	13 bw	26	12.1[a]	116%	13	11.7[a]	113%
	25	26 G	9.4	13 bw	26	8.1[b]	86%	13	7.01[b]	75%
Perri et al. (42)	15	20	9.5	None		4.1[a]	46%	None	—	—
	20	20	8.4	RP 26 bw	52	5.9	70%	None	—	—
	23	20	9.3	PST26 bw	52	10.8[b]	116%	None	—	—
Viegener et al. (43)	32	26	8.9	13 bw	26	9.0	101%	None	—	—
Wadden et al. (44)	16	26	11.9	26 wk + 13bw	52	12.2	103%	None	—	—
Wadden et al. (45)	38	20[c]	10.9	10 bw	20	12.4	113%	None	—	—
Wadden et al. (46,47)	77	26[d]	17.4	22 wk	22	15.6	90%	52	8.5	49%
Weinstock et al. (48)	45	28d	13.8	10 bw	20	15.2	110%	48	10.0	72%
Wing et al. (49)	41	26	13.5	26 wk	26	10.5	78%	52	5.7	42%
Wing et al. (50)	37	26 D	9.1	13 bw	26	5.5	56%	52	2.1	23%
	40	26 DE	10.3	13 bw	26	7.4	72%	52	2.5	24%

[a] Means with differing superscript indicate significant between-group differences ($P < .05$).

[b] Means with differing superscript indicate significant between-group differences ($P < .05$).

[c] Participants followed either a 1000 kcal per day portion controlled diet or a 1200 kcal/d balanced deficit diet.

[d] Included short-term use of a low-calorie liquid diet (925 kcal/d).

Abbreviations: bw = biweekly; D = diet; E = exercise; EF = exercise focused; WF = weight focused; H = home-based exercise; G = group-based exercise; Lb = long-bout exercise; Sb = short-bout exercise; SbE = short-bout w/home equipment; RP = relapse prevention; PST = problem-solving therapy.

Table 3 summarizes the long-term results of other strategies designed to improve long-term outcome in lifestyle interventions for weight-loss. The findings are discussed in the following sections.

B   Telephone Prompts

Considerable professional time and effort is required to provide patients with extended treatment via additional face-to-face sessions. Thus, one might consider whether telephone contact might be employed as a more efficient method for continued contact. Wing et al. (53) studied the effects of weekly posttreatment phone calls intended to prompt self-monitoring of caloric intake and body weight. The phone calls were made by interviewers who were not the participants' therapists and who offered no counseling or guidance. Although participation in the telephone contact program was positively associated with better long-term outcome, the phone prompts did not improve the maintenance of lost weight compared to a no-contact control condition.

Some studies, however, have found beneficial effects for telephone contacts during the period following initial weight loss treatment. For example, Perri et al. (39) found that patient-therapist contacts by telephone and mail significantly improved the maintenance of lost weight compared to a control condition without contact. In this study, the phone calls were made by the patients' therapists who provided counseling about ways to maintain behavioral changes in diet and exercise.

C   Skills Training

Can training in the skills needed to avoid or overcome lapses in dietary control enhance long-term outcome? Relapse prevention training (RPT) involves teaching participants how to avoid or cope with slips and relapses (55). Studies of the effectiveness of RPT on long-term weight management have revealed mixed results. Perri et al. (54) found that the inclusion of RPT during initial treatment was not effective, but that combining RPT with a posttreatment program of patient-therapist contacts by mail and telephone improved the maintenance of weight loss. Similarly, Baum et al. (55) showed that participants who received RPT combined with posttreatment therapist contacts maintained their end of treatment losses better than did participants in a minimal contact condition. In a recent study, Perri et al. (42) compared RPT and problem-solving therapy (PST) as yearlong extended treatments for weight management and found that only PST showed better long-term outcome than standard-length behavioral treatment. How-

ever, it should be noted that in this study RPT was administered in a didactic fashion as a psychoeducational program. RPT may be more effective when implemented as an individualized therapy (56).

D   Food Provision/Monetary Incentives

Jeffery and his colleagues (57) examined whether long-term weight control could be improved through the use of portion-controlled meals and monetary incentives for weight loss. During initial treatment and the year following initial treatment, the researchers provided obese patients with prepackaged, portion-controlled meals (10 per week at no cost) or with monetary incentives for weight loss or with both. The monetary incentives had no significant impact on outcome. However, participants in the food provision groups showed significantly greater weight losses than those without food provision both during initial treatment and during the subsequent 12 months. The results of an additional 12-month follow-up, without food provision, revealed a significant regaining of weight (58).

In a subsequent study (53), these researchers found that simply providing participants with the "opportunity" to purchase and use portion-controlled meals as a maintenance strategy was not effective, primarily because the participants elected not to purchase the portion-controlled meals. Collectively, this series of studies suggests that the provision of portion-controlled meals may be an effective maintenance strategy only when the meals are provided to participants at no cost. Consistent with these findings, Flechtner-Mors et al. (9) found excellent long-term maintenance of lost weight for participants who were provided with monthly clinician contacts and with no-cost portion-controlled meals and snacks (seven meals and seven snacks per week) over the course of a 48-month period.

E   Peer Support

Can social support be utilized to improve long-term outcome? The benefits of a peer support maintenance program were investigated by Perri et al. (39). After completing standard behavioral treatment, participants were taught how to run their own peer group support meetings. A meetingplace equipped with a scale was provided to the group, and biweekly meetings were scheduled over a 7-month period. Although attendance at the peer group meetings was high (67%), no advantage was observed in terms of adherence or weight change during the maintenance period compared to a control condition. The results of a long-term follow-up showed

Table 3   Randomized Trials of Maintenance Strategies Implemented or Continued After Initial Behavioral/Lifestyle Treatment

Study (Ref.)	Initial tx and length (wk)	(n)	Pre-tx weight (kg)	Mean initial weight loss (kg)	Maintenance strategies	Weeks of main.	Net loss after maintenance	Percent of initial loss maintained	Additional follow-up (wk)	Net loss at f/u (kg)	Percent of initial loss maintained
Baum et al. (55)	B	16	81.5	4.0	None	12	3.5	87%	39	1.5^a	38%
	B (26)	16	81.5	3.9	C + R	12	5.4	138%	39	3.6^b	92%
Fletchner-Mors et al. (9)	B	50	92.7	1.3^a	F 48 monthly mtgs	208	4.1^a	315%	—	—	—
	B + F (12)	50	92.6	7.1^b	F 48 monthly mtgs	208	9.5^b	134%	—	—	—
Jakicic et al. (37)	B + Lb	49	90	8.2	Lb 13 bw	26	7.0	85%	26	5.8	71%
	B + Sb	51	92	7.5	Sb 13 bw	26	5.7^a	76%	26	3.7^a	49%
	B + Sb + E (26)	48	88.3	9.3	SbE 13 bw	26	10.0^b	108%	26	7.4^b	80%
Jeffery et al. (57,58)	B	40	89.4	7.5^a	C (monthly)	52	4.4	58.6%	52	1.4	19%
	B + 1	41	92.3	7.9^a	C + 1	52	3.8	48.1%	52	1.6	20%
	B + F	40	88.1	10.0^b	C + F	52	6.7^b	67.0%	52	2.2	22%
	B + I + F (20)	41	91.1	10.2^b	C + I + F	52	6.2^b	60.8%	52	1.6	16%
Jeffery et al. (65)	B	40	86	8.3	None	52	7.6^a	92%	—	—	—
	B	41	87	6.0	Su. walks 3/wk	52	3.8^b	63%	—	—	—
	B	42	85	5.6	PT walks 5/wk	52	2.9^b	52%	—	—	—
	B	37	88	6.7	Su. walks + I	52	4.5^b	67%	—	—	—
	B (24)	36	86	7.9	PT walks + I	52	5.1^b	65%	—	—	—
Leermakers et al. (38)	B	28	94	9.6	EF 13 bw	26	7.9	82%	26	5.2	54%^{a}
	B (26)	20	94	8.7	WF 13 bw	26	8.5	98%	26	7.9	91%^{b}
Perri et al. (66)	B	17	90.9	5.6	None	65	2.1	38%	26	0.4^a	7%
	B (14)	26	84.1	6.1	C: mail + phone + peer mtg	65	5.8^c	95%	26	4.6^b	75%
Perri et al. (54)	B	21	88.6	7.5	None	26	7.6	98%	26	6.3	84%
	B + C	15	88.6	8.7	C: mail + phone	26	8.7	100%	26	5.8	66%
	B + R	15	88.6	8.5	None	26	4.9^a	58%	26	3.0^a	35%
	B + R + C (15)	17	88.6	9.7	C: mail + phone	26	10.8^b	111%	26	10.3^b	106%

Perri et al. (67)	B	16	92.1	7.5[a]	None	52	0.3[a]	4%	26	0.7[a]	9%
	B	17	92.1	8.3[a]	C: mail/phone	52	6.5[b]	78%	26	5.2[b]	63%
	B+A	16	92.1	10.3[b]	None	52	5.2[b]	50%	26	3.1[b]	30%
	B+A (20)	18	92.1	11.0[b]	C: mail/phone + peer mtg	52	9.7[c]	88%	26	7.6[c]	69%
Perri et al. (39)	B	16	88.1	10.3	None	30	7.8[a]	76%	48	3.1[a]	30%
	B	32	94.2	10.9	Peer mtg	30	9.3[a]	85%	48	6.5[b]	60%
	B (20)	27	89.8	10.7	C	30	11.5[b]	107%	48	6.4[b]	60%
Perri et al. (40)	B	16	89.0	10.8	None	52	5.7[a]	52%	26	3.6[a]	33%
	B	19	97.4	13.2	C	52	12.9[b]	97%	26	9.9[b]	98%
	B	19	95.2	11.3	C + increased A	52	13.4[b]	117%	26	8.4[b]	74%
	B	18	96.9	13.1	C + S	52	13.0[b]	99%	26	9.1[b]	70%
	B (20)	19	97.4	13.7	C + increased A + S	52	15.7[b]	114%	26	13.5[b]	99%
Perri et al. (42)	B	15	94.7	9.5	None	52	4.1[a]	46%	—	—	—
	B	20	97.0	8.4	R 26 bw	52	5.9	70%	—	—	—
	B	23	98.0	9.3	PS26 bw	52	10.8[b]	116%	—	—	—
Wadden et al. (46,47)	B	29	96.3	16.7	Bw meetings	20	14.4	86%	52	6.9	41%
	B+A	31	98.7	16.2	Aerobics 2/wk	20	13.7	85%	52	8.5	52%
	B+St	31	96.8	16.8	Strength 2/wk	20	17.2	102%	52	10.1	60%
	B+A+St (26)	< >	92.4	16.3	Aerobics and strength 2/wk	20	15.2	93%	52	8.6	53%
Wing et al. (53)	B	27	NA	14.2	None	52	8.6	60.6%	—	—	—
	B	26		12.8	Phone prompts (wkly)	52	9.3	72.7%	—	—	—
	B	22		13.4	None	52	9.2	68.7%	—	—	—
	B (26)	26		13.2	Optional FP	52	9.0	68.2%	—	—	—

[a] Different superscripts denote significant between group differences ($P < .05$).

[b] Different superscripts denote significant between group differences ($P < .05$).

Abbreviations: A = aerobic exercise; B = behavior therapy; C = therapist contact; E = exercise equipment; EF = exercise focused; F = FP = food provision; I = incentives; Lb = long-bout exercise; NA = not available; PS = problem-solving therapy; PT = personal trainer; R = relapse prevention training; S = social support; Sb = short-bout exercise; St = strength training; Su = supervised; WF = weight-focused; bw = biweekly sessions.

a trend toward better maintenance of lost weight in the peer support group compared to the control condition.

Wing and Jeffery (59) recently tested the effects of recruiting participants alone or with three friends or family members. The researchers used a partially randomized study in assigning subjects (recruited alone versus with friends) to receive either standard behavior therapy or behavior therapy with social support training. The results of a 6-month follow-up showed that participants who were recruited with friends *and* were provided social support training maintained 66% of their initial weight losses. In contrast, the individuals who entered the study alone and received standard treatment maintained only 24% of their initial losses.

F   Exercise/Physical Activity

The association between long-term weight loss and increased physical activity is a common finding in correlational studies (e.g., 60,61). Similarly, studies of obese persons who have achieved successful long-term weight losses (62) show that exercise is associated with the maintenance of lost weight. Nonetheless, an important question remains as to whether the addition of exercise or physical activity can improve long-term outcome in the treatment of obesity (63).

In a review of controlled trials of exercise in obesity treatment, Wing (64) observed that only two of 13 studies showed significantly greater initial weight losses for the combination of diet plus exercise versus diet alone. Wing also noted that only two of six studies with follow-ups of 1 year or more showed significantly better maintenance of lost weight for diet plus exercise than for diet alone. However, in all the studies reviewed, the direction of the findings favored treatment that included exercise. The short duration of treatments and the relatively low levels of exercise prescribed in many of the studies may have accounted for the modest effects of exercise on weight loss.

The maintenance of treatment integrity often poses a significant problem in controlled trials of exercise. Participants assigned to exercise conditions often vary greatly in their adherence to their exercise prescriptions, and subjects assigned to "diet only" conditions sometimes initiate exercise on their own. Poor adherence to assigned treatments can blunt or obscure the true effects of exercise interventions. For example, Wadden and his colleagues (46) examined the effects of adding aerobic exercise, strength training, and their combination, to a 48-week behavioral treatment program. None of the exercise additions improved weight loss or weight loss maintenance, compared to behavior therapy with diet

only. In all four conditions, adherence to exercise assignments was highly variable, especially during follow-up. Nevertheless, the investigators observed a positive association between exercise and long-term weight loss. Participants who indicated that they "exercised regularly" had long-term weight losses nearly twice as large as those who described themselves as "nonexercisers" ($Ms = 12.1$ vs. 6.1 kg).

Given the potential benefits of exercise for long-term management of weight, how can adherence to physical activity regimens be improved? The various strategies that have been examined include home-based exercise, the use of short bouts of exercise, the provision of home exercise equipment, monetary incentives for exercise, and posttreatment programs focused exclusively on exercise.

1   Home-Based Exercise

Although group-based exercise programs offer the opportunity for enhanced social support, over the long run such benefits may be limited by potential barriers that one must overcome in meeting up with others to exercise at a designated time and location. In contrast, home-based exercise offers a greater degree of flexibility and fewer obstacles. Perri et al. (41) investigated the use of home-based versus supervised group-based exercise programs in the treatment of obesity. After 6 months, both approaches resulted in significant improvements in exercise participation, cardiorespiratory fitness, eating patterns, and weight loss. However, over the next 6 months, participants in the home-based condition completed a significantly higher percentage of prescribed exercise sessions than subjects in the group program (83.3% vs. 62.1%, respectively). Moreover, at long-term follow-up, the participants in the home-based program displayed significantly better maintenance of lost weight than the subjects in the group-based program.

2   Personal Trainers/Financial Incentives

Jeffery and colleagues (65) studied the use of personal trainers and financial incentives as strategies to improve exercise adherence and long-term weight loss. The personal trainers exercised with participants and made phone calls reminding them to exercise. In addition, the participants could earn $1–3 per bout of walking. The use of personal trainers and financial incentives both increased attendance at supervised exercise sessions, but neither improved weight loss. In fact, participants in the control condition, which received a home-based exercise regimen, showed superior maintenance of weight loss at follow-up compared to all other conditions. These results corroborated the findings of Perri et al. (42) regarding the benefits of home-based exercise in the management of obesity.

3 Short Bouts and Home Exercise Equipment

A recent study (37) showed that the benefits of home exercise may be enhanced by providing participants with exercise equipment and by allowing them to exercise in brief bouts. Jakicic et al. (37) tested the effects of intermittent exercise (i.e., four 10-min bouts per day versus one 40-min bout per day) and the use of home exercise equipment on adherence and weight loss, and fitness. The researchers provided half of the subjects in the short-bout condition with motorized treadmills for home use. The benefits from exercise in short or long bouts were equivalent. However, participants *with* the home exercise equipment maintained significantly higher levels of long-term exercise adherence and weight loss than subjects *without* exercise equipment.

4 Exercise-Focused Maintenance Program

Leermakers and her colleagues (38) examined whether a posttreatment program focused exclusively on exercise might improve long-term outcome in obesity treatment. These researchers compared the effects of exercise-focused and weight-focused posttreatment programs. The components of the exercise-focused program included supervised exercise, incentives for exercise completion, and relapse prevention training aimed at the maintenance of exercise. The weight-focused maintenance program included problem solving of barriers to weight loss progress. The results of a long-term follow-up showed that participants in the weight-focused program had significantly greater decreases in fat intake and significantly better maintenance of lost weight, compared to subjects in the exercise-focused condition. These results highlight the necessity of focusing on dietary intake as well as exercise in the long-term management of obesity.

G Multicomponent Posttreatment Programs

A number of investigations have studied the impact of posttreatment programs with multiple components. Perri et al. (66) tested the effects of a multicomponent program that included peer group meetings combined with ongoing client-therapist contacts by mail and telephone. The multicomponent program produced significantly better maintenance of weight loss, compared to a control group that received behavioral treatment without a follow-up program. These findings were replicated in a later study (67) that employed a longer initial treatment (20 weeks rather than 14), included an aerobic exercise component, and achieved larger weight losses at posttreatment and at follow-ups.

Finally, Perri and colleagues (40) examined the effects of adding increased exercise (from 80 to 150 min/wk) and a social influence program (or both) to a posttreatment therapist contact program consisting of 26 biweekly group sessions. Compared to a control condition that received behavioral therapy without posttreatment contact, all four posttreatment programs produced significantly greater weight losses at an 18-month follow-up evaluation. The four maintenance groups succeeded in sustaining on average 83% of their initial weight losses, compared to 33% for the group without a posttreatment program. Although there were no significant between-group differences among the four maintenance conditions, only the group that received all three maintenance strategies (i.e., therapist contact + increased exercise + enhanced social support) demonstrated additional weight loss (4 kg) during the months following initial treatment (see Fig. 1).

H Pharmacotherapy

Can pharmacotherapy prevent weight regain? Haddock and colleagues (68) published a meta-analysis of randomized clinical trials of pharmacotherapy for the treatment of obesity. In studies that met their criteria for analysis, drugs produced medium effect sizes with the placebo-subtracted weight losses for single drugs versus placebo never exceeding 4.0 kg. No drug demonstrated a clear superiority as an obesity medication. Increasing

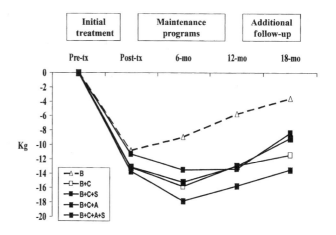

Figure 1 Effects of four maintenance programs on long-term weight management. (From Ref. 40.)

the length of drug treatment did not lead to more weight loss beyond 6 months, but longer drug treatment helped promote weight maintenance.

James and the STORM Study Group (69) reported that in a study of 605 obese patients who received sibutramine and an individualized 600 kcal/d deficit diet, 499 who completed 6 months lost an average of ~12 kg (~12% of their initial weight). The 467 patients who had lost >5% of their weight were then randomly assigned sibutramine or placebo for an additional 18 months. The dose was adjusted upward if weight gain occurred. Of 204 patients who completed the study, 43% of those receiving sibutramine maintained at least 80% of the weight lost during the initial 6 months, compared to only 16% of patients who received the placebo. In a similar study, obese patients who had lost at least 8% of their initial body weight during a 6-month low-calorie diet lead-in were randomly assigned to receive placebo, 30 mg, 60 mg, or 120 mg of orlistat three times daily for 1 year. The patients treated with 120-mg orlistat regained significantly less weight (32.8%) than those treated with placebo (58.7%) over the subsequent 1 year (70).

Wadden and colleagues (71) assessed whether adding orlistat would induce further weight losses in patients who had initially lost weight on subutramine alone. A total of 34 patients who had lost 11.6% of their weight during the prior 1 year by sibutramine combined with lifestyle modification were randomly assigned to either sibutramine plus orlistat or sibutramine plus placebo. Interestingly, the addition of the second drug did not significantly increase weight loss at the end of 16 weeks, although both groups showed excellent maintenance of the initial weight loss.

The use of a very low calorie diet (VLCD) to induce a substantial weight loss followed by a drug to help prevent the subsequent, almost inevitable weight regain is a promising idea. Apfelbaum et al. (72) randomly assigned patients who had lost 6 kg or more during a 4-week VLCD intervention to receive either sibutramine or placebo. From the 4-week time of randomization to the 1-year endpoint, patients who received sibutramine had an additional mean weight loss of 5.2 kg compared with a weight gain of 0.5 kg in those who received the placebo. A total of 75% of patients in the sibutramine group maintained at least 100% of the weight loss achieved with the VLCD, compared with 42% in the placebo group. The use of a weight loss drug following a VLCD does appear to help prevent weight regain for at least 1 year.

Surprisingly, many of the drug studies reviewed did not report the use of lifestyle strategies or did not report them in enough detail to understand exactly how lifestyle modification strategies were implemented. Poston and colleagues (73) conducted a meta-analysis of the types of lifestyle interventions that were used in randomized, placebo-controlled, double-blind obesity drug studies and assessed their contribution to weight losses associated with drug interventions. Of 108 randomized clinical trials evaluated, the authors concluded that lifestyle treatments were not widely used. Of the specific behavioral strategies, self-monitoring was reportedly used in 23.1%, eating management (i.e., techniques specifically aimed at modifying the act of eating, such as eating slowly) in 4.6%, stimulus control in 3.7%, and contingency management in 3.7% of the studies reviewed. At a minimum, the authors suggested, future studies should provide details about the nature and types of lifestyle treatments used, who provided them and how the providers were trained, the amount of time that patients received the interventions, and information about implementation and adherence.

Overall, it appears that drugs help prevent weight regain for at least 18 months. Whether or not the combination of lifestyle modification plus drugs would be even more successful at preventing regain is less clear because of the paucity of research in this area. It is likely that many patients will need both drugs and ongoing lifestyle modification to manage their weight. Research beyond 1 or 2 years is needed to assess the potential long-term benefits of the combination for prevention of weight regain.

V CONCLUSIONS

A Regaining of Lost Weight

Long-term follow-ups of behavioral interventions show a reliable pattern of gradual regaining of lost weight. Four years after the completion of behavioral treatment, a modest amount of weight loss remains evident, ~1.8 kg or 23% of initial loss. When viewed from the perspective of secular trends that show predictable weight gains for untreated obese adults, these results imply that behavioral treatment may confer some small, long-term benefit in weight management. Moreover, clinically significant, long-term losses of 5 kg or more may be sustained by as many as one in five participants in behavioral treatment. Such findings may be seen in a favorable light, particularly when one considers that the majority of intervention studies (listed in Table 1) did not provide participants with follow-up care or with strategies specifically designed to enhance the maintenance of lost weight.

B Preventing the Regaining of Lost Weight

Our review of strategies designed to improve long-term outcome in obesity treatment reveals an interesting pattern of findings. Relapse prevention training, peer group meetings, telephone prompts by nontherapists, monetary incentives for weight loss or exercise, supervised group exercise, the use of personal trainers, and the "availability" of portion-controlled meals do not appear effective in improving outcome. On the other hand, there is evidence suggesting that extending treatment beyond 6 months through the use of weekly or biweekly sessions and providing multicomponent programs with ongoing patient-therapist contact in person or via telephone and mail may improve the maintenance of lost weight. In addition, supplying patients with no-cost portion-controlled meals, implementing home-based exercise programs providing home exercise equipment, and pharmacotherapy may also contribute to improved long-term outcome.

Our review provides clear support for the proposition that extended treatment has a beneficial impact on the maintenance of lost weight. Follow-up assessments conducted on average 22 months after initiation of treatment showed that extended-treatment groups maintained mean net losses of 7 kg (66% of their initial reductions). Over the same time period, treatment groups without extended contacts showed mean net losses of 3.8 kg (38% of their initial reductions). Similarly, multicomponent approaches that combine ongoing client-therapist contacts (whether in person or by telephone and mail) with relapse prevention training or social support programs have demonstrated improved maintenance compared to behavioral treatment without such programs.

In those studies that directly tested behavior therapy with and without extended contact, greater maintenance of *behavior change* was observed in the groups with continuing contact than in those without it. Thus, continued adherene to prescribed eating and activity patterns may be responsible for the better outcomes observed in extended treatments. Indeed, ongoing professional contact typically involves prompting of "appropriate" eating and exercise behaviors. Similarly, providing patients with no-cost meals or home-based exercise equipment and home-based activity regimens represent "environmental" manipulations that also prompt adherence to behaviors required for weight management. However, extended contact with a treatment provider also allows opportunities for reinforcement of adherence and for problem solving of obstacles to continued maintenance (52).

Extended treatment is not a panacea for the problem of weight regain in the treatment of obesity. Several factors should be considered in evaluating the utility of extended treatment. Continuing therapy is labor-intensive and expensive. Yet these costs must be weighed against the alternative, namely, the seemingly inevitable weight gain that follows intervention without posttreatment care. A second issue concerns the changes in motivation of participants during extended care. As treatment duration approaches one year, session attendance becomes problematic, adherence begins to deteriorate, and participants often begin to regain weight. Furthermore, when weight loss plateaus during the course of long-term treatment, patients become disheartened and their participation in treatment flounders. Therefore, it becomes essential to address expectations about weight loss and personal goals and to have strategies available to address changes in motivation (74,75).

C Clinical Directions

Several approaches to obesity treatment may improve the maintenance of lost weight, including a comprehensive initial assessment, using multiple indicators of success, focusing on the maintenance of behavior change, and adopting a continuous care approach to obesity management.

1 Comprehensive Assessment

The long-term treatment of obesity should be preceded by a comprehensive assessment of the effects of obesity on the individual's health and emotional well-being (76). The impact of obesity on risk factors for disease (e.g., hypertension, glucose tolerance, dyslipidemia, etc.) and quality of life (e.g., emotional state, body image, binge eating, etc.) should be assessed. A careful individualized assessment will often reveal important behavioral and emotional targets for intervention, such as binge eating, body image disparagement, and anxiety or depression, problems that need to be addressed regardless of whether weight loss itself becomes an objective of treatment (52,77). For some obese individuals, self-acceptance independent of weight loss may be an important treatment objective (78).

2 Indicators of Success

Successful long-term outcome should not be viewed solely in terms of weight loss. Beneficial changes in risk factors for disease and improvements in quality of life (79) represent important indicators of success in the care of the obese person. Improvements in the quality of diet should be a component of care independent of whether weight reduction is an identified objective of care (80). Reductions in amounts of dietary fats, particularly saturated fats, can improve health as well as assist in weight loss (81). Similarly, increased physical activity and a decrease in sedentary lifestyle can represent beneficial components of long-term care irrespective of the impact of exercise on weight loss (82).

3 Maintenance of Behavior Change

Because obese persons do not have direct control over how much weight they lose, goals for the posttreatment period should be framed in terms of behaviors that they can control, such as the quantity and quality of food they consume and the amounts and types of physical activity they perform. Moreover, obese persons should be informed that significant health benefits can be derived from even modest amounts of weight loss (83,84).

4 Continuous Care Approach

Finally, clinicians and patients alike must view obesity as a chronic condition requiring continuous care (52). Short-term interventions that strive to produce reductions to "ideal" weight are doomed to long-term failure. A continuous care approach focused on the achievement of realistic long-term objectives appears more appropriate for most obese patients. Extended treatments have shown promise in promoting adherence to the behaviors required for the long-term maintenance of weight loss.

VI SUMMARY

In this chapter, we addressed the question of whether it is possible to prevent the regaining of weight that invariably seems to follow treatment-induced weight loss. Our review of long-term follow-ups of lifestyle interventions for weight loss showed a pattern of gradual regaining of weight such that 4 years after initial treatment only a modest amount of weight loss remains evident ($M = 1.8$ kg). However, as many as one in five participants in behavioral treatment may achieve clinically significant, long-term losses of 5 kg or more. The difficulty associated with maintaining lost weight appears to be the result of physiological, environmental, and psychological factors that combine to facilitate a regaining of lost weight and an abandonment of weight control efforts. A variety of methods to improve the long-term effects of treatment have been evaluated. Relapse prevention training, peer group meetings, telephone prompts by nontherapists, mone-

tary incentives for weight loss or exercise, supervised group exercise, the use of personal trainers, and the "availability" of portion-controlled meals do not appear effective in improving outcome. On the other hand, there is evidence suggesting that extending treatment beyond 6 months through the use of weekly or biweekly sessions and providing multicomponent programs with ongoing patient-therapist contact in person or via telephone and mail may improve the maintenance of lost weight. In addition, no-cost meal replacements, home-based exercise programs, the use of home exercise equipment and pharmacotherapy may enhance adherence and may contribute to improved long-term outcome. The most pressing challenge facing researchers is the improvement of programs for the long-term management of obesity. The greatest practical challenge is to convince health care professionals, obese individuals, and the general public that obesity is a complex, chronic condition that can be managed effectively through intensive programs of ongoing care.

ACKNOWLEDGMENTS

We would like to thank Joyce Corsica for her invaluable assistance in the preparation of this chapter.

REFERENCES

1. Thomas PR, ed. Weighing the Options: Criteria for Evaluating Weight-Management Programs Washington: National Academy Press, 1995.
2. Jeffery RW, Drewnowski A, Epstein LH, Stunkard AJ, Wilson GT, Wing RR, Hill DR. Long-term maintenance of weight loss: current status. Health Psychol 2000; 19(suppl 1):5–16.
3. National Heart, Lung and Blood Institute. Obesity education initiative expert panel on the identification, evaluation, and treatment of overweight and obesity in adults. Obes Res 1998; 6(suppl 2).
4. Perri MG. The maintenance of treatment effects in the long-term management of obesity. Clin Psychol Sci Pract 1998; 5:526–543.
5. Wadden TA, Brownell KD, Foster GD. Obesity: responding to the global epidemic. J Consult Clin Psychol 2002; 70:510–525.
6. Pi-Sunyer FX. A review of long-term studies evaluating the efficacy of weight loss in ameliorating disorders associated with obesity. Clin Ther 1996; 18:1006–1035.
7. Björvell H, Rössner S. Long-term treatment of severe obesity: four-year follow-up of a combined behavioural modification programme. BMJ 1985; 291:379–382.
8. Björvell H, Rössner S. A ten year follow-up of weight

change in severely obese subjects treated in a behavioural modification programme. Int J Obes Relat Metab Disord 1992; 16:623–625.

9. Flechtner-Mors M, Ditschuneit HH, Johnson TD, Suchard MA, Adler G. Metabolic and weight loss effects of long-term dietary intervention in obese patients: four-year results. Obes Res 2000; 8:399–402.

10. Gotestam KG. A three year follow-up of a behavioral treatment for obesity. Addict Behav 1979; 4:179–183.

11. Graham LE, Taylor CB, Hovell MF, Siegel W. Five-year follow-up to a behavioral weight-loss program. J Consult Clin Psychol 1983; 51:322–323.

12. Kramer FM, Jeffery RW, Forster JL, Snell MK. Long-term follow-up of behavioral treatment for obesity: patterns of weight gain among men and women. Int J Obes Relat Metab Disord 1989; 13:124–136.

13. Murphy JK, Bruce BK, Williamson DA. A comparison of measured and self-reported weights in a 4-year follow-up of spouse involvement in obesity treatment. Behav Ther 1985; 16:524–530.

14. Stalonas PM, Perri MG, Kerzner AB. Do behavioral treatments of obesity last? A five-year follow-up investigation. Addict Behav 1984; 9:175–184.

15. Stunkard AJ, Penick SB. Behavior modification in the treatment of obesity: the problem of maintaining weight loss. Arch Gen Psychiatry 1979; 36:801–806.

16. Wadden TA, Sternberg JA, Letizia KA, Stunkard AJ, Foster GD. Treatment of obesity by very low calorie diet, behavior therapy, and their combination: a five-year perspective. Int J Obes Relat Metab Disord 1989; 13(suppl 2):39–46.

17. Wadden TA, Stunkard AJ, Liebschutz. Three year follow-up of the treatment of obesity by very low calorie diet, behavior therapy, and their combination. J Consult Clin Psychol 1988; 56:925–928.

18. Brownell KD, Jeffery RW. Improving long-term weight loss: pushing the limits of treatment. Behav Ther 1987; 18:353–374.

19. Lewis CE, Jacobs DR, McCreath H, Kiefe CI, Schreiner PJ, Smith DE, Williams OD. Weight gain continues in the 1990s: 10-year trends in weight and overweight from the CARDIA study. Am J Epidemiol 2000; 151:1172–1181.

20. Shah M, Hannan PJ, Jeffery RW. Secular trends in body mass index in the adult population of three communities from the upper mid-western part of the USA: the Minnesota Heart Health Program. Int J Obes Relat Metab Disord 1991; 15:499–503.

21. Crawford D, Jeffery RW, French SA. Can anyone successfully control their weight? Findings from a three year community-based study of men and women. Int J Obes 2000; 24:1107–1110.

22. Rodin J, Schank D, Striegel-Moore R. Psychological features of obesity. Med Clin North Am 1989; 73:47–66.

23. Hill JO, Peters JC. Environmental contributors to the obesity epidemic. Science 1998; 280:1371–1374.

24. Poston WS, Foreyt JP. Obesity is an environmental issue. Atherosclerosis 1999; 146:201–209.

25. Dulloo AG, Jacquet J. Adaptive reduction in basal metabolic rate in response to food deprivation in humans: a role for feedback signals from fat stores. Am J Clin Nutr 1998; 68:599–606.

26. Ravussin E, Swinburn BA. Energy metabolism. In: Stunkard AJ, Wadden TA, eds. Obesity: Theory and Therapy. 2nd ed. New York: Raven, 1993:97–124.

27. Leibel RL, Rosenbaum M, Hirsch J. Changes in energy expenditure resulting from altered body weight. N Engl J Med 1995; 332:673–674.

28. Stock MJ. Gluttony and thermogenesis revisited. Int J Obes 1999; 23:1105–1117.

29. Rosenbaum M, Hirsch J, Leibel RL. Effects of changes in body weight on carbohydrate metabolism, catecholamine excretion, and thyroid function. Am J Clin Nutr 2000; 71:1421–1423.

30. Kern PA. Potential role of TNF alpha and lipoprotein lipase as candidate genes for obesity. J Nutr 1997; 127:1917S–1922S.

31. Kern PA, Ong JM, Saffari B, Carty J. The effects of weight loss on the activity and expression of adipose-tissue lipoprotein lipase in very obese humans. N Engl J Med 1990; 322:1053–1059.

32. Goodrick GK, Raynaud AS, Pace PW, Foreyt JP. Outcome attribution in a very low calorie diet program. Int J Eat Disord 1992; 12:117–120.

33. Jeffery RW, French SA, Schmid TL. Attributions for dietary failures: Problems reported by participants in the Hypertension Prevention Trial. Health Psychol 1990; 9:315–329.

34. Foster GD, Wadden TA, Vogt RA, Brewer G. What is a reasonable weight loss? Patients' expectations and evaluations of obesity treatment outcomes. J Consult Clin Psychol 1997; 65:79–85.

35. Cooper Z, Fairburn CG. A new cognitive-behavioural approach to the treatment of obesity. Behav Res Ther 2001; 39:499–511.

36. Perri MG, Nezu AM, Patti ET, McCann KL. Effect of length of treatment on weight loss. J Consult Clin Psychol 1989; 57:450–452.

37. Jakicic JM, Winters C, Lang W, Wing RR. Effects of intermittent exercise and use of home exercise equipment on adherence, weight loss, and fitness in overweight women: a randomized trial. JAMA 1999; 282:1554–1560.

38. Leermakers EA, Perri MG, Shigaki CL, Fuller PR. Effects of exercise-focused versus weight-focused maintenance programs on the management of obesity. Addict Behav 1999; 24:219–227.

39. Perri MG, McAdoo WG, McAllister DA, Lauer JB, Jordan RC, Yancey DZ, Nezu AM. Effects of peer support and therapist contact on long-term weight loss. J Consult Clin Psychol 1987; 55:615–617.

40. Perri MG, McAllister DA, Gange JJ, Jordan RC,

McAdoo WG, Nezu AM. Effects of four maintenance programs on the long-term management of obesity. J Consult Clin Psychol 1988; 56:529–534.

41. Perri MG, Martin AD, Leermakers EA, Sears SF, Notelovitz M. Effects of group- versus home-based exercise in the treatment of obesity. J Consult Clin Psychol 1997; 65:278–285.

42. Perri MG, Nezu AM, McKelvey WF, Shermer RL, Renjilian DA, Viegener BJ. Relapse prevention training and problem solving therapy in the long-term management of obesity. J Consul Clin Psychol 2001; 69:722–726.

43. Viegener BJ, Perri MG, Nezu AM, Renjilian DA, McKelvey WF, Schein RL. Effects of an intermittent, low-fat, low-calorie diet in the behavioral treatment of obesity. Behav Ther 1990; 21:499–509.

44. Wadden TA, Foster GD, Letizia KA. One-year behavioral treatment of obesity: comparison of moderate and severe caloric restriction and the effects of weight maintenance therapy. J Consult Clin Psychol 1994; 62:165–171.

45. Wadden TA, Considine RV, Foster GD, Anderson DA, Sarwer DB, Caro JS. Short- and long-term changes in serum leptin in dieting obese women: effects of caloric restriction and weight loss. J Clin Endocrinol Metab 1998; 83:214–218.

46. Wadden TA, Vogt RA, Andersen RE, Barlett SJ, Foster GD, Kuehnel RH, Wilk J, Weinstock R, Buckenmeyer P, Berkowitz RI, Steen SN. Exercise in the treatment of obesity: effects of four interventions on body composition, resting energy expenditure, appetite, and mood. J Consult Clin Psychol 1997; 65:269–277.

47. Wadden TA, Vogt RA, Foster GD, Anderson DA. Exercise and the maintenance of weight loss: 1-year follow-up of a controlled clinical trial. J Consult Clin Psychol 1998; 66:429–433.

48. Weinstock RS, Dai H, Wadden TA. Diet and exercise in the treatment of obesity: effects of 3 interventions on insulin resistance. Arch Intern Med 1998; 158:2477–2483.

49. Wing RR, Blair E, Marcus M, Epstein LH, Harvey J. Year-long weight loss treatment for obese patients with type II diabetes: does including an intermittent very-low-calorie diet improve outcome? Am J Med 1994; 97:354–362.

50. Wing RR, Vendetti E, Jakicic JM, Polley BA, Lang W. Lifestyle intervention in overweight individuals with a family history of diabetes. Diabetes Care 1998; 21:350–359.

51. Wilson GT. Behavioral treatment of obesity: thirty years and counting. Adv Behav Res Ther 1994; 16:31–75.

52. Perri MG, Nezu AM, Viegener BJ. Improving the Long-Term Management of Obesity: Theory, Research, and Clinical Guidelines. New York: John Wiley & Sons, 1992.

53. Wing RR, Jeffery RW, Hellerstedt WL, Burton LR. Effect of frequent phone contacts and optional food provision on maintenance of weight loss. Ann Behav Med 1996; 18:172–176.

54. Perri MG, Shapiro RM, Ludwig WW, Twentyman CT, McAdoo WG. Maintenance strategies for the treatment of obesity: an evaluation of relapse prevention training and posttreatment contact by mail and telephone. J Consult Clin Psychol 1984; 52:404–413.

55. Baum JG, Clark HB, Sandler J. Preventing relapse in obesity through posttreatment maintenance systems: comparing the relative efficacy of two levels of therapist support. J Behav Med 1991; 14:287–302.

56. Marlatt GA, George WH. Relapse prevention and the maintenance of optimal health. In: Shumaker SA, Schron EB, Ockene JK, McBee WL, eds. The Handbook of Health Behavior Change. 2nd ed. New York: Springer, 1998:33–58.

57. Jeffery RW, Wing RR, Thorson C, Burton LR, Raether C, Harvey J, Mullen M. Strengthening behavioral interventions for weight loss: a randomized trial of food provision and monetary incentives. J Consult Clin Psychol 1993; 61:1038–1045.

58. Jeffery RW, Wing RR. Long-term effects of interventions for weight loss using food provision and monetary incentives. J Consult Clin Psychol 1995; 63:793–796.

59. Wing RR, Jeffery RW. Benefits of recruiting participants with friends and increasing social support for weight loss and maintenance. J Consult Clin Psychol 1999; 67:132–138.

60. Harris JK, French SA, Jeffery RW, McGovern PG, Wing RR. Dietary and physical activity correlates of long-term weight loss. Obes Res 1994; 2:307–313.

61. Sherwood NE, Jeffery RW, French SA, Hannan PJ, Murray DM. Predictors of weight gain in the Pound of Prevention study. Int J Obes 2000; 24:395–403.

62. McGuire M, Wing R, Klem M, Lang W, Hill J. What predicts weight regain in a group of successful weight losers? J Consult Clin Psychol 1999; 67:177–185.

63. Garrow JS. Exercise in the treatment of obesity: a marginal contribution. Int J Obes 1995; 19(suppl 4): S126–S129.

64. Wing RR. Physical activity in the treatment of the adulthood overweight and obesity: current evidence and research issues. Med Sci Sports Exerc 1999; 31:S547–S552.

65. Jeffery RW, Wing RR, Thorson C, Burton LR. Use of personal trainers and financial incentives to increase exercise in a behavioral weight-loss program. J Consult Clin Psychol 1998; 66:777–783.

66. Perri MG, McAdoo WG, Spevak PA, Newlin DB. Effect of a multi-component maintenance program on long-term weight loss. J Consult Clin Psychol 1984; 52:480–481.

67. Perri MG, McAdoo WG, McAllister DA, Lauer JB, Yancey DZ. Enhancing the efficacy of behavior therapy for obesity: effects of aerobic exercise and a multi-

component maintenance program. J Consult Clin Psychol 1986; 54:670–675.

68. Haddock CK, Poston WSC, Dill P, Foreyt JP, Ericsson M. Pharmacotherapy for obesity: a quantitative analysis of four decades of published randomized clinical trials. Int J Obes 2002; 26:262–273.

69. James WPT, Astrup A, Finer N, Hilsted J, Kopelman P, Rossner S, Saris WHM, Van Gaal L, for the STORM Study Group. Effect of sibutramine on weight maintenance after weight loss: a randomised trial. Lancet 2000; 356:2119–2125.

70. Hill JO, Hauptman J, Anderson JW, Fujioka K, O'Neil PM, Smith DK, Zavoral JH, Aronne LJ. Orlistat, a lipase inhibitor, for weight maintenance after conventional dieting: a 1-y study. Am J Clin Nutr 1999; 69: 1108–1116.

71. Wadden TA, Berkowitz RI, Womble LG, Sarwer DB, Arnold ME, Steinberg CM. Effects of sibutramine plus orlistat in obese women following 1 year of treatment by sibutramine alone: a placebo-controlled trial. Obes Res 2000; 8:431–437.

72. Apfelbaum MD, Vague P, Ziegler O, Hanotin C, Thomas F, Luetenegger E. Long-term maintenance of weight loss after a very-low-calorie diet: a randomized blinded trial of the efficacy and tolerability of sibutramine. Am J Med 1999; 106:179–184.

73. Poston WSC, Haddock CK, Dill PL, Thayer B, Foreyt JP. Lifestyle treatments in randomized clinical trials of pharmacotherapies for obesity: data from 40 years of research. Obes Res 2001; 9:552–563.

74. Miller WR, Rollnick S. Motivational Interviewing. New York: Guilford Press, 1991.

75. Smith DE, Heckmeyer CM, Kratt PP, Mason DA. Motivational interviewing to improve adherence to a behavioral weight-control program for older obese women with NIDDM: a pilot study. Diabetes Care 1997; 20:52–54.

76. Beliard D, Kirschenbaum DS, Fitzgibbon ML. Evaluation of an intensive weight control program using a priori criteria to determine outcome. Int J Obes Relat Metab Disord 1992; 16:505–517.

77. Wadden TA, Foster GD. Behavioral assessment and treatment of markedly obese patients. In: Wadden TA, Van Itallie TB, eds. Treatment of the Seriously Obese Patient. New York: Guilford, 1992:290–330.

78. Wilson GT. Acceptance and change in the treatment of eating disorders and obesity. Behav Ther 1996; 27:417–439.

79. Atkinson RL. Proposed standards for judging the success of the treatment of obesity. Ann Intern Med 1993; 119:677–680.

80. Hill JO, Drougas H, Peters JC. Obesity treatment: can diet composition play a role? Ann Intern Med 1993; 119:694–697.

81. Insull W, Henderson M, Prentice R, Thompson DJ, Moskowitz M, Gorbach S. Results of a feasibility study of a low-fat diet. Arch Intern Med 1990; 150:421–427.

82. Paffenbarger RS, Lee IM. Physical activity and fitness for health and longevity. Res Q Exerc Sport 1996; 67:11–28.

83. Blackburn G. Effect of degree of weight loss on health benefits. Obes Res 1995; 3(suppl 2):211s–216s.

84. Wadden TA, Anderson DA, Foster GD. Two-year changes in lipids and lipoproteins associated with the maintenance of a 5% to 10% reduction in initial weight: some findings and some questions. Obes Res 1999; 7: 170–178.

12

Sympathomimetic and Serotonergic Drugs Used to Treat Obesity

George A. Bray and Donna H. Ryan

Pennington Biomedical Research Center, Louisiana State University, Baton Rouge, Louisiana, U.S.A.

I INTRODUCTION

The sympathomimetic and serotinergic drugs were the first groups of drugs to be approved for use in the treatment of obesity. They produce weight loss by reduction of food intake and have provided many of the lessons that have guided current efforts to develop new drugs. In this chapter, we will first comment on some of the issues in evaluating antiobesity drugs, including the process of comparison with placebo treatment. Next, we will discuss the mechanisms by which the drugs that affect monoamines produce weight loss. Finally, we will look at the pharmacology and clinical data supporting agents in these classes, including both those currently in use and those that have been withdrawn from use.

II EVALUATING ANTIOBESITY DRUGS

Following World War II, pharmaceutical companies began to evaluate potential agents for weight loss, measuring the amount of weight loss either in absolute terms or relative to initial weight, but always in comparison to the weight loss of a placebo. Weight loss in placebo-treated groups is highly variable from one study to another since the placebo effect is augmented by variations in diet, physical activity and behavioral therapy.

A number of criteria have been proposed for evaluating the response to treatment for obesity. Table 1 lists several criteria for evaluating success in treating

obesity, and readers are referred to other publications for a discussion of these approaches. Both the U.S. Food and Drug Administration (FDA) and the Committee for Proprietary Medicinal Products (CPMP) of the European Agency for the Evaluation of Medicinal Products (EMEA) have proposed criteria to be met by drugs approved for the treatment of obesity (7,8). These are summarized in Table 2. The FDA has suggested as evidence for efficacy that weight loss be more than 5% and significantly more than placebo at 12 months. The CPMP has suggested a 10% loss from baseline weight, which is significantly greater than placebo. A number of secondary criteria are also listed along with inclusion criteria and dose-ranging studies. For efficacy trials, both obese men and women should be included who are otherwise healthy with a BMI >30 kg/m^2 or >27 kg/m^2 if comorbidities such as hypertension or diabetes are present. Both agencies propose a run-in at the beginning of the trial. The CPMP encourages active placebo treatment and does not specify a difference from placebo, as long as the drug effect is significantly greater and >10% below baseline. Studies showing maintenance of weight loss are encouraged by both agencies.

Categorical analysis of the percentage of patients who have achieved more than a 5% or 10% weight loss is similar to the responder analysis used in the initial drug evaluation by Scoville (4) and has also been proposed in the FDA guidance (7) and the CPMP criteria (8). Finally, criteria for success can be based

Table 1 Some Criteria for Assessing Success in Treatment for Obesity

Author (Ref.)	Criteria
Stunkard and McLaren-Hume (1)	Percent losing >20 lb (9 kg) Percent losing >40 lb (18.1 kg)

Trulson (2)	Success: (initial wt in lb lost
	  ≤150 lb ≥10 lb,
	  151–175 lb ≥15 lb,
	  176–200 lb/ 20lb,
	  201–225 lb/25 lb,
	  225–250 lb/30 lb,
	  ≥251 lb/ 35 lb
	Failure: ≤5 lb wt loss in ≥4 months

Feinstein (3)	Reduction index = $\dfrac{\text{wt (lost)} \times \textit{Initial weight}}{(\textit{surplus wt}) \times (\textit{target wt})} \times 100$
Scoville (4)	>0.5 lb/wk more than placebo Percent losing >1 lb/wk or >3 lb/wk

Atkinson (5)	≥10% loss of excess weight for
	  >6 mo
	Loss of ≥2 BMI units for >6 mo
	Reduction in comorbidities
	  for >6 mo

Bray (6)	≥5% wt loss if BMI >27 kg/m² ≥20% loss of excess body weight >5% reduction in visceral fat Significant improvements in comorbidities

on the improvements in comorbidities that often accompany obesity (Table 2). Improvements in diabetes, fasting insulin, fasting glucose, hemoglobin A1c, insulin resistance, serum lipids, blood pressure, disappearance of sleep apnea, or an improvement in the quality of life are all criteria that can be used to evaluate treatment outcome (7,8). Criteria for evaluating weight loss drugs can calculate changes from the baseline weight (8) or as a difference from placebo (7). Figure 1 presents data from "placebo group" responses in several clinical trials lasting from 31 to 60 weeks (6). Note the diversity of responses (9–16). Most trials showed weight losses of >4 kg and one reached 14 kg. This variability in placebo response across trials of varying length reflects the inclusion of behavior therapy, diets with low or very low levels of energy, and exercise in the treatment plan in addition to the "placebo" pill. The problem with comparing a drug against these vigorous placebo effects can be appreciated from an analogy with treatment for hypertension. If patients with hypertension

are given very low energy diets with low salt intake, increased calcium and magnesium intake, and if they abstain from alcohol and eat more fiber, it would be difficult to detect an additional effect of an antihypertensive drug. Similarly, if patients are losing weight rapidly with an intensive behavioral program or a very low energy (calorie) diet, it may be difficult to see an additional effect of a medication that is designed as an appetite suppressant. Whether medications might make it easier to adhere to a very low energy diet (VLED) or a behavioral program is an unsettled question.

The multicenter trial reported by Walker et al. (17) is instructive. The trial lasted 6 weeks and compared mazindol to placebo (Fig. 2). In four of the centers (*left panel*), the placebo group lost no weight, and the effect of mazindol was readily apparent. In the fifth center (*right panel*), all patients received "behavioral therapy" in addition to their group assignment of drug or placebo. In this setting the weight loss of the "placebo group" was similar to the weight loss in the other four treatment centers, and the weight loss produced by the drug was not significantly different. Reviews of the behavior therapy literature over the past ten years indicate that effective behavioral treatment can produce a weight loss of between 9% and 10% (18). Obviously, the "vigor" used in the behavioral approaches applied to both the placebo group and the drug treatment group can make a big difference in the outcome of a weight loss trial. For this reason we prefer the CPMP criteria (8) to those of the FDA (7).

Rossner (19) has graphically summarized an approach to evaluating the success of weight loss (Fig. 3). The natural history of weight gain in the overweight is shown by the dashed line and represents an increase of ~0.25 kg/yr (20). A good population goal would be to prevent any further weight gain (pattern A). For individuals who are overweight, a sustained weight loss of 5% below baseline (pattern B) would be the minimal criterion for success in this model. Weight loss of 5–10% with or without partial normalization of risk factors would be a fair response. A sustained weight loss of >10% with improvement in risk factors would be a good response. Weight loss >15% would be excellent and normalizing of risk factors and reducing weight to a BMI <25 kg/m² (pattern C) would be ideal, but is rarely achievable.

A new approach to evaluating weight loss has recently been proposed (21). It involves pattern analysis of longitudinal data. A pattern of interest is defined at the beginning of the trial and the proportion meeting this are then evaluated. This approach has been used on one subgroup of a large multicenter drug trial (22).

Table 2 Regulatory Criteria for Establishing Efficacy of Antiobesity Drugs

	FDA Criteria (7)	CPMP Criteria (8)
Early trials	Randomized, double-blind, placebo-controlled	
Type of trial	Dose-ranging; identify lowest effective dose	Not specified
Duration	3–6 months	Not specified
Inclusion	BMI >30 kg/m^2	Not specified
Ancillary	Similar advice in diet, exercise, and behavior	Effective nonpharmacological therapy
1° Endpoint	Wt loss significantly greater than placebo	Wt loss that is fat loss
No. patients	About 200, including both sexes and minorities	Not specified
Tolerability	Yes	Yes
Mechanism of action	Yes	Yes
Pharmacokinetics	Yes	Yes
Toxicology studies	Yes	Yes
Drug interactions	Yes	Yes
Long-term	Randomized, double-blind, placebo-controlled	12 mo—open-label or random 24 hr
Type of trial	Efficacy and safety	Efficacy and safety
Duration	Year 1: double-blind	At least 1 year
	Year 2: open-label or double-blind	
Inclusion	BMI >30 kg/m^2 of otherwise healthy or BMI >27 kg/m^2 with comorbidities	BMI >30 kg/m^2 of otherwise healthy or BMI >27 kg/m^2 with comorbidities
Ancillary advice	Moderately restricted diet and exercise	Weight reducing diet; beh. mod; exercise
Run-in	Identify placebo responders; stratify; 6 wks	Yes
Measures	Body weight, body fat, and fat distribution	Body weight, body fat, and fat distribution
1° Endpoint	Wt loss significantly greater than placebo and 5% > placebo at 12 mo	Wt loss 10% below baseline and significantly > placebo at 12 mo
	Significantly greater no. 8 achieving >5% wt loss	Significantly greater no. 8 achieving >10% wt loss
	Maintenance of weight loss	Maintenance of weight loss
2° Endpoints	Significant change in body fat and fat distribution (may stratify—fat distribution risk factors, severity, duration, age)	Improved biochemical parameters
		Reduction in cardiovascular risk
		Decreased blood pressure
	Improved cardiovascular risk factor	Decreased apneic episodes
	Improved metabolic profile	Loss of body fat and/or visceral fat
	Improved quality of life	Improved joint mobility
		Improved male and female infertility
		Improved quality of life
Subjects	Male and female; minorities	Male and female
	About 1500 to complete 12 mo with 200–500 completing 2 years	

With this wide variety of criteria to assess efficacy from which to chose, we based our review of clinical studies using serotonergic and sympathomimetic agents on the calculation of the percentage of initial weight lost and whether it met the FDA criteria or the CPMP criteria. Among the clinical studies discussed later in this review, the usual pattern is active weight loss that plateaus at around 6 months. The maximal weight loss has usually been achieved by 20–24 weeks. At 6, 12, and

18 weeks, weight losses averaged 44%, 72%, and 89% of the weight loss at 24 weeks. For this reason we have rarely included studies of 6 weeks or less in the tables. We have generally included studies of more than 8 weeks that were randomized and placebo controlled. In some instances, a reported study was the first half of a 16-week or longer crossover study. We have rarely used data from the second half of crossover studies because of the carryover effects, and when this was done it will be

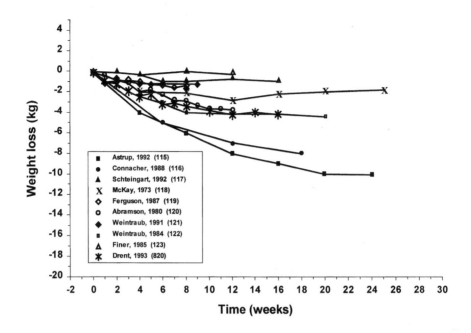

Figure 1   Weight loss of placebo-treated patients in clinical trials of antiobesity drugs lasting fewer than 30 weeks. (From Ref. 6.)

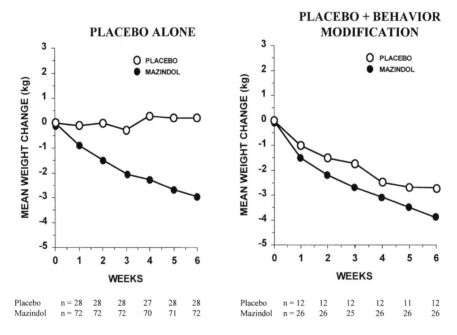

Figure 2   Comparison of mazindol against placebo (left-hand panel) or against placebo in combination with behavior modification given to all patients (right-hand panel). (From Ref. 17.)

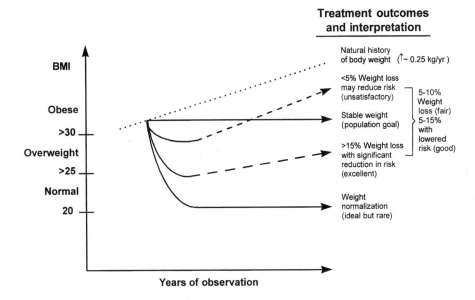

Figure 3 Evaluation of treatment outcomes in relation to the natural history of obesity and the degrees of weight loss that can be achieved. (From Ref. 19.)

noted. After a brief discussion of the mechanisms of action of the drugs under review, we will return to a review of clinical trials using these medications.

III PHYSIOLOGICAL AND PHARMACOLOGICAL MECHANISMS TO REDUCE FOOD INTAKE

A Monoamine Systems

Both norepinephrine and serotonin modulate feeding. Depending on the receptor systems activated, they can either increase or decrease food intake. Activation of the serotonin 1A receptor or the norepinephrine-activated α_2 receptor can increase feeding. Activation of the other receptors by norepinephrine or serotonin reduces food intake.

1 Norepinephrine (NE)

a. Adrenergic Receptors

The importance of central norepinephrine in the regulation of food intake is suggested by three observations. First, a lesion of the ventral noradrenergic bundle, which abolishes NE release in the perifornical areal, is associated with weight gain (23). This lesion also blocks the anorexic effect of amphetamine and diethylpropion (24). Second, blockade of tyrosine hydroxylase by injecting α-methyl-p-tyrosine into the

perifornical area increases feeding by blocking NE synthesis (25). And, finally, infusion of NE into the ventral medial nucleus (VMN) can increase food intake, decrease sympathetic activity, and produce obesity (26). This allows two strategies for drug discovery. The first is to design agonists that are specific for the desired receptor or receptors. The second is to block reuptake of norepinephrine in regions where the increased NE pool will have the desired effect on food intake.

Norepinephrine can increase or decrease food intake depending on the type of adrenergic receptors on which it acts in the brain (27). Norepinephrine acting on α_1-adrenergic receptors in the paraventricular nucleus (PVN) decreases food intake. Adrenergic agonists such as phenylpropanolamine (PPA) or metaraminol will reduce food intake (28). This effect is blocked by injection of α_1-adrenergic antagonists (28). That the α_1-adrenergic system is involved in modulating body weight in human beings is suggested by the fact that the α_1 adrenergic antagonist terazosin, which is used to treat hypertension, is associated with small weight gains relative to placebo in double-blind randomized placebo-controlled trials (29).

There are three α_2 adrenergic receptors (α_{2A}, α_{2B}, and α_{2C}) that are coupled through G-proteins to modulate cyclic AMP and calcium channels. In experimental animals, activation of α_2 adrenergic receptors in the PVN by norepinephrine or by clonidine (30,31) will stimulate food intake. This effect can be blocked by α_2

adrenergic antagonists such as yohimbine or idazoxan. Clinically, neither clonidine nor yohimbine has significant or consistent effects on body weight in humans (32).

Norepinephrine stimulation of β_2-adrenergic receptors located in the perifornical area will decrease food intake (27,31). β_2 Agonists such as clenbuterol and salbutamol will decrease food intake when injected into the central nervous system (CNS) (30). Injection of β_3 agonists into the CNS also decreases food intake (30). Whether this is through β_3 receptors in the CNS or by action on β_2 receptors in the CNS or β_3 receptors peripherally remains to be determined (33–35).

b. Mechanism of Activating Adrenergic Receptors

Receptor agonists are one mechanism to activate this system. Phenylpropanolamine is an α_1 agonist that reduces feeding (28). Clonidine is an α_2 agonist that stimulates food intake in experimental animals. A number of β_2 agonists inhibit feeding (30,33). Alternatively, drugs can block reuptake of norepinephrine (36). Mazindol is a tricyclic drug that is thought to block reuptake of NE. However, a highly specific NE reuptake inhibitor, nisoxetine, when given alone does not increase food intake, suggesting that either NE alone is insufficient to affect feeding or that the NE reuptake blocked by nisoxetine is acting in the wrong place (37). Direct application of NE to the hypothalamus is sufficient to stimulate feeding (38). The final way to enhance interneuronal norepinephrine is to enhance NE release. Amphetamine, phentermine, and diethylpropion are thought to act by this mechanism (36), but they may also act as inhibitors of NE and dopamine reuptake.

2 Serotonin

a. Serotonin Receptors

There are seven known families of serotonin (5-hydroxytryptamine; 5HT) receptors with several receptors subtypes in some of these families (39). Most of these subtypes are in the $5HT_1$ and $5HT_2$ series. These receptors may mediate the reduction of food intake that occurs when serotonin agonists such as quipazine metachlorophenylpiperazine (mCPP) and d-norfenfluramine are injected into the PVN (40). The signal transduction system for most of the serotonin receptors involves G-coupled activation or inhibition of adenylate cyclase. The $5HT_3$ receptor is the exception, acting through an ion channel (39).

Serotonin is clearly involved in regulation of food intake (41,42), and several serotonin receptors have been implicated in this process. Activation of the $5HT_{1A}$ receptor, an autocrine receptor in the dorsal raphe nucleus, acutely stimulates food intake (43). Acute administration to rats of flesinoxan, a $5HT_{1A}$ agonist in doses of 10 mg/kg, increases food intake and NPY levels in the PVN and ARC nucleus (44). However, chronic administration of $5HT_{1A}$ receptor agonists downregulates $5HT_{1A}$ receptors and no longer stimulates feeding.

Stimulation of the $5HT_{1B}$ receptor reduces food intake by acting at a postsynaptic receptor. Knockout of the $5HT_{1B}$ receptor (45) blocks the reduction of food intake by fenfluramine, suggesting that this receptor plays an important role in modulating feeding (46). A $5HT_{1B/2C}$ agonist, m-CPP, reduced food intake and NPY levels in the PVN, both acutely and after 7 days of administration to rats at 10 mg/kg (44). Stimulation of the $5HT_{2C}$ receptor through its G-protein-coupled receptor activates phospholipase-C, which produces two intracellular signals, inositol 3-phosphate (PI-3) and diacylglycerol (DAG). Transgenic mice lacking the $5HT_{2C}$ receptor (47) show increased epilepsy and weight gain, suggesting that this receptor, too, may be involved in regulating food intake (48). The $5HT_3$ receptor activates an ion channel and may be involved in the anorectic response to diets deficient in single amino acids (49). A comparison on food intake of antagonists to the $5HT_{1B}$, the $5HT_{2A/2C}$ receptor, and the $5HT_3$ receptor concluded that the $5HT_{1B}$ and the $5HT_{2A/2C}$ receptors were most involved with food intake (50).

b. Mechanisms Activating Serotonin Receptors

Drugs that block serotonin reuptake such as fluoxetine and sertraline significantly decrease food intake (51). The effect of fluoxetine on food intake is not inhibited by metergoline, suggesting that this effect may be by some other mechanism than serotonin. In a manner analogous to norepinephrine, the serotonin receptors modulating feeding can be activated by receptor agonists by enhancing serotonin release or blocking serotonin reuptake. A number of serotonin receptor agonists have been synthesized to explore the serotonin receptor system as a target for antiobesity drugs (52). So far, none have reached clinical trials.

Drugs that release serotonin and act as partial reuptake inhibitors such as dexfenfluramine also decrease food intake (53). These inhibitory effects of dexfenfluramine are attenuated by metergoline, a broad spectrum serotonin antagonist (54). The effect of dexfenfluramine can also be blocked by serotonin reuptake inhibitors.

Reduction of food intake by dexfenfluramine is also blocked by lesions in the lateral parabrachial nucleus (55).

B Pharmacology of Drugs Acting Through Central Monoamine Receptors

The pharmacology of drugs acting to reduce food intake through the monoamine system are fairly easily summarized. Some of these agents also increase thermogenesis in addition to decreasing food intake. As a class these drugs are rapidly absorbed and the duration of clinical effect depends on the metabolites. Both dexfenfluramine and sibutramine have long-lasting metabolites. The noradrenergic drugs can produce stimulation of the CNS and the cardiovascular system. A number of metabolic and endocrine effects have also been described.

1 Experimental Pharmacology

All of the centrally acting anorectic drugs, except for mazindol, are derivatives of β-phenylethylamine. The β-phenylethylamine skeleton is also the backbone for the neurotransmitters dopamine, norepinephrine, and epinephrine. These neurotransmitters are synthesized from tyrosine in the nerve terminal and stored in granules and released at the nerve ending to act on postganglionic receptors (36). After acting on these re-

ceptors they can be inactivated by catechol-O-methyl-transferase or taken back up into the nerve terminal (Fig. 4).

Amphetamine (α-methyl-β-phenethylamine) is the prototype for this group of compounds. Chemical modification of the β-phenylethylamine structure has lead to a wide range of pharmacologic responses (56–60). At one end of the spectrum are derivatives that influence dopaminergic and noradrenergic neurotransmission (amphetamine). Phentermine, diethylpropion, benzphetamine, and phendimetrazine are thought to stimulate the release of norepinephrine from the nerve terminal into the interneuronal cleft thus increasing the amount of NE interacting with postganglionic neuronal receptors (36). However, they may also stimulate dopamine release and block reuptake of NE and/or dopamine. A recent microdialysis study shows that phentermine stimulates the release of dopamine from the striatum (61). At the other end of the spectrum are drugs that affect serotonin release and reuptake such as dexfenfluramine (53). In the middle are newer drugs that block the reuptake of norepinephrine, serotonin, and dopamine (sibutramine).

Bupropion is approved by the FDA for treatment of depression. In a randomized clinical trial lasting 8 weeks, 50 overweight and obese women received either placebo or bupropion in a dose that was gradually increased from 100 mg/d to 200 mg/d. (62). Body weight loss was 4.9% in the women treated with bu-

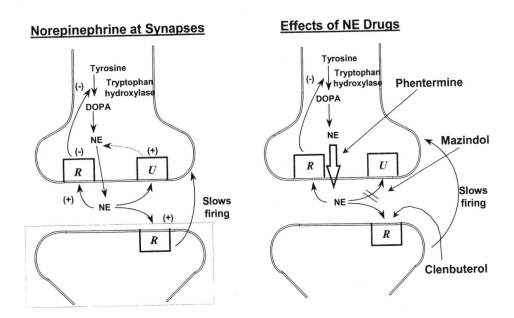

Figure 4 A model of the noradrenergic neuron showing the formation, release, and reuptake of norepinephrine.

propion against 1.3% in the women receiving placebo ($P<.0001$). A second double-blind randomized placebo-controlled trial enrolled 327 women and men with a body mass index between 30 and 40 kg/m². Subjects received an energy-deficit diet and a behavioral program. In this three-arm trial, one group received placebo and the others received either 300 or 400 mg/d of a sustained release preparation. After 6 months, weight loss was 4.9% in the placebo-treated group, 7.0% in the lower-dose bupropion group, and 9.4% in the higher-dose group (63).

a. Phenethylamine Receptors

Paul and his colleagues (64–70) explored the binding of ³H-amphetamine and ³H-mazindol to receptors in brain tissue. They demonstrated the presence of both a low- and a high-affinity saturable stereospecific protein-binding site for amphetamine and mazindol on synaptosomal membranes in the hypothalamus and corpus striatum (64). The relative binding affinities of the various phenylethylamine derivatives as measured by the inhibition of ³H-amphetamine or ³H-mazindol binding are correlated with their relative anorectic potencies but not their relative stimulant properties (Fig. 5) (67).

The amphetamine-binding sites in the hypothalamus are regulated by the levels of intracellular glucose (65,67–70). Glucose and amphetamine seem to act at the same site in the hypothalamus to stimulate a sodium-potassium ATPase, which may be involved in the glucostatic regulation of food intake (65). Mazindol

and ouabain binding are related to glucose concentration but alloxan-induced inactivation of the glucoreceptor mechanism uncouples the anorectic drug recognition site from the hypothalamic glucostat (70). Collectively these data suggest that ion channels involving ATP-dependent potassium channels may be involved in the mechanism of action of β-phenethylamine and tricyclic anorectic drugs.

b. Food Intake

In experimental animals all of the β-phenthylamine derivatives have been shown to reduce food intake, which is the primary mechanism for weight loss. In rodents, the effect is dose related and occurs rapidly after parenteral administration of the drug. In early experimental studies on dogs, Harris et al. (71) showed that weight loss only occurred if animals were allowed to reduce their food intake. Garrow et al. (72) and Petrie et al. (73) showed in human beings that weight loss with fenfluramine is not different than placebo when food intake was held constant on a metabolic unit.

The pattern of food intake differs between noradrenergic and serotonergic drugs. Amphetamine, as the prototypic drug, delays the onset of eating whereas fenfluramine does not delay the onset of eating, but hastens the termination of food ingestion (53,74,75). In experimental animals, administration of serotonin (41,75) or fenfluramine (40) reduces primarily fat intake. This occurs independently of the underlying nutrient preference of the animal. Although NE injected in the PVN is claimed to increase carbohydrate intake (76), noradrenergic drugs have not been reported to have selective effects on macronutrient intake (77).

c. Thermogenesis

Some of the β-phenethylamine drugs are thermogenic in animals. Mazindol stimulates oxygen consumption (78) and increases NE turnover in brown fat (79,80). Although mazindol seems to be the most robust stimulator of thermogenesis in rodents, other anorectics such as diethylpropion have a stimulatory effect on oxygen consumption (78). Fenfluramine, mazindol, and amphetamine, but not diethylpropion, increase the thermogenic activity of brown adipose tissue in rats (79,80). Dexfenfluramine produces a pattern of response in the experimental animal that has some similarities to a lesion in the lateral hypothalamus (LH) (81,82), although not all accept this view (83). During chronic treatment with dexfenfluramine, food intake initially falls and then gradually returns to normal, although body weight remains 10–15% below con-

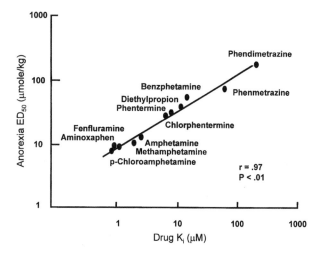

Figure 5 Relation of appetite suppressant effect and binding to hypothalamic membranes. (From Ref. 68.)

trol, probably as the result of activation of the sympathetic nervous system to brown adipose tissue (81). When animals are weight reduced before receiving the drug, dexfenfluramine does not reduce food intake (83). In addition, the animal lesioned in the lateral hypothalamus (LH) is more sensitive to fenfluramine (84), suggesting that stimulating factors for feeding from the LH (possibly orexins; see below) and the serotonin system affected by fenfluramine may both be feeding into the same CNS elements. Sibutramine, which blocks reuptake of NE, serotonin, and dopamine, reduces food intake and also stimulates thermogenesis in brown fat of experimental animals (85).

2 Clinical Pharmacology

a. Pharmacokinetics

Table 3 summarizes pharmacokinetic information on the drugs under discussion. The noradrenergic appetite suppressant drugs are generally well absorbed from the gastrointestinal tract (86,87). Peak blood levels occur within the first 1–2 hr for most of them (Table 3). Removal from the blood occurs by metabolism or conjugation in the liver, which produces active metabolites from some drugs (fenfluramine, sibutramine) and

inactivates others. The excretion of unmetabolized drugs and their metabolites into the urine is accelerated when the urine is acidified. The plasma half life is long for fenfluramine, dexfenfluramine, and for the metabolites of sibutramine (88). For the other drugs it is shorter. Obesity can affect the metabolism of appetite suppressant drugs (88). Dexfenfluramine has a high clearance and large tissue distribution in both excess lipid and lean tissues (88). There are similar data for the other sympathomimetic drugs (89–91).

b. Food Intake

A documented reduction in food intake of human beings occurs after the administration of several of the appetite suppressing drugs (74,77,92–96). The noradrenergic drugs reduce food intake without specific effects on macronutrient selection (77). Effects of d-amphetamine on food intake are attenuated by odensatron, a $5HT_3$ antagonist suggesting that a serotonin pathway may be involved in the response to noradrenergic drugs (97).

The serotonergic drugs (fenfluramine and dexfenfluramine) have been reported to reduce food intake of carbohydrate cravers (98). The design of the experi-

Table 3 Pharmacokinetic Data on Anorectic Drugs

	Time to peak (hr)	$T_{1/2}$	DEA schedule	Self-admin.	Anorectic reinforcing ratio[a]	Dose
Amphetamine[b]	1–2	10–30	II	+	1.0	5–30 mg/d
Dextroamhetamine[b]	1–2	10–12	II	+	1.0	5–30 mg/d
Metamphetamine[b]	1–2	4–5	II	+	1.0	15 mg/d
Phenmetrazine[b]	1–2	2–10	II	+	.41	75 mg/d
Benzphetamine	1–2	6–12	III	+	70	25–150 mg/d
Phendimetrazine	1–2	2–10	III	+	NA	70–210 mg/d
Chlorphentermine[c]	1–2		III	±	.23	65 mg/d
Chlortermine[c]	1–2		III	±	.19	50 mg/d
Diethylpropion	1–2	4–6	IV	+	1.22	75 mg/d
Mazindol	1–2	10	IV	+	70	1–3 mg/d
Phentermine	4–8	19–24	IV	+	.21	15–37.5 mg/d
Fenfluramine[c]	2–4	11–30	IV	–	0	60–120 mg/d
Dexfenfluramine[c]	1–8	17–20	IV	–	0	30 mg/d
Sibutramine[d]	1–3	1–16	IV	–	0	5–30 mg/d
Phenylpropanolamine[c]	1–2	3–4	OTC	–	0	75 mg/d
Ephedrine[e]	1–2	3–6	OTC	±	NA	75 mg/d

[a] Anorectic/reinforcing ratio: Dose of medication supressing baboon food intake 50% (mg/kg/d). Lowest reinforcing dose in baboon (mg/kg/infusion).
[b] Drugs in Schedule II are not approved for use in obesity.
[c] No longer marketed.
[d] Not yet marketed.
[e] Usually used in combination with caffeine for treatment of obesity.
NA = Not available; OTC = over-the-counter.

ments on which this conclusion is based used snack foods that contained both carbohydrate and fat, making it difficult to separate macronutrient intake when snack intake was suppressed. Much of the rest of the literature suggests that serotonin and dexfenfluramine reduce fat and protein intake (74,77,92,94,99) or all nutrients (96). Studies in humans suggest that dexfenfluramine decreases food intake by a selective effect on dietary fat (101). In a double-blind placebo-controlled, latin square trial in 12 healthy men, Goodall et al. (102) showed that 30 mg of dexfenfluramine significantly reduced fat intake. Dexfenfluramine is nearly twice as potent in reducing food intake as its active metabolite, d-norfenfluramine (100). Dexfenfluramine inhibits total food intake more than l-fenfluramine (93). Combining d-amphetamine with d-fenfluramine was not more effective in reducing food intake than d-amphetamine alone (93) but the combination did reduce intake of sweet tasting foods more than the individual compounds. Dexfenfluramine decreases meal size and nearly eliminates snacking (99). When administered for three days d-fenfluramine also significantly reduced the intake of a test meal, more so when the preload meal was high in protein as compared to carbohydrate (103).

Ritanserin, a putative $5HT_{2C}$ antagonist, abolished the reduction in food intake by dexfenfluramine and also abolished the rise in prolactin and temperature (102). Meta-chlorophenylpiperazine (m-CPP), a $5HT_{2C}$ agonist, decreased feeding in human beings (104). The hypophagic, endocrine, and subjective responses to m-CPP in healthy men and women suggest that $5HT_{2C}$ receptors may mediate some of the effects of serotonin on feeding (104). On the other hand, sumatriptan, a selective $5HT_{1B/D}$ receptor agonist, reduced food intake in a double-blind placebo-controlled crossover study in 15 healthy females. The major reduction was in fat intake (105). In addition to decreasing food intake, sumatriptan also increased plasma growth hormone in healthy women (105). Thus, both $5HT_{1B/D}$ and $5HT_{2C}$ are still candidates for the anorectic effects of serotonin in human beings.

c. Cardiovascular Effects

Since β-phenethylamine is the backbone for the available appetite suppressing drugs as well as for dopamine, NE, and epinephrine, one might expect that the noradrenergic appetite-suppressant drugs would be sympathomimetic and affect the cardiovascular system. These noradrenergic appetite suppressant drugs have small stimulatory effects on heart rate and blood pres-

sure after acute administration. Relative to amphetamine set at 1 mg, phenmetrazine required 2–4 mg to produce the same effect on blood pressure and benzphetamine and diethylpropion 8–10 mg (106). In one study of normal men, fenfluramine, in contrast to amphetamine, had essentially no effect on blood pressure, temperature, or sleep but caused reduction in food intake and a greater dysphoria than amphetamine (107). In most reports, the pulse and blood pressure return to normal with chronic administration, which may be partly the result of weight loss that lowers blood pressure (108–113).

Blood pressure drops with weight loss in most but not all patients (114). Pulse rate also drops with weight loss but stabilizes by the third week of treatment (103,112,115). During treatment with most appetite-suppressant drugs or with diet alone (110), blood pressure and pulse rate dropped to or below baseline by 8–12 weeks (111–113). Sibutramine appears to be an exception to this rule. This drug produces a small dose-related rise in diastolic and systolic blood pressure of 3–5 mm Hg and a rise in pulse of 2–4 beats per minute, which does not return to baseline even during 2.5 years of treatment (22).

Dexfenfluramine and fenfluramine lower blood pressure in normotensive (116,117) and hypertensive (118) obese patients. Blood pressure is also reduced in short-term studies when weight loss is prevented (119,120). Using ambulatory blood pressure monitoring equipment the reduction in blood pressure during treatment with dexfenfluramine occurred during the day with no change at night (120). In a 4-day crossover trial in which food intake was held constant, supine and standing systolic and diastolic blood pressure were decreased by dexfenfluramine (119). Plasma noradrenaline and renin were also decreased independent of weight loss during short-term treatment with dexfenfluramine (119).

d. Metabolic and Endocrine Effects

Weight loss itself corrects many of the metabolic abnormalities associated with obesity (121–125). Early studies showed that fenfluramine, independent of weight loss, acutely increased glucose disposal (125, 126) and had a hypoglycemic action in diabetes mellitus. In contrast, Petrie et al. (73) did not find that fenfluramine lowered blood glucose, and Larsen et al. (127) found the glucose lowering effect initially but after 7 days of dexfenfluramine, there was no residual effect on an IV GTT. In a double-blind crossover study of 10 overweight women who received placebo and dexfenfluramine (15 mg BID) body weight remained constant. During the treatment period with dexfen-fluramine serum insulin, serum C-peptide and total cholesterol were significantly reduced compared to the placebo period. Dexfenfluramine also significantly reduced glucose oxidation in the basal state and tended to increase glucose disposal during an euglycemic hyper-insulinemic clamp (128). Dexfenfluramine administered to weight stable subjects on a metabolic ward also showed that insulin requiring diabetics needed 21% less insulin while taking fenfluramine as compared to placebo. Dexfenfluramine treatment has been associated with a selective reduction of visceral fat during weight loss that correlates with improved insulin resistance and a reduction of hepatic fat (129,130). Dexfenfluramine increases fatty acid turnover and oxidation while reducing serum glucose in diabetic subjects independent of weight loss (130).

Endocrine changes have been reported with some appetite suppressants. Dolecek (131) evaluated a battery of endocrine tests in subjects taking mazindol or placebo. Mazindol lowered insulin and growth hormone but increased T_4 during an oral glucose tolerance test. There were no changes in FSH, LH, testosterone, renin, angiotensin II, or growth hormone (GH) during an insulin tolerance test, ^{131}I uptake, basal metabolic rate, Achilles' tendon reflexes, T_3 RIA, or urinary 17-ketosteroids after testing with metyrapone or after stimulation with ACTH. Mazindol also delayed gastric emptying significantly (132). Another appetite suppressant, fenfluramine, changed ACTH patterns to a more circadian rhythm while GH secretion diminished at night (133).

The serotonergic drugs fenfluramine and dexfenfluramine also affect the endocrine system. Dexfenfluramine is a more potent stimulus for prolactin secretion than 1-fenfluramine (134) and amphetamine had no significant effect. The rise in prolactin produced by dexfenfluramine can be attenuated in lean women by naloxone, an opioid antagonist, but in obese women naloxone had no effect on the rise in prolactin (135). In contrast, the rise in ACTH and cortisol following naloxone was significantly higher in obese than in lean women and 7 days of treatment with dexfenfluramine attenuated the response to naloxone (136). The response to corticotrophin-releasing hormone (CRH) was similar in lean and obese women, and was unaffected by dexfenfluramine. In a 7-day crossover study, the cortisol and ACTH response to naloxone was higher in the obese than in control women and was reduced by dexfenfluramine. In contrast, ACTH and cortisol responses to CRH were not different in obese and control women and were unaffected by dexfenfluramine (136). When healthy men were given dexfenfluramine and d-amphet-

amine, the rise in cortisol was greater than with either one alone (137).

Dexfenfluramine was also found to enhance release of the growth hormone following administration of GH-releasing hormone (GHRH) (138,139). The rise of GH after injecting GHRH was significantly higher, and the insulin levels lower in dexfenfluramine-treated subjects than in the placebo-treated group, probably reflecting their different central monoamine response system, but this result may have been influenced by diet (138). Kars et al. (140) found no effect of dexfenfluramine on galanin or GHRH stimulation of growth hormone release in a double-blind placebo-controlled 6-day randomized crossover trial. Dexfenfluramine increased prolactin levels in subjects with endogenous depression, obsessive-compulsive disorder, and panic disorder but less so than in normal controls (141–143). The prolactin response to fenfluramine improves after depression remits (144). Fenfluramine (60 mg) increases prolactin 42% and decreases cortisol 33% in depressed subjects compared to an 80% increase in prolactin and a 94% increase in cortisol in the normal controls (145). The prolactin response to dexfenfluramine improved with treatment of depression but the cortisol response remained blunted (145–147).

e. Thermogenesis

A thermogenic effect for many appetite suppressing drugs is clear from the animal data (79,80). Human data are less clear-cut. The potential thermic response to dexfenfluramine was examined in several studies. Using a calorimeter Breum et al. (148) measured energy expenditure in patients before and after 13 months of treatment with dexfenfluramine or placebo and found no differences in thermogenesis. These subjects were treated with a very low calorie diet (VLCD) and had lost weight, which may contribute to the findings. Van Gaal et al. (149) reported that resting metabolic rate (RMR) fell less during three months of treatment with dexfenfluramine (30 mg/d) and a VLCD compared to placebo in 32 obese postmenopausal women. In an acute study using a double-blind crossover protocol, Scalfi et al. (150) found that RMR in the fasting state was increased by dexfenfluramine compared to placebo. Postprandial thermogenesis was also increased in these obese males confirming the data of Levitsky et al. (151,152). In contrast, Lafreniere et al. (101) found no effect at 1 week or 3 months in a study comparing placebo- and dexfenfluramine-treated men and women. One difference between the paper by Lafreniere et al. (101) and the one by Scalfi et al. (150) is the heterogeneity of the patients whose variance may have swamped small effects.

Sibutramine is thermogenic in animals (85), but the human data are contradictory. Seagle et al. (153) conducted a randomized clinical trial and measured RMR at baseline and 3 hr after the first dose of sibutramine or placebo and again after 8 weeks of treatment with sibutramine. They detected no difference between placebo and drug at any time point (153). Hansen et al. (154) conducted a double-blind latin square study in which healthy men received sibutramine or placebo either fasting or with a meal. Energy expenditure was measured over 5 hr. They reported that over the last 3.5 hr, sibutramine increased energy expenditure in both the fed and fasted states (154). It is the late effect that was probably lost in the first trial. Energy expenditure is not increased by PPA (155).

IV CLINICAL TRIALS WITH SYMPATHOMIMETIC AND SEROTONERGIC DRUGS THAT REDUCE FOOD INTAKE

Both short-term and long-term clinical trials have established the effectiveness of sympathomimetic and serotinergic drugs. Weight loss was significantly greater than placebo in most trials, but the magnitude of the weight loss has been variable. We review below the short-term, then long-term studies that meet our criteria for efficacy outlined earlier in Section II.

A Short-Term Clinical Studies of 3 Months' Duration with Single Drugs

In 1976 Scoville (4) summarized studies submitted to the FDA to support new drug applications for appetite-suppressing drugs (Table 4). There were over 200 double-blind controlled studies in this database in which subjects were measured serially and in which the data had been submitted to the FDA. These studies involved a number of different anorectic drugs including amphetamine, methamphetamine, phenmetrazine, benzphetamine, phendimetrazine, phentermine, chlorphentermine, chlortermine, mazindol, fenfluramine, and diethylpropion. There were 4542 subjects on active medication and 3182 subjects on placebo. More than 90% of these studies demonstrated more weight loss on active medication. The dropout rate was ~24.3% at 4 weeks and 47.9% at the end of studies that lasted from 3 to 8 weeks or more. Subjects on active medication lost 0.23 kg/wk (0.5 lb/wk) more than placebo, were twice as

Table 4 Summary of Results on Patients Treated with Placebo or Active Drug

	Placebo	Active drug
Number of patients	4543	3182
Dropouts (percent)		
4 weeks of treatment	18.5%	24.3%
End of study	49.0%	47.9%
Weight loss achieved		
(percent)		
1 lb/wk	26%	44%
3 lb/wk	1%	2%
Percent achieving		
a given weight loss		
over 4 weeks		
1 lb/wk	46%	68%
3 lb/wk	4%	10%

Source: Ref. 4.

likely to lose 0.45 kg/wk (1 lb/wk) as the placebo subjects (44% vs. 26%), and lost approximately twice as much weight as the placebo subjects. Administration of the appetite-suppressing drugs included in this review produced comparable weight loss. Since there was no difference in the weight loss produced by the various agents, the choice between them would seem to hinge on their respective side effects and potential for abuse (see below).

Figure 6 uses data from one of the clinical trials submitted to the FDA (156). It was selected since it was one of the longest in this set, lasting 20 weeks. All 15 patients in the control group and 30 patients in the drug-treated group completed the trial. It is clear that the patients who received biphetamine (a mixture of d-amphetamine and l-amphetamine) lost significantly more weight, and that the difference from placebo continued to widen through the entire 20-week trial, although a plateau at approximately 10 kg was evident in the drug-treated patients (Fig. 6) (156).

Tables 5 and 6 list the short-term studies that met our criteria. To be selected for inclusion in this table studies had to be published in English and had to be double-blind controlled trials lasting 8 weeks or more or the first half of a crossover study lasting 16 weeks or more. Only studies that included the initial body weight, number of subjects, and final weights were used. This allowed us to calculate the percentage weight loss and to evaluate "success" using the US FDA-drafted criteria (7) or the European CPMP criteria. The short-term studies have been subdivided into two tables, one including noradrenergic drugs (Table 5) and the other the serotonergic drugs fenfluramine and dex-

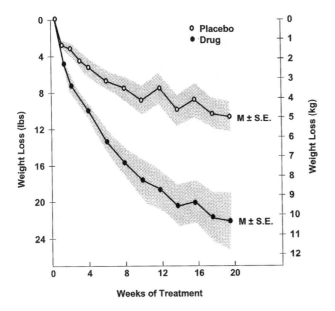

Figure 6 Comparison of placebo and biphetamine-like drug. The drug-treated group consisted of 30 patients and the placebo group consisted of 15 patients, all of whom finished the 20-week trial. (From Ref. 156.)

fenfluramine (Table 6). Several drugs are not available on the U.S. market or elsewhere, but were reviewed to see if they had any unexpected lessons [aminorex (194–198); benfluorex (199–201); flutiorex (202); oborex (203); Ro4-5282 (204–206)]. Some studies on drugs in U.S. Drug Enforcement Agency Schedule II (d-amphetamine, methamphetamine, phenmetrazine) were also reviewed. d-Amphetamine is the prototypic sympathomimetic appetite suppressant drug that has provided much insight into the biology and pharmacology of nonadrenergic drugs as well as the problems of drug addiction. The following studies were reviewed, but not used [d-amphetamine (204,207,208); phenmetrazine (209–214); chlorphentermine (208,210,215)].

1 Noradrenergic Drugs

Several features of Table 5 deserve comment. First, few studies met either the proposed FDA or CPMP criteria, even though studies lasting 3 months (12 weeks) would produce 75% or so of the maximal expected weight loss. Two drugs, mazindol and phentermine, had a number of trials meeting these criterion. It is also noteworthy that neither criterion was clearly superior. All groups treated with sympathomimetic drugs (Table 6) lost weight except the study of pregnant women (160). This

ranged from a low of 2.1 kg to a high of 16.0 kg. In all but two studies (157,159), the placebo-treated patients lost weight. In the review by Scoville (4), the mean effect size for rate of weight loss (difference between drug effect and placebo effect) was 0.25 kg/wk.

Intermittent therapy has been reported with several drugs (14,161,163,164,216–220). Only one of these trials lasted >12 weeks (14). Four of the trials showed no difference in weight loss between the fenfluramine-d-amphetamine (221) mazindol/d-amphetamine (218) diethylpropion/mazindol (222) or mazindol/fenfluramine (164), but a small trial comparing mazindol and d-amphetamine (163) favored mazindol.

Several multicenter trials have been reported (17,173,218,223–226). Three multicenter trials in general practice (173,218,224) provide information on real world uses of appetite suppressants over a short time period. One group of investigators compiled data on several agents administered over 12 weeks to patients defined as having "refractory" obesity or the inability to lose weight on a prescribed diet (227). The weight losses were modest, only 1–4 kg, and with three of the six drugs (diethylpropion, mazindol, and chlorphentermine) were almost identical.

Sympathomimetic appetite suppressant drugs have been tested in many different patient populations, including children who were treated with diethylpropion (157,228,229), mazindol (165,222), and phentermine (230). The responses in children were, in general, similar to those of adults. These drugs have also been used in patients with hypertension (231,232) and with cardiovascular disease (233,234) without reported ill effects.

Since appetite suppressants do not cure obesity, one would expect an effective drug to lower body weight and to have weight return to control when the drug was stopped. Although we have not included the crossover data in our analysis, they are instructive in many instances in showing weight regain or slower weight loss after the medication is changed to placebo. In one study of 21 patients, weight loss occurred with diet but no medication. On subsequent occasions when placebo or no medication was given, subjects gained weight (213). While receiving drugs, patients lost weight. This response to effective drugs with weight regain when they are discontinued is the expected result from withdrawing an effective therapeutic agent.

Studies comparing two active agents with or without placebo have been reported for most of the drugs (210, 216,217,219,231,235–241). As noted by Scoville (4), there was no consistent effect of one drug over the other.

Plasma concentrations of medications have been used to test predictability of weight loss (242,243). The

Table 5 Short-Term Studies with Noradrenergic Drugs

Author (Ref.)	Year	No. subjects Start P/D	No. subjects Complete P/D	Dose (mg/d)	Duration of study (weeks)	Initial wt (kg) Placebo	Initial wt (kg) Drug	Wt loss (kg) Placebo	Wt loss (kg) Drug	Wt loss (%) Placebo	Wt loss (%) Drug	Met criteria FDA	Met criteria CPMP	Comments
Diethylpropion														
Andelman (157)	1967	46/51	10/37	75	11	82.2	84.7	+0.3	−5.1	+0.3%	−5.1%	Yes	Yes	Adolescents
Bolding (158)	1968	25/27	18/17	75	12	78.0	85.8	−4.9	−8.1	−6.3%	−9.4%	No	No	Women
Boileau (159)	1968	53/53	52/53	75	13	67.1	70.5	+3.2	+0.5	+4.8%	+0.7%	No	No	Pregnant
Bolding (160)	1974	25/25	20/21	75	12	87.0	81.2	−4.5	−6.6	−5.0%	−8.3%	No	No	Women
McQuarrie (161)	1975	19/22	18/22	75	12	74.4	84.3	−1.5	−4.4	−2.1%	−5.5%	No	No	4-Wk run-in; Intermittent Rx group
Abramson (162)	1980	40/40	28/32	75	12	82.5	80.3	−3.7	−6.6	−4.4%	−8.0%	No	No	With behavior therapy
Mazindol														
Hadler (163)	1972	20/40	19/27	2	12	107.6	93.7	−4.4	−5.4	−4.1%	−5.8%	No	No	Skinfold decreased more with mazindol; wt loss not different
Kornhaber (164)	1973	15/15	12/14	3	12	73.3	74.9	−2.4	−8.5	−3.3%	−11.3%	Yes	Yes	Compared to d-amphetamine
Sharma (165)	1973	58/58	43/50	2	12	77.6	78.6	−5.4	−8.6	−7.0%	−10.9%	No	Yes	Children (11–18 yrs)
Vernace (166)	1974	33/32	30/30	2	12	83.3	83.9	−2.5	−6.4	−3.0%	−7.7%	No	No	Compared to d-amphetamine
Bauta (167)	1974	20/20	11/12	2	12	79.4	78.9	−3.8	−13.8	−2.2%	−8.0%	Yes	No	Adolescents (12–18 yrs)
Crommelin (168)	1974	20/20	18/18	1	12	82.1	87.9	−2.5	−4.5	−3.0%	−5.1%	No	No	Diabetics
Elmaleh (169)	1974	20/40	17/33	2	12	80.7	79.8	−0.4	−2.2	−0.5%	−2.7%	No	No	Wt Δ sig $P<.01$
Heber (170)	1975	25/25	20/20	2	12	77.5	84.6	−1.6	−6.9	−2.1%	−8.1%	Yes	No	Difference significant $P<.001$
Sedgwick (171)	1975	30/30	24/27	2	12	84.8	82.0	−6.6	−8.4	−7.7%	−10.3%	No	No	

Author (Ref)	Year													Comments
Woodhouse (172)	1975	9/12	7/11	3	12	82.6	76.4	-0.5	-0.5	-0.6%	-6.5%	Yes	No	Significant ↓ in cholesterol
Maclay (173)	1977	207/207	137/155	2	12	83.0	80.8	-4.6	-7.2	-5.5%	-8.9%	No	No	Δ wt P<.001
Slama (174)	1978	24/22	18/19	2	12	81.0	84.9	-4.2	-13.5	-5.2%	-15.9%	Yes	Yes	Diabetics
Yoshida (175)	1994	18/18	14/18	1.5	12	97.8	97.8	-4.5	-13.5	-4.6%	-13.8%	Yes	Yes	Δ Wt sig P<.01
Phendimetrazine														
Hadler (176)	1968	42/45	35/36	105	12	92.1	96.7	-0.5	-3.4	-0.5%	-7.5%	No	No	Δ Wt P<.01
Phentermine														
Cohen (177)	1968	40	37/39/39	20 (10 phentermine compound)	12 Females	81.8	88.2	-4.0	-2.6	-8.9%	-2.9%	Yes	Yes	Prisoners phentermine compound = (20 mg phentermine + 5 mg d, l-amphetamine, 5 mg d-amphetamine)
		40			Males	85.5	90.9	-9.5	-6.0	-11.1%	-6.6%	No	No	
Truant (178)	1972	36/34	16/22	30	16	80.0	79.5	-5.2	-9.2	-6.5%	-11.4%	Yes	Yes	Intermittent Rx group too
Gershberg (179)	1977	11/11	10/10	30	16	84.1	85.0	-2.9	-7.8	-3.4%	-9.1%	Yes	No	Diabetics 1000-kcal diet
Phenylpropanolamine														
Weintraub (180)	1986	53/53	38/40	75	12	78.2	76.3	-4.3	-6.1	-5.5%	-8.0%	No	No	
Greenway (181)	1989	51/51	40/45	75	12	80.6	78.3	-1.1	-2.7	-1.4%	-3.4%	No	No	
Scheingart (182)	1992	51/51	7/10	75	20	83.4	78.9	-0.8	-5.1	-0.5%	-6.5%	Yes	No	After 6 wks subjects were given option to continue double-blind study to 20 wks; 24 PPA and 12 placebo did so

Table 6   Short-Term Studies with the Serotenergic Drugs Dexfenfluramine and Fenfluramine

Author (Ref.)	Year	No. subjects Start P/D	No. subjects Complete P/D	Dose (mg/d)	Duration of study (weeks)	Initial wt. (kg) Placebo	Initial wt. (kg) Drug	Wt. loss (kg) Placebo	Wt. loss (kg) Drug	Wt. loss (%) Placebo	Wt. loss (%) Drug	Met criteria FDA	Met criteria CPMP	Comments
Dexfenfluramine														
Finer (183)	1985	24/26 20/19		30	12	81.9 86.6	81.7 91.5	−1.4 +1.7	−5.3 −2.8	−1.7	−6.5	No	No	General practice Hospital
Enzi (116)	1988	69/64	68/59	60	12 (90d)	87.2	84.0	−3.5	−8.1	−4.0%	−9.6%	Yes	No	
Goodall (184)	1988	16/17	7/9	30	12	92.4	91.9	−2.8	−5.4	−3.0%	−5.8%	No	No	Schizophrenic on neuroleptic meds
Kolanowski (118)	1991	14/16		30	12	101.0	95.4	−1.4	−6.0	−1.3%	−6.3%	Yes	No	Borderline hypertensives
Willey (185)	1992	24/25	23/22	30	12	87.7	98.7	−0.6	−3.8	−0.7%	−3.9%	No	No	Diabetics on oral agents
Lafreniere (101)	1993	15/15	15/15	30	12	91.9	93.2	+0.4	−4.6	−0.4%	−4.9%	No	No	Measured TEF too
Stewart (186)	1993	20/20	18/20	30	12	101.5	94.3	+0.4	−3.7	−0.4%	−3.9%	No	No	Diabetic diet and/or sulfonylurea; 4-wk run-in
Bremer (187)	1994	14/15	14/12	30	12	86.8	79.3	+0.4	−2.1	−0.5%	−2.6%	No	No	Dyslipidemia 8-wk run-in
Willey (188)	1994	11/9	11/9	30	12	86.6	94.7	−2.0	−1.1	−2.3%	−1.1%	No	No	Diabetics insulin and metformin
Drent (139)	1995	58/54	52/51	30	9	93.6	93.7	+0.2	−3.1	+0.2%	−3.3%	No	No	↓ Fat and CHO intake
Van Gaal (149)	1995	15/11		30	12 wks	94.5	96.6	−12.8	−16.0	−13.5%	−16.5%	No	No	VLCD; Dexfen prevented drop in RMR
Swinburn (189)	1996	42/42	39/38	30	12 wks	95.5	93.1	−0.3	−4.2	−0.3%	−4.4%	No	No	12-Wk run-in low-fat diet
Galletly (190)	1996	11/10	16	not given	12 wks		100.3	−3.3	−3.2	−3.3%	−3.2%	No	No	Half of a 24-wk crossover trial
Fenfluramine														
Munro (191)	1966	30/30	25/25	80	12 wks	89.0	90.9	+0.2	−4.2	+0.2%	−4.6%	No	No	
Weintraub (192)	1983	25/26	19/18	60	8 wks	85.3	88.7	−3.3	−5.9	−5.5%	−8.0%	No	No	Slow release, 2-wk run-in 8 wk Rx
Brun (193)	1988	22/22	22/18	60	12 wks	85.6	85	−0.0	−3.0	0%	−3.5%	No	No	Dyslipidemics

initial data were promising, but two other studies failed to find plasma levels to predict success. However, in the International Dexfenfluramine (INDEX) trial of fenfluramine, Guy-Grand et al. (244,245) reported a good relationship between plasma fenfluramine and weight loss. Patients assigned to medication but who had none in their serum lost only as much weight as the placebo-treated patients.

PPA is an α_1-adrenergic agonist of the propanolamine group. It was an over-the-counter preparation with a provisional FDA approval for weight loss until it was removed from the market in early 2001. The three published double-blind controlled clinical trials of PPA lasting 8 weeks or more are included in Table 5. In reviews by Weintraub (246) and Greenway (247), including published and unpublished studies obtained from the manufacturer, 1439 subjects were on active medication and 1086 on placebo. At the end of the studies, which were up to 12 weeks in length and performed before 1985, subjects on PPA lost ~0.27 kg/wk more than subjects on placebo. This was similar to the results reported by Scoville (4). In the studies performed after 1985, the rate of weight loss over 4 weeks was 0.21 kg/wk more than in the placebo-treated subjects. The rate of weight loss slowed after the first 4 weeks and at the end of the studies subjects on PPA had lost only 0.14 kg/wk more than placebo. These findings are consistent with the small number of studies that have directly compared PPA with prescription anorectic medication. Although there was no statistically significant difference between PPA and mazindol, dextroamphetamine and diethylpropion in studies lasting 4–8 weeks, the mean weight loss for the prescription anorectics was 0.86 kg/wk in 123 subjects compared to 0.64 kg/wk for 121 subjects on PPA (247).

There is only one controlled trial of PPA that lasted 20 weeks. In this double-blind placebo-controlled trial (182), 101 subjects were treated with placebo or PPA for 6 weeks with an optional double-blind extension to week 20 (182). At 6 weeks the PPA-treated group had lost 2.4 kg (0.43 kg/wk) compared to 1.1 kg (0.18 kg/wk) in the placebo group. In the optional extension, 24 subjects on PPA lost 5.1 kg (6.5%) compared to 12 subjects treated with placebo who lost 0.4 kg/wk (.5%) of initial body weight ($P < .05$).

In a study comparing PPA 75 mg/d alone and benzocaine gum 96 mg/d alone, the combination of PPA 75 mg/d and benzocaine gum 96 mg/d against placebo in 40 obese women over 8 weeks, the PPA-treated group lost twice as much weight as the placebo-treated group (247). The group receiving the benzocaine lost essentially no weight, and the difference in weight loss between benzocaine and PPA was significant in favor of PPA. The group on combined PPA and benzocaine was equal to the placebo group.

2 Serotonergic Drugs

The short-term studies with dexfenfluramine and fenfluramine are presented in Table 6. In this group of studies, two using dexfenfluramine (118,180) met the FDA criteria but none met the CPMP criteria. However, the duration these studies were all of 12 weeks or less. Weight losses in the drug-treated patients ranged from −2.6 kg (−3.3%) to −16.0 kg (−16.5%). One study was done in borderline hypertensives (118), two in diabetics (185,186,188), and two in dyslipidemics (187,189).

B Clinical Studies of 14 or More Weeks' Duration

1 Noradrenergic Drugs

The longer-term double-blind placebo-controlled studies with sympathomimetic appetite suppressants are summarized in Table 7. For the purpose of this table, long term is defined as trials of >14 weeks. Included in this table are studies with diethylpropion and phentermine. The criteria for inclusion in Table 7 were the same as for short-term studies, except for the requirement that the treatment exceed 14 weeks.

a. Diethylpropion

There are two long-term placebo-controlled studies evaluating diethylpropion for weight loss (249,250), one of which meets FDA and CPMP criteria for success and a trial comparing continuous and intermittent use of diethylpropion (220). Silverstone and Solomon (249) compared diethylpropion 75 mg/d every other month against placebo over a 1-year period in 32 subjects. The five subjects on diethylpropion who completed the study lost 11% of their body weight compared to a slightly but not significantly greater 13.3% for the six subjects on placebo. The small number of subjects completing the trial make it difficult to interpret the study and probably reflect a high dropout rate in patients who were not losing weight. In the other study, McKay et al. (250) compared diethylpropion 75 mg/d to placebo treatment in a 6-month trial including 20 subjects. The group on diethylpropion lost 12.3% of their initial body weight, compared to 2.8% in the placebo group. Blood pressure was reduced in proportion to the amount of weight lost. When diethylpropion was used continuously versus every other month for 24 weeks, those on continuous

Table 7 Long-Term Studies with Noradrenergic Drugs

Author (Ref.)	Year	No. subjects Start P/D	No. subjects Complete P/D	Dose (mg/d)	Duration of study (weeks)	Initial wt. (kg) Placebo	Initial wt. (kg) Drug	Wt. loss (%) Placebo	Wt. loss (%) Drug	Wt. loss (%) Placebo	Wt. loss (%) Drug	Met criteria FDA	Met criteria CPMP	Comments
Diethylpropion														
Silverstone (249)	1965	16/16	6/5	75	52	78.8	80.7	−10.5	−8.9	−13.3%	−11.0%	No	No	Medication given on alternate months
McKay (250)	1973	10/10	6/10	75	24	84.5	92.3	−2.5	−11.7	−2.8%	−12.3%	Yes	Yes	
Phentermine														
Munro (14)	1968	36/36 (36)	25/17 (22)	30	36	63	60	−4.8	−12.3	−7.6%	−20.5%	Yes	Yes	Intermittent; Rx group lost like continuous Rx
Langlois (251)	1974	29/30	23/26	30	14	85.1	84.8	−1.7	−7.4	−2.0%	−8.7%	Yes	No	
Williams (252)	1981	15/15	11/11	30	24	73.6	73.6	−4.5	−6.3	−9.2%	−12.6%	No	Yes	Osteoarthritis

therapy lost a larger percentage of their goal weight. However, 82% dropped out in this trial making it difficult to interpret (220).

b. Phentermine

There are three long-term studies using phentermine (14,251,252), as illustrated in Table 7. In the first study (14), one group of patients received placebo, the second group phentermine resin 30 mg/d, and the third group phentermine resin alternating with placebo at 1-month intervals (Fig. 7) (14). The two groups given intermittent therapy with phentermine lost an average of 13.4% of initial body compared, the group given continuous therapy with phentermine lost 13.0% of initial body weight compared to 5.1% loss of initial body weight with placebo. The group treated intermittently nicely illustrates the change in rate of weight loss when transferring from active drug to placebo. At each transition weight loss accelerated or slowed relative to the continuously treated patients. These authors concluded that intermittent phentermine was preferable because it was cheaper, gave equivalent weight loss, and reduced exposure to medication. In the second study, Williams and Foulsham (252) treated 30 osteoarthritic subjects for 6 months with phentermine resin 30 mg/d or placebo. The authors reported that the group treated with phentermine lost 12.6% of their body weight, compared to 9.2% for the group receiving placebo. In the third study (251), 59 subjects were treated for 14 weeks with phentermine 30 mg/d or placebo. Subjects in the phentermine group lost 8.7% of their body weight compared to 2.0% for placebo.

2 Serotonergic Drugs

Most of the data on serotonergic drugs have been collected using fenfluramine (the racemic mixture that contains nor- and dexfenfluramine) or dexfenfluramine, both of which have been removed from the market because of valvular problems (discussed later). The fenfluramines block serotonin reuptake and stimulate its release. The INDEX trial with dexfenfluramine was groundbreaking as the first yearlong multicenter trial of any appetite-suppressing drug. In this trial, weight loss in the drug-treated group was significantly greater than with placebo, although the placebo lost 7.5% below the baseline compared to over 9% for the drug-treated group. The studies with fluoxetine and sertraline, selective serotonin reuptake inhibitors, show a modest effect on weight loss. With fluoxetine, weight is regained even while therapy is continued.

a. Dexfenfluramine

The largest number of long-term double-blind placebo-controlled trials have been done with dexfenfluramine and are summarized in Table 8. The criteria for inclusion in Table 8 are similar to those in Tables 5–7; double-blind randomized controlled trials containing initial and final weights. Trials not meeting these criteria, such as trials that gave weight loss without initial weights, were not included. In the randomized, placebo-controlled multicenter INDEX trial reported by Guy-Grand et al. (12), 404 subjects were randomized to the placebo group, and 418 received 15 mg of dexfenfluramine twice daily for 1 year with a 2-month posttreat-

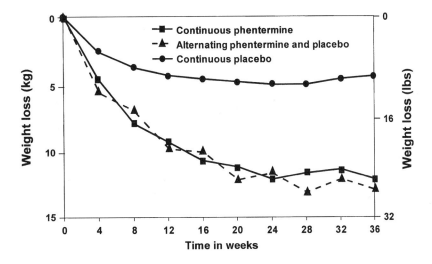

Figure 7 Comparison of intermittent and continuous phentermine with placebo in patients refractory obesity. (From Ref. 14.)

Table 8 Long-Term Studies with Dexfenfluramine

Author (Ref.)	Year	No. subjects Start P/D	Complete P/D	Dose (mg/d)	Duration of study (Weeks)	Initial wt. (kg) Placebo	Drug	Wt. loss (%) Placebo	Drug	Wt. loss (%) Placebo	Drug	Met criteria FDA	CPMP	Comments
Guy-Grand (12)	1989	418/404	229/254	30	52	98	96.6	−7.15	−9.82	−7.3%	−10.0%	No	Yes	INDEX trial
Noble (117)	1990	30/30	23/19	30	24	100.8	90.0	−1.8	−6.2	−1.8%	−6.9%	Yes	No	
Andersen (16)	1992	21/21	13/17	30	52	106.6	92.5	−9	−10	−8.4%	−10.8%	No	No	INDEX substudy with VLCD
Finer (253)	1992	22/23	16/16	30	26	107.3	107.9	+2.9	−5.8	−2.7%	−5.3%	No	No	Wt maintenance study after wt. loss on VLCD
Mathus-Vliegen (15)	1992	39/36	36/29	30	52	110.3	111.2	−8.0	−10.7	−7.3%	−9.6%	No	No	INDEX substudy
Mathus-Vliegen (254)	1993	21/21	17/18	30	52	111.9	107.8	−8.6	−12.8	−7.8%	−11.9%	No	No	INDEX substudy
Tauber-Lassen (255)	1990	20/20	17/15	30	52	94.9	98.6	−2.7	−5.7	−2.9%	−6.3%	No	No	Diabetics, probably INDEX substudy
Pfohl (256)	1994	24/24	15/19	30	52	88	94	−9.6	−10.9	−9.1%	−11.2%	No	No	INDEX substudy
Ditschuneit (257)	1996	12/13	12/13	30	52	96.9	95.1	−2.8	−13.5	−2.9%	−14.2	Yes	Yes	INDEX substudy
O'Connor (258)	1995	30/30	24/27	30	24	100	93.6	−4.9	−9.7	−4.9%	−10.4%	Yes	Yes	1000–12,000 kcal/d

ment follow-up. Diet decisions were left to individual centers. More subjects dropped out from the placebo group for ineffectiveness (36%) than defaulted from the dexfenfluramine group for adverse events (27%). The dexfenfluramine-treated group lost >9% of initial body weight, compared to >7% in the placebo group, which was statistically significant based on subjects completing the study. The percentage of subjects completing the trial and losing >5%, 10%, and 15% of their initial weight in the dexfenfluramine and placebo groups, respectively, was 72% versus 50%, 53% versus 30%, and 29% versus 16% (Fig. 8). When these percentages were recalculated on the basis of all subjects entering the trial, the percentages were approximately one-quarter to one-third less, but the dexfenfluramine group maintained an efficacy ratio of about 2:1 relative to the placebo group.

The results of weight loss in the INDEX trial were reanalyzed by Sandage et al. (259) and published in the package insert during the time the drug was marketed in the United States. This reanalysis revealed that of subjects who lost >1.8 kg (4 lb) in the first 4 weeks of treatment, 60% went on to lose >10% of their initial body weight at 1 year of treatment, an amount that should result in health benefits. Subjects who lost <1.8 kg (4 lb) in the first 4 weeks of treatment lost a mean of 2.7 kg at 1 year of treatment and only 9% lost >10% of body weight.

Seven of the trials in Table 8 (15,16,96,254–257) and one not included in the table (94) are substudies in the INDEX trial (12). Andersen et al. (16) followed 42

obese women who were treated with a VLCD and either dexfenfluramine or placebo for 1 year as part of the INDEX trial. These same patients appear to have been used by Breum et al. (96,148). Of this group, 71% completed the trial and there was no significant difference in weight loss between placebo- and drug-treated groups: both groups lost about 10% of initial body weight. In most of these trials except the one by Finer (253), the drug-treated patients lost 6.9–11.9% of their initial body weight, compared to 1.8–10.0% for the placebo-treated groups. Breum et al. (96,148) reported two substudies from the INDEX trial. In one (203) study, 10 obese females were used to examine energy expenditure. The 10 subjects in the dexfenfluramine group lost 16.4% of their initial body weight in comparison to the placebo group that lost 8.8% of their initial body weight. The other study (96) reported that neither food selection nor serum amino acids were predictors of weight loss.

One report followed up some of the participants of one site in the INDEX trial for up to 3 years (94). At the end of the drug treatment period there was some initial weight regain. With the relatively small numbers of patients, the authors were able to show that weight loss was better maintained in the drug-treated patients than in those on placebo.

Mathus-Vliegen et al. (149) reported on 42 obese subjects from one site in the INDEX trial. Seven subjects dropped out. At the end of 1 year of treatment with dexfenfluramine, the drug-treated group had lost 11.9% of their initial body weight compared to 7.8% of initial body weight in the placebo-treated group. Because of the small numbers, this difference was not significant. Fifty-three percent of the dexfenfluramine group, however, lost >10% of their initial body weight, which was significantly greater than the 28% for the placebo group.

Noble (117) studied 60 obese subjects that had lost >4.5 kg but were unable to lose further. He enrolled them into 6-month double-blind, randomized, controlled study of dexfenfluramine (30 mg/d) or placebo. Weight loss at 6 months in the dexfenfluramine group was 7% of initial body weight, compared to 2% of initial body weight in the placebo group.

O'Connor et al. (258) reported a 6-month double-blind study of 58 subjects randomized to dexfenfluramine (15 mg BID) or placebo. The dexfenfluramine group lost 10% of their initial body weight compared to 5% of initial body weight lost in the placebo group. Not only was there a significantly greater weight loss in the dexfenfluramine-treated group but the dexfenfluramine-treated group also had a significant improvement in lipid and insulin profile in comparison to the

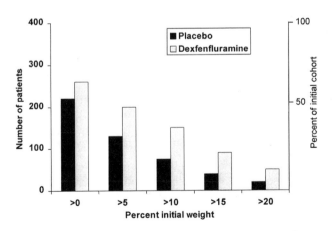

Figure 8 Responder analysis for dexfenfluramine. These data from the International Dexfenfluramine (INDEX) trial show the percentage of patients treated with placebo or active drug who lost more than various levels of initial body weight. (From Ref. 12.)

control group. Fifty percent of the dexfenfluramine group lost 10% or more of their initial body weight, which was significantly more than 14.3% of the placebo-treated group.

Weight loss in patients treated with dexfenfluramine occurs over a period of 3–6 months and then remains stable during the remainder of the 1–1.5 years over which it has been tested. Weight regain at the end of studies with dexfenfluramine is generally faster in those who lost most weight, which suggests that the drug remained effective until discontinued. The addition of dexfenfluramine to regimens of metformin or metformin with sulfonylureas in obese type 2 diabetics using a double-blind design caused greater weight loss, better diabetic control, and lower blood pressure than in the placebo group (260).

b.   Fenfluramine

There are five long-term studies with d,1-fenfluramine that are worthy of discussion, although none of them met the criteria for inclusion into Table 8. Steel et al. (219), in a study lacking a placebo control group, divided 175 obese women into five groups of 35 women for a 9-month trial. This included: (1) continuous fenfluramine (60 mg/d); (2) intermittent fenfluramine; (3) alternating fenfluramine and phentermine every other month (30 mg/d); (4) intermittent fenfluramine alternating with intermittent phentermine; and (5) intermittent phentermine. The group treated continuously with fenfluramine lost 13.7% of initial body weight, which was not significantly different from the intermittent phentermine treatment group, who lost 12.8% of initial body weight. The groups that had intermittent periods on fenfluramine had a higher incidence of side effects, especially depression. The authors concluded that intermittent phentermine was equally as effective as continuous fenfluramine, and that fenfluramine should not be used intermittently due to an increased risk of depression when it is discontinued. Weintraub also concluded that intermittent therapy with fenfluramine and phentermine had more side effects than continuous therapy (11,261).

Two open-label studies are particularly instructive. In one of these, Hudson (262) treated 176 subjects for 1 year followed by a second year with no drug treatment. His three treatment groups during the first year were: (1) normotensive subjects treated with d,1-fenfluramine (80–120 mg/d); (2) hypertensive subjects treated with d,1-fenfluramine; and (3) normotensive and hypertensive subjects treated with diet. The maximum reduction of blood pressure was seen in the first 4 weeks of the study and the drop was greatest in the hypertensive

group on fenfluramine and least in the hypertensive and normotensive subjects on diet. The group treated with fenfluramine lost 10% of initial body weight over the first 6 months and maintained it for the remainder of the year, while the placebo group lost 6% of initial body weight. Over the year of follow-up off medication, subjects regained almost all of the weight they had lost, showing that this drug was effective when used but that it did not cure obesity and did not leave any "residual," thus in effect allowing subjects to regain the weight they had lost.

In the second open-label study, Stunkard et al. (263) divided 120 women into three groups for 6 months of treatment and 6 months of follow-up. The treatment groups were: (1) behavior modification; (2) fenfluramine (120 mg/d); and (3) behavior modification plus fenfluramine and an observation group. The groups on fenfluramine lost ~15% of initial body weight at 6 months compared to 12% treated with behavior modification alone. At 6 months of follow-up, the groups on fenfluramine were 6% below baseline while the behavior modification group was 10% below baseline. These differences were significant ($P < .05$), and the authors concluded that fenfluramine gave greater weight loss but that weight was more easily regained after the medication was stopped than with behavior modification alone, probably because the "treatment effects" of behavior modification were continuing to be used.

The only trial with d,1-fenfluramine that failed to show an effect of drug was an open-label study that lasted 9 months and randomized 156 patients into one of four groups who received d,1-fenfluramine 60 mg/d; d,1-fenfluramine 40 mg/d; d,1-fenfluramine 20 mg/d; or placebo and diet. The groups lost between 4% and 11% of initial body weight, but there was no significant difference between groups (264).

c.   Fluoxetine and Sertraline

Fluoxetine and sertraline are selective serotonin reuptake inhibitors (SSRIs) that are approved for use as antidepressants, but not for the treatment of obesity. Both fluoxetine (264,265) and sertraline (266) reduce food intake in experimental animals. During clinical trials to approve these drugs as antidepressants, weight loss was observed. Table 9 summarizes data on clinical trials with fluoxetine. Effects on food intake have been reported (267,268).

Wise (278) reviewed six short-term double-blind placebo-controlled studies with fluoxetine of 6–8 weeks' duration, only three of which are published elsewhere (268). He found that fluoxetine (60 mg/d) produced a loss of 0.23 kg/wk more than placebo.

Table 9 Clinical Trials with Fluoxetine

Author (Ref.)	Year	No. of subjects Placebo	No. of subjects Drug	Dose of medication (mg/d)	Duration (wks)	Initial weights (kg) Placebo	Initial weights (kg) Drug	Weight changes (kg) Placebo	Weight changes (kg) Drug	Met criteria FDA	Met criteria CPMP	Comments, conclusion
Ferguson (269)	1987	50	50	40 60 80	8	93	93	−1.7	−4.8	No	No	Benzphetamine as comparison lost −4.0 kg
Levine (270)	1989	131	131 131 131 131	10 20 40 60	8	97	95 92 94 95	−0.54	−0.94 −1.93 −2.16 −3.91	No	No	Multicenter dose-ranging study
Marcus (13)	1990	No binge Binge	10/13 12/10	60	52	110.0	92.8	+0.6	−17.1	Yes	Yes	Binge eaters— 10 centers
Darga (9)	1991	22	23	60	52	94.7	103.9	−4.6	−8.4	No	No	Type 2 diabetics
Gray (10)	1992	24	24	60	24	102.9	105.8	−0.8	−8.2	No	No	Crossover
Fernandez-Soto (271)	1995	19	23	60	12	107.3	105.5	−8.6	−4.2 −7.3	No	No	
Connolly (272)	1994	11	13	60	24	36.8 (BMI) 92.0	35.1 (BMI) 85.1	0.0	−3.9	No	No	Elderly >60 yrs type 2 diabetics
O'Kane (273)	1993	9	10	60	52	97.5	97.8	+1.5	−4.3	Yes	No	Type 2 diabetics
Visser (274)	1993	20	18	60	12	89.1	87.7	−2.4	−5.9	No	No	MRI of visceral fat
Goldstein (275)	1993	107 106	104 106	20 60	48	89.1	89.2 84.9	−2.0	−1.7 −3.1	No	No	Multicenter, entry after >3.6 kg wt loss on fluoxetine
Goldstein (276)	1994	228	230	60	52	99.2	100.3	−2.1	−1.7	No	No	Multicenter
Daubresse (277)	1996	43	39	60	8	93.0	90.9	−0.9	−3.1	No	No	Multicenter, type 2 diabetics

Levine et al. (270) reported a dose response to fluoxetine over the dose range 10–80 mg/d. In a study of binge eaters, Marcus et al. (13) reported that binge eaters responded as well as nonbinge eaters over the 1-year trial. In a study of diabetics (10,279) the fluoxetine-treated patients lost more weight and reduced their requirement for insulin.

The principal problem with fluoxetine as an antiobesity agent was the regain in weight observed in long-term clinical trials (9,275,276). Darga et al. (9) noted a weight loss of 11.7% by 29 weeks, but by the end of 1 year, the weight loss was only 7.8% and not significantly different from placebo. In an analysis of these long-term studies Sayler et al. (280) found that the 504 patients treated with placebo lost 2.1% at 6 months, compared with a 5.3% loss in the 522 subjects treated with fluoxetine. By the end of 12 months of treatment, however, the group taking fluoxetine had lost only 2.7% of their baseline weight, compared to 1.6% in the placebo group.

In an 8-month study comparing fluoxetine 40 mg/d with the combination of fluoxetine 40 mg/d and dexfenfluramine 15 mg/d, Pedrinola et al. (281) demonstrated that the combination doubled the weight loss seen with fluoxetine alone. A secondary prevention study is the only controlled weight loss trial with sertraline, and sertraline was not different from placebo (282).

We conclude that SSRIs, per se, do not appear to be efficient medications for weight loss, but for those patients who are obese as well as depressed, these agents may be a more appropriate treatment than other antidepressants that are known to be associated with weight gain, such as some of the tricyclic antidepressants. Both sertraline and fluoxetine lose their effectiveness as weight loss drugs with continued administration. This loss of effectiveness is not seen with other drugs, and the basis for this effect is unknown.

3 Clinical Trials with Serotonin-Norepinephrine Reuptake Inhibitor

a. Sibutramine

Sibutramine is a selective reuptake inhibitor that is most potent for serotonin and norepinephrine, but it also blocks dopamine reuptake. Like the drugs acting on individual receptors, sibutramine reduces food intake and probably increases thermogenesis. In clinical trials, the drug (at doses >5 mg/d) produces dose-related weight loss that is significantly greater than placebo. Its side effects are similar to noradrenergic drugs. Patients should be watched carefully during early therapy in case they have an unexpectedly high rise in

blood pressure. Sibutramine has not been reported to produce cardiac valvular insufficiency (283).

In experimental animals the inhibition of food intake by sibutramine is duplicated by combining a noradrenergic reuptake inhibitor (nisoxetine) with a serotonin reuptake inhibitor (fluoxetine) (284). Sibutramine produces the behavioral sequence of satiety (285). Sibutramine does not bind to any one of the wide variety of receptors on which it has been tested. In addition to the inhibition of food intake (286), sibutramine also stimulates thermogenesis in experimental animals (85) and may block the weight loss effect of slowed thermogenesis in human beings, but as noted above, the human data are contradictory (153,154,287–289).

Both short-term (290–295) and long-term (296–305) clinical trials have been reported with sibutramine, and these are summarized in Table 10 and elsewhere (285, 306). In an 8-week trial comparing placebo with 5 and 20 mg/d of sibutramine, Weintraub et al. (290) noted a weight loss of 1.4 ± 2.1 kg in placebo group, 2.9 ± 2.3 kg in the group treated with 5 mg/d, and 5.0 ± 2.7 kg in the group treated with 20 mg/d.

Data from a multicenter 6-month trial (300) show a dose-related weight loss lasting up to 6 months (Fig. 9). A total of 1024 patients were randomized to receive placebo, 1, 5, 10, 15, 20, or 30 mg/d of sibutramine (300). There was a clear dose response with the placebo group losing 1% and the 30 mg/d group losing 9.5% of initial body weight. By the end of the 6 months, patients receiving the lower doses had plateaued in their weight loss, but the 15-, 20-, and 30-mg/d dose groups were still losing weight.

An abstract of a 1-year trial with sibutramine compared placebo with 10 and 15 mg/d. There was a significantly greater weight loss in the 10- and 15-mg/d group than in the placebo-treated group but no difference between doses (297). Similarly, in a short-term (12 week) study using 235 obese patients, Hanotin et al. (299) demonstrated significant dose-related weight loss compared to placebo and for 5-mg, 10-mg, and 15-mg doses of sibutramine. Of particular note are the studies (304, 307,308) that demonstrate the long-term efficacy of sibutramine in not only producing but also maintaining weight loss. The Sibutramine Trial in Obesity Reduction and Maintenance (STORM) trial (304) provides evidence of sibutramine's use for 2 years. Another study (307) observes sibutramine-treated patients for 68 weeks. The pattern from these studies is that weight loss occurs in the first six months, and if the medication is maintained, weight loss is maintained.

Sibutramine has also been evaluated in patients with type 2 diabetes (294,302) in patients with controlled

Table 10 Clinical Trials with Sibutramine

Author (Ref.)	Year	No. subjects Start P/D	No. subjects Completers P/D	Dose (mg/d)	Duration of study (wks)	Initial wt. (kg) Placebo	Initial wt. (kg) Drug	Wt. loss (kg) Placebo	Wt. loss (kg) Drug	Wt. loss (%) Placebo	Wt. loss (%) Drug	Met criteria FDA	Met criteria CPMP	Comments
Weintraub (290)	1991	20 20 20	19 18 18	5 20	8	97	97.9 102.4	−1.4	−2.9 −5.0	−1.3	3.0 5.1	No No	No	Dose-ranging phase II
Jones (297)	1995	163 161 161	76 80 93	10 15	52	87	87 87	−2.2	−6.2 −6.9	−2.5	−7.1 −7.9	No Yes	No No	Abstract
Bray (298)	1996	24 23 24 25 25 24 26		1 5 10 15 20 30	24	92.0	95.8 90.9 87.2 89.7 90.9 91.4	−0.75	−2.96 −2.87 −6.19 −6.89 −7.30 −8.24	−0.77	−3.20 −3.07 −6.91 −7.77 −8.06 −9.17	No No Yes Yes Yes Yes	No	Part of multicenter study. Data on completing women
Hannotin (299)	1998	59 56 59 62	47 47 49 52	5 10 15	12	84	83.3 85.0 88.3	−1.4	−2.4 −5.1 −4.9	−1.7	−2.9 −6.0 −5.5	No No No	No	Multicenter trial
Bray (300)	1999	148 149 151 150 152 146 151	87 95 107 99 98 96 101	0 1 5 10 15 20 30	24	95	94 94 91 93 93 95	−1.3	−2.4 −3.7 −5.7 −7.0 −8.2 −9.0	−1.2	−2.7 −3.9 −6.1 −7.4 −8.8 −9.4	No No Yes Yes Yes Yes	No	Multicenter phase III trial
Apfelbaum (296)	1999	181 82	48 60	10	52	97.7	95.7	+0.2	−6.1	+0.2	−6.4	Yes	No	Multicenter wt. loss ≥6 kg on 4 wk VLCD randomized
Finer (294)	2000	44/47	40/43	15	12	82.5	84.6	0.1	2.4	.12	2.8	No	No	Type 2 diabetes; 2 centers
Fanghanel (301)	2000	54/55	44/40	10	24	86.4	87.5	3.6	7.5	5.4	8.7	No	Yes	Monocenter
Cuellar (292)	1999	34/35	9/22	15	24	90.1	86.0	1.3	10.3	1.4	11.8	Yes	Yes	Hispanic population; monocenter
Hazenberg (293)	2000	59/54	50/56	10	12	97.0	93.6	2.2	4.4	2.3	4.7	No	No	Hypertensive subjects; 3-wk placebo run-in
Fujioka (302)	2000	86/89	62/58	20	24	98.2	99.3	0.4	4.3	0.5	4.5	No	No	Type 2 diabetes; multicenter; 5-wk placebo run-in
McMahon (303)	2000	74/150	69/142	20	52	95.5	97.0	0.5	4.4	0.7	4.7	No	No	Multicenter; 2–10 wk run-in; hypertensive patients controlled with CA channel blockers ± thiazide diuretic

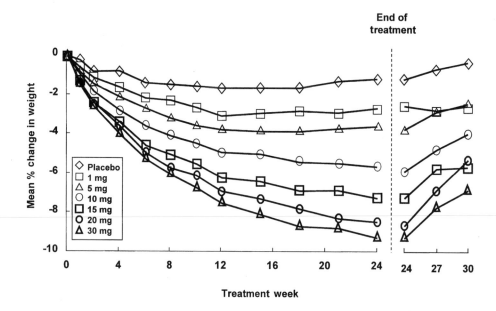

Figure 9 Effect of sibutramine on body weight. There was a dose-dependent reduction in body weight over the 24 weeks of the trial. (From Ref. 300.)

hypertension (293,295,303,305) and in Hispanics (292, 301). Finer et al. (294) report a 12-week placebo-controlled study using sibutramine 15 mg in 91 obese patients with type 2 diabetes. The completion rate was 91% in both groups. The mean weight loss was significantly greater in the sibutramine group (−2.4 vs. 0.1 kg), and 19% of sibutramine-treated patients lost 15% from baseline compared to 0% of the placebo-treated patients. Improvements in glycosylated hemoglobin and fasting glucose were seen with sibutramine treatment and were consistent with weight loss. Fujioka et al. (302) studied 175 obese patients with type 2 diabetes. Following a 5-week placebo run-in, patients were randomly assigned to sibutramine 5–20 mg daily or placebo for 24 weeks. The completion rates were 67% for sibutramine treatment and 71% for placebo. Mean weight loss was greater in sibutramine-treated patients (−4.3 kg) than in those on placebo (−0.4 kg). Weight loss ≥5% from baseline was achieved by 33% of sibutramine-treated patients but by 0% of those on placebo. Improvements in glycemic control correlated with weight loss.

There are four studies documenting sibutramine use in obese patients with hypertension controlled mainly with calcium channel blockers, β-blockers, or angiotensin-converting enzyme (ACE) inhibitors. A 12-week study from nine clinics (293) describes sibutramine 10 mg versus placebo in 127 patients with stabilized hypertension. Mean weight loss in the sibutramine-treated patients (−4.7%) was significantly greater than those on placebo (−2.3%). Reduction in weight was associated with reduction in blood pressure in both groups. McMahon et al. (303) describe a 1-year double-blind, placebo-controlled trial of sibutramine 5–20 mg/d in obese hypertensives controlled on calcium channel blocker ± diuretic. Mean weight loss at one year was −4.4 kg (−4.7%) for sibutramine-treated patients and −0.5 kg (−0.7%) for the placebo-treated patients. Weight loss of ≥5% from baseline was achieved by 40.1% of sibutramine-treated patients compared to only 8.7% of those on placebo. Sibutramine-treated patients had small but significant mean increases in diastolic blood pressure (+2.0 mmHg) compared to placebo-treated patients (−1.3 mmHg).

As with dexfenfluramine, the initial weight loss in patients treated with sibutramine predicts long-term response. Of those losing >2 kg in 4 weeks, only 20% of those on placebo versus 49% of those on sibutramine lost >10% of initial body weight in 12 months (300). Weight loss with sibutramine or placebo produces a graded decrease in triglycerides and LDL cholesterol.

Sibutramine has been compared to other medications in double-blind studies. Hanotin et al. (299) compared dexfenfluramine 30 mg/d against sibutramine 10 mg/d in 226 subjects in a double-blind multicenter study and found no difference in effectiveness or tolerability (299). Hanotin also compared dexfenfluramine

30 mg/d against sibutramine 10 mg/d in 226 subjects (296,309). The subjects on fenfluramine in this 12-week double-blind study lost 3.6 kg compared to 4.7 kg in the sibutramine group ($P < .05$). Although there was more weight loss in the sibutramine group, adverse events were similar.

Sibutramine has substantial clinical data documenting its efficacy. The amount of weight loss is related to the dose of medication and the intensity of the behavioral intervention. Intensive lifestyle interventions combined with the drug have been shown to produce ~16% weight loss from baseline (296,310). Less intensive lifestyle approaches are associated with more modest losses and one can expect the "drug effect" when used with no behavioral intervention to be ~ −4% (310). Most important is the finding of long-term weight control for up to 2 years if sibutramine is continued. The chief concern with sibutramine is the increase in blood pressure and pulse associated with its use. The drug is contraindicated in those with cardiovascular disease. We discuss the issue of blood pressure effects later in this review. Since weight loss can produce benefits in glycemic control, lipid profiles, and other cardiovascular risk factors, the prudent approach to sibutramine use would be to closely observe blood pressure changes and to use clinical judgement of risk versus benefit in continuing the drug. A placebo-controlled trial compared sibutramine 15 mg/d given intravenously for 48 weeks to sibutramine given intermittently during weeks 1–12, weeks 19–30, and weeks 37–48, and to placebo. Sibutramine treatment produced significantly more weight loss than did placebo, and the two treatment arms produced similar weight losses (311).

b. Bupropion

Bupropion is a monoamine reuptake inhibitor with actions primarily targeting norepinephrine and serotonin. The drug is marketed as an antidepressant and as an aid to smoking cessation.

There are two published reports (62,63) of bupropion as an agent for inducing weight loss in overweight women. In a randomized, double-blind placebo controlled comparison, 50 overweight and obese subjects received a lifestyle modification program and either placebo or bupropion 100 mg/d increasing to 200 mg/d for up to 24 weeks. After 8 weeks, the 25 patients in the bupropion group lost −4.9% body weight compared to −1.3% for the 25 patients in the placebo group. Those patients who responded were allowed to continue treatment, and after 16 more weeks the weight loss was −6.2% (N = 18) versus −1.6% (N = 13). Bupropion is

currently undergoing further clinical testing for weight loss.

V CLINICAL TRIALS USING TWO APPROVED DRUGS IN COMBINATION

Since phentermine causes weight loss through noradrenergic mechanisms and fenfluramine through serotonergic mechanisms, Weintraub et al. (312) reasoned that combining the two medications might improve the treatment of obesity by increasing weight loss or reducing symptoms (Table 11). In an initial 6-month study, 81 subjects were divided into four groups to compare phentermine 30 mg/d, fenfluramine 60 mg/d, and the combination of phentermine 15 mg/d and fenfluramine 30 mg/d against placebo. The three drug-treated groups lost significantly more weight than the placebo-treated group, but were not different from one another. The side effects of the combination were less than those of any of the single-medication groups alone, presumably because the combination of a stimulant with a depressant may cancel some of the side effects. Encouraged by this experience, Weintraub et al. designed a 4-year study that they published as a series of articles in 1992 (313–319).

The trial consisted of several phases. Phase 1 was a randomized double-blind placebo controlled study lasting 34 weeks (314). During the first 6 weeks a single-blind placebo period used active treatment with diet, exercise, and behavior therapy (Fig. 10). Weight loss in these 6 weeks averaged 4.2 kg (4.5 ± 0.3 in active treatment group and 3.9 ± 0.4 in placebo group). The 121 subjects were then randomized using minimization techniques to receive either placebo or fenfluramine (60 mg/d) and phentermine (15 mg/d) for 28 weeks in a double-blind trial along with continued diet, exercise, and behavior modification. At the end of 34 weeks the 58 placebo-treated patients had lost 4.6 ± 0.8 kg (4.9 ± 0.9%) of their initial body weight, and the 54 patients remaining in the medication group had lost 14.2 ± 0.9 kg (15.9 ± 0.9%). Nine of the 121 subjects (7.5%) who entered the study dropped out before the conclusion of the 34-week treatment period. The main adverse effect was dry mouth.

Phase 2 of the study (weeks 34–104) explored intermittent versus continuous effect of active therapy for those initially randomized to drug, and open-label drug treatment for the initial placebo group (315). The effectiveness of an augmented dose was evaluated in 12 patients who did not respond to the initial treatment. Subjects gained weight during the times that they were

Table 11 Clinical Trials Using Two Approved Drugs

Author (Ref.)	Year	Total subjects	Drug	Dose (mg/d)	Comments
Weintraub (312)	1984	81	Phentermine Fenfluramine Phentermine + fenfluramine	30 60 15 30	4-Arm study; 3 drug-treated groups lost significantly more than placebo; side effects were less with combination than any single drug group.
Weintraub (313–319)	1992	121	Phentermine + fenfluramine	15 60	5-Phase study over 3.5 years of phentermine + fenfluramine vs. placebo.
Atkinson (320)	1995	1197	Phentermine + fenfluramine	15–30 20–60	Open-label, uncontrolled, observational study in private practice.
Spitz (321)	1997	96	Phentermine + fenfluramine	15 60	Drug treatment following VLCD for an average of 16.5 weeks.
Wadden (307)	2000	34	Sibutramine + orlistat Sibutramine + placebo	10–15 120 10–15	Randomization after 1-yr treatment with sibutramine and 11.6% weight loss; no change in mean body weight during 16 weeks of study.

VLCD, very low calorie diet.

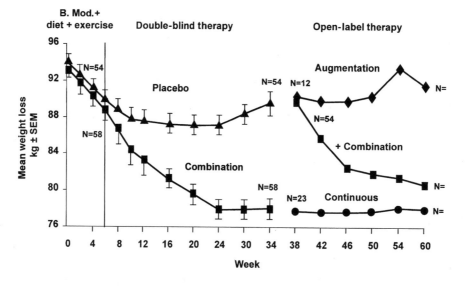

Figure 10 Effect of fenfluramine and phentermine on weight loss. Participant body weight (kg) by study week. In the first 34 weeks, closed triangles represent placebo group mean ± SEM (n = 54). Closed squares represent fenfluramine plus phentermine group mean ± SEM (n = 58). (From Refs. 367, 368.)

off medication and lost weight to the level of the continuous medication group when they were on medication. By the end of phase 2 (week 104), 83 (68%) of the initial patients were still in the program. At the end of phase 2, average weight loss was 10.8 ± 0.7 kg ($11.6 \pm 0.8\%$). Intermittent and continuous therapy produced identical weight loss (11.6 kg), whereas those on augmented therapy were less successful (-6.5 ± 1.5 kg wt loss). Augmentation of the medication dose did not seem to improve weight loss in this subgroup.

Phase 3 (week 104–156) was an open-label dose adjustment phase (316). Those who completed this phase (N = 59) had regained 2.7 ± 0.5 kg, but were nonetheless 9.4 ± 0.8 kg below baseline. Phase 4 was a second double-blind randomized trial (weeks 156–190) (317). Here again the drug-treated patients maintained weight loss better than the placebo-treated group who regained weight. Those treated with drug (N = 27) gained significantly less (4.4 ± 0.5 kg or $5.3 \pm 0.5\%$) than the placebo-treated patients (N = 24) (6.9 ± 0.8 kg or $8.5 \pm 1.1\%$). At week 190, the beginning of phase 5, medication was discontinued (318). After >3.5 years of treatment with fenfluramine and phentermine, there was some weight regain in all the groups, but the group receiving two medications maintained a lower weight (-5.0 ± 1.4 kg) than those on placebo (-2.1 ± 1.2 kg) (318). There were 51 subjects remaining in the study at the end of 190 weeks, for a dropout rate of 58% over > 3.5 years. When medication was stopped the group that had been on medication regained weight faster than the group that had been on placebo showing that the drugs were effective when used but that they did not cure obesity. Lipids and blood pressure improved in those who lost weight (319). This study demonstrated that two medications could achieve medically significant weight loss with few side effects over 3.5 years. There was a slow, upward creep of weight in both the drug- and placebo-treated groups over this period, but this may represent the natural history of obesity. No other controlled trials with two drugs have yet been published.

Two additional open-label, uncontrolled studies of fenfluramine and phentermine in a private practice have been published (see Table 11). Atkinson et al. (320) reported a 16.5-kg weight loss in 1197 patients at 6 months. This weight loss was maintained at 18 months. Of this cohort, 298 had a BMI >40 kg/m². Approximately one-half completed 1 year of treatment while only one-third completed 2 years. Weight loss was 17.9% of initial body weight at both time points (320). In a second study, 96 subjects that were treated with fenfluramine and phentermine after losing weight during treatment with a VLCD for an average of 16.5 weeks

(321). These subjects lost 16.2% of initial body weight on the VLCD and 9 months after starting drugs had lost an additional 2.9% of initial body weight. Because one-third to one-half of the weight loss was regained at 3 years in the study by Weintraub et al. (317) and because a double-blind randomized placebo-controlled study with phentermine and fenfluramine after 3 years of treatment with that same combination of medication demonstrated a slower weight regain on the medication, it is reasonable to conclude that the medication does not lose its effectiveness and that obesity is a slowly progressive disease.

Studies using other combinations of therapeutic agents do not show additive effects on weight loss. Wadden et al. (307) studied the effectiveness of a combination that included a centrally acting agent, sibutramine, with orlistat, a pancreatic lipase inhibitor. In this study, 34 women who had taken sibutramine 10–15 mg for 1 year and had lost an average of 11.6% of initial weight were randomized to orlistat 120 mg TID or placebo, both continued with sibutramine. In the 16 weeks of observation, there was no additional weight loss in either group. Thus, despite earlier experiences in which combination therapy produced additive effects, this small study raises the question of utility of some combinations. Certainly, before we can adequately assess the efficacy of combination chemotherapy for obesity, we must have a larger pharmacopeia of safe and effective individual agents.

VI PREVENTION OF WEIGHT REGAIN (SECONDARY PREVENTION)

Several double-blind, randomized, placebo-controlled studies have compared the effect of drugs or placebo in helping maintain weight loss induced in an initial open-label therapy (see Table 12). These studies have used d,1-fenfluramine, dexfenfluramine, fluoxetine, sertraline, and sibutramine. In the first reported study of this type, Douglas et al. (322) treated a group of obese women with d,1-fenfluramine for up to 26 weeks. The women who lost 6 kg or more in 26 weeks were randomized to receive either d,1-fenfluramine 60 mg/d or placebo for a further 26 weeks. Of the group treated with d,1-fenflurmine, 38% maintained their weight loss, compared to only 9.5% of those treated with placebo.

Finer et al. (253) used a similar design, but induced the initial weight loss with a VLCD for 8 weeks before beginning the randomized placebo-controlled trial of dexfenfluramine for 6 months in 45 subjects. During 8 weeks on the VLCD, patients lost 11–12% of initial

Table 12 Secondary Prevention

Author (Ref.)	Year	Total subjects	Duration of study (wks)	Weight loss phase	Weight maintenance phase	Comments
Douglas (322)	1983		26	Weight loss ≥6 kg after treatment with fenfluramine for 26 weeks	Fenfluramine 60 mg/d vs. placebo	38% Maintained loss with drug treatment compared to 9.5% with placebo.
Finer (253)	1992	45	35	Very-low-calorie diet for 8 weeks	Dexfenfluramine 15 mg/d vs. placebo for 6 months	Placebo-treated subjects regained 2.9%; drug-treated subjects lost an additional 5.8%.
Wadden (282)	1995	53	80	Very-low-calorie diet combined with behavior therapy for 26 weeks	Sertraline 200 mg/d vs. placebo for 54 weeks	At 54 weeks, placebo-treated subjects were 11.7% below initial weight compared to 8.2% in the drug-treated group.
Goldstein (275)	1993	317	48	Fluoxetine 60 mg/d for 8 weeks	Fluoxetine 20 mg/d vs. fluoxetine 60 mg/d vs. placebo for 40 weeks	No difference in the 3 groups at the end of 40 weeks.
Apfelbaum (296)	1999	159	56	Weight loss ≥6 kg after 4-week treatment with very-low-calorie diet	Sibutramine 10 mg/d for 52 weeks vs. placebo	At month 12, 75% of sibutramine-treated subjects maintained at least 100% of the weight loss achieved with a VLCD, compared to 42% in the placebo group.
James (304)	2000	605	108	Sibutramine 10 mg/d in a 6-month open-label, multicenter trial	Sibutramine 10 mg/d (n = 352) vs. placebo (n = 115) for 18 months	43% of sibutramine-treated subjects maintained 80% of original weight loss compared with 16% of the 57 placebo-treated subjects.

body weight. The patients randomized to placebo maintained their weight loss for a few weeks, but by the end of the trial had regained 2.9% of their initial body weight. In contrast, the patients randomized to dexfenfluramine lost an additional 5.8% of their initial body weight. The study by Noble (Table 8) (117) used subjects who lost >4.5 kg prior to randomization and might also be considered a secondary prevention trial.

A secondary prevention trial with sertraline, an SSRI, failed to prevent weight regain (282). Wadden et al. studied a group of 53 women who had lost an average of 22.9 ± 7.1 kg while adhering to a VLCD. They were then randomized to receive either placebo or sertraline 200 mg/d for 54 weeks. During the first 6 weeks, sertraline-treated patients lost an additional 5.1% (1.0 kg) of their body weight. Thereafter, the body weight of both groups rose. At the end of 54 weeks the placebo group were still 11.7% below their initial starting weight, compared to 8.2% in the sertraline-treated group.

Goldstein et al. (275) reported a multicenter trial in which 317 subjects were treated with fluoxetine 60 mg/d for 8 weeks and achieved a 7.2% loss of initial body weight. He then randomized the patients into three groups that were treated for 40 weeks. Of these subjects, 107 received placebo, 104 received fluoxetine 20 mg/d, and 106 received fluoxetine 60 mg/d. At the end of the study the weight loss was ~2.1% below initial body weight in the three groups and was not significantly lower in those treated with fluoxetine.

A secondary prevention trial of sibutramine has been reported by Apfelbaum et al. (296). Obese patients who initially lost 6 kg with a very low calorie liquid diet (VLCLD) for 4 weeks were randomly assigned to placebo (n = 78) or sibutramine (n = 81) for 12 months. At the end of the 1-month VLCD phase, weight loss was −7.4 kg for the placebo-treated groups. After 1 year of treatment, the sibutramine-treated group had continued to lose weight for the first 6 months and maintained that loss, while the placebo group demonstrated weight regain. The sibutramine-treated patients maintained an additional loss of 5.2 kg, while the placebo group regained 0.5 kg. Thus, following a VLCLD, sibutramine was effective in improving and maintaining weight loss for up to 1 year.

James et al. (304) reported a large multicenter study of sibutramine in weight maintenance. In this study, 605 obese patents patients (mean BMI 36.7 kg/m^2) enrolled in the first phase, which was a 6-month open-label period of treatment with sibutramine 10 mg/d. There were 106 patients who withdrew and 32 patients who

did not achieve 5% weight loss at 6 months. Thus, 467 (77%) of enrollees were randomized to receive sibutramine 10–20 mg/d (n = 352) or placebo (n = 115). After 18 months of further treatment, 42% of sibutramine-treated patients and 50% of placebo-treated patients had dropped out. The weight loss at 24 months was maintained at 80% or more of that loss achieved in the first 6 months in the 43% who received sibutramine compared with only 16% of the placebo group. At the end of 24 months, the mean loss from baseline was −10.2 kg for the sibutramine-treated group compared to −4.7 kg for the placebo-treated group. This study demonstrates both the utility of long-term drug therapy for maintenance of weight loss as well as the difficulty in achieving medication compliance (42% dropouts over 18 months).

VII PREDICTION OF RESPONSE TO MEDICATION

There is a wide spectrum of response to antiobesity drugs. This variability of weight loss may reflect differences in patient adherence as well as individual differences in response to the medication (323).

Comparing identical diets given to inpatient and outpatient groups, the rate of weight loss in the outpatients is slower than observed with the inpatients, in spite of the greater activity associated with being an outpatient subject. This implies a reduction in adherence to the diet in outpatients (324,325). Variable adherence was also noted in the INDEX study (244,245). Patients randomized to dexfenfluramine treatment with no measurable d-fenfluramine and d-norfenfluramine in their plasma at the 6-month visit had weight losses identical with the placebo-treated patients. Increasing blood levels were associated with increasing weight loss. Innes et al. (326) reported similarly that women with plasma fenfluramine and norfenfluramine levels of 200 ng/mL lost a mean of 8.8 kg compared to a loss of 2.1 kg in women with concentrations <100 ng/mL (326). Phentermine blood levels, on the other hand, did not correlate with weight loss (242).

Initial rate of weight loss has been a frequently noted predictor of subsequent weight loss (259,300). Those who lose >2 kg in the first month are more likely to succeed. Age is another predictor, with each additional 10 years of age being associated with an increased weight loss over 3 months of ~1 kg (190). Weintraub et al. (327) also identified a number of predictors of success including weight loss during the 3-week dietary run-in period, the physician estimate of patient motivation, presence of binge eaters who lost more weight, adherence to treatment, and the type of treatment employed.

The issue of how to assess the amount of weight loss that an individual drug might produce has been addressed briefly in a discussion of the placebo effect relative to obesity trials. The intensity of the behavioral approach influenced the observed drug effect, as is nicely illustrated in a recent publication by Wadden et al. (310). In that 1-year study, all patients received sibutramine 5–15 mg/d, but were randomized to receive one of the following three behavioral approaches: no behavioral intervention, a lifestyle counseling group, or the same group setting with a 16-week portion-controlled diet (four liquid supplements + one meal daily). The mean weight change at one year is illustrated in Figure 11.

VIII   SAFETY OF NORADRENERGIC AND SEROTONINERGIC MEDICATIONS

A number of safety problems have arisen with medications for obesity. As shown in Table 13, noradrenergic and serotonergic agents have contributed to the unfortunate history of drug therapy for obesity. Amphetamine is an addictive drug that should not be used for treating obesity, but the other appetite-suppressing drugs have little (benzphetamine, diethylpropion, mazindol, phentermine, or phendimetrazine) or no (sibutramine, fenfluramine, PPA) abuse potential. Neu-

Table 13   History of Drug Treatments for Obesity

Date	Drug	Outcome
1893	Thyroid	Hyperthyroidism
1934	Dinitrophenol	Cataracts; neuropathy
1937	Amphetamine	Addiction
1967	Rainbow pills (digitalis; diuretics)	Deaths
1971	Aminorex	Pulmonary hypertension
1978	Collagen-based VLCD	Deaths
1997	Fenfluramine/ phentermine	Valvular insufficiency
2001	Phenylpropanolamine	Stroke in women

roanatomic changes have been reported when high doses of fenfluramine or dexfenfluramine have been given parenterally, but comparable data in humans do not exist. Primary pulmonary hypertension is a rare disease initially reported with use of aminorex, which led to its recall more than 25 years ago. Rare cases of pulmonary hypertension have been reported in association with fenfluramine. The major problem in recent years with the noradrenergic and serotonergic drugs has been the appearance of cardiac valvular insufficiency in patients treated with fenfluramine and dexfenfluramine (discussed in detail below). Most recently, phenylpropanolamine was removed from the over-the-counter market resulting in a recall of both weight loss and cold preparations (see below).

A   Side-Effects Profile

From the clinical trials in which placebo groups are included, it is possible to identify the side-effects profile for the sympathomimetic appetite suppressants. Dry mouth, asthenia, reduced appetite, and insomnia are the principal reported side effects. The effect on sleep of the serotonergic drug fenfluramine and the sympathomimetic drugs differ. Diethylpropion was clearly a stimulant producing frequent awakenings, delay of paradoxical (REM) sleep, and increased time in stage 1 (drowsiness) (328). The same is true of d-amphetamine (329–331) and phentermine (331). Fenfluramine, on the other hand, did not affect awakenings or REM sleep, but did cause frequent shifts into stage 1 sleep (328).

Emotional symptomatology, such as anxiety or anxious-depressive symptoms, were more effectively allevi-

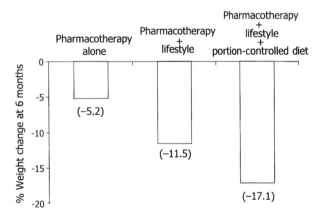

Figure 11   Comparison of lifestyle and lifestyle plus a portion-controlled diet added to pharmacotherapy. Pharmacotherapy consisted of daily treatment with sibutramine 10–15 mg/d. The lifestyle consisted of weekly sessions using the LEARN Manual. The portion-controlled diet using four servings of Optifast and 1 frozen entree each day. (From Ref. 310.)

ated by fenfluramine or by d-amphetamine than by placebo (332). These are usually mild and rarely lead to termination of treatment. For the sympathomimetic agents (benzphetamine, phendimetrazine, phentermine, diethylpropion, mazindol, and sibutramine), constipation is a common complaint. For the serotonergic drugs (d,1-fenfluramine and dexfenfluramine) the incidence of diarrhea or loose bowels is reported. Among the other side effects are abdominal pain, anxiety, delusions, and dizziness.

B Serious Side Effects

Seven issues of a more serious nature must also be included in decisions to use medications. These are the reports of drug abuse and addiction, of neuronal changes, of the serotonin syndrome, of primary pulmonary hypertension, of valvular heart damage, and of blood pressure elevations and increased risk for stroke.

1 Abuse Potential

Evaluation of abuse potential can be done with several techniques (333). The reinforcing properties of anorectic drugs have been one of the techniques used to evaluate abuse potential. In rats phenmetrazine, diethylpropion, and phentermine have reinforcing properties as assessed by self-administration of these drugs. Fenfluramine, on the other hand, is not reinforc-

ing (334–336). In baboons, cocaine, chlorphentermine, and diethylpropion are reinforcing, but fenfluramine is not (337). Amphetamine and diethylpropion also reduced food and maintained responding in rhesus monkeys (338,339).

For regulatory purposes, the U.S. government divides sympathomimetic drugs into categories purported to represent their potential for central nervous system stimulation and abuse. Compounds in category II, amphetamine, methamphetamine, and phenmetrazine, have clearly been abused (337). Table 14 lists the rank order in 1988 and 1994 of some abused substances derived from the Drug Abuse Warning Network (DAWN). The DAWN listing of various anorectic drugs is compiled from emergency room visits and does not list either benzphetamine or phendimetrazine as abused drugs in the last 10 years (340,341) (Table 15). Seven of the drugs discussed in this review appear on the list. Methamphetamine, d-amphetamine, and PPA appear in both years. Figure 12 compares the ratio of the 50% reduction in food intake to the lowest reinforcing dose in baboons. Two drugs, fenfluramine and PPA, are not abused in this baboon model (342,343).

Abuse potential has also been studied in people. d,1-Fenfluramine and d-amphetamine have been compared in eight postaddict volunteers. Fenfluramine overall was unpleasant and sedative, although it produced euphoria in some subjects. Amphetamine and fenfluramine were qualitatively different, leading Grif-

Table 14 Changes in Weight and Blood Pressure During Weight Loss with Diet, Sibutramine, and Orlistat

Clinical trial (Ref.)	Duration (Months)	Drug or diet		Placebo or control	
		ΔWt (%)	ΔDBP (mmHg)	Δ Wt (%)	ΔDBP (mmHg)
Hypertensive patients					
Sibutramine (Ca channel blockers) (357)	12	−4.7%	+2.0	−0.7%	−1.3
Sibutramine (ACE inhibitors) (307)	12	−4.8%	+3.0	−0.3%	−0.1
Sibutramine (β-blockers) (308)	3	−4.5%	+1.7	−0.4%	+1.3
HPT (383)	12	−4.7%	−4.3	+0.4%	−3.1
TOHP (384,385)	12	−3.6%	−5.8	+0.4%	−3.8
Normotensive patients					
Sibutramine (299)	6	−5.8%	+3.4	−0.9%	+1.7
Sibutramine (304)	6	−8.7%	+0.8	−4.2%	−1.1
Orlistat (387)	12	−10.2%	−2.1	−6.1%	+0.2
Orlistat (388)	12	−9.7%	−0.9	−6.6%	−1.3
Orlistat (389)	12	−8.8%	−1.0	−5.8%	+1.3
Orlistat (390)	12	−7.9%	−1.0	−4.2%	+2.0

Table 15 Relative Frequency of Various Drugs Mentioned by Emergency Rooms in the 1994 Drug Abuse Warning Network

Drug	1988		1994	
	Rank	%	Rank	%
Alcohol in combination			1	31
Cocaine	1	38.80	2	27.55
Aspirin	8	3.46	6	3.73
Ibuprofen			7	3.67
Methamphetamine/speed	11	1.89	8	3.41
Amphetamine	22	0.82	14	1.86
Fluoxetine			17	1.76
Caffeine	44	0.32	35	.61
Ephedrine			48	.46
OTC diet aids	52	0.27	52	.37
Theophylline			55	.32
Phenylpropanolamine	116	0.06	105	.09
Diethylpropion	223	0.01		

fith et al. (107) and Locke et al. (344) to conclude that fenfluramine does not have abusive properties. Sibutramine is a Schedule IV drug, but in experimental animals, it does not have reinforcing properties (345). Sibutramine was also studied for abuse potential in 12 polydrug users (346). A dose of 25 mg produced subjective effects indistinguishable from placebo and at 75 mg produced unpleasant effects such as anxiety, confusion, and decreased vigor. The drug was also compared to d-amphetamine and showed no reinforcing efficacy while d-amphetamine did. Sibutramine was also evaluated alone and with alcohol in a placebo-controlled trial in 20 healthy volunteers (347). There were no adverse effects on cognitive function either with or without alcohol. In fact, the single statistically significant interaction was an improvement in cognitive function rather than a worsening of the effects of alcohol (346,347). PPA has no potential for abuse and the abuse potential of caffeine is equivocal. The abuse potential for ephedrine, while low, does exist (Table 15). In studies with self-administration, d-amphetamine is preferred more than diethylpropion and both more than placebo (348). Although abuse in humans is clear, particularly with d-amphetamine, methamphetamine, and phenmetrazine (349), it is unclear whether overweight individuals treated with these drugs are as likely to become addicted as individuals of normal weight (350).

2 Serotonin Syndrome

Combination of fenfluramine or dexfenfluramine with other serotonergic drugs such as serotonin reuptake

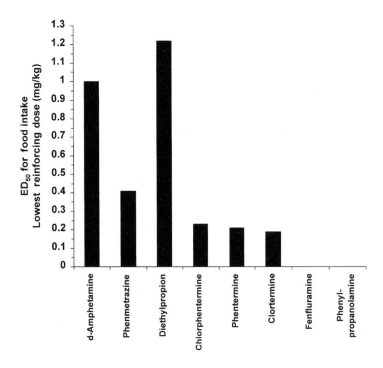

Figure 12 Ratio of ED_{50} for food intake to lowest reinforcing dose. (From Ref. 342.)

inhibitors, sumatriptan, dihydroergotamine, or melatonin can produce the "serotonin syndrome" (351). The serotonin syndrome may also occur with sibutramine treatment (352,353). This consists of one or more of the following symptoms: excitement, hypomania, restlessness, loss of consciousness, confusion, disorientation, anxiety, agitation, motor weakness, myoclonus, tremor, hemiballismus, hyperreflexia, ataxia, dysarthria, incoordination, hyperthermia, shivering, pupillary dilatation, diaphoresis, emesis, and tachycardia. Treatment consists in appropriate support and withdrawing the drug (351).

3 Neuroanatomic Changes

In animal studies, acute doses of dexfenfluramine that produce 10 times the brain concentrations seen in humans have been associated with decreased brain serotonin concentrations that last for weeks to months (354–360). However, studies of neuronal function that used techniques that are independent of serotonin content such as retrograde transport, silver staining, and glial fibrillary acidic protein content did not detect neuronal damage using doses of dexfenfluramine that resulted in decreased brain serotonin content (358). In squirrel monkeys (355) brain serotonin content was decreased for 14–17 months following a 4-day treatment regimen that achieved brain serotonin concentrations 35 times those seen in obese humans taking usual therapeutic doses. Fenfluramine caused marked reductions in serotonin-specific binding in regions of the baboon brain on positron emission tomography, a method that could be applied to living humans (356). Although all animal species tested by all routes of administration have shown decreased brain serotonin concentrations with acute high-dose administration of dexfenfluramine, the same is not true for escalating dose regimens. A 2-year study in mice achieving brain concentrations of serotonin 12 times that seen in humans produced no change in brain serotonin concentration or in the number of serotonin transporters (358). Although reductions in brain serotonin concentrations are usually reversible, this may depend in part on the dose (359). There were no changes in animal behavior associated with decreased brain serotonin concentrations, and clinical use has not been associated with reported changes in behavior.

4 Primary Pulmonary Hypertension

An outbreak of cases of pulmonary hypertension following the introduction of aminorex (Menocil) to treat obesity in 1967–1972 was the first documentation of a relationship between β-phenethylamines and primary pulmonary hypertension (plexogenic arteriopathy) (360). Primary pulmonary hypertension (PPH) is a rare disease that occurs with a frequency of about 1–2 per million persons per year (361). Obesity increases the risk by two to three times and it is further increased with anorectic medication. A retrospective case control study including 95 cases from several European centers and 355 matched controls estimated that the use of appetite-suppressant medications may have increased the odds ratio to between 10 and 23 for an incidence to 28–43 cases per million exposures per year (361). Kramer and Lane (362) reexamined the data from the aminorex cases to provide a comparison with fenfluramine. They estimate the odds ratio for developing PPH after exposure to aminorex was 97.8 (95% CI = 78.9–121.3) and that nearly 80% of the cases of PPH in the affected countries could be attributed to aminorex. Using the French and Belgian cases in the dexfenfluramine study (361), they estimated the odds ratio for developing PPH after exposure to dexfenfluramine to be 3.7 (95% CI = 1.9–7.2) for 3 months or more exposure and 7.0 (95% CI = 2.8–17.6) for exposures lasting >12 months (361). Dexfenfluramine, in contrast to aminorex, was estimated to increase the background rate by 20% or less.

Dexfenfluramine has been demonstrated to increase pulmonary vascular resistance in dogs similar to the effect of hypoxia but separate from it (363). Aminorex, fenfluramine, and dexfenfluramine also inhibit potassium current in rat pulmonary vascular smooth muscle causing pulmonary vasoconstriction. Inhibition of nitric oxide production enhances vasoconstriction, suggesting that susceptibility to primary pulmonary hypertension may be associated with decreased endogenous nitric oxide production (364). Following the release of dexfenfluramine in the United States, one fatal case of pulmonary hypertension was reported (365). Based on an evaluation of the risk-benefit ratio at the time of release, Manson and Faich (366) concluded the balance was tipped in favor of the drug when used appropriately.

5 Valvulopathy in Patients Treated with Fenfluramine and Dexfenfluramine

The association of valvular heart disease and appetite-suppressant use was unsuspected until July 1997, when an article (367) posted on the Internet described 24 women who had taken phentermine and fenfluramine together and who had echocardiographic demonstration of unusual heart valve morphology with predominantly aortic regurgitation. In September 1997, fenfluramine and its isomer, dexfenfluramine, were voluntarily removed from the market. Since then, the clinical manifestations of valvulopathy associated with the fenfluramines and phentermine have emerged through studies taking various approaches to the problem.

Khan et al. (368) conducted a case control study (257 patients, 239 controls) of patients who had participated in clinical trials using dexfenfluramine alone, dexfenfluramine and phentermine, or fenfluramine and phentermine for various periods. Echocardiographic analysis demonstrated that 1.3% of control subjects compared with 22.7% of patients met the case definition for regurgitation (≥mild aortic or ≥moderate mitral regurgitation). A similar approach was taken by Weissman et al. (369), who modified an ongoing trial of dexfenfluramine versus sustained-release dexfenfluramine versus placebo. The average duration of treatment was only 71–72 days in each group, yet there was still a small increase in prevalence of aortic or mitral regurgitation in patients treated with the dexfenfluramine preparations, though the degree of regurgitation was mild in most cases.

A population-based, nested case-control study (370) was conducted in the General Practice Research Database located in the United Kingdom. It compared 6532 patients who received dexfenfluramine, 2371 who received fenfluramine, 862 who received phentermine, and 9281 control subjects. There were 11 cases of newly diagnosed cardiac valve disorders in those who used fenfluramine or dexfenfluramine, in contrast to none in the control subjects who had not taken medication. In that study, duration of exposure beyond 4 months was a risk factor. Wadden et al. (371) reported that six of 20 patients who completed 2 years of treatment with fenfluramine and phentermine had echocardiographic evidence of ≤mild aortic and/or ≤moderate mitral regurgitation. A sample of 412 subjects (372), including 172 patients who took dexfenfluramine (mean duration 6.9 months), were studied. The prevalence of FDA-grade regurgitation was 7.6% in those taking dexfenfluramine and 2.1% in controls.

Two incidence studies have been reported (373,374) and are important because they document the development of abnormalities in patients who had echocardiograms before exposure to fenfluramine or dexfenfluramine. Wee et al. (373) studied 46 patients who took either drug for 14 or more days. Eight had regurgitation at baseline and two developed regurgitation after exposure. In a larger study, Ryan et al. (374) studied 86 patients who fortuitously had echocardiography at the

start of a weight loss program. Seven had aortic or mitral regurgitation on echocardiography at baseline. There were 13 new cases of echocardiographic regurgitation, and the development of new regurgitation was correlated with the duration of exposure to fenfluramine or dexfenfluramine (Fig. 13).

What is apparent from the cited studies is that the degree of valvular regurgitation is not as severe as one might have guessed from the initial 1997 report. Rather, most cases of regurgitation are discovered by highly sensitive echocardiography in asymptomatic patients. Most of those qualifying as cases are mild aortic regurgitation. Only 30 cases have involved valve operations (375). Furthermore, dose of medication predicts severity of valvulopathy (376), and only patients exposed for >4 months (370,374) to fenfluramine or dexfenfluramine seem to have increased risk for regurgitation.

Perhaps the most encouraging aspect of the anorexiant valvulopathy episode is that the mild valve regurgitation may remit. Thus far, only small numbers of patients and early reports have appeared (372,377–379), but the evidence is strong enough to advise caution in advancing too rapidly to surgery for patients with valvulopathy; it may be best to observe for improvement prior to surgery (375). Most interestingly, a retrospective study (380) in the Fargo, ND, clinical site that was the scene of the original 1997 observation, evaluated serial echocardiograms in 43 patients with aortic regurgitation. There was improvement in 19, no change in 22, and worsening in two. Results were similar for other heart valves.

6 Blood Pressure Elevation

A positive relationship of blood pressure and overweight has been demonstrated in most studies (381, 382). Moreover, weight loss induced by nonpharmacologic means reduces blood pressure (383–385) and this reduction is maintained while the blood pressure remains down (386). However, a note of caution was recently raised by the Swedish Obese Subjects study where weight loss of 20% from baseline was induced by gastric surgical operations. Although body weight and blood pressure initially fell as expected, by the fourth year of postoperative follow-up blood pressure had returned to control levels, even though body weight remained reduced from baseline (387).

Three studies (303,308,309) that used sibutramine to treat the obesity in patients whose blood pressure was controlled with calcium channel blockers, with beta blockers, or with ACE inhibitors provide insight into

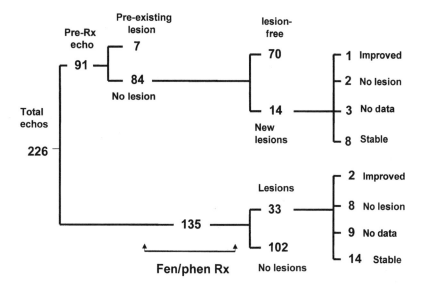

Figure 13 Echocardiographic findings on patients treated with fenfluramine/phentermine or fenfluramine/mazindol at the Pennington Biomedical Research Center. One group of patients (upper series) had echocardiograms prior to beginning treatment and after a period of treatment. The patients in the lower half received echocardiograms only after the potential effects of fenfluramine/phentermine were recognized. The overall percentages of positive echocardiograms were similar, but there was a significant baseline presence of abnormalities. (From Ref. 374.)

the problem of blood pressure effects of sibutramine. A rise in heart rate is characteristic of patients treated with sibutramine and might be a response to the sympathomimetic properties of this drug. That this rise was not attenuated by the beta blockers, however, suggests that a "sympathomimetic" mechanism may not be the explanation for the rise in heart rate. The other possible, and untested, hypothesis would be that sibutramine had lowered vagal activity to the heart leading to the rise in heart rate.

The failure of blood pressure to fall with weight loss in normotensive and hypertensive patients treated with sibutramine (295,305) differs from the decline seen with orlistat (388–392) or weight loss induced by lifestyle (383–385) (Table 15). In the 18-month trial with sibutramine (304), the 4.5% weight loss in the placebo-treated patients was associated with a 1.6 mmHg decrease in diastolic blood pressure in contrast to the 2.3 mmHg increase in the sibutramine-treated patients, even though they lost more weight (10.0%). From epidemiological studies Stamler et al. (393) have estimated that for each 3 mmHg decrease in diastolic blood pressure there is a 4–8% reduction in cardiovascular mortality. In the case with sibutramine, the potentially detrimental effect due to the failure of blood pressure to fall with weight loss that might occur with continued use of sibutramine may be offset by the reduction in lipids,

insulin, and uric acid that do occur with weight loss (300,304). A sound clinical strategy for sibutramine rise would be to identify those patients who respond to sibutramine with weight loss but who have minimal change in blood pressure. This too could serve to reduce the concerns about using a drug that otherwise has a good safety record and is effective in maintaining weight reductions for 12–18 months (294,304).

7 Stroke

PPA is an α_1-agonist and as such can cause vasoconstriction and increase blood pressure. Clinical trials (394,395) show this to be a small problem when the drug is used at recommended levels. In October 2000, the FDA announced the withdrawal of all products containing phenylpropanolamine, including appetite suppressants and cough and cold formulations (396). This decision was based on the results of the Hemorrhagic Stroke Project (397), a case control study of men and women, ages 18–49 years, recruited from 43 hospitals. The 702 patients had subarachnoid hemorrhage or intracerebral hemorrhage and were compared to 1376 matched control subjects. Of the 383 women patients, 21 had been exposed to PPA, six as appetite suppressants. Of the 319 men patients, six had been exposed to PPA, all as cold preparations. For women, the adjusted odds ratio was 16.58 (1.51–182.21) for association with use of appetite suppressants containing PPA and 3.13 (0.86–11.46) for first use of PPA-containing cough or cold medication. The finding of increased risk with PPA exposure was not found in the analysis of men (n = 319). The authors concluded that for women, exposure to PPA in appetite suppressants was an independent risk factor and calculated that the risk of stroke would be one woman for every 107,000–3,268,000 women who use the products within a 3-day window.

IX CONCLUSION

Several comments are appropriate after preparing and writing this review. First, the quality of clinical trials that evaluated antiobesity drugs in the last quarter of the 20th century are much improved over those conducted during the third quarter of the century. In this earlier period, the trials were generally of short duration, were often crossover in design, had small numbers of subjects that underpowered them, and the reports were often lacking in detail. Between the approval of chlorphentermine, clortermine, mazindol, and fenfluramine in 1973 and the approval of dexfenfluramine in 1996, the clinical trials had increased in length, were more often multicenter, used many more subjects to provide the needed power, and sometimes used stratification to balance the groups. All of these procedures have greatly improved the data available for review. At hearings before the FDA in 1995, one of us (G.A.B.) had expressed doubts about the possibility of conducting 2-year trials because the placebo group would have a tendency to drop out because of inadequate weight loss. This has been disproven by the 2-year double-blind randomized placebo-controlled trial of orlistat (388–391) and the STORM trial (304).

The basis for short-term trials earlier in this century was the belief that if patients lost weight they would be able to keep it off; that is, there was an underlying assumption that obesity could be cured. This has proven wrong, and obesity is now viewed as other chronic diseases that require long-term treatment when the risk is sufficiently high. This changing attitude is reflected in the need for longer-term efficacy and safety data. Adding to this need for long-term data was the regain in weight of many patients treated with fluoxetine and sertraline after their initial weight loss. These drugs became ineffective in chronic treatment, indicating the need to document chronic effectiveness for any drug that would be used.

The third important message we obtained from reviewing this literature was the importance of a drug's safety profile in medicating for obesity. Historically, sympathomimetic and serotonergic drugs have been associated with a series of debacles that threatened patient safety and further reinforced negative attitudes among physicians about pharmacotherapy for at-risk individuals. The current emphasis on safety and on efficacy over the long term is appropriate. With perseverance and with advances in the expanding knowledge base of body weight regulation mechanisms, we are likely to see new and innovative strategies for treatment of obesity. We anticipate that the 21st century will yield safe and effective agents to the benefit of those at health risk from obesity.

REFERENCES

1. Stunkard AJ, McLauren-Hume M. The results of treatment for obesity. Arch Intern Med 1959; 103:79–85.
2. Trulson MF, Wasloh ED, Caso EK. A study of obese patients in a nutrition clinic. JAMA 1947; 23:941–946.
3. Feinstein AR. The treatment of obesity: an analysis of methods, results and factors which influence success. J Chron Disord 1960; 11:349–393.
4. Scoville BA. Review of amphetamine-like drugs by the Food and Drug Administration: clinical data and value judgments. In: Obesity in Perspective DHEW, Publ No. (NIH) 75–708, 1975:441–443.
5. Atkinson RL. Proposed standards for judging the success of the treatment of obesity. Ann Intern Med 1993; 119:677–680.
6. Bray GA. Evaluation of drugs for treating obesity. Obes Res 1995; 3:425S–434S.
7. Food and Drug Administration. Guidance for the Clinical Evaluation of Weight Control Drugs. Rockville, MD: Food and Drug Administration, 1996.
8. European Agency for the Evaluation of Medicinal Products Committee for Proprietary Medicinal Products. Clinical Investigation of Drugs Used in Weight Control, 1997.
9. Darga LL, Carroll-Michals L, Botsford SJ, Lucas CP. Fluoxetine's effect on weight loss in obese subjects 1–3. Am J Clin Nutr 1991; 54:321–325.
10. Gray DS, Fujioka K, Devine W, Bray GA. Fluoxetine treatment of the obese diabetic. Int J Obes 1992; 16: 193–198.
11. Weintraub M, Sundaresan PR, Schuster B, Cox C, Averbuch M, Stein EC, Byrne L, Moscucci M, Balder A, Madan M, Lasagna L. Long term weight control: the National Heart, Lung and Blood Institute funded multimodal intervention study. I–VII. Clin Pharmacol Ther 1992; 51:581–646.

12. Guy-Grand B, Apfelbaum M, Crepaldi G, Gries A, Lefebvre P, Turner P. International trial of long-term dexfenfluramine in obesity. Lancet 1989; 2:1142–1144.

13. Marcus MD, Wing RR, Ewing L, Kern E, McDermott M, Gooding W. A double-blind, placebo-controlled trial of fluoxetine plus behavior modification in the treatment of obese binge-eaters and non-binge-eaters. Am J Psychol 1990; 147:876–881.

14. Munro JF, MacCuish AC, Wilson EM, Duncan LJP. Comparison of continuous and intermittent anorectic therapy in obesity. BMJ 1968; 1:352–356.

15. Mathus-Vliegen EM, Van de Voorde K, Kok AM, Res AM. Dexfenfluramine in the treatment of severe obesity: a placebo-controlled investigation of the effects on weight loss, cardiovascular risk factors, food intake and eating behavior. J Intern Med 1992; 232:112–119.

16. Andersen T, Astrup A, Quaade F. Dexfenfluramine as adjuvant to low-calorie formula diet in the treatment of obesity: a randomized clinical trial. Int J Obes 1992; 16:35–40.

17. Walker BR, Ballard IM, Gold JA. A multicenter study comparing mazindol and placebo in obese patients. J Int Med Res 1977; 5:85–89.

18. Williamson DA, Perrin LA. Behavioral therapy for obesity. Endocrinol Metab Clin North Am 1996; 25:943–954.

19. Rossner S. Factors determining the long-term outcome of obesity treatment. In: Bjorntorp P, Brodoff BN, eds. Obesity. New York: JB Lippincott, 1992:712–719.

20. Williamson DF. Dietary intake and physical activity as "predictors" of weight gain in observational, prospective studies. Nutr Rev 1996; 54:S101–S109.

21. Holman SL, Goldstein DJ, Enas GG. Pattern analysis method for assessing successful weight reduction. Int J Obes 1994; 18:281–285.

22. Ryan DH, Bray GA, Wilson JK, Machiavelli RE, Heidingsfelder S, Greenway FL, Gordon DL, Williamson DA, Champagne CM. A 2 1/2 year study of weight loss and maintenance with sibutramine. Obes Res 1997; 5:56S. abstract.

23. Ahlskog JE, Hoebel BG. Overeating and obesity from damage to a noradrenergic system in the brain. Science 1982; 182:166–169.

24. Borsini F, Bendotti C, Carli M, Poggesi E, Cohen H. The roles of brain noradrenaline and dopamine in the anorectic activity of diethylpropion in rats: a comparison with d-amphetamine. Res Commun Chem Pathol Pharmacol 1992; 26:3–11.

25. Leibowitz SF, Brown LL. Histochemical and pharmacological analysis of catecholaminergic projections to the periformical hypothalamus in relation of feeding inhibition. Brain Res 1980; 201:315–345.

26. Shimazu T, Noma M, Saito M. Chronic infusion of norepinephrine into the ventromedial hypothalamus induces obesity in rats. Brain Res 1986; 369:215–223.

27. Leibowitz SF. Reciprocal hunger-regulating circuits involving alpha- and beta-adrenergic receptors located, respectively, in the ventromedial and lateral hypothalamus. Proc Natl Acad Sci USA 1970; 67:1063–1070.

28. Wellman PJ. Norepinephrine and the control of food intake. Nutrition 2000; 16:837–842.

29. Anonymous. Physicians Desk Reference. Montvale, NJ: Medical Economics Co, 1997:435. Terazosin.

30. Tsujii S, Bray GA. Food intake of lean and obese Zucker rats following ventricular infusions of adrenergic agonists. Brain Res 1992; 587:226–232.

31. Leibowitz SF. Brain monoamines and peptides: role in the control of eating behavior. Fed Proc 1986; 45:1396–1403.

32. Sax L. Yohimbine does not affect fat distribution in men. Int J Obes 1991; 15:561–565.

33. Yamashita J, Onai T, York DA, Bray GA. Relationship between food intake and metabolic rate in rats treated with β-adrenergic agonists. Int J Obes 1994; 18:429–433.

34. Tsujii S, Bray GA. B$_3$ adrenergic agonist (BRL-37344) decreases food intake. Physiol Behav 1998; 63:723–728.

35. Susulic VS, Frederic RC, Lawitts J, Tozzo E, Kahn BB, Harper ME, Himms-Hagen J, Flier JS, Lowell BB. Targeted disruption of the β(3) adrenergic receptor gene. J Biol Chem 1995; 270:9483–9492.

36. Samanin R, Garattini S. Neurochemical mechanism of action of anorectic drugs (review). Pharmacol Toxicol 1993; 73(2):63–68.

37. Heal DJ, Aspley S, Prow MR, Jackson HC, Martin KF, Cheetham SC. Sibutramine: a novel anti-obesity drug. A review of the pharmacological evidence to differentiate it from d-amphetamine and d-fenfluramine. Int J Obes 1998; 22:S18–S28.

38. De Lecea L, Kilduff TS, Peyron C, Gao XB, Foye PE, Danielson PE, Fukuhara C, Battenberg ELF, Gautvik VT, Bartlett FS, Frankel WN, Van den Pol AN, Bloom FE, Gautvik KM, Sutcliffe JG. The hypocretins: hypothalamus-specific peptides with neuroexcitatory activity. Proc Natl Acad Sci USA 1998; 95:322–327.

39. Baez M, Kursar JD, Helton LA, Wainscott DB, Nelson DLG. Molecular biology of serotonin receptors. Obes Res 1995; 3:441–447.

40. Smith BK, York DA, Bray GA. Chronic d-fenfluramine treatment reduces fat intake independent of macronutrient preference. Pharmacol Biochem Behav 1998; 60:105–114.

41. Blundell JE, Lawton CL, Halford JCG. Serotonin, eating behavior, and fat intake. Obes Res 1995; 3:471–476.

42. Leibowitz SF, Weiss GF, Shor-Posner G. Hypothalamic serotonin: pharmacological, biochemical, and behavioral analyses of its feeding-suppressive action. Clin Neuropharmacol 1988; 11(suppl 1):S51–S71.

43. Dourish CT. Multiple serotonin receptors: opportu-

nities for new treatments for obesity? Obes Res 1995; 3(suppl 4):449S–462S.

44. Dryden S, Wang Q, Frankish HM, Williams G. Differential effects of the 5-HT$_{1B/2C}$ receptor agonist mCPP and the 5-HT$_{1A}$ agonist flesinoxan on hypothalamic neuropeptide Y in the rat: evidence that NPY may mediate serotonin's effects on food intake. Peptides 1996; 17(6):943–949.

45. Lucas JL, Yamamoto A, Scearce-Levie K, Saudou F, Hen R. Absence of fenfluramine-induced anorexia and reduced c-fos induction in the hypothalamus and central amygdaloid complex of serotonin 1B receptor knock-out mice. J Neurosci 1998; 18:5537–5544.

46. Kennett GA, Dourish CT, Curzon G. 5-HT1B agonists induce anorexia at a postsynaptic site. Eur J Pharmacol 1987; 141:429–435.

47. Tecott LH, Sun LM, Skana SF, Strack AM, Lowenstein DH, Dallman MF, Julius D. Eating disorder and epilepsy in mice lacking the 5-HT2C serotonin receptor. Nature 1995; 374:542–546.

48. Halford JCG, Lawton CL, Blundell JE. The 5-HT2 receptor agonist MK-212 reduces food-intake and increases resting but prevents the behavioral satiety sequence. Pharmacol Biochem Behav 1997; 56:41–46.

49. Hammer VA, Gietzen DW, Beverly JL, Rogers QR. Serotonin3 receptor antagonists block anorectic responses to amino acid imbalance. Am J Physiol 1990; 259:R627–R636.

50. Bovetto S, Richard D. Functional assessment of the 5-HT$_{1A-,1B-,2A/2C-}$ and $_3$-receptor subtypes on food intake and metabolic rate in rats. Am Physiol Soc 1995; 268:R14–R20.

51. Stark P, Fuller RW, Wong DT. The pharmacologic profile of fluoxetine. J Clin Psychiatry 1985; 46:7–13.

52. Blundell JE, Halford JCG. Serotonin and appetite regulation-implications for the pharmacological treatment of obesity (review). Int J Eat Disord 1998; 9(6): 473–495.

53. Garattini S. Biological actions of drugs affecting serotonin and eating. Obes Res 1995; 3:463–470.

54. Goodall E, Silverstone T. The interaction of methergoline, A 5-HT receptor blocker, and dexfenfluramine in human feeding. Clin Neuropharmacol 1988; 11(1): S135–S138.

55. Li BH, Spector AC, Rowland NE. Reversal of dexfenfluramine-induced anorexia and c-Fos/c-Jun expression by lesion in the lateral parabrachial nucleus. Brain Res 1994; 640:255–267.

56. Clare BW. Structure-activity correlations for psychotomimetics. 1. Phenylalkylamines: electronic, volume, and hydrophobicity parameters. J Med Chem 1990; 33:687–702.

57. Nichols DE. Studies of the relationship between molecular structure and hallucinogenic activity. Pharmacol Biochem Behav 1986; 24:335–340.

58. Lemaire D, Jacob P, Shulgin AT. Ring-substituted β-methoxyphenethylamines: a new class of psychotomimetic agents active in man. J Pharm Pharmacol 1985; 37:575–577.

59. Dunn WJ, Wold S. Structure-activity study of β-adrenergic agents using the SIMCA method of pattern recognition. J Med Chem 1978; 21:922–930.

60. Beregi SL, Duhault J. Structure-anorectic activity relationships in substituted phenethylamines. Arzneimittelforschung 1977; 27:116–118.

61. Balcioglu A, Wurtman RJ. Effects of phentermine on striatal dopamine and serotonin and serotonin release in conscious rats: in vivo microdialysis study. Int J Obes 1998; 22:325–328.

62. Gadde KM, Parker CB, Maner LG, Wagner HR 2nd, Logue EJ, Drezner MK, Krishnan KR. Bupropion for weight loss: an investigation of efficacy and tolerability in overweight and obese women. Obes Res 2001; 9:544–551.

63. Anderson JW, Greenway FL, Fujioka K, Gadde KM, McKenney J, O'Neil PM. Bupropion SR enhances weight loss: a 48-week double-blind, placebo-controlled trial. Obes Res 2002 Jul; 10:(7)633–641.

64. Paul SM, Hulihan-Giblin B, Skolnick P. (+)-Amphetamine binding to rat hypothalamus: relation to anorexic potency of phenylethylamines. Science 1982; 218:487–490.

65. Angel I, Hauger RL, Luu MD, Giblin B, Skolnick P, Paul SM. Glucostatic regulation of (+)-[^{3}H]amphetamine binding in the hypothalamus: correlation with Na$^+$, K$^+$-ATPase activity. Proc Natl Acad Sci U S A 1985; 82:6320–6324.

66. Angel I, Kiss A, Stivers JA, Skirboll L, Crawley JN, Paul SM. Regulation of [^{3}H]mazindol binding to subhypothalamic areas: involvement in glucoprivic feeding. Brain Res Bull 1986; 17(6):873–877.

67. Hauger R, Hulihan-Giblin B, Angel I, Luu MD, Janowsky A, Skolnick P, Paul SM. Glucose regulates [^{3}H](+)-amphetamine binding and Na$^+$K$^+$ATPase activity in the hypothalamus: a proposed mechanism for the glucostatic control of feeding and satiety. Brain Res Bull 1986; 16(2):281–288.

68. Angel I, Luu MD, Paul SM. Characterization of [^{3}H]mazindol binding in rat brain: sodium-sensitive binding correlates with the anorectic potencies of phenethylamines. J Neurochem 1987; 48(2):491–497.

69. Angel I, Janowsky A, Paul SM. The effects of serotonergic and dopaminergic lesions on sodium-sensitive [3H] mazindol binding in rat hypothalamus and corpus striatum. Brain Res 1989; 503(2):339–341.

70. Angel I, Hauger RL, Giblin BA, Paul SM. Regulation of the anorectic drug recognition site during glucoprivic feeding. Brain Res Bull 1992; 28(2):201–207.

71. Harris SC, Ivy AC, Searle LM. The mechanism of amphetamine-induced loss of weight. JAMA 1947; 134: 1468–1475.

72. Garrow JS, Belton EA, Daniel A. A controlled inves-

tigation of the "glycolytic" action of fenfluramine. Lancet 1972; 2:559–561.

73. Petrie JC, Bewsher PD, Mowat JA, Stowers JM. Metabolic effects of fenfluramine—a double-blind study. Postgrad Med J 1975; 51:139–144.

74. Blundell JE, Hill AJ. Serotonergic drug potentates the satiating capacity of food—action of d-fenfluramine in obese subjects. Ann NY Acad Sci 1989; 575:493–495.

75. Orthen-Gambill N, Kanarek RR. Differential effects of amphetamine and fenfluramine on dietary self-selection in rats. Pharmacology 1982; 16:303–309.

76. Leibowitz SF, Weiss GF, Yee F, Tretter JB. Noradrenergic innervation of the paraventricular nucleus: specific role in control of carbohydrate ingestion. Brain Res Bull 1985; 14:561–567.

77. Foltin RW, Kelly TH, Fischman MW. Effect of amphetamine on human macronutrient intake. Physiol Behav 1995; 58(5):899–907.

78. Lang SS, Danforth E Jr, Lien EL. Anorectic drugs which stimulate thermogenesis. Life Sci 1983; 33:1269–1275.

79. Yoshida T, Umekawa T, Wakabayashi Y, Yoshimoto K, Sakane N, Kondo M. Anti-obesity and anti-diabetic effects of mazindol in yellow KK mice: its activating effect on brown adipose tissue thermogenesis. Clin Exp Pharmacol Physiol 1996; 23:476–482.

80. Lupien JR, Bray GA. Effect of mazindol, d-amphetamine and diethylpropion on purine nucleotide binding to brown adipose tissue. Pharmacol Biochem Behav 1986; 25(4):733–738.

81. Arase K, Sakaguchi T, Bray GA. Lateral hypothalamic lesions and activity of the sympathetic nervous system. Life Sci 1987; 41:657–662.

82. Levitsky DA, Strupp BJ, Lupoli J. Tolerance to anorectic drugs: pharmacological or artifactual. Pharmacol Biochem Behav 1981; 14:661–667.

83. Carlton J, Rowland NE. Effects of initial body weight on anorexia and tolerance to fenfluramine in rats. Pharmacol Biochem Behav 1985; 23:551–554.

84. Blundell JE, Leshem MB. The effects of 5-hydroxytryptophan on food intake and on the anorexic action of amphetamine and fenfluramine. J Pharm Pharmacol 1975; 27:31–37.

85. Stock MJ. Sibutramine: a review of the pharmacology of a novel anti-obesity agent. Int J Obes 1997; 21:S25–S29.

86. Hinsvark ON, Truant AP, Jenden DJ, Steinborn JA. The oral bioavailability and pharmacokinetics of soluble and resin-bound forms of amphetamine and phentermine in man. J Pharmacokinetic Biopharm 1973; 1:319–328.

87. Groenewoud G, Schall R, Hundt HKL, Müller FO, Van Dyk M. State pharmacokinetics of phentermine extended-release capsules. Int J Clin Pharmacol Ther Toxicol 1993; 31:368–372.

88. Cheymol G, Weissenburger J, Poirier JM, Gellee C. The pharmacokinetics of dexfenfluramine in obese and non-obese subjects. Br J Clin Pharmacol 1995; 39:684–687.

89. Brown NJ, Ryder D, Branch RA. A Pharmacodynamic interaction between caffeine and phenylpropanolamine. Clin Pharmacol Ther 1991; 50:363–371.

90. Johnson DA, Hricik JG. The pharmacology of α-adrenergic decongestants. Pharmacotherapy 1993; 13:110S–115S.

91. Kanfer I, Dowse R, Vuma V. Pharmacokinetics of oral decongestants. Pharmacotherapy 1993; 13:116S–128S.

92. Silverstone T, Goodall E. Serotonergic mechanisms in human feeding: the pharmacological evidence. Appetite 1986; 7(suppl):85–97.

93. Goodall E, Feeney S, McGuirk J, Silverstone T. A comparison of the effects of d- and l-fenfluramine and d-amphetamine on energy and macronutrient intake in human subjects. Psychopharmacology 1992; 106(2):221–227.

94. Mathus-Vliegen LMH, Res AMA. Dexfenfluramine influences dietary compliance and eating behavior, but dietary instruction may overrule its effect on food selection in obese subjects. J Am Diet Assoc 1993; 93:1163–1165.

95. Silverstone JT, Turner P, Humpherson PL. Direct measurement of the anorectic activity of diethylpropion (Tenuate Dospan). J Clin Pharmacol 1968; 8:172–179.

96. Breum L, Moller SE, Andersen T, Astrup A. Long-term effect of dexfenfluramine on amino acid profiles and food selection in obese patients during weight loss. Int J Obes 1996; 20:147–153.

97. Silverstone PH, Oldman D, Johnson B, Cowen PJ. Ondansetron, a 5-HT$_3$ receptor antagonist, partially attenuates the effects of amphetamine: a pilot study in healthy volunteers. Int Clin Psychopharm 1992; 7:37–43.

98. Wurtman JJ. Carbohydrate craving. Relationship between carbohydrate intake and disorders of mood. Drugs 1990; 39:49–52.

99. Blundell JE, Hill AJ. Serotonin modulation of the pattern of eating and the profile of hunger-satiety in humans. Int J Obes 1987; 11:141–153.

100. McTavish D, Heel RC. Dexfenfluramine. A review of its pharmacological properties and therapeutic potential in obesity. Drugs 1992; 43:713–733.

101. Lafreniere F, Lambert J, Rasio E, Serri O. Effects of dexfenfluramine treatment on body weight and postprandial thermogenesis in obese subjects. A double-blind placebo-controlled study. Int J Obes 1993; 17:25–30.

102. Goodall EM, Cowen PJ, Franklin M, Silverstone T. Ritanserin attenuates anorectic, endocrine and thermic responses to d-fenfluramine in human volunteers. Psychopharmacology 1993; 112:461–466.

103. Hill AJ, Blundell JE. Sensitivity of the appetite control

system in obese subjects to nutritional and serotonergic challenges. Int J Obes 1990; 14:219–233.

104. Cowen PJ, Sargent PA, Williams C, Goodall EM, Orlikov AB. Hypophagic, endocrine and subjective responses to m-chlorophenylpiperazine in healthy men and women. Hum Psychopharmacol 1995; 10:385–391.

105. Boeles S, Williams C, Campling GM, Goodall EM, Cowen PJ. Sumatriptan decreases food intake and increases plasma growth hormone in healthy women. Psychopharmacology 1997; 129:179–182.

106. Griffith JD. Structure-activity relationships of several amphetamine drugs in man. In: Ellinwood EH Jr, Kiloey MN, eds. Cocaine and Other Stimulants. New York: Plenum Press, 1977:705–715.

107. Griffith JD, Nutt JG, Jasinski DR. A comparison of fenfluramine and amphetamine in man. Clin Pharmacol Ther 1975; 18:563–570.

108. Chaing BN, Perlman LV, Epstein FH. Overweight and hypertension: a review. Circulation 1969; 39:403–421.

109. Treatment of Mild Hypertension Research Group. A randomized, placebo-controlled trial of a nutritional-hygienic regimen along with various drug monotherapies. Arch Intern Med 1991; 151:1413.

110. Davis BR, Blaufox MD, Oberman A, Wassertheil-Smoller S, Zimbaldi N, Cutler JA, Kirchner K, Langford HG. Reduction in long-term antihypertensive medication requirements. Arch Intern Med 1993; 153:1773–1782.

111. MacMahon S, Cutler J, Brittain E, Higgins M. Obesity and hypertension: epidemiological and clinical issues (review). Eur Heart J 1987; 8:S57–S70.

112. Sowers JR, Whitfield LA, Catania RA, Stern N, Tuck ML, Dornfeld L, Maxwell M. Role of the sympathetic nervous system in blood pressure maintenance in obesity. J Clin Endocrinol Metab 1982; 54:1181–1186.

113. Dornfeld LP, Maxwell MH, Waks A, Tuck M. Mechanisms of hypertension in obesity. Kidney Int Suppl 1987; 22:S254–S258.

114. Tuck ML, Sowers J, Dornfeld L, Kledzik G, Maxwell M. The effect of weight reduction on blood pressure, plasma renin activity, and plasma aldosterone levels in obese patients. N Engl J Med 1981; 304:930–933.

115. Zwiauer K, Schmidinger H, Klicpera M, Mayr H, Widhalm K. 24 Hours electrocardiographic monitoring in obese children and adolescents during a 3 weeks low calorie diet (500 kcal). Int J Obes Relat Metab Disord 1989; 13:101–105.

116. Enzi G, Crepaldi G, Inelman EM, Bruni R, Baggio B. Efficacy and safety of dexfenfluramine in obese patients: a multicenter study. Clin Neuropharmacol 1988; 11(1):S173–S178.

117. Noble RE. A six-month study of the effects of dexfenfluramine on partially successful dieters. Curr Ther Res 1990; 47:612–619.

118. Kolanowski J, Younis LT, Vanbutsele R, Detry JM. Effect of dexfenfluramine treatment on body weight, blood pressure and noradrenergic activity in obese hypertensive patients. Eur J Clin Pharmacol 1992; 42:599–606.

119. Andersson B, Zimmermann ME, Hedner T, Bjorntorp P. Hemodynamic, metabolic and endocrine effects of short-term dexfenfluramine treatment in young, obese women. Eur J Clin Pharmacol 1991; 40(3):249–254.

120. Flechtner Mors M, Ditschuneit HH, Yip I, Adler G. Blood pressure and plasma norepinephrine responses to dexfenfluramine in obese postmenopausal women. Am J Clin Nutr 1998; 67:611–615.

121. National Heart, Lung and Blood Institute. Clinical guidelines on the identificastion, evaluation, and treatment of overweight and obesity in adults—the evidence report. Obes Res 1998; 6(suppl 2):51S–210S.

122. Prentice AM, Jebb SA. Obesity in Britain: gluttony or sloth? BMJ 1995; 311(7002):437–439.

123. World Health Organization. Obesity: Preventing and Managing the Global Epidemic. Geneva: World Health Organization, 1997.

124. Goldstein DJ. Beneficial health effects of modest weight-loss. Int J Obes Relat Metab Disord 1992; 16(6):397–415.

125. Burland WL. A review of experience with fenfluramine. In: Bray G, ed. Obesity in Perspective. A conference sponsored by the John E. Fogarty International Center for Advanced Study in the Health Sciences. National Institutes of Health, Bethesda, MD, Oct 1–3, 1973. Washington: DHEW Publication No. (NIH) 75–708, 1975:429–440.

126. Turtle JR, Burgess JA. Hypoglycemic action of fenfluramine in diabetes mellitus. Diabetes 1973; 22:858–867.

127. Larsen S, Vejtorp L, Hornnes P, Bechgaard H, Sestoft L, Lyngsoe J. Metabolic effects of fenfluramine in obese diabetics. Br J Clin Pharm 1977; 4:529–533.

128. Andersen PH, Richelsen B, Bak J, Schmitz O, Sorensen NS, Lavielle R, Pedersen O. Influence of short-term dexfenfluramine therapy on glucose and lipid metabolism in obese non-diabetic patients. Acta Endocrinol (Copenh) 1993; 128:251–258.

129. Marks SJ, Moore NR, Clark ML, Strauss BJ, Hockaday TD. Reduction of visceral adipose tissue and improvement of metabolic indices: effect of dexfenfluramine in NIDDM. Obes Res 1996; 4(1):1–7.

130. Marks SJ, Moore NR, Ryley NG, Clark ML, Pointon JJ, Strauss BJ, Hockaday TD. Measurement of liver fat by MRI and its reduction by dexfenfluramine in NIDDM. Int J Obes 1997; 21(4):274–279.

131. Dolecek R. Endocrine studies with mazindol in obese patients. Pharmatherapeutica 1980; 2:309–316.

132. Jonderko K, Kucio C. Extra-anorectic actions of mazindol. Isr J Med Sci 1989; 25:20–24.

133. Ditschuneit HH, Flechtner-Mors M, Dolderer M, Fulda U, Ditschuneit H. Endocrine and metabolic

effects of dexfenfluramine in patients with android obesity. Horm Metab Res 1993; 25:573–578.

134. Feeney S, Goodall E, Silverstone T. The prolactin response to *d*- and l-fenfluramine and to d-amphetamine in human subjects. Int Clin Psychopharmacol 1993; 8:49–54.

135. Argenio GF, Bernini GP, Vivaldi MS, Del Corso C, Santoni R, Franchi F. Naloxone does not modify fenfluramine-induced prolactin increase in obese patients. Clin Endocrinol 1991; 35(6):505–508.

136. Boushaki FZ, Rasio E, Serri O. Hypothalamic-pituitary-adrenal axis in abdominal obesity: effects of dexfenfluramine. Clin Endocrinol 1997; 46:461–466.

137. Feeney S, Goodall E, Silverstone T. The effects of d- and l-fenfluramine (and their interactions with d-amphetamine) on cortisol secretion. Int Clin Psychopharmacol 1993; 8:139–142.

138. Medeiros-Neto G, Lima N, Perozim L, Pedrinola F, Wajchenberg BL. The effect of hypocaloric diet with and without D-fenfluramine treatment on growth hormone release after growth hormone-releasing factor stimulation in patients with android obesity. Metabolism 1994; 43:969–973.

139. Drent ML, Ader HJ, Van der Veen EA. The influence of chronic administration of the serotonin agonist dexfenfluramine on responsiveness to corticotropin releasing hormone and growth hormone-releasing hormone in moderately obese people. J Endocrinol Invest 1995; 18:780–788.

140. Kars ME, Pijl H, Cohen AF, Frolich M, Schoemaker HC, Brandenburg HC, Meinders AE. Specific stimulation of brain serotonin mediated neurotransmission by dexfenfluramine does not restore growth hormone responsiveness in obese women. Clin Endocrinol 1996; 44(5):541–546.

141. Lichtenberg P, Shapira B, Gillion D, Kindler S, Cooper TB, Newman ME, Lerer B. Hormone responses to fenfluramine and placebo challenge in endogenous depression. Psychol Res 1992; 43:136–146.

142. Hewlett WA, Vinogradov S, Martin K, Berman S, Csernansky JG. Fenfluramine stimulation of prolactin in obsessive-compulsive disorder. Psychiatry Res 1992; 42(1):81–92.

143. Apostolopoulos M, Judd FK, Burrows GD, Norman TR. Prolactin response to dl-fenfluramine in panic disorder. Psychoneuroendocrinology 1993; 18:337–342.

144. Shapira B, Cohen J, Newman ME, Lerer B. Prolactin response to fenfluramine and placebo challenge following maintenance pharmacotherapy withdrawal in remitted depressed patients. Biol Psychiatry 1993; 33:531–535.

145. Weizman A, Mark M, Gil-Ad I, Tyano S, Laron Z. Plasma cortisol, prolactin, growth hormone, and immunoreactive B-endorphin response to fenfluramine challenge in depressed patients. Clin Neuropharmacol 1988; 11:250–256.

146. Coccaro EF, Klar H, Siever LJ. Reduced prolactin response to fenfluramine challenge in personality disorder patients is not due to deficiency of pituitary lactotrophs. Biol Psychiatry 1994; 36:344–346.

147. Maes M, D'Hondt P, Suy E, Minner B, Vandervorst C, Raus J. Hpa-axis hormones and prolactin responses to dextro-fenfluramine in depressed patients and healthy controls (review). Prog Neuropsychopharmacol Biol Psychiatry 1991; 15:781–790.

148. Breum L, Astrup A, Andersen T, Lambert O, Nielsen E, Garby L, Quadde F. The effect of long-term dexfenfluramine treatment on 24-hour energy-expenditure in man—a double-blind placebo controlled study. Int J Obes 1990; 14:613–621.

149. Van Gaal LF, Vansant GA, Steijaert MC, De Leeuw IH. Effects of dexfenfluramine on resting metabolic rate and thermogenesis in premenopausal obese women during therapeutic weight reduction. Metabolism 1995; 44:42–45.

150. Scalfi L, D'Arrigo E, Carandente V, Coltorti A, Contaldo F. The acute effect of dexfenfluramine on resting metabolic rate and postprandial thermogenesis in obese subjects: a double-blind placebo-controlled study. Int J Obes 1993; 17:91–96.

151. Levitsky DA, Schuster JA, Stallone D, Strupp BJ. Modulation of the thermic effect of food by fenfluramine. Int J Obes 1986; 10:169–173.

152. Levitsky DA, Stallone D. Enhancement of the thermic effect of food by d-fenfluramine. Clin Neuropharmacol 1988; 11:S90–S92.

153. Seagle HM, Bessesen DH, Hill JO. Effects of sibutramine on resting metabolic rate and weight loss in overweight women. Obes Res 1998; 6(2):115–121.

154. Hansen DL, Toubro S, Stock MJ, Macdonald IA, Astrup A. Thermogenic effects of sibutramine in humans. Am J Clin Nutr 1998; 68:1180–1186.

155. Alger S, Larson K, Boyce VL, Seagle H, Fontvieille AM, Ferraro RT, Rising R, Ravussin E. Effect of phenylpropanolamine on energy expenditure and weight loss in overweight women. Am J Clin Nutr 1993; 57:120–126.

156. Bray GA. The Obese Patient. Philadelphia: W.B. Saunders, 1976.

157. Andelman MB, Jones C, Nathan S. Treatment of obesity in underprivileged adolescents: Comparison of diethylpropion hydrochloride with placebo in a double-blind study. Clin Pediatr 1967; 6:327–330.

158. Bolding OT. Diethylpropion hydrochloride: an effective appetite suppressant. Curr Ther Res 1974; 16:40–48.

159. Boileau PA. Control of weight gain during pregnancy: use of diethylpropion hydrochloride. Appl Ther 1968; 10:763–765.

160. Bolding OT. A double-blind evaluation of tenuate dospan in overweight patients from a private gynecologic practice. J Med Assoc State Alabama 1968; 38:209–212.

161. McQuarrie HG. Clinical assessment of the use of an anorectic drug in a total weight reduction program. Curr Ther Res 1975; 17:437–443.

162. Abramson R, Garg M, Cioffari A, Rotman PA. An evaluation of behavioral techniques reinforced with an anorectic drug in a double-blind weight loss study. J Clin Psychiatry 1980; 41:234–237.

163. Hadler AJ. Mazindol, a new non-amphetamine anorexigenic agent. J Clin Pharm 1972; 12:453–458.

164. Kornhaber A. Obesity: depression: clinical evaluation with a new anorexigenic agent. Psychsomatics 1973; 14(3):162–167.

165. Sharma RK, Collipp PJ, Rezvani I, Strimas J, Maddaih VT, Rezvani E. Clinical evaluation of the anorexic activity and safety of 42–548 in children. Clin Pediatr 1973; 12(3):145–149.

166. Vernace BJ. Controlled comparative investigators of mazindol, d-amphetamine and placebo. Obes Bariatric Med 1974; 3:124–127.

167. Bauta HP. Evaluation of a new anorexic agent in adolescence. Conn Med 1974 Sep; 38(9):460–463.

168. Crommelin RM. Nonamphetamine, anorectic medication for obese diabetic patients: controlled and open investigations of mazindol. Clin Med 1974; 81: 20–24.

169. Elmaleh MK, Miller J. Controlled clinical of a new anorectic. Pennsylvania Med 1974; 77(9):46–50.

170. Heber KR. Double-blind trial of mazindol in overweight patients. Med J Aust 1975; 2:566–567.

171. Sedgwick JP. Mazindol in the treatment of obesity. Practitioner 1975; 214:418–420.

172. Woodhouse SP, Nye ER, Anderson K, Rawlings J. A double-blind controlled trial of a new anorectic agent AN448. N Z Med J 1975; 81(542):546–549.

173. Maclay WP, Wallace MG. A multi-center general practice trial of mazindol in the treatment of obesity. Practitioner 1977; 218:431–434.

174. Slama G, Selmi A, Hautecouverture M, Tchobroutsky G. Double-blind clinical trial of mazindol on weight loss blood glucose, plasma insulin and serum lipids in overweight diabetic patients. Diabete Metab 1978; 4:193–199.

175. Yoshida T, Sakane N, Umekawa T, Yoshioka K, Kondo M, Wakabayashi Y. Usefulness of mazindol in combined diet therapy consisting of a low-calorie diet and optifast in severely obese women. Int J Clin Pharm 1994; 104(4):125–132.

176. Hadler AJ. Sustained-action phendimetrazine in obesity. J Clin Pharmacol 1968; 8:113–117.

177. Cohen A, DeFelice EA, Leb SM, Fuentes JG, Rothwell KG, Truant AP. Double-blind comparison of efficacy, safety, and side effects of bionamin, phentermine compound, and placebo in the treatment of exogenous obesity. Curr Ther Res Clin Exp 1968; 10:323–334.

178. Truant AP, Olon LP, Cobb S. Phentermine resin as an adjunct in medical weight reduction: a controlled randomized, double-blind prospective study. Curr Ther Res 1972; 14:726–738.

179. Gershberg H, Kane R, Hulse M, Pensgen E. Effects of diet and an anorectic drug (phentermine resin) in obese diabetics. Curr Ther Res 1977; 22:814–820.

180. Weintraub M, Ginsberg G, Stein EC, Sundaresan PR, Schuster B, O'Connor P, Byrne LM. Phenylpropanolamine OROS (Acutrim) vs placebo in combination with caloric estriction and physician-managed behavior modification. Clin Pharm Ther 1986; 39:501–509.

181. Greenway F. A double-blind clinical evaluation of the anorectic activity of phenylpropanolamine versus placebo. Clin Ther 1989; 11:584–589.

182. Schteingart DE. Effectiveness of phenylpropanolamine in the management of moderate obesity. Int J Obes 1992; 16:487–493.

183. Finer N, Craddock D, Lavielle R, Keen H. Dextrofenfluramine in the treatment of refractory obesity. Curr Ther Res 1985; 38:847–854.

184. Goodall E, Oxtoby C, Richards R, Watkinson G, Brown D, Silverstone T. A clinical trial of the efficacy and acceptability of d-fenfluramine in the treatment of neuroleptic-induced obesity. B J Psychiatry 1988; 153:208–213.

185. Willey KA, Molyneaux LM, Overland JE, Yue DK. The effects of dexfenfluramine on blood glucose control in patients with type 2 diabetes. Diabetic Med 1992; 9:341–343.

186. Stewart GO, Stein GR, Davis T, Findlater P. Dexfenfluramine in type II diabetes: effect on weight and diabetes control. Med J Aust 1993; 158:167–169.

187. Bremer JM, Scott RS, Lintott CJ. Dexfenfluramine reduces cardiovascular risk factors. Int J Obes 1994; 18:199–205.

188. Willey KA, Molyneaux LM, Yue DK. Obese patients with type 2 diabetes poorly controlled by insulin and metformin: effects of adjunctive dexfenfluramine therapy on glycaemic control. Diabet Med 1994; 11:701–704.

189. Swinburn BA, Carmichael HE, Wilson MR. Dexfenfluramine as an adjunct to a reduced-fat, ad libitum diet: effects on body composition, nutrient intake and cardiovascular risk factors. Int J Obes 1996; 20:1033–1040.

190. Galletly C, Clark A, Tomlinson L. Evaluation of dexfenfluramine in a weight loss program for obese infertile women. Int J Eat Disord 1996; 19:209–212.

191. Munro JF, Seaton DA, Duncan LJP. Treatment of refractory obesity with fenfluramine. BMJ 1966; 2: 624–625.

192. Weintraub M, Sriwatanakul K, Sundaresan PR, Weis OF, Dorn M. Extended-release fenfluramine: patient acceptance and efficacy of evening dosing. Clin Pharmacol Ther 1983; 33(5):621–627.

193. Brun LD, Bielmann P, Gagne C, Moorjani S, Nadeau A, Lupien PJ. Effects of fenfluramine in hypertriglyceridemic obese subjects. Int J Obes 1988; 12:423–431.

194. Carlstrom H, Reizenstein P. A new appetite reductant tested by a new method. Acta Med Scand 1967; 181:291–295.
195. Hadler AJ. Further studies of aminorex, a new anorexigenic agent. Curr Ther Res 1970; 12(10):639–644.
196. Kew MC. Aminorex fumarate: a double-blind trial and examination for signs of pulmonary arterial hypertension. S Afr Med J 1970; 44(14):421–423.
197. Sandoval RG, Wang RIH, Rimm AA. Body weight changes in overweight patients following an appetite suppressant in a controlled environment. J Clin Pharmacol 1971; 11(2):120–124.
198. Wood LC, Owen JA. Clinical evaluation of a new anorexigenic drug, aminoxaphen, in obese diabetics. J New Drugs 1965; 5(3):181–185.
199. Bianchi R, Bongers V, Bravenboer B, Erkelens DW. Effects of benfluorex on insulin resistance and lipid metabolism in obese type II diabetic patients. Diabetes Care 1993; 16:557–559.
200. Bianchi R, Bongers V, Bravenboer B, Erkelens DW. Benfluorex decreases insulin resistance and improves lipid profiles in obese type 2 diabetic patients. Diabetes/Metab Rev 1993; 9:29S–34S.
201. De Feo P, Lavielle R, De Gregoris P, Bolli GB. Antihyperglycemic mechanisms of benfluorex in type II diabetes mellitus. Diabetes Rev 1993; 9:35S–41S.
202. Giudicelli JF, Richer C, Berdeaux A. Preliminary assessment of flutiorex, a new anorectic drug, in man. Br J Clin Pharmacol 1976; 3:113–121.
203. Bjurulf P, Carlstrom S, Rorsman G. Oborex, a new appetite-reducing agent. Acta Med Scand 1967; 182:273–280.
204. Benjamin JM. A new anorectic drug. Br J Clin Pract 1968; 22:350–352.
205. Feldman HS. Preliminary clinical evaluation of a new appetite suppressant: a double-blind study. J Med Soc NJ 1996; 63:454–457.
206. Silverstone JT, Solomon T, Ross M, Kelly T. Controlled trial of a new anorectic drug in the treatment of obesity. Br J Clin Pract 1967; 21:337–339.
207. Reus VI, Silberman E, Post RM, Weingartner H. d-Amphetamine: effects on memory in a depressed population. Biol Psychiatry 1979; 14(2):345–356.
208. Delamonica E, Shaffer JW, Brown CC, Kurland AA. Effects of dextroamphetamine, pentobarbital, chlorphentermine, and placebo on the alpha blocking response in normal subjects. J New Drugs 1966; 6(4):224–228.
209. Hadler AJ. Weight reduction with phenmetrazine: a double-blind study. Curr Ther Res 1967; 9:462–467.
210. Hadler AJ. Weight reduction with phenmetrazine and chlorphentermine: a double-blind study. Curr Ther Res 1967; 9:563–569.
211. Hadler AJ. Reduced-dosage sustained-action phenmetrazine in obesity. Curr Ther Res 1968; 10:255–259.
212. Hadler AJ. Phenmetrazine vs. phenmetrazine with amobarbital for weight reduction: a double-blind study. Curr Ther Res 1969; 11:750–754.
213. Huston JR. Phenmetrazine effect without dietary restriction. Ohio Med J 1966; 62:805–807.
214. Jenner EB. The effectiveness of phenmetrazine in obesity. N Z Med J 1968; 67:147–149.
215. Rauh JL, Lipp R. Chlorphentermine as an anorexigenic agent in adolescent obesity. Clin Pediatr 1968; 7:138–140.
216. Silverstone T. Intermittent treatment with anorectic drugs. Practitioner 1974; 213(1274):245–252.
217. Allen GS. A double-blind clinical trial of diethylpropion hydrochloride, mazindol and placebo in the treatment of exogenous obesity. Curr Ther Res 1977; 22:678–684.
218. Gomez G. Obese patients in general practice: a comparison of the anorectic effects of mazindol, fenfluramine and placebo. Clin Trials 1975; 12:38–43.
219. Steel JM, Munro JF, Duncan LJ. A comparative trial of different regimens of fenfluramine and phentermine in obesity. Practitioner 1973; 211:232–236.
220. LeRiche WH, Csima A. A long-acting appetite suppressant drug studied for 24 weeks in both continuous and sequential administration. Can Med Assoc J 1967; 97:1016–1020.
221. Stunkard A, Rickels K, Hesbacher P. Fenfluramine in the treatment of obesity. Lancet 1973; 1(802):503–505.
222. Rosenberg BA. A double-blind study of diethylpropion in obesity. Am J Med Sci 1961; 242:201–206.
223. Defelice EA, Chaykin LB, Cohen A. Double-blind clinical evaluation of mazindol, dextroamphetamine, and placebo in treatment of exogenous obesity. Curr Ther Res 1973; 15(7):358–366.
224. Evans ER, Wallace MG. A multi-center trial of mazindol (Teronac) in general practice in Ireland. Curr Med Res Opin 1975; 3(3):132–137.
225. Inoue S, Egawa M, Satoh S, Saito M, Suzuki H, Kumahara Y, Abe M, Kumagai A, Goto Y, Shizume K, Shimizu N, Naito C, Onishi T. Clinical and basic aspects of an anorexiant, mazindol, as an antiobesity agent in Japan. Am J Clin Nutr 1992; 55(1):199S–202S.
226. Elliott BW. A collaborative investigation of fenfluramine: anorexigenic with sedative properties. Curr Ther Res 1970; 12(8):502–515.
227. Munro JF, ed. The Treatment of Obesity Baltimore: MTP Press Limited, 1979.
228. Stewart DA, Bailey JD, Patell H. Tenuate dospan as an appetite suppressant in the treatment of obese children. Appl Ther 1970; 12(5):34–36.
229. Shutter L, Garell DC. Obesity in children and adolescents: a double-blind study with cross-over. J Sch Health 1966; 36(6):273–275.
230. Lorber J. Obesity in childhood: a controlled trial of anorectic drugs. Arch Dis Child 1966; 41:309–312.
231. Follows OJ. A comparative trial of fenfluramine and

diethylpropion in obese, hypertensive patients. Br J Clin Prac 1971; 25:236–238.

232. Miach PJ, Thomson W, Doyle AE, Louis WJ. Double-blind cross-over evaluation of mazindol in the treatment of obese hypertensive patients. Med J Aust 1976; 2:378–380.

233. Evangelista I. Management of the overweight patients with cardiovascular disease: double-blind evaluation of an anorectic drug, diethylpropion hydrochloride. Curr Ther Res 1968; 10:217–222.

234. Russek HI. Control of obesity in patients with angina pectoris: a double-blind study with diethylpropion hydrochloride. Am J Med Sci 1966; 251(4):461–464.

235. Atkinson RL, Greenway FL, Bray GA, Dahms WT, Molitch M, Hamilton K, Rodin J. Treatment of obesity: comparison of physician and nonphysician therapists using placebo and anorectic drugs in a double blind trial. Int J Obes 1977; 1(5):113–120.

236. Silverstone JT, Cooper RM, Begg RR. A comparative trial of fenfluramine and diethylpropion in obesity. Br J Clin Pract 1970; 24(10):423–425.

237. Dykes MH. Evaluation of three anorexiants. Clortermine hydrochloride (Voranil), fenfluramine hydrochloride (Pondimin), and mazindol (Sanorex). JAMA 1974; 230(2):270–272.

238. Goldrick RB, Nestel PJ, Havenstein N. Comparison of a new anorectic agent AN 448 with fenfluramine in the treatment of refractory obesity. Med J Aust 1974; 1:882–885.

239. Stahl KA, Imperiale TF. An overview of the efficacy and safety of fenfluramine and mazindol in the treatment of obesity. Arch Fam Med 1993; 2:1033–1038.

240. Murphy JE, Donald JF, Molla AL, Crowder D. A comparison of mazindol (Teronac) with diethylpropion in the treatment of exogenous obesity. J Int Med Res 1975; 3(3):202–206.

241. Kesson CM, Ireland JT. Phenformin compared with fenfluramine in the treatment of obese diabetic patients. Practitioner 1976; 216(1295):577–580.

242. Douglas A, Douglas JG, Robertson CE, Munro JF. Plasma phentermine levels, weight loss and side-effects. Int J Obes 1983; 7(6):591–595.

243. Hossain M, Campbell DB. Fenfluramine and methylcellulose in the treatment of obesity: the relationship between plasma drug concentrations and therapeutic efficacy. Postgrad Med J 1975; 51(1):178–182.

244. Guy-Grand B. Clinical studies with dexfenfluramine: from past to future. Obes Res 1995; 3:491S–496S.

245. Guy-Grand B. Clinical studies with d-fenfluramine. Am J Clin Nutr 1992; 55:173S–176S.

246. Weintraub M. Phenylpropanolamine as an anorexiant agent in weight control: a review of published and unpublished studies. In: Morgan JP, Kagan DV, Brody JS, eds. Phenylpropanolamine: Risks, Benefits and Controversies, 5th ed. New York: Praeger Publishers, Clinical Pharmacology and Therapeutics Series, 1985:53–79.

247. Greenway F. Clinical studies with phenylpropanolamine: a meta-analysis. Am J Clin Nutr 1992; 55:203S–205S.

248. Bess BE, Marlin RL. A pilot study of medication and group therapy for obesity in a group of physicians. Hillside J Clin Psychiatry 1984; 6:171–187.

249. Silverstone JJ, Solomon T. The long-term management of obesity in general practice. Br J Clin Pract 1965; 19:395–398.

250. McKay RHG. Long-term use of diethylpropion in obesity. Curr Med Res Opin 1973; 1:489–493.

251. Langlois KJ, Forbes JA, Bell GW, Grant GF Jr. A double-blind clinical evaluation of the safety and efficacy of phentermine hydrochloride (Fastin) in the treatment of exogenous obesity. Curr Ther Res 1974; 16:289–296.

252. Williams RA, Foulsham BM. Weight reduction in osteoarthritis using phentermine. Practitioner 1981; 225(1352):231–232.

253. Finer N. Body weight evolution during dexfenfluramine treatment after initial weight control. Int J Obes 1992; 16:S25–S29.

254. Mathus-Vliegen EMH. Prolonged surveillance of dexfenfluramine in severe obesity. Neth J Med 1993; 43:246–253.

255. Tauber-Lassen E, Damsbo P, Henriksen JE, Palmvig B, Beck-Nielsen H. Improvement of glycemic control and weight loss in type 2 (non-insulin-dependent) diabetics after one year of dexfenfluramine treatment. Diabetologia 1990; 33(suppl):A124.

256. Pfohl M, Luft D, Blomberg I, Schmulling RM. Long-term changes of body weight and cardiovascular risk factors after weight reduction with group therapy and dexfenfluramine. Int J Obes 1994; 18:391–395.

257. Ditschuneit HH, Flechtner-Mors M, Adler G. The effects of dexfenfluramine on weight loss and cardiovascular risk factors in female patients with upper and lower body obesity. J Cardiovasc Risk 1996; 3:397–403.

258. O'Connor HT, Richman RM, Steinbeck KS, Caterson ID. Dexfenfluramine treatment of obesity: a double blind trial with post trial follow-up. Int J Obes 1995; 19:181–189.

259. Sandage BWJ, Loar SB, Cary M, Cooper GL. Predictors of therapeutic success with dexfenfluramine. Obes Res 1995; 3:355S.

260. Wales JK. The effect of fenfluramine on obese, maturity-onset diabetic patients. Acta Endocrinol 1979; 90:616–623.

261. Weintraub M. Long-term weight control: conclusions. Clin Pharmacol Ther 1992; 51(5):642–646.

262. Hudson KD. The anorectic and hypotensive effect of fenfluramine in obesity. J R Coll Gen Pract 1977; 27:497–501.

263. Stunkard AJ, Craighead LW, O'Brien R. Controlled trial of behavior therapy, pharmacotherapy and their combination in the treatment of obesity. Lancet 1980; 2(8203):1045–1047.

264. Sensi S, Della Loggia F, Del Ponte A, Guagnano MT. Long-term treatment with fenfluramine in obese subjects. Int J Clin Pharmacol Res 1985; 5:247–253.

265. O'Keane V, McLoughlin D, Dinan TG. D-fenfluramine-induced prolactin and cortisol release in major depression: response to treatment. J Affect Disord 1992; 26:143–150.

266. Nathan C. Dextrofenfluramine and body weight in overweight patients. In: Vague IJ, ed. Metabolic Complications of Human Obesity. Amsterdam: Elsevier Science, 1985:229–234.

267. McGuirk J, Silverstone T. The effect of the 5-HT reuptake inhibitor fluoxetine on food intake and body weight in healthy male subjects. Int J Obes 1990; 14:361–372.

268. Levine LR, Rosenblatt S, Bosomworth J. Use of serotonin re-uptake inhibitor, fluoxetine, in the treatment of obesity. Int J Obes 1987; 11:185S–190S.

269. Ferguson JM, Feighner JP. Fluoxetine-induced weight loss in overweight non-depressed humans. Int J Obes 1987; 11:163–170.

270. Levine LR, Enas GG, Thompson WL, Byyny RL, Dauer AD, Kirby RW, Kreindler TG, Levy B, Lucas CP, McIlwain HH, Nelson EB. Use of fluoxetine, a selective serotonin-uptake inhibitor, in the treatment of obesity: a dose-response study. Int J Obes 1989; 13:635–645.

271. Fernandez-Soto ML, Gonzalez-Jimenez A, Barredo-Acedo F, Luna del Castillo JD, Escobar-Jimenez F. Comparison of fluoxetine and placebo in the treatment of obesity. Ann Nutr Metab 1995; 39:159–163.

272. Connolly VM, Gallagher A, Kesson CM. A study of fluoxetine in obese elderly patients with type 2 diabetes. Diabetic Med 1995; 12:416–418.

273. O'Kane M, Wiles PG, Wales JK. Fluoxetine in the treatment of obese type 2 diabetic patients. Diabetic Med 1994; 11:105–110.

274. Visser M, Seidell JC, Koppeschaar PF, Smits P. The effect of fluoxetine on body weight, body composition and visceral fat accumulation. Int J Obes 1992; 17:247–253.

275. Goldstein DJ, Rampey AH, Dornseif BE, Levine LR, Potvin JH, Fludzinski LA. Fluoxetine: a randomized clinical trial in the maintenance of weight loss. Obes Res 1993; 1(2):92–98.

276. Goldstein DJ, Enas GG, Potvin JH, Fludzinski LA, Levine LR. Fluoxetine: a randomized clinical trial in the treatment of obesity. Int J Obes 1994; 18:129–135.

277. Daubresse JC, Kolanowski J, Krzentowski G, Kutnowski M, Scheen A, Van Gaal L. Usefulness of fluoxetine in obese non-insulin dependent diabetics: a multicenter study. Obes Res 1996; 4:391–396.

278. Wise SD. Clinical studies with fluoxetine in obesity. Am J Clin Nutr 1992; 55:181S–184S.

279. Gray DS, Fujioka K, Devine W, Bray GA. A randomized double-blind clinical trial of fluoxetine in obese diabetics. Int J Obes 1992; 16(suppl 4):S67–S72.

280. Sayler ME, Goldstein DJ, Roback PJ, Atkinson RL. Evaluating success of weight-loss programs, with an application to fluoxetine weight-reduction clinical trial data. Int J Obes 1994; 18:742–751.

281. Pedrinola F, Sztejnsznajd C, Lima N, Halpern A, Medeiros-Neto G. The addition of dexfenfluramine to fluoxetine in the treatment of obesity: a randomized clinical trial. Obes Res 1996; 4:549–554.

282. Wadden TA, Bartlett SJ, Foster GD, Greenstein RA, Wingate BJ, Stunkard AJ, Letizia KA. Sertraline and relapse prevention training following treatment by very-low-calorie diet: a controlled clinical trial. Obes Res 1995; 3:549–557.

283. Bach DS, Rissanen AM, Mendel CM, Shepherd G, Weinstein SP, Kelly F, Seaton TB, Patel B, Pekkarinen TA, Armstrong WF. Absence of cardiac valve dysfunction in obese patients treated with sibutramine. Obes Res 1999; 7(4):363–369.

284. Halford JCG, Heal DJ, Blundell JE. Investigation of a new potential anti-obesity drug, sibutramine, using the behavioral satiety sequence. Appetite 1994; 23(3):306–307.

285. Ryan DH, Kaiser P, Bray GA. Sibutramine: a novel new agent for obesity treatment. Obes Res 1995; 3:553–559.

286. Heal DJ, Frankland AT, Gosden J, Hutchins LJ, Prow MR, Luscombe GP, Buckett WR. A comparison of the effects of sibutramine hydrochloride, bupropion and methamphetamine on dopaminergic function: evidence that dopamine is not a pharmacological target for sibutramine. Psychopharmacology 1992; 107: 303–309.

287. Hansen DL, Toubro S, Stock MJ, Macdonald IA, Astrup A. The effect of sibutramine on energy expenditure and appetite during chronic treatment without dietary restriction. Int J Obes Relat Metab Disord 1999; 23(10):1016–1024.

288. Walsh KM, Leen E, Lean ME. The effect of sibutramine on resting energy expenditure and adrenaline-induced thermogenesis in obese females. Int J Obes Relat Metab Disord 1999; 23(10):1009–1015.

289. Danforth E. Sibutramine and thermogenesis in humans (review). Int J Obes Relat Metab Disord 1999; 23(10):1007–1008.

290. Weintraub M, Rubio A, Golik A, Byrne L, Scheinbaum ML. Sibutramine in weight control: a dose-ranging, efficacy study. Clin Pharmacol Ther 1991; 50:330–337.

291. Rolls BJ, Shide DJ, Thorwart ML, Ulbrecht JS. Sibutramine reduces food intake in non-dieting women with obesity. Obes Res 1998; 6:1–11.

292. Cuellar GE, Ruiz AM, Monsalve MC, Berber A. Six-month treatment of obesity with sibutramine 15 mg; a double-blind, placebo-controlled monocenter clinical trial in a Hispanic population. Obes Res 2000; 8(1):71–82.

293. Hazenberg BP. Randomized, double-blind, placebo-controlled, multicenter study of sibutramine in obese hypertensive patients. Cardiology 2000; 94(3):152–158.

294. Finer N, Bloom SR, Frost GS, Banks LM, Griffiths J. Sibutramine is effective for weight loss and diabetic control in obesity with type 2 diabetes: a randomised, double-blind, placebo-controlled study. Diabetes Obes Metab 2000; 2(2):105–112.

295. Sramek JJ, Leibowitz MT, Weinstein SP, Rowe ED. Efficacy and safety of sibutramine for weight loss in obese patients with hypertension well controlled by β-adrenergic blocking agents: a placebo-controlled, double-blind, randomised trial. J Hum Hypertens 2002; 16(1):13–19.

296. Apfelbaum M, Vague P, Ziegler O, Hanotin C, Thomas F, Leutenegger E. Long-term maintenance of weight loss after a VLCD: sibutramine vs placebo. Am J Med 1999; 106:179–184.

297. Jones SP, Smith IG, Kelly F, Gray JA. Long-term weight loss with sibutramine. Int J Obes 1995; 19(suppl 2):40.

298. Bray GA, Ryan DH, Gordon D, Heidingsfelder S, Cerise F, Wilson K. A double-blind randomized placebo-controlled trial of sibutramine. Obes Res 1996; 4:263–270.

299. Hanotin C, Thomas F, Jones SP, Leutenegger E, Drouin P. Efficacy and tolerability of sibutramine in obese patients: a dose-ranging study. Int J Obes 1998; 22:32–58.

300. Bray GA, Blackburn GL, Ferguson JM, Greenway FL, Jain AK, Mendel CM, Mendels CM, Mendels J, Ryan D, Schwartz SL, Scheinbaum ML, Seaton TB. Sibutramine produces dose-related weight loss. Obes Res 1999; 7:189–198.

301. Fanghanel G, Cortinas L, Sanchez-Reyes L, Berber A. A clinical trial of the use of sibutramine for the treatment of patients suffering essential obesity. Int J Obes Relat Metab Disord. 2000; 24(2):144–150.

302. Fujioka K, Seaton TB, Rowe E, Jelinek CA, Raskin P, Lebovitz HE, Weinstein SP. Sibutramine/Diabetes Clinical Study Group. Weight loss with sibutramine improves glycaemic control and other metabolic parameters in obese patients with type 2 diabetes mellitus. Diabetes Obes Metab 2000; 2(3):175–187.

303. McMahon FG, Fujioka K, Singh BN, Mendel CM, Rowe E, Rolston K, Johnson F. Efficacy and safety of sibutramine in obese white and African American patients with hypertension: a 1-year, double-blind, placebo-controlled, multicenter trial. Arch Intern Med. 2000;24;160(14):2185–2191.

304. James WP, Astrup A, Finer N, Hilsted J, Kopelman P, Rossner S, Saris WH, Van Gaal LF. Effect of sibutramine on weight maintenance after weight loss: a randomised trial. STORM Study Group. Sibutramine Trial of Obesity Reduction and Maintenance. Lancet 2000; 356(9248):2119–2125.

305. McMahon FG, et al. Sibutramine is safe and effective for weight loss in obese patients whose hypertension is well controlled with angiotensin-converting enzyme inhibitors. J Hum Hypertens 2002; 16:5–11.

306. Lean MEJ. Sibutramine—a review of clinical efficacy. Int J Obes 1997; 21:S30–S36.

307. Wadden TA, Berkowitz RI, Womble LG, Sarwer DB, Arnold ME, Steinberg CM. Effects of sibutramine plus orlistat in obese women following 1 year of treatment by sibutramine alone: a placebo-controlled trial. Obes Res 2000; 8(6):431–437.

308. Ryan DH. Use of sibutramine and other noradrenergic and serotonergic drugs in the management of obesity (review). Endocrine 2000; 13(2):193–199.

309. Hanotin C, Thomas F, Jones SP, Leutenegger E, Drouin P. A comparison of sibutramine and dexfenfluramine in the treatment of obesity. Obes Res 1998; 6:285–291.

310. Wadden TA, Berkowitz RI, Sarwer DB, Prus-Wisniewski R, Steinberg C. Benefits of lifestyle modification in the pharmacologic treatment of obesity: a randomized trial. Arch Intern Med 2001; 161(2):218–227.

311. Wirth A, Krauss J. Long-term weight loss with sibutramine: a randomised controlled trial. JAMA 2001; 286:1331–1339.

312. Weintraub M, Hasday JD, Mushlin AI, Lockwood DH. A double blind clinical trial in weight control. Use of fenfluramine and phentermine alone and in combination. Arch Intern Med 1984; 144:1143–1148.

313. Weintraub M. Long-term weight control: the National Heart, Lung and Blood Institute funded multimodal intervention study. Clin Pharmacol Ther 1992; 51(5):581–585.

314. Weintraub M, Sundaresan PR, Schuster B, Ginsberg G, Madan M, Balder A, Lasagna L, Cox C. Long-term weight control study. 1. (weeks 0 to 34)—the enhancement of behavior-modification, caloric restriction, and exercise by fenfluramine plus phentermine versus placebo. Clin Pharmacol Ther 1992; 51:586–594.

315. Weintraub M, Sundaresan PR, Schuster B, Ginsberg G, Madan M, Balder A, Stein EC, Byrne L. Long-term weight control study. 2. (weeks 34 to 104)—an open-label study of continuous fenfluramine plus phentermine versus targeted intermittent medication as adjuncts to behavior-modification, caloric restriction, and exercise. Clin Pharmacol Ther 1992; 51(5):595–601.

316. Weintraub M, Sundaresan PR, Schuster B, Moscucci M, Stein EC. Long-term weight control study. 3. (weeks 104 to 156)—an open-label study of dose adjustment of fenfluramine and phentermine. Clin Pharmacol Ther 1992; 51(5):602–607.

317. Weintraub M, Sundaresan PR, Schuster B, Moscucci M, Stein EC. Long-term weight control study. 4. (weeks 156 to 190)—the 2nd double-blind phase. Clin Pharmacol Ther 1992; 51(5):608–614.

318. Weintraub M, Sundaresan PR, Schuster B, Averbuch M, Stein EC, Byrne L. Long-term weight control study. 5. (weeks 190 to 210)—follow-up of participants after cessation of medication. Clin Pharmacol Ther 1992; 51(5):615–618.

319. Weintraub M, Sundaresan PR, Schuster B. Long-term

weight control study. 7. (weeks 190 to 210)—serum-lipid changes. Clin Pharmacol Ther 1992; 51(5):634–646.

320. Atkinson RL, Blank RC, Loper JF, Schumacher D, Lutes RA. Combined drug treatment of obesity. Obes Res 1995; 3:497S–500S.

321. Spitz AF, Schumacher D, Blank RC, Dhurandhar NV, Atkinson RL. Long-term pharmacologic treatment of morbid obesity in a community practice. Endocr Pract 1997; 3:269–275.

322. Douglas JG, Gough J, Preston PG, Frazer I, Haslett C, Chalmers SR, Munro JF. Long-term efficacy of fenfluramine in treatment of obesity. Lancet 1983; 1:384–386.

323. Campbell DB, Gordon BH, Ings RMJ, Richards R, Taylor DW. Factors that may effect the reduction of hunger and body weight following d-fenfluramine administration. Clin Neuropharmacol 1988; 11:S160–S172.

324. Inoue S. Clinical studies with mazindol. Obes Res 1995; 3:S549–S552.

325. Bray GA. Obesity: a human energy problem. In: Beecher GR, ed. Beltsville, Symposia in Agricultural Research. Granada: Allanheld, Osmun and Co. 1981; 4:95–112.

326. Innes JA, Watson ML, Ford MJ, Munro JF, Stoddart ME, Campbell DB. Plasma fenfluramine levels, weight loss and side effects. BMJ 1977; 2:1322–1325.

327. Weintraub M, Taves DR, Hasday JD, Mushlin AI, Lockwood DH. Determinants of response to anorexiants. Clin Pharmacol Ther 1981; 30:528–533.

328. Oswald I, Jones HS, Mannerheim JE. Effects of two slimming drugs on sleep. BMJ 1968; 1:796–799.

329. Newhouse PA, Belenky G, Thomas M, Thorne D, Sing HC, Fertig J. Effects of d-amphetamine on arousal, cognition, and mood after prolonged total sleep deprivation. Neuropsychopharmacology 1989; 2:153–164.

330. Baranski JV, Pigeau RA. Self-monitoring cognitive performance during sleep deprivation: effects of modafinil, d-amphetamine and placebo. J Sleep Res 1997; 6:84–91.

331. Waters WF, Magill RA, Bray GA, Volaufova J, Smith SR, Lieberman HR, Rood J, Hurry M, Anderson T, Ryan DH. A comparison of tyrosine against phentermine caffeine and D-amphetamine during sleep deprivation. Nutritional Neurosci 2003. In press.

332. Rickels K, Hesbacher P, Fisher E, Perloff MM, Rosenfeld H. Emotional symptomatology in obese patients treated with fenfluramine and dextroamphetamine. Psychol Med 1976; 6:623–630.

333. Foltin RW, Fischman MW. Methods for the assessment of abuse liability of psychomotor stimulants and anorectic agents in humans. Br J Addict 1991; 86:1633–1640.

334. Götestam KG, Andersson BE. Assessment of reinforcing properties of amphetamine analogues in self-administering rats. Postgrad Med J 1975; 51:80–83.

335. Götestam KG. The discriminative properties of amphetamine analogues tested in self-administering rats under maintained stimulus control. Addict Behav 1977; 2:27–33.

336. Papasava M, Singer G, Papasava CL. Phentermine self-administration in naive free-feeding and food-deprived rats: a dose response study. Psychopharmacology 1985; 85:410–413.

337. Griffiths RR, Brady JV, Bigelow GE. Predicting the dependence liability of stimulant drugs. NIDA Res Monogr 1981; 37:182–196.

338. Johanson CE. Effects of intravenous cocaine, diethylpropion, d-amphetamine and perphenazine on responding maintained by food delivery and shock avoidance in rhesus monkeys. J Pharmacol Exp Ther 1978; 204:118–129.

339. Corwin RL, Woolverton WL, Schuster CR, Johanson CE. Anorectics: effects on food intake and self-administration in rhesus monkeys. Alcohol Drug Res 1987; 7:351–361.

340. US Department of Health and Human Services, Public Health Service, Alcohol, Drug Abuse, and Mental Health Administrion. National Institute on Drug Abuse, Statistical Series. Washington: PHS, Annual Data, Ser 1, No. 8, 1988.

341. US Department of Health and Human Services, Drug Abuse Warning Network. Annual Emergency Department data Washington: PHS, Annual Data, 1994.

342. Griffiths RR, Brady JV, Snell JD. Progressive-ratio performance maintained by drug infusions: comparison of cocaine, diethylpropion, chlorphentermine, and fenfluramine. Psychopharmacology 1978; 56:5–13.

343. Griffiths RR, Brady JV, Snell JD. Relationship between anorectic and reinforcing properties of appetite suppressant drugs: implications for assessment of abuse liability. Biol Psychiatry 1978; 13:283–290.

344. Locke KW, Levesque TR, Nicholson KL, Balster RL. Dexfenfluramine lacks amphetamine-like abuse potential. Prog Neuropsychopharmacol Biol Psychiatry 1996; 20(6):1019–1035.

345. Heal DJ, Cheetham SC, Prow MR, Martin KF, Buckett WR. A comparison of the effects on central 5-HT function of sibutramine hydrochloride and other weight-modifying agents. Br J Pharmacol 1998; 125(2):301–308.

346. Schuh LM, Schuster CR, Hopper JA, Mendel CM. Abuse liability assessment of sibutramine, a novel weight control agent. Psychopharmacology 2000; 147:339–346.

347. Wisnes KA, Garratt C, Wickens Gudgeon A, Oliver S. Effects of sibutramine alone and with alcohol on cognitive function in healthy volunteers. Br J Clin Pharmacol 2000; 49:110–117.

348. Johanson CE, Uhlenhuth EH. Drug self-administration in humans. NIDA Res Monogr 1978:68–85.

349. Ladewig D, Battegay R. Abuse of anorexics with special reference to newer substances. Int J Addict 1971; 6:167–172.

350. Angle HV, Carroll JA, Ellinwood EH. Psychoactive drug use among overweight psychiatric patients: problem aspect of anorectic drugs. Chem Depend 1980; 4:47–55.

351. Lane R, Baldwin D. Selective serotonin reuptake inhibitor–induced serotonin syndrome: review. J Clin Psychopharmacol 1997; 17(3):208–221.

352. Trakas K, Shear NH. Serotonin syndrome risk with antiobesity drug. Can J Clin Pharmacol 2000; 7(4): 216.

353. Giese SY, Neborsky R. Serotonin syndrome: potential consequences of Meridia combined with Demerol or fentanyl. Plas Reconstruct Surg 2001; 107(1):293–294.

354. Westphalen RI, Dodd PR. The regeneration of d,1-fenfluramine-destroyed serotonergic nerve terminals. Eur J Pharmacol 1993; 238:399–402.

355. Ricaurte GA, Molliver ME, Martello MB, Katz JL, Wilson MA, Martello AL. Dexfenfluramine neurotoxicity in brains of non-human primates. Lancet 1991; 338:1487–1488.

356. Scheffel U, Szabo Z, Matthews WB, Finley PA, Yuan J, Callahan B, Hatzidimitriou G, Dannals RF, Ravert HT, Ricaurte GA. Fenfluramine-induced loss of serotonin transporters in baboon brain visualized with PET. Synapse 1996; 24:395–398.

357. McCune U, Hatzidim G, Ridenour A, Fischer C, Yuan J, Katz J, Ricaurte G. Dexfenfluramine and serotonin neurotoxicity—further preclinical evidence that clinical caution is indicated. J Pharmacol Exp Ther 1994; 269:792–798.

358. Miller DB, O'Callaghan JP. The interactions of MK-801 with the amphetamine analogues d-methamphetamine (d-METH), 3,4-methylenedioxymethamphetamine (d-MDMA) or d-fenfluramine (d-FEN): neural damage and neural protection. Ann NY Acad Sci 1993; 679:321–324.

359. Invernizzi R, Berettera C, Garattini S, Samanin R. d- and l-Isomers of fenfluramine differ markedly in their interaction with brain serotonin and catecholamines in the rat. Eur J Pharmacol 1986; 120:9–15.

360. McCann UD, Seiden LS, Rubin LJ, Ricaurte GA. Brain serotonin neurotoxicity and primary pulmonary hypertension from fenfluramine and dexfenfluramine: a systematic review of the evidence. JAMA 1997; 278:666–672.

361. Abenhaim L, Moride Y, Brenot F, Rich S, Benichou J, Kurz X, Higenbottam T, Oakley C, Wouters E, Aubier M, Simonneau G, Begaud B. Appetite-suppressant drugs and the risk of primary pulmonary hypertension. International Primary Pulmonary Hypertension Study Group. N Engl J Med 1996; 335:609–616.

362. Kramer MS, Lane DA. Aminorex, dexfenfluramine, and primary pulmonary hypertension. J Clin Epidemiol 1998; 51:361–364.

363. Naeije R, Maggiorini M, Delcroix M, Leeman M, Melot C. Effects of chronic dexfenfluramine treatment on pulmonary hemodynamics in dogs. Am J Respir Crit Care Med 1996; 154:1347–1350.

364. Weir EK, Reeve HL, Huang JM, Michelakis E, Nelson DP, Hampl V, Archer SL. Anorexic agents aminorex, fenfluramine, and dexfenfluramine inhibit potassium current in rat pulmonary vascular smooth muscle and cause pulmonary vasoconstriction. Circulation 1996; 94:2216–2220.

365. Mark EJ, Patalas ED, Chang HT, Evans RJ, Kessler SC. Fatal pulmonary hypertension associated with short-term use of fenfluramine and phentermine. N Engl J Med 1997; 337:602–606.

366. Manson JE, Faich GA. Pharmacotherapy for obesity: do the benefits outweigh the risks? N Engl J Med 1996; 335:659–660.

367. Connolly HM, Crary JL, McGoon MD, Hensrud DD, Edwards BS, Edwards WD, Schaff HV. Valvular heart disease associated with fenfluramine-phentermine. N Engl J Med 1997; 337:581–588.

368. Khan MA, Herzog CA, St Peter JV, Hartley GG, Madlon-Kay R, Dick CD, Asinger RW, Vessey JT. The prevalence of cardiac valvular insufficiency assessed by transthoracic echocardiography in obese patients treated with appetite-suppressant drugs. N Engl J Med 1998; 339(11):713–718.

369. Weissman NJ, Tighe JF Jr, Gottdiener JS, Gwynne JT. Sustained-Release Dexfenfluramine Study Group. An assessment of heart-valve abnormalities in obese patients taking dexfenfluramine, sustained-release dexfenfluramine, or placebo. N Engl J Med 1998; 339(11):725–732.

370. Jick H, Vasilakis C, Weinrauch LA, Meier CR, Jick SS, Derby LE. A population-based study of appetite-suppressant drugs and the risk of cardiac-valve regurgitation. N Engl J Med 1998; 339(11):719–724.

371. Wadden TA, Berkowitz RI, Silvestry F, Vogt RA, St. John Sutton MG, Stunkard AJ, Foster GD, Aber JL. The fen-phen finale: a study of weight loss and valvular heart disease. Obes Res 1998; 6:278–284.

372. Shively BK, Roldan CA, Gill EA, Najarian T, Loar SB. Prevalence and determinants of valvulopathy in patients treated with dexfenfluramine. Circulation 1999; 100(21):2161–2167.

373. Wee CC, Phillips RS, Aurigemma G, Erban S, Kriegel G, Riley M, Douglas PS. Risk for valvular heart disease among users of fenfluramine and dexfenfluramine who underwent echocardiography before use of medication. Ann Intern Med 1998; 129(11):870–874.

374. Ryan DH, Bray GA, Helmcke F, Sander G, Volaufova J, Greenway F, Subramaniam P, Glancy DL. Serial echocardiographic and clinical evaluation of valvular regurgitation before, during and after treatment with fenfluramine or dexfenfluramine and mazindol or phentermine. Obes Res 1999; 7(4):313–322.

375. Connolly HM, McGoon MD. Obesity drugs and the heart (review). Curr Prob Cardiol 1999; 24(12):745–792.

376. Li R, Serdula MK, Williamson DF, Bowman BA, Graham DJ, Green L. Dose-effect of fenfluramine use on the severity of valvular heart disease among fen-phen patients with valvulopathy. Int J Obes Relat Metab Disord 1999; 23(9):926–928.

377. Cannistra LB, Cannistra AJ. Regression of multi-valvular regurgitation after the cessation of fenfluramine and phentermine treatment. N Engl J Med 1998; 339(11):771.

378. Asinger RW. The fen-phen controversy: is regression another piece of the puzzle? Mayo Clin Proc 1999; 74(12):1302–1304.

379. Ryan DH, Bray GA, Greenway FL, Helmcke F. Prevalence, incidence and natural history of echocardiographic valvulopathy in patients treated with appetite suppressants. Obes Res 1999; 7(suppl 1):50S.

380. Mast ST, Jollis JG, Ryan T, Anstrom KJ, Crary JL. The progression of fenfluramine-associated valvular heart disease assessed by echocardiography. Ann Intern Med 2001; 134(4):261–266.

381. MacMahon S, Cutler J, Brittain E, Higgins M. Obesity and hypertension: epidemiological and clinical issues (review). Eur Heart J 1987; 8(suppl B):57–70.

382. Cutler JA. Randomized clinical trials of weight reduction in nonhypertensive persons (review). Ann Epidemiol 1991; 1:363–370.

383. Stamler R, et al. Primary prevention of hypertension by nutritional-hygienic means. JAMA 1987; 262:1801–1807.

384. Hypertension Prevention Trial. Three-year effects of dietary changes on blood pressure. Hypertension Prevention Trial Research Group. Arch Intern Med 1990; 150:153–162.

385. Stevens VJ, et al. Weight loss intervention in phase 1 of the Trials of Hypertension Prevention. The TOHP Collaborative Research Group. Arch Intern Med 1993; 153:849–858.

386. Stevens VJ, Obarzanek E, Cook NR, Lee IM, Appel LJ, Smith West D, Milas NC, Mattfeldt-Beman M, Belden L, Bragg C, Millstone M, Raczynski J, Brewer A, Singh B, Cohen J. Trials for the Hypertension Prevention Research Group. Long-term weight loss and changes in blood pressure: results of the Trials of Hypertension Prevention, phase II. Ann Intern Med 2001; 134(1):1–11.

387. Sjostrom CD, Lissner L, Wedel H, Sjostrom L. Reduction in incidence of diabetes, hypertension and lipid disturbances after intentional weight loss induced by bariatric surgery: the SOS Intervention Study. Obes Res 1999; 7:477–484.

388. Sjostrom L, et al. Randomised placebo-controlled trial of orlistat for weight loss and prevention of weight regain in obese patients. European Multicentre Orlistat Study Group. Lancet 1998; 352:167–172.

389. Rossner S, et al. Weight loss, weight maintenance, and improved cardiovascular risk factors after 2 years treatment with orlistat for obesity. European Orlistat Obesity Study Group. Obes Res 2000; 8:49–61.

390. Davidson MH, et al. Weight control and risk factor reduction in obese subjects treated for 2 years with orlistat: a randomized controlled trial. JAMA 1999; 281:235–242.

391. Hauptman J, et al. Hauptman Orlistat in the long-term treatment of obesity in primary care settings. Arch Fam Med 2000; 9:160–167.

392. Bray GA, et al. Sibutramine produces dose-related weight loss. Obes Res 1999; 7:189–198.

393. Stamler J, et al. INTERSALT study findings. Public health and medical care implications. Hypertension 1989; 14:570–577.

394. Blackburn GL, Morgan JP, Lavin PT, Noble R, Funderburk FR, Istfan N. Determinants of the pressor effect of phenylpropanolamine in healthy subjects. JAMA 1989; 261(22):3267–3272.

395. Morgan JP, Funderburk FR. Phenylpropanolamine and blood pressure: a review of prospective studies. Am J Clin Nutr 1992; 55:206S–210S.

396. Safety issues of phenylpropanolamine (PPA) in over-the-counter drug products. Meeting of the Nonprescription Drugs Advisory Committee of the Food and Drug Administration, Center for Drug Evaluation and Research, Gaithersburg, MD, Oct 19, 2000.

397. WN Jerner, CM Viscoli, LA Brass, et al. Phenylpropanolamine and the risk of hemorrhagic stroke. N Engl J Med 343:1826–1832.

13

Drugs That Modify Fat Absorption and Alter Metabolism

Luc F. Van Gaal

University of Antwerp and University Hospital Antwerp, Antwerp, Belgium

George A. Bray

Pennington Biomedical Research Center, Louisiana State University, Baton Rouge, Louisiana, U.S.A.

I INTRODUCTION

There is growing evidence that obesity, particularly central obesity, has an important impact on predisposing risk factors for coronary heart disease, including dyslipidemia, glucose intolerance, insulin resistance, and elevated blood pressure. Reversal of these metabolic abnormalities associated with obesity is one of the most important targets in the actual clinical management of obesity (1,2).

Although diet and lifestyle remain the cornerstones of therapy for obesity (3,4), weight losses are often small, and long-term success is extremely disappointing. Despite the availability of a variety of dietary manipulations ranging from calorie restriction to fat restriction and very low calorie diets (VLCD), the long-term maintenance of clinically significant weight loss defined as a loss of 5–10% of initial body weight remains uncommon (3). Over the past decade obesity research has been focused on the exploration of new biochemical pathways and on new pharmacological intervention possibilities.

The use of pharmacological agents for long-term treatment of obesity may play a useful role as part of an overall weight reduction program that includes diet, physical exercise and behavioral support (5). The use of drugs to treat obesity may be considered for people with BMI >30 kg/m^2, or BMI >27 kg/m^2, when additional complicating factors are present. Although not endorsed by American or European drug agencies, subjects with a recent onset of obesity and a rather sudden weight gain of 10–15 kg may also qualify for pharmacological treatment.

Large-scale, long-term clinical trials lasting up to 2 years have demonstrated that pharmacological agents, including orlistat, sibutramine, and d-fenfluramine, are able to induce significant weight loss over and above that produced in the control group. Important reductions of comorbidities are usually observed as well. These drugs allow the maintenance of the reduced body weight for at least 1–2 years. The weight loss that can be attributed to these drugs is in general modest, i.e., up to 10% weight loss. However, the reduction of up to 25% in most of the well-known co-morbid risk factors can be more than the magnitude of the weight loss.

From a consideration of the components involved in regulation of body weight, three different mechanisms may be used to classify pharmacological treatment of obesity (6): drugs that reduce appetite and food intake; drugs that increase energy expenditure; and drugs that affect metabolism or nutrient partitioning. This chapter will deal with drugs in the third category.

II PREABSOPTIVE DRUGS

A Orlistat

Because of their high energy content and low potential for inducing satiety, high-fat diets are conducive to overconsumption and weight gain, particularly in individuals who are relatively inactive. Indeed, humans are much more likely to become obese through the excessive consumption of dietary fat than by excess consumption of carbohydrate (7). It is therefore reasonable to decrease the proportion of fat as well as the total number of calories. By reducing fat absorption after ingestion, a continued calorie deficit may be maintained more easily over the long term than by dieting alone. Lipase inhibition may help in this strategy to reduce fat absorption.

1 Pharmacology

Orlistat is the hydrogenated derivative of lipstatin that is produced by the bacterium *Streptococcus toxytricini* (8,9). It has an α-lactone ring structure that is essential for activity, since opening this ring destroys it. This compound is highly lipophilic and is a potent inhibitor of most if not all mammalian lipases (8–10). Pancreatic lipase is a 449–amino acid enzyme that shares with other lipases a folded structure that is inactive. In the folded state, the N-terminal domain contains the catalytic site that includes serine, histidine, and aspartate. Binding of the enzyme to triglyceride is facilitated by colipase in the presence of bile salts. This interaction serves to expose the active site by opening the lid. One view of this is as though a lid were moved away from the active site by the interaction of the colipase and triglyceride in the bile salt milieu. Orlistat attaches to the active site of the lipase once the lid is opened and in so doing creates an irreversible inhibition at this site. In contrast to its inhibition of lipases, orlistat does not inhibit other intestinal enzymes, including hydrolases, trypsin, pancreatic phospholipase A2, phosphoinositol-specific phospholipase C, acetylcholinesterase, or nonspecific liver carboxyesterase. Because of its very small absorption (11, 12), it has no effect on systemic lipases (Fig. 1).

During short-term treatment with orlistat, fecal fat loss rises during the days of treatment and then returns to control levels after the medication is discontinued, as would be expected from an inhibitor of intestinal lipase (11,13,14). With volunteers eating a 30% fat diet, there is a dose-related increase in fecal fat loss that increases rapidly with doses up to 200 mg/d and then reaches a plateau with doses >400–600 mg/d. The plateau is at ~32% of dietary fat lost into the stools. Because the drug partially inhibits triglyceride digestion, it is possible

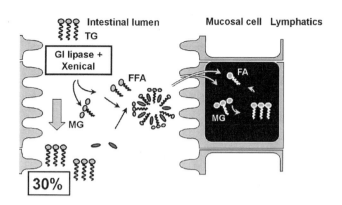

Figure 1   Mechanism of action of orlistat. (From Refs. 11, 12.)

that nutrients or drugs might be less well absorbed (11). Because of its lipid solubility, <1% of an oral dose is absorbed and degraded into two major metabolites (15).

Pharmacodynamic studies suggest that orlistat does not affect the pharmacokinetic properties of digoxin (16), phenytoin (16), warfarin (17), glyburide (17), oral contraceptives (18), or alcohol (8). Orlistat also did not affect a single dose of four different antihypertensive drugs—furosemide, captopril, nifedipine (16), or atenolol (19). Absorption of vitamins A, E, and β-carotene may be slightly reduced (15,16), and this may require vitamin therapy in a small number of patients. After oral administration of a single dose of 360 mg ^{14}C-labeled orlistat to healthy or obese volunteers, peak plasma radioactivity levels were reached ~6–8 hr after the dose (15,20). Plasma concentrations of intact orlistat were small, indicating negligible systemic absorption of the drug (15). Pooled data from five long-term clinical trials with orlistat lasting 6 months to 2 years at doses of 180–720 mg/d in obese patients indicated that there was a dose-related increase in plasma concentrations of orlistat. However, these plasma concentrations were low and generally below the level of assay detection (21).

2 Clinical Trials

a. Short-Term Clinical Trials

A number of initial short-term trials have revealed that orlistat promotes weight loss and improves hypercholesterolemia in obese patients. The weight-reducing effect of orlistat was further confirmed in another short-term dose-ranging study involving almost 200 healthy obese subjects. Weight reduction was statistically significant in those subjects receiving orlistat 120 mg TID compared to those receiving diet and placebo (22,23). Initial studies on healthy volunteers have shown that the maximum amount of fat excreted in the feces following doses of orlistat at 400 mg/d is ~32% of ingested fat.

A European dose-ranging study indicated that among 676 obese male and female subjects orlistat treatment resulted in a dose-dependent reduction in body weight with doses ranging from 30 to 240 mg TID. Orlistat 120 mg TID represents the optimal dosage regimen (24). In absolute terms mean weight loss reached 9.8% in the 120 mg/d orlistat group. More orlistat than placebo treated patients lost >10% of initial body weight (37% of the 120 mg group vs. 19% of the placebo group) (25). Daily fecal fat excretion also increased from the baseline value in a dose-dependent manner up to 18.5 g/d in those treated with 120 mg/d.

b. Long-Term Clinical Trials

Several double-blind randomized placebo-controlled trials lasting 1 and 2 years have been conducted and the data published in papers or in abstract form. Table 1 summarizes the available data. A 1-year multicenter placebo-controlled study, designed to assess the efficacy and tolerability of orlistat administered for 52 weeks, indicated that at 6 months the orlistat-treated patients lost 8.6 kg, versus 5.5 kg on placebo, a net additional loss of body weight of 0.13 kg/wk (25).

The design of the trials lasting 2 years followed two formats. They both included a 4- to 5-week single-blind run-in period after which subjects were stratified into those losing ≥2 kg or <2 kg. Orlistat was given at a dose of 60 or 120 mg before each of three meals. The diet contained 30% fat and was designed to produce a mild hypocaloric deficit of 500–600 kcal/d during the first year. During the second year patients were placed on a "eucaloric" diet to evaluate the effect of orlistat on weight maintenance. Weight loss at 1 year varied from 5.5% to 6.6% of initial body weight in the placebo group and from 8.5% to 10.2% in the orlistat-treated group. During the second year patients were kept on the same drug regimen as in the first year in two trials (26), and in the other two trials (27,28) patients were rerandomized to placebo or active drug in a crossover design. The percentage of patients losing >5% ranged from 23% to 49.2% in the placebo-treated group and from 49% to 68.5% in those treated with orlistat. Using a criterion of >10% weight loss, 17.7–25% of placebo-treated patients reached this goal compared to the more successful 38.8–43% among those treated with orlistat. Nearly two-thirds of the enrolled patients completed year 1.

Data on the second year of treatment are available from four studies. In one study (26), subjects remained on the same treatment for 2 years. At the end of the second year weight loss from baseline was −7.6% ± 7.0% for those receiving orlistat compared to −4.5% ± 7.6% for the placebo-treated group. At one year the corresponding losses were −9.7 ± 6.3% and −6.6 ± 6.8%. In the two other studies the orlistat subjects were rerandomized at the end of 1 year to placebo or orlistat 60–120 mg TID (25,28). One of these is shown in Figure 2 (27).

Those remaining on orlistat for 2 years regained 32.5% from the end of year 1 to the end of year 2 but were still −8.8 ± 7.6% below baseline. The patients who continued on orlistat with the maintenance diet regained half as much weight (2.5 kg or 2.6%) as those switched from orlistat to placebo (5.7 kg or 52% regain). In this trial subjects who received orlistat in the second year and placebo in the first year lost an average of 0.9 kg more. These data show that initial weight loss is greater and that weight regain is slowed by orlistat. The 2-year U.S. Prevention of Weight Regain Study treated patients who had lost >8% of their initial weight by dieting with orlistat 30, 60, or 120 mg TID (28). At the end of 1 year the placebo-treated group had regained 56% of the weight they had lost, in contrast to a regain of 32.4% in the group treated with orlistat 120 mg TID.

Initial successful weight loss, both during the initial 4 weeks run-in phase and during the active treatment period of 8–12 weeks, predicted the final outcome. Subjects who were not able to lose significant amounts of weight during these periods were considered as nonresponders whereas those who lost >5% of initial body weight after 3 months of therapy lost >16% of body weight after 1 year (29).

c. Effects of Orlistat on Lipids and Lipoproteins

The modest weight reduction observed with orlistat treatment may have a beneficial effect on lipids and lipoproteins (30). A 10% weight loss usually results in modest improvement of total and LDL cholesterol (−5 to 10%), a reduction of up to 30% in triglycerides, and a favorable increase of 8–10% in HDL cholesterol. In addition a beneficial effect has been observed in concentrations of small dense lipoprotein particles (31).

These improvements in lipid profile are in agreement with a meta-analysis conducted by Dattilo and Kris-Etherton (32) on the effects of weight loss on plasma lipids and lipoproteins. It was estimated that for every 1 kg reduction in body weight there is 0.05, 0.02,

Table 1   Effect of Orlistat in Clinical Trials of 1 and 2 Years' Duration

Author	Year	No. subjects Placebo	No. subjects Drug	Dose mg/tid	Duration of study (wks)	Run-in (wks)	Diet	Initial wt. (kg) Placebo	Initial wt. (kg) Drug	Wt. loss (kg or %) Placebo	Wt. loss (kg or %) Drug	Met criteria FDA	Met criteria CPMP	Comments
Drent (22)	1993	19	20	50	12	4	500 kcal/d deficit	81.9	85.5	−2.1kg	−4.3 kg	No	No	Single site
Drent (23)	1995	46	48 45 47	30 60 120	12	4	500 kcal/d deficit	90.0	92.1 92.6 94.1	−2.98kg	−3.61kg −3.69kg −4.74kg	No No No	No No No	Multicenter, dose-ranging
Drent (137)	1995	7	7	120	12	4	500 kcal/d deficit	86.8	89.8	−2.8kg	−4.2kg	No	No	Substudy of 821
James (25)	1997	23	23	120	52	4	600 kcal/d deficit	99	100	−2.6kg −2.6kg	−8.4kg −8.4kg	Yes	No	Wt. loss at 12 mos.
Finer (36)	1997	108	110		52	4	600 kcal/d deficit	98.4	97.9	−5.4%	−8.5%	No	No	British, 1 year
Van Gaal (24)	1998	125	122 124 122 120	30 60 120 240	24	4	500 kcal/d deficit	35 BMI	35 34 35 34	−6.5%	−8.5% −8.8% −9.8% −9.3%	No No No No	No No ± ±	Multicenter, dose-ranging
Sjostrom (27)	1998	340	343	120	104	4	600 kcal/d deficit (yr 1) maintenance (yr 2)	99.8	99.1	−6.1kg −6.1%	−10.3 kg −10.2%	No	Yes	European multicenter, crossover 52-wk data
Hollander (44)	1998	159	162	120	52	5	500 kcal/d deficit 30% fat	99.7	99.6	−4.3kg −4.3%	−6.2kg −6.2%	No	No	U.S., diabetic study
Davidson (28)	1999	223	657	120	104	4	600 kcal/d deficit (yr 1) maintenance (yr 2) 30% fat	100.6	100.7	−5.8kg −5.8%	−8.8 kg −8.7%	No	No	U.S., multicenter crossover 52-wk data

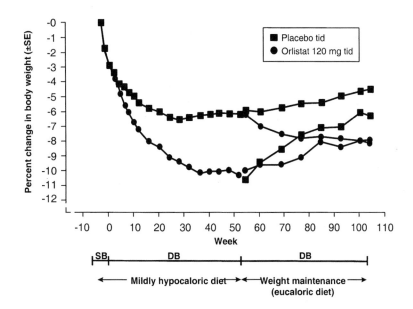

Figure 2 Effect of placebo and orlistat on body weight during 2 years. Subjects were rerandomized at the end of year 1. (From Ref. 23.)

and 0.015 mmol/L decrease in TC, LDL-C and TG, respectively. In addition, for every 1 kg decrease in body weight, a 0.007 mmol/L increase in HDL-C occurred in subjects at stabilized, reduced body weight. Baseline risk factors, the magnitude of weight loss, and exercise can influence the degree of change in lipid profile.

Orlistat seems to have an independent effect on LDL cholesterol. From a meta-analysis of the data relating orlistat to lipids, orlistat-treated subjects had almost twice as much reduction in LDL cholesterol as their

placebo-treated counterparts for the same weight loss category reached after 1 year (Fig. 3).

One study was designed to evaluate the effects of orlistat on weight loss and on cardiovascular risk factors, particularly serum lipids, in obese patients with hypercholesterolemia (33). The main findings were that orlistat promoted clinically significant weight loss and reduced LDL-C in obese patients with elevated cholesterol levels more than could be attributed to weight loss alone. These data support the conclusions of previous

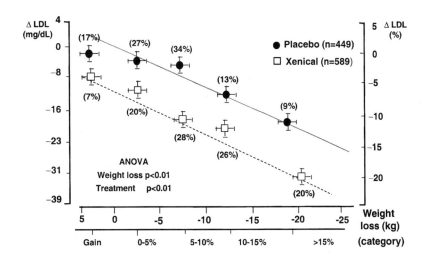

Figure 3 Incremental effect on LDL-cholesterol beyond weight loss. (From Ref. 33.)

controlled trials that partial inhibition of dietary fat absorption with the gastrointestinal lipase inhibitor, in conjunction with a hypocaloric diet, promotes weight loss of 6–10% in at risk patients (34–37).

Weight loss and modification of dietary fat appear to have independent and additive effects on the reduction in serum lipids: The net favorable effect of weight loss seems to be greater than that of dietary fat modification, as weight loss per se is responsible for ~60% and 70% of the fall in LDL-C and TG, respectively. The ObelHyx study extends these beneficial effects of orlistat on cardiovascular risk and demonstrates an additional 10% LDL-C lowering in obese subjects with baseline elevated LDL-C levels compared to placebo (33).

Figure 4 provides mean percentage changes in LDL-C after 24 weeks of double-blind treatment in three 2-year controlled trials, where the majority of patients were normocholesterolemic at baseline. These data indicate that the difference in mean percentage change in LDL-C between orlistat and placebo is ~10–12% in all studies, whether this difference is computed as change from the start of the single-blind placebo dietary run-in or from the start of double-blind treatment. It is noteworthy that LDL-C levels continued to decline after the start of double-blind treatment in orlistat-treated subjects in all trials, but that LDL-C either remained largely unchanged or increased during double-blind therapy in placebo-treated recipients, despite further weight loss. These data are in agreement with the 10% LDL-C decrease previously seen with orlistat 120 mg TID in nonobese patients with primary hyperlipidemia, who were kept on a weight maintenance diet. This independent cholesterol-lowering effect probably reflects a reduction in intestinal absorption of cholesterol. Since lipase inhibition by orlistat prevents the absorption of ~30% of dietary fat, the prescribed diet of 30% of energy from fat would thus become in effect a

20–24% of available fat in the diet when associated with orlistat treatment. It has been hypothesized that inhibition of gastrointestinal lipase activity may lead to retention of cholesterol in the gut through a reduction in the amount of fatty acids and monoglycerides absorbed from the gut, and/or may lead to sequestration of cholesterol within a more persistent oilphase in the intestine. Partial inhibition of intestinal fat and cholesterol absorption probably leads to decreased hepatic cholesterol and saturated fatty acid concentration, upregulation of hepatic LDL receptors, and decreased LDL-C levels. The decrease in LDL-C observed in the study with hypercholesterolemic subjects (33) is comparable to the 14% LDL-C reduction that was previously achieved with a plant stanol ester-containing margarine but of a lesser magnitude than the LDL-C lowering effects that are commonly observed with fibrate or statin drugs (38,39).

d. Effects of Orlistat on Glucose Tolerance and Diabetes

Weight gain is a known risk factor for the development of type 2 (non-insulin-dependent) diabetes, and even modest weight reduction can reduce the risk of the development of diabetes; controlling body weight is therefore an important public health goal in the fight against diabetes and its comorbidities. Weight reduction is also a cornerstone in the management of diabetes, improving glycemic control and reducing other risk factors associated with this disease. Pharmacotherapy such as orlistat can contribute to the prevention of diabetes and to the management of type 2 diabetes in overweight and obese patients.

Preventive strategies designed to reduce excess weight can have an impact on the risk for diabetes. Even modest weight loss (i.e., 5–10% body weight reduction) can reduce the risk of type 2 diabetes as much as 50% (40). The benefits of weight loss have been observed in different studies regardless whether the weight is lost through diet, exercise, or a combination of the two. Furthermore, if weight loss can be sustained, there may be further reductions in the relative risk of type 2 diabetes. A study by Moore et al. (41), looking at weight loss maintained over two consecutive 8-year periods, noted that individuals who sustained weight loss (3.6–6.8 kg) enjoyed a 33% reduction in the risk of diabetes. Greater weight losses (>6.8 kg) maintained for the same time period gave a 51% reduction in the risk of diabetes.

The recent report from the Finnish Diabetes Prevention study revealed that lifestyle intervention can lead to

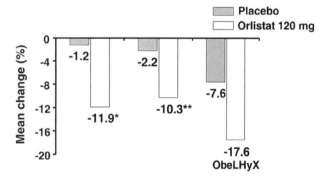

Figure 4 Effect on LDL-cholesterol. Comparison with previous studies. (From Refs. 27, 138.)

a substantial reduction (up to 58%) in the onset of type 2 diabetes in high-risk individuals with impaired glucose tolerance after a minimal weight reduction (42). These lifestyle strategies include eating a healthy (low-fat) diet and physical exercise.

The orlistat-treated subjects in trials lasting for at least 1 year were analyzed by Heymsfield and coworkers (43), who found that orlistat reduced the conversion of impaired glucose tolerance (IGT) to diabetes and that the transition from normal to impaired glucose tolerance was also reduced in subjects treated with orlistat for 1 year. In orlistat-treated subjects the conversion from normal glucose tolerance to diabetes occurred in 6.6% of patients, whereas ~11% of placebo-treated patients had a similar worsening of glucose tolerance. Conversion from IGT to diabetes was less frequent in orlistat-treated patients than in placebo-treated obese subjects by 3.0% and 7.6%, respectively (43). Although these data are based on a retrospective analysis of 1-year trials in which data on glucose tolerance were available, it shows that modest weight reduction—with pharmacotherapy—may lead to an important risk reduction for the development of type 2 diabetes. Only prospective information such as in the ongoing Xendos study can definitively confirm these preliminary data.

There are many studies among >2500 diabetic subjects treated for 6 months to 1 year with orlistat who received different anti-diabetic medications. Orlistat has been proven, in spite of the limited weight loss in diabetics (44), to improve metabolic control with a reduction of up to 0.53% in hemoglobin A1c (HbA_{1c}) and a decrease in the concomitant ongoing antidiabetic therapy. More patients treated with orlistat achieve clinically beneficially changes in HbA_{1c}, particularly in those with baseline levels of HbA_{1c} >8%. Concomitant reduction in the requirement for antidiabetic medication was also observed. Independent effects of orlistat on lipids were also shown in this study (44). Orlistat also has an acute effect on postprandial lipemia in overweight patients with type 2 diabetes (45). By lowering both remnantlike particle cholesterol and free fatty acids in the postprandial period, orlistat may contribute to a reduction in atherogenic risk (46).

The efficacy of orlistat in patients with type 2 diabetes has been demonstrated in three 6-month and four 1-year studies (44–49). One study randomized 550 insulin-treated patients to receive either placebo or orlistat 120 mg TID for 1 year. Weight loss in the orlistat-treated group was $-3.9 \pm 0.3\%$ compared to $-1.3 \pm 0.3\%$ in the placebo-treated group. Hemoglobin A1c was reduced -0.62% in the orlistat-treated group, but only -0.27% in the placebo group. The required dose

of insulin decreased more in the orlistat group, as did plasma cholesterol (47). Among data from a retrospective analysis of seven multicenter, double-blind trials enrolling overweight or obese patients (BMI 28–43 kg/m²) with type 2 diabetes and treated with metformin, sulfonylurea (SU), and/or insulin, orlistat-treated patients had significantly greater improvements in HbA_{1c} and fasting plasma glucose than placebo (48). The improvements in HbA_{1c} and FPG achieved with orlistat were similar across the diabetic medication subgroups. Orlistat-treated patients had least square mean differences from placebo in HbA1c of -0.34% ($P = .0007$), -0.42% ($P < .0001$), and -0.35% ($P = .002$) in the metformin, SU, and insulin groups, respectively. Orlistat, in combination with diet, represents a clinically beneficial adjunct to antidiabetic therapy for overweight or obese patients with type 2 diabetes (48).

Diabetic subjects reaching the target of 1% reduction in HbA_{1c} will benefit from the important risk reduction in all diabetes-related complications (21%) and diabetic microangiopathy (35%), as was shown in the UKPDS study (50).

Orlistat may have an independent effect on metabolic glycemic control. In a meta-analysis of four multicenter, double-blind 1-year trials in overweight/obese type 2 diabetics, much of the glycemic improvements in orlistat compared to placebo-treated patients seem to be independent of weight loss (49). The mechanisms behind these findings are still unknown, although fat intake may influence both insulin sensitivity and insulin secretion by the β-cells. It is, however, unclear how a lesser absorption of fat may have such an independent effect on glucose homeostasis.

The phenomenon of insulin resistance, known to be a triggering factor of the origin of diabetes and its complications, seems to be of specific importance. Related to this insulin resistance, Després et al. (51) have shown that orlistat reduces hyperinsulinemia in obese men with abdominal fat accumulation.

3   Side Effects and Safety of Orlistat

No pharmacodynamic or pharmacokinetic interactions were observed with orlistat 360 mg/d and warfarin (15) or glyburide (20) in healthy volunteers or with pravastatin in patients with mild hypercholesterolemia (52). No pharmacokinetic interactions were reported with orlistat and digoxin (16), nifedipine (53), or phenytoin (54). Orlistat did not interfere with oral contraceptive medication in healthy women (55). Orlistat had no clinically significant effects on the pharmacokinetics of captopril, nifedipine, atenolol, or furosemide in healthy volunteers (56). Short-term treatment with orlistat had no effect on ethanol pharmacokinetics, nor did ethanol interfere with the ability of orlistat to inhibit dietary fat absorption in healthy male volunteers (21,56).

Other pivotal functions such as blood pressure and heart rate are influenced in a positive way by orlistat. The most reported adverse effects consisted of abdominal pain, liquid stools, fecal incontinence with oily stools, nausea, vomiting, and flatulence, but these symptoms were in general mild and transient. Fecal fat loss and related gastrointestinal symptoms are common initially, but subside as the patients learn to use the drug.

In the 6-month European dose-ranging study, mean levels of vitamins A, D, E, and β-carotene were evaluated; the results showed that vitamin levels remained within the clinical reference range in all treatment groups and rarely required supplementation (24). Some patients need supplementation with fat-soluble vitamins that can be lost in the stools. Because it is impossible to predict which patients will need such supplements, a multivitamin can be provided with instructions to take it before bedtime. Absorption of other drugs does not seem to be significantly affected by orlistat (6). In some studies there was some trend toward a decrease in lipid-soluble vitamin levels, but only the decrease in vitamin E levels was statistically significant, while remaining within normal windows.

B   Amylase Inhibitors

Obese individuals have impaired starch tolerance due to their insulin resistance. Berchtold and Kiesselbach (57) reported that an amylase inhibitor, BAY e 4609, improved insulin and glucose during a starch tolerance test but did not cause weight loss in a controlled trial of 59 obese humans. Nevertheless, commercial preparations of amylase inhibitors were sold in the early 1980s with the claim that when taken in tablet form 10 min before meals, they would block the digestion of 100 g starch in the diet. Garrow (58) tested this claim with starch enriched with carbon 13 and found that these "starch blockers" do not affect starch digestion or absorption in vivo.

In 1979 Hillebrand et al. (59,60) reported that acarbose, an alpha-glucosidase inhibitor, reduced the insulin and glucose response to a mixed meal. Puls (61) reported a dose-related inhibition of weight gain in both Wistar and Zucker rats. Similar findings and a reduction in visceral adipose tissue was demonstrated with another alpha-glucosidase inhibitor, AO-128 or voglibose, suggesting that these effects are related to

this class of compounds (62–64). William-Olsson (65) treated 24 weight-reduced women with acarbose, showing that such treatment was able to inhibit weight regain. Wolever (66) has recently reported a 1-year double-blind, randomized, placebo-controlled study in 354 type 2 diabetic subjects. Subjects on acarbose lost 0.46 kg while the placebo group gained 0.33 kg, which was statistically significantly different ($P = .027$).

We conclude that alpha amylase inhibitors usually have no place in the treatment of obesity without concomitant diabetes. Acarbose gives only a small weight loss and is not indicated as an obesity treatment, but it certainly deserves consideration in treating obese type 2 diabetic subjects who have failed treatment with diet and exercise. Also the more recent molecule miglitol, an α-glucosidase inhibitor of second generation, has been shown to improve metabolic control in type 2 diabetics. In a combination trial with metformin, in patients insufficiently treated with the biguanide alone, addition of miglitol led to an improvement of metabolic control (placebo subtracted, -0.43% in HbA_{1c}) but also to a weight reduction of 2.5 kg over 28 weeks of treatment (67). Although this was not significant when compared to placebo, weight reduction during active therapy for glucose control always has to be considered as a success, in view of the known weight effects in UKPDS.

C   Olestra

Acylation of sucrose with five or more fatty acids produces a molecule that has the physical characteristics of triglyceride but which cannot be digested by pancreatic lipase. Olestra (Olean) is a commercially available form of sucrose polyester that is largely solid at body temperature. This fat substitute cannot be digested and is currently being used to cook snack foods. Short-term studies substituting olestra for triglyceride in the diet show two patterns of adaptation. When olestra (sucrose polyester) was substituted in a single breakfast meal, there was energy compensation over the next 24–36 hr in healthy young males (68). Substitution with olestra at the noon or evening meal lowered digestible fat from 40% to 30% of the fat, and there was no energy or nutrient compensation over the next 24 hr (69). However, when the olestra substitution lowered the fat intake from 30% to nearly 20% of energy over three meals, healthy subjects felt less satisfied at the end of the substitution and compensated for nearly 75% of the energy deficit over the next day (70).

Both short-term and long-term clinical trials have been done with olestra in obese and normal-weight individuals. In two short-term trials, one-third of dietary fat was replaced with olestra, thus reducing calories from 2000 to 1750 kcal/d. In each experiment there was only partial compensation, suggesting that when the energy density of the diet changed, the subjects continued to eat the same mass of food, even though it provided fewer metabolizable calories. Weight loss in the two-week experiment was 1.5 kg and in the 3-month experiment was > 5 kg, which was significantly greater than the control group (69–73).

In a 9-month parallel arm trial, three groups of 45 overweight men were divided into three equal groups matched for initial cholesterol, BMI, and age. One group received a 33% fat diet, a second group ate a 25% reduced-fat diet, and the third group ate a diet with 25% of the dietary fat replaced with olestra. All subjects ate their dinner 5 days a week at the center and were given takeout food for breakfast and lunch and for their weekend meals. Body fat was measured by dual energy x-ray absorptiometry at baseline and at 3, 6, and 9 months. Changes in visceral fat were tracked from baseline to 3, 6, and 9 months. The two measures of fat provided a similar conclusion, and the data for total abdominal fat are shown in Figure 5.

During the first 3 months there was a decrease in total body fat and in the total abdominal cross-sectional fat area, probably reflecting the fact that the available food was less than the subjects would normally have eaten. During the next 6 months there was a clear divergence

of fat in the three groups. The control group eating a 33% fat diet did not show any further significant change in their total and visceral fat. The group for whom dietary fat was replaced by olestra continued to lose body weight and by 9 months were 5.85% below baseline. The group eating the 25% reduced-fat diet did not lose more fat, but actually had a significant increase over the last 6 months of the trial indicating the difficulty of adhering to a low-fat diet over extended periods of time (74).

III POSTABSORPTIVE MODIFIERS OF NUTRIENT METABOLISM

A Growth Hormone

Human growth hormone is a 191–amino acid peptide composed of a single chain with two disulfide bonds (75). It is of interest in relation to obesity because obese individuals secrete less growth hormone (76), because growth hormone enhances lipolysis (77), because it increases metabolic rate and leads to changes in fat patterning in hypopituitary children treated with growth hormone (78). Based on these observations, early studies with growth hormone showed that it would enhance mobilization of fat, stimulate oxygen consumption (79), and lead to reduced protein loss in obese people (80). When given to fasting obese subjects on a metabolic ward, it accelerated ketosis by increasing

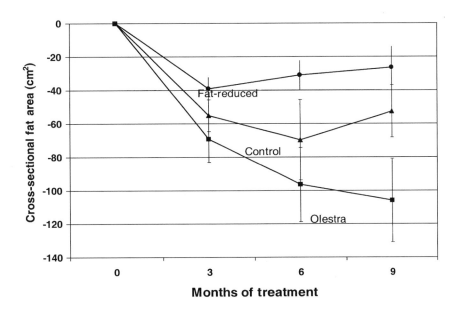

Figure 5 Change in total abdominal fat area during the 9 months of treatment. (From Ref. 74.)

Table 2 Clinical Studies with Growth Hormone in Obesity

Author (Ref.)	Year	No. subjects P	No. subjects D	Dose of medication	Duration (wks)
Bray (80)	1971	4F (hGH—N = 2) (hGH + T3 N = 4)		5 mg/d	hGH alone—30 d; hGH + T₃—15 d
Clemmons (84)	1987	5F 3M		0.1 mg/kg IBW every other day wks 3–5 wks 8–10	11 wks
Snyder (85)	1988	8F 2M	8F 2M	0.1 mg/kg IBW every other day wks 2–12	13 wks
Snyder (86)	1989	11F		0.1 mg/kg IBW every other day wks 2–4	Two 5-wk periods 5-wk washout
Snyder (87)	1990	8F		0.1 mg/kg daily	Two 5-week periods 5-week washout
Richelson (88)	1994	9F Premenopausal		0.03 mg/kg IBW/d	Two 5-week periods 5-week washout
Jorgensen (89)	1994	10 F Premenopausal		0.03 mg/kg IBW/d	Two 5-week periods 5-week washout 5 weeks
Snyder (90)	1995	11		0.05 mg/kg	4 weeks
Drent (91)	1995	6F 2M	7F	6µg/d	8 weeks
Johannsson (92)	1997	15M	15M	9.5 µg/kg daily	39 weeks
Karlsson (93)	1998	15M	15M	9.5 µg/kg daily	39 weeks
Thompson (94)	1998	7	9 9 10	GH 0.025 mg/kg BW/d IGI1 0.015 mg/kg/d GH + IGFI	12 weeks

Diet	Weight loss (kg)		Fat loss (kg or %)		Comments
	P	D	P	D	
900 kcal/d formula diet	211 g/d 523 g/d 550 g/d T_3	337 g/d 240 g/d 380 g/d T_3+hGH			Metabolic ward
24 kcal/kg IBW 1.0 prot/kg IBW	−4.16	−3.42	−2.64 ± 1.08	−3.06 ± 1.39	Metabolic ward, crossover study or IGF1↑; nitrogen balance improved
18 kcal/kg IBW 1.2 g prot/kg IBW	−15.2 ± 3.8	−13.9 ± 3.0	−7.5 ± 1.5%	−8.1 ± 2.4%	Metabolic ward parallel arm study; nitrogen balance positive but less with time. IGF-1↑; FFA↑
12 kg kcal/kg IBW 1.0 g prot/kg IBW Diet I—72% carb Diet II—20% carb	−8.5 ± 1.7 −8.2 ± 0.7	−7.4 ± 1.9 −7.5 ± 1.8	−2.8 ± 0.7%	−3.7 ± 1.0% −3.8 ± 0.9% −3.6 ± 1.2%	Metabolic unit study; GH↑ fat loss as % wt loss from 64% to 81%
12 kcal/kg IBW	−7.2 ± 2.3 6.3 ± 5.0	—	−3.6 ± 1.1%	−3.5 ± 1.1%	Crossover; improved N_2 balance; ↑ IGF-I
Not specified		+3.0 ± .13		−2.1 ± .06 kg	Crossover; visceral fat. LPL↓; FFA↑; C-peptide↑
Not specified	Data not given. Subjects may overlap with paper above.		Data not given. Subjects may overlap with paper above		Crossover T_3↑; EE↑; FFA↑; RER↓; IGF-I↑
15 kcal/kg	−8.4 ± 1.4 7.3 ± 1.4	—	−2.6 ± 1.0%	−3.4 ± 0.9%	Crossover IGF-I↑
VLCD + exercise	−12.8 ± 5.0 13.8 ± 4.0	—			IGF-I↑; IGFBP-3↑
Not specified	FFM +0.7	+2.0		−9.2 ± 2.4%	Parallel arm
Not specified	+0.5	−1.0	−0.1kg	−3.0kg	Parallel arm Same patients as in report. BMR↑; leptin↓; visceral fat↓ 68.1%
500 kcal/d deficit	−3.7	−4.2 −3.5 −5.6	−3.5kg	−6.3kg −4.0kg −8.4kg	Parallel arm

fatty acid mobilization (81). More recently, treatment of adult growth hormone deficiency has been shown to reduce body fat (82), whereas treatment of acromegaly in which growth hormone secretion is high, increases fat (83).

The nitrogen-sparing effects of growth hormone in human subjects on a reduced-calorie diet were investigated in a series of studies using different levels of caloric restriction (84–91). In all of these studies, growth hormone increased the concentration of free fatty acids (FFA) in the circulation, increased IGF-1, and increased insulin and C-peptide. In most studies it preserved nitrogen and increased fat loss or the loss of fat relative to body weight loss.

Table 2 summarizes these data and other clinical trials in obese subjects. Most of the studies have been relatively short term with treatment lasting from 21 days to 5 weeks (81,86,90), but few have lasted from 11 to 39 weeks (84,85,92–94). Most of the subjects were women. Metabolic rate is increased where measured, and respiratory exchange rate (RER) is reduced, indicating that more fat is being oxidized. IGF-I increased FFA and the rate of fat loss relative to protein loss increased. A number of side effects were noted (91) that reduce the enthusiasm for long-term trials. The only long-term study lasted 9 months and used continuous daily injections of growth hormone. There were 15 men in each arm of the randomized double-blind placebo-controlled clinical trial (93). In these men, growth hormone enhanced fat loss with a larger percentage of this fat coming from the visceral than from the subcutaneous compartment (Table 2).

B Metformin

Metformin is a biguanide that is approved for the treatment of diabetes mellitus, a disease that is exacerbated by obesity and weight gain. Although the cellular mechanisms for the effects of metformin are poorly understood, it has three effects at the clinical level (95–101). First, it reduces hepatic glucose production, which is a major source of circulating glucose. Mainly among overweight and obese subjects, metformin also reduces intestinal absorption of glucose, which is an additional source of circulating glucose. Finally, metformin increases the sensitivity to insulin, mainly in obese individuals, thus increasing peripheral glucose uptake and utilization.

Metformin has been associated with significant weight loss when compared to sulfonylureas or placebo. Campbell et al. (97) compared metformin and glipizide in a randomized double-blind study of type 2 diabetic individuals who had failed on diets. The 24 subjects on metformin lost weight and had better diabetic control of fasting glucose and glycohemoglobin than did the glipizide group. The glipizide group gained weight, and the difference in weight between the two groups at the end of the study was highly significant. In a double-blind placebo-controlled trial in subjects with the insulin resistance syndrome, metformin also increased weight loss. Fontbonne et al. (98) reported the results from the BIGPRO study, a 1-year French multicenter study that compared metformin with placebo in 324 middle-aged subjects with upper-body obesity and the insulin resistance syndrome. The subjects on metformin lost significantly more weight (1–2 kg) than the placebo group, and the study concluded that metformin may have a role in the primary prevention of type 2 diabetes mellitus. The package insert for metformin (99) describes a 29-week double-blind study comparing glyburide 20 mg/d with metformin 2.5 g/d and their combination in 632 type 2 diabetic subjects who had inadequate glucose control. The metformin group lost 3.8 kg compared to a loss of 0.3 kg in the glyburide group and a gain of 0.4 kg in the combined group.

The package insert also describes a double-blind controlled study in poorly controlled type 2 diabetic subjects comparing metformin 2.5 g/d to placebo. Weight loss in the placebo group was 1.1 kg, compared to 0.64 kg in the metformin group. Lee and Morley (100), however, compared 48 type 2 diabetic women in a double-blind controlled trial, randomizing subjects to metformin 850 mg BID or placebo. Subjects on metformin lost 8.8 kg over 24 weeks compared to only 1.0 kg in the placebo group, a highly significant difference ($P < .001$).

The Diabetes Prevention Program trial to prevent or delay the conversion of individuals with impaired glucose tolerance to diabetes mellitus is the most recent and largest trial with metformin. Of the slightly more than 2000 individuals treated with medication, half received metformin and the other half took placebo. Nearly 75% of each group took their pills for the average 2.8 years of follow-up. Weight loss in the metformin group was significantly greater than placebo with a nadir at 6 months, but with weight remaining below baseline for the remainder of the trial. Metformin was effective in men and women and all ethnic groups (Fig. 6). It was more effective in younger individuals and in those who were more overweight (101). Although metformin may not give enough weight loss to receive an indication from the U.S. Food and Drug Administration for treating obesity, it certainly deserves consideration in

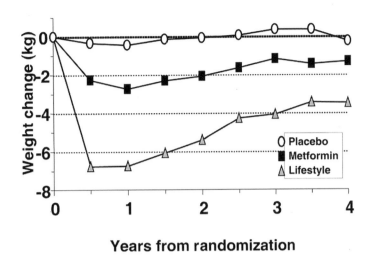

Figure 6 Weight change from placebo, metformin, and lifestyle intervention. (From Ref. 101.)

obese type 2 diabetic individuals who have failed diet and exercise treatment for their diabetes, and it has been used in children (100).

C Hydroxycitrate

Another compound, (-)-hydroxycitrate, inhibits citrate lyase, the first extramitochondrial step in fatty acid synthesis from glucose. This compound causes weight loss by decreasing calorie intake (103). Although the mechanism of this inhibition of food intake is not clear, studies by Hellerstein and Xie (104) suggest that it may be through trioses like pyruvate. In a double-blind trial of 60 subjects who were randomized to hydroxycitric acid 1320 mg/d or placebo and a 1200-calorie diet for 8 weeks, the hydroxycitrate group lost 6.4 kg whereas the placebo group lost only 3.8 kg ($P < .001$) (105). *Garcinia cambogia*, an herbal product containing hydroxycitrate, has been compared to placebo in a double-blind randomized clinical trial (106). The herbal product was given TID in a dose to provide 500 mg each time. The subjects treated with hydroxycitrate lost no more weight than placebo.

D Human Chorionic Gonadotropin

Injection of small doses of human chorionic gonadotropin (HCG) daily for 6 weeks or more has been widely used in the treatment of obesity following the introduction of this treatment for undescended testes and its use with alleged success in patients with what was termed Frohlich's syndrome. A number of controlled clinical trials have been done to evaluate the

use of HCG and these have recently been reviewed (107,108) (Table 3).

Lijesen et al. (108) evaluated 16 uncontrolled and eight controlled studies found through a literature search. All studies were graded on a 100-point scale, and those making a score of 50 or greater were evaluated. Of these studies only one concluded that HCG was a useful adjunct to a weight loss program compared to a placebo. Table 3 is a summary of the double-blind placebo-controlled randomized trials that have been published in the past 25 years (109–118). We conclude that HCG is no more effective than placebo, but we also note that all of these studies used a very low calorie diet that gave a significant weight loss in both groups.

E Androgens

For this discussion, androgens will be divided into two groups, the "weak" androgenic compounds including androsterone, dehydroepiandrosterone, Δ^4-androstenedione, and anabolic steroids, and the potent androgens, testosterone and dihydrotestosterone.

1 Dehydroepiandrosterone

Dehydroepiandrosterone (DHEA = Δ^5-androsten-3-β-ol-17-one) is a product of the adrenal gland. In human beings, this steroid and its sulfated derivative are the most abundant steroids produced by the adrenal. In experimental animals the quantities are much lower, and in rodents they are just above the threshold for detection. In spite of their high concentration in the circulation and abundance as adrenal products, no

Table 3 Clinical Trials with HCG Injections for the Treatment of Obesity

Author (Ref.)	Year	Number of subjects Placebo	Number of subjects Drug	Diet (kcal/d)	Design	Wt. loss (kg) Placebo	Wt. loss (kg) Drug	Wt. loss (%) Placebo	Wt. loss (%) Drug	Comments
Carne (109)	1961	12/10 11/8 10/7	13/12	500	Diet + HCG Diet + vehicle Diet + vehicle Diet only	-8.6 -10.1 -8.0	-9.5	-10.3 -12.2 -11.3	-12.5	Injections were better than no injections, but HCG not better than saline.
Craig (110)	1963	11/9		550	Randomized double-blind	-3.0	-4.0			HCG had no demonstrable effect. Weight loss due to diet.
Frank (111)	1964	63/30		500	Double-blind; 3 injections/week	-5.6	-5.2			Changes in body measurements and rating of hunger were the same in both groups. HCG had no effect.
Asher (113)	1973	20/13	20/17	500	Modified double-blind (3 patients from each vial)	-9.0	-5.0	-6.8	-11.5	HCG possibly effective. Five of placebo group and none of HCG group received <21 injections.
Stein (114)	1976	26/21	25/20	500	Double-blind, randomized, placebo-controlled	-7.0	-7.2	-9.3	-9.5	No difference in weight loss, waist or hip circumference, or hunger rating between HCG and placebo.
Greenway and Bray (108)	1977	20/20		500	Double-blind, randomized, placebo-controlled	-8.1	-8.8	-10.2	-10.9	No difference in weight loss, hunger rating, mood or body circumference between HCG and placebo.
Shetty (115)	1977	5/5	6/6	500	Double-blind inpatient study lasting 30 d	-9.4	-9.3	-9.5	-9.1	No difference in weight loss, fat redistribution, hunger, or well-being.
Bosch (116)	1990	20/16	20/17	1190 (5000 kJ)	Double-blind, randomized	-4.6	-3.2	-4.9	-3.4	No difference in weight loss, fat redistribution, hunger, or well-being.

clear function has been identified. DHEA levels decline with age in both men and women (119). With very high BMI values of 40–60 kg/m², on the other hand, there was a significant negative correlation. In contrast with the limited effect relationship between DHEA and body weight or total fat, there is a clearer relation with fat distribution (120) and hyperinsulinemia (119). Animal studies have shown that DHEA may be immunosuppressive and have antiatherogenic and antitumor effects (121). It is the fact that mice, rats, cats, and dogs fed DHEA lose weight that has led to its evaluation as a potential treatment for obesity. A recent structure function analysis by Lardy et al. (122) showed that the biological effect on body fat of DHEA related steroids was greatest with 7-oxo-DHEA derivatives.

Several clinical studies with DHEA have been done and are reviewed by Clore (121). In a study lasting 28 days with 10 normal-weight volunteers, DHEA at 1600 mg/d, near the limit where hepatic toxicity is a risk, had no effect on body weight or on insulin sensitivity as assessed by the euglycemic-hyperinsulinemic clamp (123). A similar study showed no effect of DHEA on energy expenditure, body composition, or protein turnover (124). After 28 days of treatment with DHEA, obese male volunteers showed no improvement in body fat or insulin sensitivity (125). In obese female volunteers there was likewise no change in body fat, but there was a decrease in insulin sensitivity (126). Based on these negative studies in both lean and obese human subjects, it would appear that DHEA is ineffective in human obesity. A steroid derivative of DHEA called etiocholanedione has been suggested to reduce body weight in one preliminary study (127). More data are awaited.

2 Testosterone and Dihydrotesterone

Testosterone is the principal product of the testis and is responsible for masculinization. Testosterone is converted to dihydrotesterone (DHT) in peripheral androgenic tissues and converts the "soft" hair to the terminal hair in male androgenic areas. Testosterone can also be produced by the adrenal, the ovary, and by conversion in peripheral tissues (128). In females, 25% of testosterone comes from the ovary, 25% from the adrenal, and 50% from peripheral conversion. In human subjects, the concentration of testosterone is positively related to the level of visceral fat in women, and negatively correlated with visceral fat in men (129,130). A recent report suggests that androstane-3-β, 17-α-diol may be a correlate of visceral obesity (131).

The inverse relationship between testosterone and visceral fat in men suggested that visceral fat might be reduced by treatment with testosterone. Marin et al. (132–134) have evaluated this in two trials using men with low-normal circulating testosterone levels (< 20 nmol/L) and a BMI > 25 kg/m². In the first trial, testosterone 80 mg BID was given orally as the undecenoate. The 11 men who received testosterone had a significant decrease of visceral fat mass as measured by computed tomography compared to the 12 men who received placebo for 8 months. There were no changes in body mass, subcutaneous fat mass, or lean body mass. Insulin sensitivity was improved (134).

In a second trial (133), 31 men were randomly allocated to three groups receiving either placebo, testosterone, or dihydrotestosterone. The testosterone was given as a gel with 5 g containing 125 mg testosterone applied to the arms daily. The DHT was applied in a similar gel at the same dose. The placebo group received only the gel. After 9 months, the testosterone-treated group showed a significant decrease in waist circumference and visceral fat. The DHT-treated group, on the other hand, showed an increase in visceral fat. Testosterone was increased in the group treated with the testosterone. Treatment with DHT reduced testosterone and increased DHT levels. Insulin sensitivity was also improved by treatment with testosterone (134,135).

Two additional studies have examined the effects of anabolic steroids in men and women (135,136). The first was a 9-month trial on 30 healthy overweight men with mean BMI values of 33.8–34.5 kg/m² and testosterone values between 2 and 5 ng/mL (136). During the first 3 months, when an oral anabolic steroid (oxandrolone) was given daily, there was a significantly greater decrease in subcutaneous fat and a greater fall in visceral fat than in the groups treated with placebo or testosterone enanthate injected every 2 weeks. Because of the drop in HDL cholesterol, which is a known side effect of oral anabolic steroids (135), the anabolic steroid group was changed to an injectable drug, nandrolone decanoate. The effects were similar to those of testosterone enanthate. The data with testosterone given as a biweekly injection did not replicate the data of Marin et al. (132,133), and the biweekly injections of nandrolone failed to maintain the difference seen with daily treatment with oxandrolone. This suggests that to obtain the visceral effects with steroids, frequent if not daily administration may be needed.

In a second 9-month trial with 30 postmenopausal overweight women, Lovejoy et al. (136) randomized subjects to nandrolone decanoate, spironolactone, or placebo. The weight loss was comparable in all three groups, but the women treated with nandrolone decanoate gained lean mass and visceral fat and lost more total body fat. Women treated with the antiandrogen spironolactone lost significantly more visceral fat. The conclusions from the four studies described above are that visceral and total body fat can be manipulated separately, and that testosterone plays an important role in this differential fat distribution in both men and women.

REFERENCES

1. Després JP, Lemieux S, Lamarche B, Prud'homme D, Moorjani S, Brun LD, Gagne C, Lupien PJ. The insulin resistance-dyslipidemic syndrome: contribution to visceral obesity and therapeutic implications. Int J Obes Relat Metab Disord 1995; 19:S76–S86.

2. Van Gaal LF, Mertens IL. Effects of obesity on cardiovascular system and blood pressure control, digestive disease and cancer. In: Kopelman P, Stock M, eds. Clinical Obesity. Oxford: Blackwell Science, 1998: 205–225.

3. Van Gaal LF. Dietary treatment of obesity. In: Bray GA, Bouchard C, James WPT, eds. Handbook of Obesity. New York: Marcel Dekker, 1998:875–890.

4. Vansant G, Muls E. New directions in public health approach to obesity management. Acta Clin Belg 1999; 54:151–153.

5. Scheen AJ, Lefèbvre PJ. Pharmacological treatment of obesity: present status. Int J Obes Relat Metab Disord 1999; 23(suppl 1):47–53.

6. Bray GA, Greenway FL. Current and potential drugs for treatment of obesity. Endocr Rev 1999; 20:805–875.

7. Lissner L, Heitman BL. Dietary fat and obesity: evidence from epidemiology. Eur J Clin Nutr 1995; 49:79–90.

8. Guerciolini R. Mode of action of orlistat. Int J Obes Relat Metab Disord 1997; 21(suppl 3):S12–S23.

9. Hadvary P, Lengsfield H, Wolfer H. Inhibition of pancreatic lipase in vitro by the covalent inhibitor tetrahydrolipstatin. Biochem J 1988; 256:357–361.

10. Lookene A, Skottova N, Olivecrona G. Interactions of lipoprotein lipase with the active-site inhibitor tetrahydrolipstatin (orlistat). Eur J Biochem 1994; 222:395–403.

11. Zhi J, Melia AT, Guerciolini R, Chung J, Kinberg J, Hauptman JB, Patel IH. Retrospective population-based analysis of the dose-response (fecal fat excretion) relationship of orlistat in normal and obese volunteers. Clin Pharmacol Ther 1994; 56:82–85.

12. Reitsma JB, Castro Cabezas M, De Bruin TW, Erkelens DW. Relationship between improved postprandial lipemia and low-density lipoprotein metabolism during treatment with tetrahydrolipstatin, a pancreatic lipase inhibitor. Metabolism 1994; 43:293–298.

13. Hauptman JB, Jeunet FS, Hartmann D. Initial studies

14. Hussain Y, Guzelhan C, Odink J, Van der Beek EJ, Hartmann D. Comparison of the inhibition of dietary fat absorption by full versus divided doses of orlistat. J Clin Pharmacol 1994; 34:1121–1125.

15. Zhi J, Melia AT, Funk C, Viger-Chougnet A, Hopfgartner G, Lausecker B, Wang K, Fulton JS, Gabriel L, Mulligan TE. Metabolic profiles of minimally absorbed orlistat in obese/overweight volunteers. J Clin Pharmacol 1996; 36:1006–1011.

16. Melia AT, Zhi J, Koss-Twardy SG, Min BH, Smith BL, Freundlich NL, Arora S, Passe SM. The influence of reduced dietary fat absorption induced by orlistat on the pharmacokinetics of digoxin in healthy volunteers. J Clin Pharmacol 1995; 35:840–843.

17. Zhi J, Melia AT, Koss-Twardy SG, Min B, Guerciolini R, Freundlich NL, Milla G, Patel IH. The influence of orlistat on the pharmacokinetics and pharmacodynamics of glyburide in healthy volunteers. J Clin Pharmacol 1995; 35:521–525.

18. Guzelhan C, Odink J, Niestijl Jansen-Zuidema JJ, Hartmann D. Influence of dietary composition on the inhibition of fat absorption by orlistat. J Int Med Res 1994; 22:255–265.

19. Weber C, Tam YK, Schmidtke-Schrezenmeier G, Jonkmann JH, Van Brummelen P. Effect of the lipase inhibitor orlistat on the pharmacokinetics of four different antihypertensive drugs on healthy volunteers. Eur J Clin Pharmacol 1996; 51:87–90.

20. Zhi J, Melia AT, Eggers H, Joly R, Patel IH. Review of limited systemic absorption of orlistat, a lipase inhibitor, in healthy human volunteers. J Clin Pharmacol 1995; 35:1103–1108.

21. Hvizdos KM, Markham A. Orlistat: a review of its use in the management of obesity. Drugs 1999; 58:743–760.

22. Drent ML, Van der Veen EA. Lipase inhibition: a novel concept in the treatment of obesity. Int J Obes Relat Metab Disord 1993; 17:241–244.

23. Drent ML, Larsson I, William-Olsson T, Quadde F, Czubayko F, Von Bergmann K, Strobel W, Sjostrom L, Van der Veen EA. Orlistat (Ro18-0647), a lipase inhibitor, in the treatment of human obesity: a multiple dose study. Int J Obes Relat Metab Disord 1995; 19:221–226.

24. Van Gaal LF, Broom JI, Enzi G, Toplak H. Efficacy and tolerability of orlistat in the treatment of obesity: a 6-month dose-ranging study. Eur J Clin Pharmacol 1998; 54:125–132.

25. James WP, Avenell A, Broom J, Whitehead J. A one-year trial to assess the value of orlistat in the management of obesity. Int J Obes Relat Metab Disord 1997; 21(suppl 3):S24–S30.

26. Noack R. Two-year study of orlistat in the treatment of obesity. Endocrine Society 79th Annual Meeting, June 11–14, 1997.

in humans with the novel gastrointestinal lipase inhibitor Ro 18-0647 (tetrahydrolipstatin). Am J Clin Nutr 1992; 55(suppl 1):309S–313S.

27. Sjostrom L, Rissanen A, Andersen T, Boldrin M, Golay A, Koppeschaar HP, Krempf M. Randomized placebo-controlled trial of orlistat for weight loss and prevention of weight regain in obese patients. European Multicentre Orlistat Study Group. Lancet 1998; 352: 167–172.

28. Davidson MH, Hauptman J, DiGirolamo M, Foreyt JP, Halsted CH, Heber D, Heimburger DC, Lucas CP, Robbins DC, Chung J, Heymsfield SB. Long-term weight control and risk factor reduction in obese subjects treated with orlistat, a lipase inhibitor. JAMA 1999; 281:235–242.

29. Rissanen A, Lean M, Rossner S, Segal K, Sjostrom L. Predictive value of early weight loss in obesity management with orlistat: an evidence based assessment of prescribing guidelines. Int J Obes Relat Metab Disord 2003; 27:103–109.

30. Tonstad S, Pometta D, Erkelens DW, Ose L, Moccetti T, Schouten JA, Golay A, Reitsma J, Del Bufalo A, Pasotti E. The effects of gastrointestinal lipase inhibitor, orlistat, on serum lipids and lipoproteins in patients with primary hyperlipidaemia. Eur J Clin Pharmacol 1994; 46:405–410.

31. Van Gaal LF, Wauters M, De Leeuw IH. The beneficial effects of modest weight loss on cardiovascular risk factors. Int J Obes 1997; 21(suppl 1):S5–S9.

32. Dattilo AM, Kris-Etherton PM. Effects of weight reduction on blood lipids and lipoproteins: a meta-analysis. Am J Clin Nutr 1992; 56:320–328.

33. Muls E, Kolanowski J, Scheen A, Van Gaal LF. The effects of orlistat on weight and on serum lipids in obese patients with hypercholesterolemia: a randomized, double-blind, placebo-controlled, multicenter study. Int J Obes Relat Metab Disord 2001; 25:1713–1721.

34. Davidson MH, Hauptman J, DiGirolamo M, Foreyt JP, Halsted CH, Heber D, Heimburger DC, Lucas CP, Robbins DC, Chung J, Heymsfield SB. Weight control and risk factor reduction in obese subjects treated for 2 years with orlistat: a randomized controlled trial. JAMA 1999; 281:235–242.

35. Rössner S, Sjöstrom L, Noack R, Meinders E, Noseda G. Weight loss, weight maintenance and improved cardiovascular risk factors after 2 years treatment with orlistat for obesity. European Orlistat Obesity Study Group. Obes Res 2000; 8:49–61.

36. Finer N, James WP, Kopelman PG, Lean ME, Williams G. One-year treatment of obesity: a randomized, double-blind, placebo-controlled, multicentre study of orlistat, a gastrointestinal lipase inhibitor. Int J Obes Relat Metab Disord 2000; 24:306–313.

37. Zavoral JH. Treatment with orlistat reduces cardiovascular risk in obese patients. J Hypertens 1998; 16: 2013–2017.

38. Linton MF, Fazio S. Re-emergence of fibrates in the management of dyslipidemia and cardiovascular risk. Curr Atheroscler Rep 2000; 2:29–35.

39. Maron DJ, Fazio S, Linton MF. Current perspectives on statins. Circulation 2000; 101:207–213.

40. Wing RR, Venditti E, Jakicic JM, Polley BA, Lang W. Lifestyle intervention in overweight individuals with a family history of diabetes. Diabetes Care 1998; 21: 350–359.

41. Moore LL, Visioni AJ, Wilson PW, D'Agostino RB, Finkle WD, Ellison RC. Can sustained weight loss in overweight individuals reduce the risk of diabetes mellitus? Epidemiology 2000; 11:269–273.

42. Tuomilehto J, Lindstrom J, Eriksson JG, Valle TT, Hamalainen H, Ilanne-Parikka P, Keinanen-Kiukaanniemi S, Laakso M, Louheranta A, Rastas M, Salminen V, Uusitupa M. Prevention of type 2 diabetes mellitus by changes in lifestyle among subjects with impaired glucose tolerance. N Engl J Med 2001; 344:1343–1350.

43. Heymsfield SB, Segal KR, Hauptman J, Lucas CP, Boldrin MN, Rissanen A, Wilding P, Sjöström L. Effects of weight loss with orlistat on glucose tolerance and progression to type 2 diabetes in obese adults. Arch Intern Med 2000; 160:1321–1326.

44. Hollander PA, Elbein SC, Hirsch IB, Kelley D, McGill J, Taylor T, Weiss SR, Crockett SE, Kaplan RA, Comstock J, Lucas CP, Lodewick PA, Canovatchel W, Chung J, Hauptman J. Role of orlistat in the treatment of obese patients with type 2 diabetes. A 1-year randomized double-blind study. Diabetes Care 1998; 21: 1288–1294.

45. Tan MH. Current treatment of insulin resistance in type 2 diabetes mellitus. Int J Clin Pract Suppl 2000; 113:54–62.

46. Ceriello A. The postprandial state and cardiovascular disease: relevance to diabetes mellitus. Diabetes Metabol Res Rev 2000; 16:125–132.

47. Kelley D, Bray G, Pi-Sunyer FX, Klein S, Hill J, Miles J, Hollander P. Clinical efficacy of orlistat therapy in overweight and obese patients with insulin-treated type 2 diabetes mellitus: a one-year, randomized, controlled trial. Diab Care 2002; 25:1033–1041.

48. Hollander P, Van Gaal L. Orlistat consistently improves glycemic control in patients with type 2 diabetes. Submitted.

49. Hauptman J. The effect of orlistat on glycemic control is independent of weight loss. Submitted.

50. Turner R, Cull C, Holman R. United Kingdom Prospective Diabetes Study. A 9-year update of a randomized controlled trial on the effect of improved metabolic control on complications in non-insulin dependent diabetes mellitus. Ann Intern Med 1996; 124:136–145.

51. Despres JP. The impact of orlistat on the multifactorial risk profile of abdominally obese patients. Diabetes 1999; (suppl 1):A307.

52. Oo CY, Akbari B, Lee S, Nichols G, Hellmann CP. Effect of orlistat, a novel anti-obesity agent, on the pharmacokinetics and pharmacodynamics of prava-

statin in patients with mild hypercholesterolaemia. Clin Drug Invest 1999; 17:217–223.

53. Melia AT, Mulligan TE, Zhi J. Lack of effect of orlistat on the bioavailability of a single dose of nifedipine extended-release tablets (Procardia XL) in healthy volunteers. J Clin Pharmacol 1996; 36:352–355.

54. Melia AT, Mulligan TE, Zhi J. The effect of orlistat on the pharmacokinetics of phenytoin in healthy volunteers. J Clin Pharmacol 1996; 36:654–658.

55. Hartmann D, Guzelhan C, Zuiderwijk PB, Odink J. Lack of interaction between orlistat and oral contraceptives. Eur J Clin Pharmacol 1996; 50:421–424.

56. Melia AT, Zhi J, Zelasko R, Hartmann D, Guzelhan C, Guerciolini R, Odink J. The interaction of the lipase inhibitor orlistat with ethanol in healthy volunteers. Eur J Clin Pharmacol 1998; 54:773–777.

57. Berchtold P, Kiesselbach NHK. The clinical significance of the alpha-amylase inhibitors Bay d 7791 and Bay e 4609. In: Berchtold P, Cairella M, Jacobelli A, Silano V, eds. Regulators of Intestinal Absorption in Obesity, Diabetes and Nutrition. Proceedings of Satellite Symposium No. 7: Third International Congress on Obesity. Siena, Italy: Oct 13–15, 1980. Vol. I. Rome: Societa Editrice Universo, 1998:181–200.

58. Garrow JS, Scott PF, Heels S, Nair KS, Halliday D. A study of 'starch blockers' in man using ^{13}C-enriched starch as a tracer. Hum Nutr Clin Nutr 1983; 37:301–305.

59. Hillebrand I, Boehme K, Frank G, Fink H, Berchtold P. The effects of the alpha-glucosidase inhibitor BAY g 5421 (acarbose) on meal-stimulated elevations of circulating glucose, insulin, and triglyceride levels in man. Res Exp Med (Berl) 1979; 175:81–86.

60. Hillebrand I, Boehme K, Frank G, Fink H, Berchtold P. The effects of the alpha-glucosidase inhibitor BAY g 5421 (acarbose) on postprandial blood glucose, serum insulin, and triglyceride levels: dose-time-response relationships in man. Res Exp Med (Berl) 1979; 175: 87–94.

61. Puls W, Keup U, Krause HP, Thomas G. Pharmacological significance of glucosidase inhibitors (acarbose). In: Berchtold P, Cairella M, Jacobelli A, Silano V, eds. Regulators of Intestinal Absorption in Obesity, Diabetes and Nutrition. Proceedings of Satellite Symposium No. 7: Third International Congress on Obesity. Siena, Italy: October 13–15, 1980, Rome: Societa Editrice Universo, 1981; 1:231–260.

62. Goto Y, Yamada K, Ohyama T, Matsuo T, Odaka H, Ikeda H. An alpha-glucosidase inhibitor, AO-128, retards carbohydrate absorption in rats and humans. Diabetes Res Clin Pract 1995; 28:81–87.

63. Ikeda H, Odaka H. AO-128, alpha-glucosidase inhibitor: antiobesity and antidiabetic actions in genetically obese diabetic rats, Wistar family. Obes Res 1995; 3 (suppl 4):617S–621S.

64. Kobatake T, Matsuzawa Y, Tokunaga K, Fujioka S, Kawamoto T, Keno Y, Inui Y, Odaka H, Matsuo T, Tarui S. Metabolic improvements associated with a reduction of abdominal visceral fat caused by a new alpha-glucosidase inhibitor, AO-128, in Zucker fatty rats. Int J Obes 1989; 13:147–154.

65. William-Olsson T. Alpha-glucosidase inhibition in obesity. Acta Med Scand Suppl 1985; 706:1–39.

66. Wolever TM, Chiasson JL, Josse RG, Hunt JA, Palmason C, Rodger NW, Ross SA, Ryan EA, Tan MH. Small weight loss on long-term acarbose therapy with no change in dietary pattern or nutrient intake of individuals with non-insulin-dependent diabetes. Int J Obes Relat Metab Disord 1997; 21:756–763.

67. Van Gaal L, Maislos M, Schernthaner G, Rybka J, Segal P. Miglitol combined with metformin improves glycaemic control in type 2 diabetes. Diabetes Obes Metab 2001; 3:326–331.

68. Rolls BJ, Pirraglia PA, Jones MB, Peters JC. Effects of olestra, a noncaloric fat substitute, on daily energy and fat intakes in lean men. Am J Clin Nutr 1992; 56:84–92.

69. Cotton JR, Burley VJ, Weststrate JA, Blundell JE. Fat substitution and food intake: effect of replacing fat with sucrose polyester at lunch or evening meals. Br J Nutr 1996; 75:545–556.

70. Cotton JR, Weststrate JA, Blundell JE. Replacement of dietary fat with sucrose polyester: effects on energy intake and appetite control in nonobese males. Am J Clin Nutr 1996; 63:891–896.

71. Hill JO, Seagle HM, Johnson SL, Smith S, Reed GW, Tran ZV, Cooper D, Stone M, Peters JC. Effects of 14d of covert subsitution of olestra for conventional fat on spontaneous food intake. Am J Clin Nutr 1998; 67: 1178–1185.

72. Bray GA, Sparti A, Windhauser MM, York DA. Effects of two weeks fat replacement by olestra on food intake and energy metabolism. FASEB J 1995; 9:A439.

73. Roy HJ, Most MM, Sparti A, Lovejoy JC, Volaufova J, Peters JC, Bray GA. Effect on body weight of replacing dietary fat with olestra for two or ten weeks in healthy men and women. J Am Coll Nutr 2002; 21:259–267.

74. Bray GA, Lovejoy JC, Most-Windhauser M, Smith SR, Volaufova J, Denkins Y, De Jonge L, Roos J, Lefevre M, Eldridge AL, Peters JC. A nine-month randomized clinical trial comparing a fat-substituted and fat-reduced diet in healthy obese men: the Ole Study. Am J Clin Nutr 2002; 76:928–934.

75. Daughaday WH. Growth hormone, insulin-like growth factors, and acromegaly. In: DeGroot LJ, Besser M, Burger HG, Jameson JL, Loriaux DL, Marshall JC, Odell WC, Potts JT, Rubenstein AH, eds. Endocrinology, 3rd ed. Philadelphia: W.B. Saunders, 1995:303–329.

76. Veldhuis JD, Liem AY, South S, Weltman A, Weltman J, Clemmons DA, Abbott R, Mulligan T, Johnson ML, Pincus S, Straume M, Iranmanesh A. Differential impact of age, sex steroid hormones, and obesity on basal versus pulsatile growth hormone secretion in men as

assessed in an ultrasensitive chemiluminescence assay. J Clin Endocrinol 1995; 80:3209–3222.

77. Gertner JM. Effects of growth hormone on body fat in adults. Horm Res 1993; 40:10–15.

78. Gertner JM. Growth hormone actions on fat distribution and metabolism. Horm Res 1992; 38(suppl 2):41–43.

79. Bray GA. Calorigenic effect of human growth hormone in obesity. J Clin Endocrinol Metab 1969; 29:119–122.

80. Bray GA, Raben MS, Londono J, Gallagher TF Jr. Effects of triiodothyronine, growth hormone and anabolic steroids on nitrogen excretion and oxygen consumption of obese patients. J Clin Endocrinol Metab 1971; 33:293–300.

81. Felig P, Marliss EB, Cahill GF Jr. Metabolic response to human growth hormone during prolonged starvation. J Clin Invest 1971; 50:411–421.

82. Bengtsson BA, Eden S, Lonn L, Kvist H, Stokland A, Lindstedt G, Bosaeus I, Tolli J, Sjostrom L, Isaksson OG. Treatment of adults with growth hormone (GH) deficiency with recombinant human GH. J Clin Endocrinol Metab 1993; 76:309–317.

83. Brummer RJ, Lonn L, Kvist H, Grandgard U, Bengtsson BA, Sjostrom L. Adipose tissue and muscle volume determination by computed tomography in acromegaly, before and 1 year after adenomectomy. Eur J Clin Invest 1993; 23:199–205.

84. Clemmons DR, Snyder DK, Williams R, Underwood LE. Growth hormone administration conserves lean body mass during dietary restriction in obese subjects. J Clin Endocrinol Metab 1987; 64:878–883.

85. Snyder DK, Clemmons DR, Underwood LE. Treatment of obese, diet-restricted subjects with growth hormone for 11 weeks: effects on anabolism, lipolysis, and body composition. J Clin Endocrinol Metab 1988; 67:54–61.

86. Snyder DK, Clemmons DR, Underwood LE. Dietary carbohydrate content determines responsiveness to growth hormone in energy-restricted humans. J Clin Endocrinol Metab 1989; 69:745–752.

87. Snyder DK, Underwood LE, Clemmons DR. Anabolic effects of growth hormone in obese diet-restricted subjects are dose dependent. Am J Clin Nutr 1990; 52:431–437.

88. Richelsen B, Pederson SB, Borglum JD, Moller-Pedersen T, Jorgensen J, Jorgensen JO. Growth hormone treatment of obese women for 5 wk: effect on body composition and adipose tissue LPL activity. Am J Physiol 1994; 266:E211–E216.

89. Jorgensen JO, Pedersen SB, Borglum J, Moller N, Schmitz O, Christiansen JS, Richelsen B. Fuel metabolism, energy expenditure, and thyroid function in growth hormone–treated obese women: a double-blind placebo-controlled study. Metabolism 1994; 43:872–877.

90. Snyder DK, Underwood LE, Clemmons DR. Persis-

tent lipolytic effect of exogenous growth hormone during caloric restriction. Am J Med 1995; 98:129–134.

91. Drent ML, Wever LD, Ader HJ, Van der Veen EA. Growth hormone administration in addition to a very low calorie diet and an exercise program in obese subjects. Eur J Endocrinol 1995; 132:565–572.

92. Johannsson G, Marin P, Lonn L, Ottosson M, Stenlof K, Bjorntorp P, Sjostrom L, Bengtsson BA. Growth hormone treatment of abdominally obese men reduces abdominal fat mass, improves glucose and lipoprotein metabolism, and reduces diastolic blood pressure. J Clin Endocrinol Metab 1997; 82:727–734.

93. Karlsson C, Stenlof K, Johannsson G, Marin P, Bjorntorp P, Bengtsson BA, Carlsson B, Carlsson LM, Sjostrom L. Effects of growth hormone treatment on the leptin system and on energy expenditure in abdominally obese men. Eur J Endocrinol 1998; 138:408–414.

94. Thompson JL, Butterfield GE, Gylfadottir UK, Yesavage J, Marcus R, Hintz RL, Pearman A, Hoffman AR. Effects of human growth hormone, insulin like growth factor, and diet and exercise on body composition of obese postmenopausal women. J Clin Endocrinol Metab 1998; 83:1477–1484.

95. McAlpine LG, McAlpine CH, Waclawski ER, Storer AM, Kay JW, Frier BM. A comparison of treatment with metformin and gliclazide in patients with non-insulin-dependent diabetes. Eur J Clin Pharmacol 1988; 34:129–132.

96. Josephkutty S, Potter JM. Comparison of tolbutamide and metformin in elderly diabetic patients. Diabetes Med 1990; 7:510–514.

97. Campbell IW, Menzies DG, Chalmers J, McBain AM, Brown IR. One year comparative trial of metformin and glipizide in type 2 diabetes mellitus. Diabetes Metab 1994; 20:394–400.

98. Fontbonne A, Charles MA, Juhan-Vague I, Bard JM, Andre P, Isnard F, Cohen JM, Grandmottet P, Vague P, Safar ME, Eschwege E. The effect of metformin on the metabolic abnormalities associated with upper-body fat distribution. BIGPRO Study Group. Diabetes Care 1996; 19:920–926.

99. Scheen AJ, Letiexhe MR, Lefebvre PJ. Short administration of metformin improves insulin sensitivity in android obese subjects with impaired glucose tolerance. Diabetes Med 1995; 12:985–989.

100. Lee A, Morley JE. Metformin decreases food consumption and induces weight loss in subjects with obesity with type II non-insulin-dependent diabetes. Obes Res 1998; 6:47–53.

101. Knowler WC, Barrett-Connor E, Fowler SE, Hamman RF, Lachin JM, Walker EA, Nathan DM. Reduction in the incidence of type 2 diabetes with lifestyle intervention or metformin. N Engl J Med 2002; 346:393–403.

102. Lutjens A, Smit JL. Effect of biguanide treatment in obese children. Helv Paediatr Acta 1977; 31:473–480.

103. Sullivan AC, Triscari J, Hamilton JG, Miller ON. Effect of (-)-hydroxycitrate upon the accumulation of lipid in the rat. II. Appetite. Lipids 1974; 9:129–134.

104. Hellerstein MK, Xie Y. The indirect pathway of hepatic glycogen synthesis and reduction of food intake by metabolic inhibitors. Life Sci 1993; 53:1833–1845.

105. Thom E. Hydroxycitrate in the treatment of obesity. Int J Obes Relat Metab Disord 1996; 20(suppl 4):75.

106. Heymsfield SB, Allison DB, Vasselli JR, Pietrobelli A, Greenfield D, Nunez C. Garcinia cambogia (hydroxycitric acid) as a potential antiobesity agent: a randomized controlled trial. JAMA 1998; 280:1596–1600.

107. Lijesen GK, Theeuwen I, Assendelft WJ, Van der Wal G. The effect of human chorionic gonadotropin (HCG) in the treatment of obesity by means of the Simeons therapy: a criteria-based meta-analysis. Br J Clin Pharmacol 1995; 40:237–243.

108. Greenway FL, Bray GA. Human chorionic gonadotropin (HCG) in the treatment of obesity: a critical assessment of the Simeons method. West J Med 1977; 127:461–463.

109. Carne S. The action of chorionic gonadotrophin in the obese. Lancet 1961; ii:1282–1284.

110. Craig LS, Ray RE, Waxler SH, Madigan H. Chorionic gonadotropin in the treatment of obese women. Am J Clin Nutr 1963; 12:230–234.

111. Frank BW. The use of chorionic gonadotropin hormone in the treatment of obesity. A double-blind study. Am J Clin Nutr 1964; 14:133–136.

112. Lebon P. Treatment of overweight patients with chorionic gonadotropin: follow-up study. J Am Geriatr Soc 1966; 14:116–125.

113. Asher WL, Harper HW. Effect of human chorionic gonadotrophin on weight loss, hunger and feeling of well-being. Am J Clin Nutr 1973; 26:211–218.

114. Stein MR, Julis RE, Peck CC, Hinshaw W, Sawicki JF, Deller JJ Jr. Ineffectiveness of human chorionic gonadotropin in weight reduction: a double-blind study. Am J Clin Nutr 1976; 29:940–948.

115. Shetty KR, Kalkhoff RK. Human chorionic gonadotropin (HCG) treatment of obesity. Arch Intern Med 1977; 137:151–155.

116. Bosch B, Venter I, Stewart RI, Bertram SR. Human chorionic gonadotrophin and weight loss. A double-blind, placebo-controlled trial. S Afr Med J 1990; 77:185–189.

117. Young RL, Fuchs RJ, Woltjen MJ. Chorionic gonadotropin in weight control. A double-blind crossover study. JAMA 1976; 236:2495–2497.

118. Miller R, Schneiderman LJ. A clinical study of the use of human chorionic gonadotropin in weight reduction. J Fam Pract 1977; 4:445–448.

119. Svec F, Porter JR. The actions of exogenous dehydroepiandrosterone in experimental animals and humans. Proc Soc Exp Biol Med 1998; 218:174–191.

120. Williams DP, Boyden TW, Pamenter RW, Lohman TG, Going SB. Relationship of body fat percentage and fat distribution with dehydroepiandrosterone sulfate in premenopausal females. J Clin Endocrinol Metab 1993; 77:80–85.

121. Clore JN. Dehydroepiandrosterone and body fat. Obes Res 1995; 3(suppl 4):613S–616S.

122. Lardy H, Kneer N, Wei Y, Partridge B, Marwah P. Ergosteroids. II. Biologically active metabolites and synthetic derivatives of dehydroepiandrosterone. Steroids 1998; 63:158–165.

123. Nestler JE, Barlascini CO, Clore JN, Blackard WG. Dehydroepiandrosterone reduces serum low density lipoprotein levels and body fat but does not alter insulin sensitivity in normal men. J Clin Endocrinol Metab 1998; 66:57–61.

124. Welle S, Jozefowicz R, Statt M. Failure of dehydroepiandrosterone to influence energy and protein metabolism in humans. J Clin Endocrinol Metab 1990; 71:1259–1264.

125. Usiskin KS, Butterworth S, Clore JN, Arad Y, Ginsberg HN, Blackard WG, Nestler JE. Lack of effect of dehydroepiandrosterone in obese men. Int J Obes 1990; 14:457–463.

126. Mortola JF, Yen SS. The effects of oral dehydroepiandrosterone on endocrine-metabolic parameters in postmenopausal women. J Clin Endocrinol Metab 1990; 71:696–704.

127. Zumoff B, Strain GW, Heymsfield SB, Lichtman S. A randomized double-blind crossover study of the antiobesity effects of etiocholanedione. Obes Res 1994; 2:13–18.

128. Handelsman DJ. Testosterone and other androgens: physiology, pharmacology and therapeutic use. Endocrinology 1995; 3:2351–2361.

129. Evans DJ, Hoffmann RG, Kalkoff RK, Kissebah AH. Relationship of androgenic activity to body fat topography, fat cell morphology, and metabolic aberrations in premenopausal women. J Clin Endocrinol Metab 1983; 57:304–310.

130. Seidell JC, Bjorntorp P, Sjostrom L, Sannerstedt R, Krotkiewski M, Kvist H. Regional distribution of muscle and fat mass in men—new insight into the risk of abdominal obesity using computed tomography. Int J Obes 1989; 13:289–303.

131. Tchernof A, Labrie F, Belanger A, Prud'homme D, Bouchard C, Tremblay A, Nadeau A, Despres JP. Androstane-3-α,17-β-diol glucuronide as a steroid correlate of visceral obesity in men. J Clin Endocrinol Metab 1997; 82:1528–1534.

132. Marin P, Holmang S, Jonsson L, Sjostrom L, Kvist H, Holm G, Lindstedt G, Bjorntorp P. The effects of testosterone treatment on body composition and metabolism in middle-aged obese men. Int J Obes Relat Metab Disord 1992; 16:991–997.

133. Marin P, Holmang S, Gustafsson C, Jonsson L, Kvist H, Elander A, Eldh J, Sjostrom L, Holm G, Bjorntorp

P. Androgen treatment of abdominally obese men. Obes Res 1993; 1:245–251.

134. Marin P. Testosterone and regional fat distribution. Obes Res 1995; 3(suppl 4):609S–612S.

135. Lovejoy JC, Bray GA, Breeson CS, Klemperer M, Morris J, Partington C, Tulley R. Oral anabolic steroid treatment, but not parenteral androgen treatment, decreases abdominal fat in obese, older men. Int J Obes Relat Metab Disord 1995; 19:614–624.

136. Lovejoy JC, Bray GA, Bourgeois MO, Macchiavelli R, Rood JC, Greeson C, Partington C. Exogenous andro-

gens influence body composition and regional body fat distribution in obese postmenopausal women—a clinical research center study. J Clin Endocrinol Metab 1996; 81:2198–2203.

137. Drent ML, Van der Veen EA. First clinical studies with orlistat: a short review. Obes Res 1995; 3:S623–S625.

138. Rossner S, Sjostrom L, Noack R, Meinders AE, Noseda G. Weight loss, weight maintenance, and improved cardiovascular risk factors after 2 years treatment with orlistat for obesity. European Orlistat Obesity Study Group. Obes Res 2000; 8:49–61.

14

Leptin: From Laboratory to Clinic

José F. Caro

Lilly Research Laboratories, Eli Lilly and Company, Indianapolis, Indiana, U.S.A.

Robert V. Considine

Indiana University School of Medicine, Indianapolis, Indiana, U.S.A.

I INTRODUCTION

Body weight and body composition in humans are determined by the complex interaction of genetic, environmental, behavioral, and social factors. The central nervous system, primarily through hypothalamic centers, is responsible for integrating the input of these various factors to maintain a reasonably stable body weight. For the hypothalamic centers to maintain body weight efficiently, information concerning the amount of energy intake, energy expenditure, and energy stores would be needed. The adipose tissue hormone leptin provides a signal to the central nervous system of energy intake and energy stored in the body as adipose tissue. For this reason leptin has been viewed, since its discovery, as a potential therapuetic agent that could be used to regulate body weight and treat obesity. Although leptin is very effective in regulating body weight in rodent models, results in human studies have been mixed. Despite this, the study of leptin biology has provided novel insights into the mechanisms through which body weight is regulated.

A Leptin Is Predicted by the Lipostasis Theory

Kennedy (1) first articulated the existence of a leptinlike satiety factor in the lipostasis theory. He proposed that a peripheral signal is produced in proportion to the amount of adipose tissue in the body. This signal would then be compared to a "setpoint" by the appropriate brain area(s), including but not limited to the hypothalamus, and changes in energy intake (food consumption) and energy expenditure (physical activity, thermogenesis) initiated to maintain the energy stores in the adipose tissue at the predetermined amount. Compelling evidence in support of the lipostasis theory prior to the discovery of leptin was obtained from parabiosis of lean and obese animals. Hervey (2) observed that the parabiotic union of a normal weight rat with an obese rat, made so by lesion of the ventromedial hypothalamus, resulted in hypophagia and weight loss in the normal-weight animal. Hervey interpreted this finding to suggest that the unlesioned animal was responding to an increased serum concentration of a "satiety signal" from the obese animal. In contrast, Coleman (3) found that the union of the genetically obese *ob/ob* mouse with a wild-type lean animal led to a reduction in appetite and weight loss in the obese mouse. This experiment suggested that the *ob/ob* mouse was obese because it lacked an adipose related "satiety factor," which was provided by the lean mouse. Parabiosis of an *ob/ob* mouse with a *db/db* obese mouse resulted in weight loss and death by starvation of the *ob/ob* mouse. This finding provided further evidence that the *ob/ob* mouse lacked an adipose signal that was supplied in even greater quantities by the obese *db/db* mouse than a lean mouse. Furthermore, it appeared that the obesity of the *db/db* mouse resulted from a defect similar to that in rats with ventromedial lesions, i.e., the central nervous system could not respond to the satiety signal (3).

The observation that obesity resulted from a heritable defect in *ob/ob* and *db/db* mice, which appeared to involve the signalling components hypothesized in the lipostasis theory, prompted a molecular genetics approach to find the defective genes that resulted in obesity in these mice. The subsequent discovery of the *Lep* gene (originally termed *ob* gene) and its protein product leptin by Friedman and colleagues in 1994 (4) identified the circulating factor predicted in the lipostasis theory. The discovery shortly thereafter that the *db* gene encoded a receptor for leptin that was primarily expressed in the brain (5–7) completed the identification of the major components of the signal pathway originally hypothesized by Kennedy (1) as a means for the adipose tissue to communicate with the central nervous system.

B Leptin and the Leptin Receptor

The gene for leptin in both humans (*LEP*) and rodents (*Lep*) encodes a 167 amino acid protein with an amino terminal secretory signal sequence of 21 amino acids (4). The signal sequence is cleaved during protein processing and leptin circulates in the blood as a 16-kDa protein (Fig. 1) (8). Leptin release from the adipocyte appears to follow a constituitive secretory pathway as a significant number of leptin-containing granules have not been detected within the adipocyte. However, observations from two studies suggest that a small amount of leptin may be stored in the adipocyte since insulin can acutely (within minutes) increase leptin release (9,10). In these studies insulin appears to increase the rate of transport of leptin-containing granules from the endoplasmic reticulum to the plasma membrane. In vivo, insulin has not been shown to acutely stimulate leptin release. Therefore, leptin synthesis and release from adipocytes appears to be primarily regulated by transcriptional mechanisms as most studies in vivo and in vitro find that changes in leptin release are associated with parallel changes in the amount of *Lep* gene expression (11).

The leptin receptor is a member of the class I cytokine receptor family (12). These cytokine receptors do not possess endogenous kinase activity within the intracellular domain but instead associate with a janus kinase (JAK). Binding of leptin to its receptor activates JAK, which phosphorylates tyrosines within the leptin receptor itself. JAK also phosphorylates signal transducer

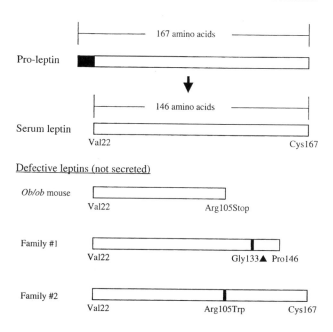

Figure 1 Stucture of leptin and defective leptin proteins. The gene for leptin in both humans and rodents encodes a 167–amino acid protein with an amino terminal secretory signal sequence of 21 amino acids (4). The signal sequence is cleaved during protein processing and leptin circulates in the blood as a 16 kDa protein. In C57BL/6J *ob/ob* mice a T to C substitution in the first position of codon 105 changes an arginine to a premature stop codon. Two families with mutations in the *LEP* gene have been identified. In family No. 1, a guanine nucleotide in codon 133 is deleted, which results in a frameshift and the synthesis of a truncated leptin protein (91). In the second family a C to T substitution in the first base of codon 105 changes arginine to tryptophan (92). The mutant leptin protein in the *ob/ob* mouse and in both families is not secreted but is degraded in the adipocyte.

and activator of transcription (STAT) proteins associated with the leptin receptor. The STAT proteins then dimerize and translocate to the nucleus to initiate gene transcription. STAT-3 is the major STAT protein activated by the hypothalamic leptin receptor in mice (13). The leptin receptor has also been observed to initiate JAK-dependent signaling to other pathways including MAP kinase in transfected cell lines, but the relevance of this pathway to leptin action is not yet understood (14).

In addition to the hypothalamic leptin receptor (Ob-Rb or long receptor isoform) described above, five other leptin receptor isoforms have been identified (Ob-Ra, Ob-Rc, Ob-Rd, Ob-Re, Ob-Rf), all of which are encoded by alternative splicing of the same gene (7,15). The extracellular domain of each of these receptors is identical to Ob-Rb; however, the intracellular domains terminate at different lengths (Fig. 2). Owing to the

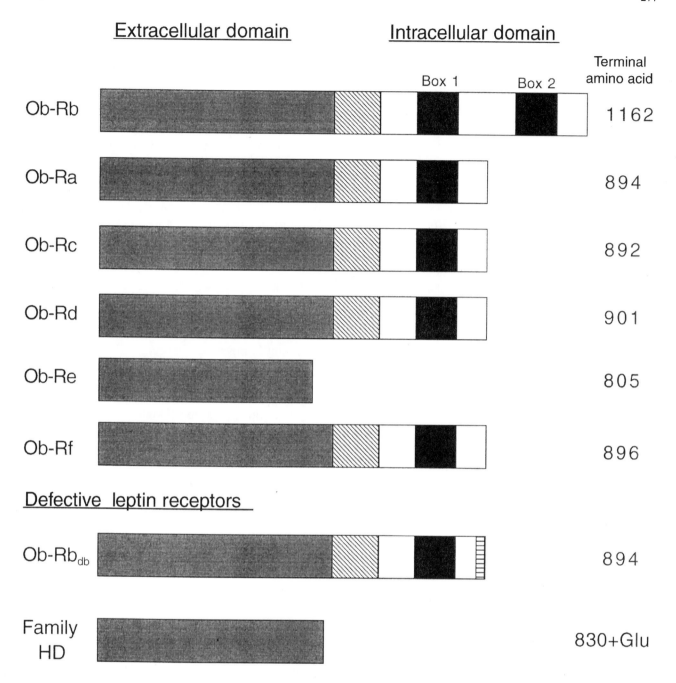

Figure 2 Structure of the leptin receptor isoforms. All isoforms share an identical extracellular leptin-binding domain (12,15). Ob-Rb contains both a box 1 sequence for JAK association and a box 2 motif for STAT protein binding. The remaining receptors lack the STAT protein association sequence. Ob-Re lacks the transmembrane domain (denoted by the hatched box) and is released to the circulation to act as a leptin-binding protein (19,20). Ob-Rb in *db/db* mice lacks the STAT interaction site and does not activate JAK/STAT signalling (6,7). A mutation in the leptin receptor gene in a human family (HD) results in a truncated leptin receptor that acts as binding protein in the serum (93).

truncated intracellular domain, these short leptin receptors lack the Box 2 motif at which STAT proteins bind and these leptin receptors do not activate STAT signaling. The short receptor isoform Ob-Ra, present in most cells and tissues examined, activates JAK2 and MAPK in transient transfection models, but the physiologic significance of this observation is not yet known (14). Ob-Ra is highly expressed in the choroid plexus, where it functions to transport leptin across the blood/cerebrospinal fluid barrier (5,16–18).

The Ob-Re receptor isoform lacks both the intracellular and transmembrane domain and circulates in the blood as a leptin binding protein (19,20). This leptin-binding protein functions like other binding proteins to prolong the half-life of the hormone (21). Increased Ob-Re synthesis by the placenta, resulting in a longer half-life for leptin, has been suggested to explain the greater serum leptin in pregnant mice (22). An increase in soluble leptin receptor during pregnancy has been observed in women with type 1 diabetes, but there was no significant change in serum Ob-Re in the nondiabetic controls in this study (23).

C   Mutations in the Leptin and Leptin Receptor Genes Cause Obesity in Rodents

Two separate mutations in the *Lep* gene that block the synthesis of leptin have been identified in *ob/ob* mice (4). In C57BL/6J *ob/ob* mice a T to C substitution in the first position of codon 105 changes an arginine to a premature stop codon (Fig. 1). In *ob²ʲ/ob²ʲ* mice no mRNA is synthesized owing to the insertion of a transposon in the first intron of the gene (24). Both strains of mice lack circulating leptin. *Ob/ob* mice are hyperphagic, cold intolerant, and morbidly obese. No *Lep* gene mutations resulting in defective leptin synthesis or release have been reported in other animals.

In C57BL/KsJ *db/db* mice a point mutation in the hypothalamic leptin receptor has been identified (6,7). As discussed above, differential splicing of the leptin receptor message yields the long and short forms of the leptin receptor. In *db/db* mice, a G to T substitution generates a new splice donor within the exon of the shorter receptor. This new splice donor competes with the upstream splice donor of the long form of the receptor for the same downstream splice acceptor. This alternative splicing of the receptor coding region adds the first 106 bp of the short-form exon and a premature termination signal to the long form of the receptor (Fig. 2). This defect in the message for the leptin receptor results in synthesis of a truncated long receptor which in unable to activate STAT proteins (25). The inability of the long receptor to signal after leptin binding is the cause of obesity in *db/db* mice. Two other mutations have been identified in *db^{Pas}/db^{Pas}* and *db^{3J}/db^{3J}* mice that result in receptors lacking transmembrane and cytoplasmic domains (26).

In the Zucker *fatty* (*fa/fa*) rat an A to C substitution at nucleotide 880 in the leptin receptor changes glutamine-269 to a proline (27,28). This mutation reduces the amount of leptin receptor on the cell surface and the capacity of the receptor to signal (28,29). In obese Koletsky rats, no leptin receptor mRNA is detectable in the brain due to a point mutation (T2349A) in codon 763 which creates a premature stop codon just before the transmembrane domain (30,31). The lack of functional leptin receptors results in obesity in both Zucker and Koletsky rats.

D   Leptin Causes Weight Loss in Mice

Shortly following the discovery of leptin the ability of the hormone to cause weight loss was demonstrated in mice. Daily intraperitoneal injection of leptin in C57BL/6J *ob/ob* mice resulted in a dose- and time-dependent decrease in body weight (32–37). Leptin also reduced body weight in C57BL/6J heterozygotes (+/?) and wild-type mice, although at much higher doses (32–34). No weight loss was induced by leptin in C57BL/6J *db/db* mice at any concentration tested (33–35,37). Leptin-induced weight loss in *ob/ob* mice resulted from an increase in oxygen consumption, body temperature, and locomotor activity, as well as a reduction in food intake (32). In lean mice leptin had no effect on body temperature or locomoter activity but did reduce food intake. Leptin treatment also lowered insulin and glucose in *ob/ob* mice, a finding discussed in greater detail below (32,36). Early experiments also demonstrated that the hypothalamus was the major site through which leptin acted to regulate body weight since administration of leptin directly into the lateral or third ventricle was sufficient to inhibit food intake in both obese and lean mice (34). Since these initial experiments, many investigators have observed that leptin, administered either peripherally or centrally, effectively reduces food intake to stimulate weight loss in most animal models of obesity with the exception of those with inactivating leptin receptor mutations.

II   PHYSIOLOGY OF LEPTIN IN HUMANS

A   Determinants of Serum Leptin

1   Adiposity and Gender

The primary determinant of serum leptin under conditions of consistent food intake is the amount of body fat. Leptin is highly correlated with fat mass in adults (38,39), children (40–43), and newborns (44–46). As such, serum leptin is elevated in obesity (Fig. 3) and significantly reduced in lipodystrophic states (38–47). The elevation in serum leptin in obesity appears to result from both increased fat mass and an increased leptin release from larger adipocytes in obese subjects. *LEP* gene expression is greater in larger adipocytes than in smaller adipocytes isolated from the same piece of adipose tissue (48), and leptin secretion is strongly correlated with fat cell volume (49).

Serum leptin is significantly greater in women than in men with equivalent body fat mass (50,51). One explanation for this finding is that women have a significantly greater subcutaneous adipose tissue mass relative to omental adipose mass than men (52). Studies using adipose tissue obtained from females have observed that *LEP* gene expression/leptin production is greater in subcutaneous than omental adipocytes from the same individual (53–55). In markedly obese subjects the subcutaneous adipocytes of females are significantly larger than omental adipocytes in the same subject (56, 57). Cell size may therefore explain in part the greater leptin production in subcutaneous versus omental adipose tissue and the gender effect on serum leptin.

Reproductive hormones also influence leptin production. Testosterone therapy reduces serum leptin in hypogonadal men, and leptin levels decrease as serum testosterone increases during pubertal development in boys (58–60). Estrogen, in combination with antiandrogens, increases leptin in male-to-female transsexuals,

and testosterone decreases leptin in female-to-male transsexuals, independent of changes in adipose tissue mass (61). In vitro, estradiol stimulates, and dihydrotestosterone inhibits, leptin production in human omental adipose tissue pieces cultured for 48 hr (62,63). Although these in vitro experiments suggest that the reproductive hormones exert direct effects on leptin synthesis, the mechanism is not yet elucidated.

Changes in the amount of adipose tissue alter leptin mRNA levels in the adipocyte and the circulating concentration of the hormone. A decrease in adipose tissue with weight loss results in a decrease in leptin. An increase in the adipose tissue with weight gain significantly increases circulating leptin (26,64). The mechanism for changes in leptin with weight change likely involves both changes in adipose tissue mass as well as adipocyte size.

2 Nutrition

Caloric intake influences serum leptin independently of changes in adipose tissue mass. However, with regular daily food intake (three meals per day in humans), leptin levels are fairly constant, exhibiting a maximal daily variation of ~30% (65). Several studies in vivo and in vitro suggest that glucose and insulin are the signal linking energy intake and leptin synthesis in the adipocyte.

Serum leptin falls with short-term fasting (24 hr) and will increase within 4–5 hr of refeeding. Maintenance of euglycemia prevents the fasting-induced drop in leptin, implicating insulin or glucose as the nutritional signal that is recognized by the adipocyte for leptin synthesis (66,67). In a prolonged study of energy restriction (moderate and severe), changes in serum leptin were best correlated with changes in glycemia (68).

The diurnal profile in serum leptin is entrained to food intake. The peak in serum leptin occurs at ~0200 hr both lean and obese subjects under normal living conditions. Day/night reversal shifts the peak in serum leptin by 12 hr. A meal shift of 6.5 hr without changing light or sleep cycles shifts the leptin peak 5–7 hr, suggesting that the nocturnal rise in leptin may represent a delayed postprandial response induced by the after meal excusions in glucose and insulin (69).

The macronutrient content of the diet can also influence serum leptin. Consumption of high-fat/low-carbohydrate meals (60%/20%) over the course of 1 day reduces leptin levels (70). High-fat/low-carbohydrate meals induce smaller insulin and glucose excursions than meals of standard fat/carbohydrate content, again implicating insulin and glucose in the nutritional regulation of leptin production.

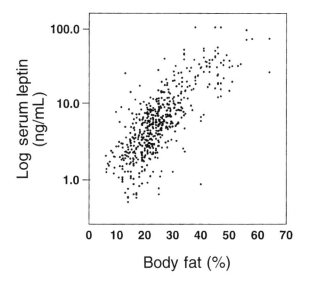

Figure 3 Relation between percent body fat and serum leptin in adults. (From Ref. 64.)

Direct evidence that glucose and insulin regulate leptin production has been obtained with euglycemic-hyperinsulinemic clamp techniques. Serum leptin is elevated by the end of prolonged (9-hr) euglycemic-hyperinsulinemic clamps at physiologic insulin (71) or within 4–8 hr with supraphysiologic insulin concentrations (72). In cultured rat adipocytes leptin release is highly dependent on the extent of glucose metabolism (73,74).

Hexosamine biosynthesis is one link between glucose metabolism and leptin production (75). Approximately 1–3% of glucose taken into the cell enters the hexosamine biosynthetic pathway. The endproduct of the pathway, UDP-N-acetylglucosamine (UDP-GlcNAc), is utilized in O-linked glycosylation reactions that modify several proteins including transcription factors (76). In rodents, infusion of glucosamine, uridine, or free fatty acids during a 3-hr euglycemic hyperinsulinemic clamp increased tissue UDP-GlcNAc, muscle *Lep* gene expression, and serum leptin compared to saline-infused controls clamped under identical conditions (77). In transgenic mice overexpressing glutamine:fructose-6-phosphate amidotransferase (GFAT), the rate-limiting enzyme in hexosamine biosynthesis, serum leptin, and adipose tissue *Lep* gene expression is significantly increased (78).

UDP-GlcNAc in the subcutaneous adipose tissue of obese humans is elevated 3.2-fold compared to lean subjects and a significant positive relationship between adipose tissue UDP-GlcNAc and BMI is present (79). In cultured subcutaneous adipocytes an increase in hexosamine biosynthesis increased leptin release to the medium and inhibition of GFAT activity reduced glucose-stimulated leptin release. These observations suggest that hexosamine biosynthesis may be the link glucose metabolism to leptin production. However, these findings do not rule out the possibility that other pathways for glucose metabolism, including ATP synthesis (80), may also regulate leptin release.

3 Sympathetic Nervous System

The sympathetic nervous system can influence adipose tissue metabolism through direct innervation of the tissue or by the release of catecholamines from the adrenal. To mimic activation of the sympathetic nervous system, several groups have infused isoproterenol and observed a significant reduction in serum leptin (81–83). These observations are in agreement with animal data that catecholamines inhibit leptin production (84–87), although the mechanism through which this occurs has not been elucidated. In vitro, catecholamines inhibit leptin production from 3T3-L1 cells (88) and cultured human adipose tissue pieces (89).

B Mutations in Leptin and the Leptin Receptor in Humans

Mutations in the *LEP* gene have been found in two families (Fig. 1). The first two cases were identified in children of a consanguineous Pakastani family (90). In these subjects a guanine nucleotide in codon 133 is deleted, which results in a frameshift and the synthesis of a truncated leptin protein. The truncated protein is degraded by the proteosome and not released into the blood (91). The lack of circulating leptin in these children resulted in hyperphagia and extreme early-onset morbid obesity; however, as discussed below, leptin therapy has been very successful in these patients. A second *LEP* gene mutation was identified in a Turkish family (92). In these three subjects a C to T substitution in the first base of codon 105 changes arginine to tryptophan. In the *ob/ob* mouse this same mutation results in a premature STOP codon (4). Serum leptin was very low but detectable in all three subjects homozygous for the mutation. No leptin was synthesized in COS-1 cells expressing the mutant gene. The lack of leptin in these subjects results in hyperphagia, morbid obesity, and hypogonadism. One subject also exhibited low sympathetic tone.

As with mutations in the *LEP* gene, mutations in the leptin receptor in humans are rare. A G to A substitution in the splice donor site of exon 16 has been identified in three sisters of a Kabilian family (93). This mutation results in a truncated leptin receptor that lacks the transmembrane and intracellular domains (Fig. 2). The mutant extracellular domain circulates in the blood at high concentrations and acts as a leptin binding protein greatly elevating serum leptin concentrations (94). As observed with leptin gene mutations, this leptin receptor mutation results in early-onset morbid obesity, hyperphagia, and hypothalamic hypogonadism. The inability of leptin to prevent the morbid obesity in these individuals suggests that they are "leptin resistant."

C Leptin Resistance

As discussed above, inactivating mutations in the human leptin and leptin receptor gene are rare and not the cause of obesity in the general population. Rather, it has been observed that serum leptin levels are elevated in obese subjects (Fig. 3). This observation has led to the hypothesis, based on the tenets of the lipostasis theory, that obese individuals are resistant to the weight-reducing actions of leptin (64). Leptin resistance, as defined by the lipostasis theory, is dependent on the premise that the major function of leptin is to oppose changes in body weight and that leptin is equally effective in altering metabolism to oppose both weight loss and weight gain. From an evolutionary perspective, it is difficult to conceive of a mechanism that would limit food intake in times of excess. Flier and colleagues (95,96) have therefore hypothesized that the major function of leptin is to signal the reduction in energy intake associated with fasting rather than the excess storage of energy in times of food abundance. The reduction in leptin with fasting is associated with metabolic, hormonal, and behavioral changes designed to conserve energy and increase energy intake. Administration of leptin to prevent the fasting-induced fall in endogenous hormone levels prevents the adaptations to food restriction, thus implicating leptin as the signal of food deprivation (97). The concept of leptin resistance is compatible with the role of leptin as a signal of energy deprivation. It is possible that the central nervous system in obese individuals does not properly receive or process the leptin signal generated by the adipose tissue, despite the elevated serum leptin levels. This would result in metabolic adaptations to conserve energy and increase energy intake. It is therefore useful to examine the leptin signal pathway for defects other than those in leptin or its receptor that would impair leptin signalling.

The leptin endocrine pathway is illustrated in Figure 4. In the first step leptin is released from the adipose tissue. As previously discussed, defects in the human leptin gene that impair leptin synthesis or secretion are rare. In the general population leptin gene expression is positively correlated with the amount of adipose tissue (39). *LEP* transcription and leptin secretion by the adipose tissue increase with weight gain and decrease with weight loss (38,39,97,98). These observations indicate that a major defect in leptin production in the adipose tissue is unlikely to be the cause of obesity in humans. However, it is important to note that leptin levels lower than would be predicted by the amount of body weight have been associated with greater weight gain at follow-up in Pima Indians (99). This finding suggests that low leptin levels signal for increased energy intake in humans. Although some individuals from cross-sectional examinations of the population have been observed to have disproportionately low leptin (Fig. 3), a finding of low serum leptin following the overnight fast appears to be the exception rather than the rule. In contrast, the synthesis and release of leptin from the adipose tissue in response to a specific

stimulus has not been examined in great detail. It is possible that insufficient leptin release from the adipose tissue—for example, as observed in response to a high fat meal (70)—could result in weight gain. Further studies are needed to fully address this point.

Leptin circulates in the blood in association with several binding proteins, one of which is the extracellular domain of the leptin receptor Ob-Re (19,20,94). Ob-Re acts in a traditional manner to prolong the half-life of leptin (21,94). Most of the leptin in the blood of lean subjects is bound. In contrast, there is much more free leptin in the circulation of obese subjects. The amount of binding protein appears to be similar in lean and obese subjects, so the greater leptin production in obese subjects results in more free leptin in this population (19). In the case of most hormones, the "free" hormone is biologically active. It is therefore unlikely that leptin binding proteins impair leptin action in obese subjects. Neutralizing leptin antibodies, an additional possible defect in obese humans, have not been reported.

Leptin is cleared from the circulation by the kidney (100,101). There is no difference in the rate of clearance of leptin in lean and obese subjects indicating that circulating leptin is determined by its rate of synthesis. Serum leptin is elevated in end-stage renal disease (101,102).

Prior to leptin binding to its receptor in the hypothalamus, it must first gain access to the brain. To do this the hormone must cross the blood brain barrier from the circulation to the cerebrospinal fluid either by transcytosis or through the median eminence in which the capillaries lack tight junctions. Banks et al. (103) originally demonstrated that ^{125}I-labeled leptin is transported across the blood brain barrier in rodents by a saturable system. Leptin reached the brain intact and the entry rate was comparable to other factors of similar size. The transport of leptin across the blood brain barrier is facilitated by the Ob-Ra leptin receptor isoform (104), and human brain microvessels actively bind and internalize leptin in vitro (17).

Intact leptin is detectable in human cerebrospinal fluid (CSF) by Western blot (105), and the amount of leptin in the CSF is positively correlated with BMI (105,106). The ratio of CSF to serum leptin decreases with increasing BMI indicating that leptin transport into the CSF in humans is limited (105,106). CSF leptin is proportional to serum leptin up to a serum concentration of ~20 ng/mL, above which further increases in serum leptin do not directly increase CSF leptin. Limited transport of leptin into the CSF may impair leptin action in extremely obese subjects; however, it is unlikely to be an initiating cause of the obesity. Saturation

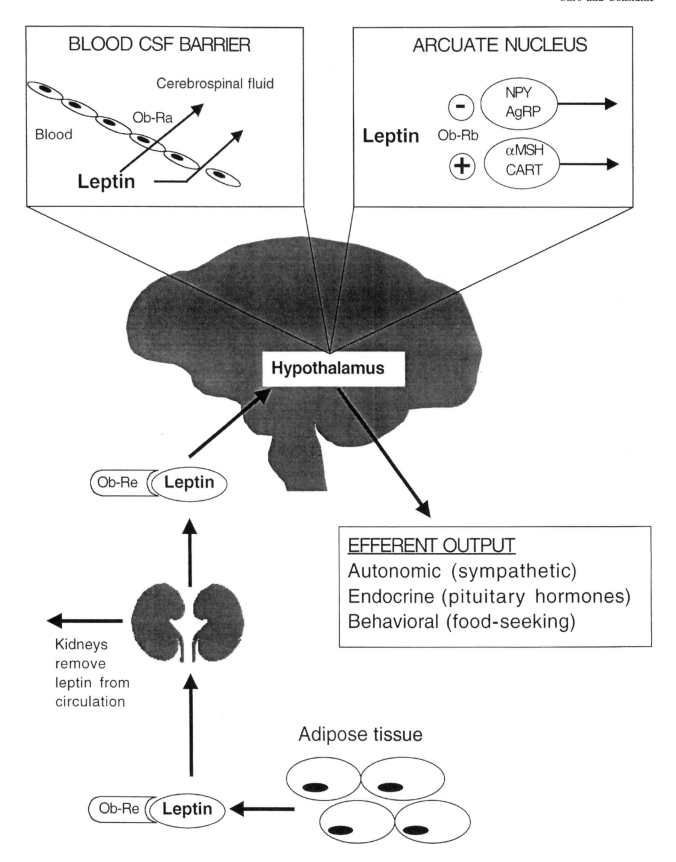

of leptin transport occurs at a serum concentration of ~ 20 ng/mL, which is three times greater than the average for lean subjects. Therefore, moderate increases in leptin that would occur as weight was gained should have access to the hypothalamus and signal the weight gain prior to the development of obesity. Interestingly, high-fat diets have been shown to decrease the effectiveness of peripherally injected leptin to induce weight loss and the defect appears to involve access of leptin to the brain (107,108). This implies that defective leptin transport into the brain, induced by diet, could contribute to the development of obesity in humans. Further work is needed to resolve this issue.

The leptin receptor is detectable in several areas of the CNS but is highly expressed in the arcuate, paraventricular, ventromedial, and dorsomedial nuclei of the hypothalamus (109). Leptin likely accesses the arcuate nucleus directly from the blood within the median eminence, which lacks the tight junctions characteristic of the blood brain barrier. Leptin binding to its receptor in the arcuate nucleus reduces the expression of neuropeptides that stimulate food intake and increases expression of neuropeptides that inhibit feeding. As such, leptin suppresses neuropeptide Y (NPY) and agouti-related peptide (AgRP) expression in one type of neuron and induces the expression of alpha melanocyte-stimulating hormone (α-MSH) and cocaine- and amphetamine-regulated transcript (CART) in a second set of neurons (109). These neurons innervate several other nuclei within the hypothalamus and also communicate with other areas of the brain (110). These leptin responsive neurons in the arcuate also mediate the effects of leptin on the sympathetic nervous system and hypothalamic pituitary axes.

Suppressors of cytokine signalling (SOCS) are a group of early genes activated by the JAK/STAT signal transduction pathway. The SOCS proteins are inhibitors of cytokine signaling which act in a negative feedback loop to limit cytokine signaling (111). SOCS-3 is a potent inhibitor of leptin receptor initiated JAK/

STAT signaling in cultured cell lines, and leptin induces SOCS-3 mRNA in the hypothalamus (112). Interestingly, SOCS-3 message is increased in leptin-responsive hypothalamic neurons in Agouti mice. Agouti mice are resistant to central leptin administration suggesting that the increased SOCS-3 expression could cause leptin resistance in these animals (112). Furtherwork will be needed to fully understand the importance of this observation and its relevance to obesity in humans.

III LEPTIN THERAPY IN HUMANS

The administration of leptin to obese humans has clearly demonstrated two points: (1) leptin is an important hormone in the regulation of body weight. Congenital leptin deficiency is characterized by early childhood obesity, which is markedly improved by low amounts of daily injectable leptin. (2) Human obesity is characterized by leptin resistance. Large amounts of leptin, injected daily to treat common obesity, results in a variable and only modest decrease in body weight

A Recombinant Leptin Therapy in a Child with Congenital Leptin Deficiency

As described above, O'Rahilly's laboratory identified two cousins with severe, early-onset obesity and undetectable serum leptin concentrations that were homozygous for a frameshift mutation in the leptin gene (90). The older of these children, a 9-year-old girl, was the first patient to be treated with recombinant human leptin (113).

The patient had normal weight at birth but began gaining weight excessively at about 4 months of age. She had marked hyperphagia, and was disruptive when denied food. As a result of her severe obesity, valgus deformities of the legs developed, for which she required bilateral proximal tibial osteotomies.

Figure 4 The leptin signal pathway. Leptin is secreted from the adipocytes through constitutive pathways and circulates in the blood in association with binding proteins including the extracellular domain of the leptin receptor Ob-Re (19,20,94). Leptin is cleared from the circulation by the kidneys (100,101). Leptin accesses its receptor in the hypothalamus through a saturable transport system across the epithelium of the blood brain barrier (103,104). Leptin also reaches the hypothalamus via diffusion through the more porous capillary epithelium within the median eminence (109). First-order neurons that respond to leptin binding are of two types. Neurons containing neuropeptide Y (NPY) and agouti-related peptide (AgRP) stimulate feeding and are inhibited by leptin binding. Neurons expressing alpha melanocyte stimulating hormone (α-MSH) and cocaine- and amphetamine-regulated transcript (CART) inhibit feeding and are activated by leptin binding (CART) (110). Efferent output resulting from leptin binding in the hypothalamus is mediated by the autonomic nervous system, pituitary hormones, and behavioral changes (160).

The patient was treated with recombinant methionyl leptin, administered subcutaneously once daily at 8AM, in a dose of 0.028 mg/kg lean mass, for 12 months. The dose was calculated to achieve a peak serum leptin concentration equivalent to 10% of the child's predicted normal serum leptin concentration (70 ng/mL), calculated on the basis of age, sex, and body composition. At baseline and every 2 months thereafter, her height was measured and her body composition determined by dual-energy x-ray absorptiometry. Spontaneous energy intake was measured with the use of a standardized test meal and the amount of food consumed was measured covertly. The patient's sleeping metabolic rate was measured by whole-body indirect calorimetry, and her basal metabolic rate was estimated as the sleeping metabolic rate × 1.05. The patient's total energy expenditure was measured with the use of doubly labeled water ($^2H^{18}O$) at baseline and at 6 and 12 months. The physical-activity level was calculated as the patient's total energy expenditure divided by her basal metabolic rate.

At baseline the patient weighed 94.4 kg (>99.9th centile for age) and her height (140 cm) was at the 91st centile (Fig. 5A). On clinical examination, the patient was prepubertal and had no evidence of acanthosis nigricans; her temperature and blood pressure were normal. The patient lost weight within 2 weeks after the initiation of leptin treatment. Weight loss continued over the 12-month period of treatment, during which she lost a total of 16.4 kg at a rate of approximately

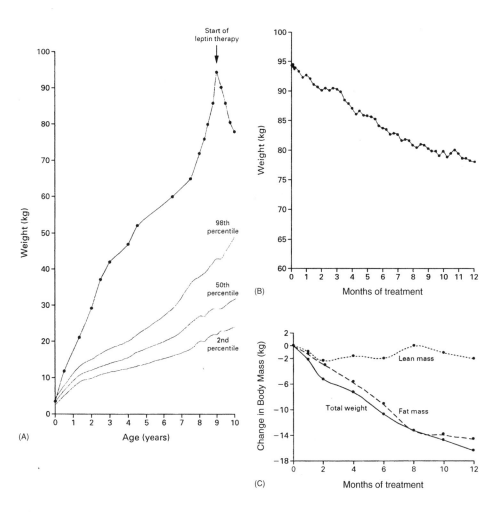

Figure 5 Weight in the first patient with congenital leptin deficiency before and in response to leptin treatment. Panel A shows the changes in weight from birth to the age of 10 years and the 2nd, 50th, and 98th centiles for weight among girls. Panel B shows the weight during leptin treatment. Panel C shows the changes in body composition during treatment. (From Ref. 113.)

1–2 kg per month (Fig. 5B). The injections of leptin were well tolerated with no systemic or local reactions.

At baseline, 59% of the patient's body weight was fat. After 12 months of leptin treatment, the amount of body fat decreased by 15.6 kg. At baseline, the patient rapidly consumed almost all of the test meal. Within seven days after the initiation of leptin treatment, a marked change in the patient's eating behavior was reported by her mother and observed by the investigating physician.

At baseline, the patient's basal metabolic rate and total energy expenditure were higher, in absolute terms, than those of a typical 9-year-old girl weighing 28 kg. However, when expressed per unit lean mass, both her basal metabolic rate and her total energy expenditure were the same as the expected values (both for the patient and for a normal 9-year-old girl). In response to leptin treatment, the patient's basal metabolic rate decreased progressively to 1500 kcal/d at 12 months. At 6 months, her total energy expenditure had decreased by 10% to 2650 kcal/d, but by 12 months it had returned to near the baseline value. Her physical-activity level increased from 1.6 at baseline to 1.9 at 12 months, which is consistent with the observed improvement in her mobility.

At baseline, the patient was normoglycemic but had high plasma insulin and nonesterified fatty acid concentrations while fasting. Her serum cholesterol and triglyceride concentrations were normal. Following 12 months of treatment, nonesterified fatty acids were reduced to just above the normal range. The patient's serum concentrations of estradiol, follicle-stimulating hormone, and luteinizing hormone were consistent with her prepubertal status at baseline. After 12 months of leptin treatment, the nocturnal pattern of gonadotropin secretion was pulsatile, which is consistent with early puberty.

The clinical features of congenital leptin deficiency, as previously described in this patient and her cousin, are marked hyperphagia, excessive weight gain in early life, and severe obesity (113). Although there are no normative data for a child of this weight, there was no evidence of substantial impairment in her basal or total energy expenditure. Thus, leptin may be less central to the regulation of energy expenditure in humans than in mice. A further difference between *ob/ob* mice and all humans reported to have either leptin or leptin-receptor mutations thus far relates to the consistently normal glucocorticoid concentrations in humans, in contrast to the marked excess in *ob/ob* mice (113).

Recombinant leptin treatment of this 9-year-old patient with congenital leptin deficiency led to a sus-tained reduction in weight, predominantly as a result of a loss of fat. The chief effect of leptin on energy balance was through its suppressive effects on food intake. The patient's total energy expenditure was similar before and after 12 months of leptin therapy. Thus, the therapeutic effects of leptin were largely attributable to changes in energy intake.

In summary, the therapeutic response to leptin in this child with leptin deficiency confirms the importance of leptin in the regulation of body weight in humans and establishes an important role for this hormone in the regulation of appetite.

B Recombinant Leptin Therapy in Obese Adults Without Leptin Deficiency

Serum concentrations of leptin increase in parallel with body fat in every obese person who does not have a mutation in the leptin gene. This apparent "resistance" to the weight-reducing effects of endogenously produced leptin could mean that exogenous leptin administration would be ineffective in decreasing body weight. However, it has been demonstrated in a randomized, double-blind, placebo-controlled, escalating-dose cohort trial in lean and obese adult subjects that exogenously administered recombinant human leptin can induce modest weight loss (114).

Leptin therapy was tested by monitoring body weight and composition changes among 54 lean and 73 obese, predominantly white men and women with a mean age of 39 years. Subjects were randomly assigned to escalating dose groups (0.01, 0.03, 0.10, or 0.30 mg/kg) of recombinant methionyl human leptin (rL) (Amgen Inc., Thousand Oaks, CA) or matching placebo. Recombinant methionyl human leptin was self-administered by daily morning subcutaneous injection. The study was conducted in two parts. Both lean and obese subjects participated in Part A, which lasted for 4 weeks. Obese subjects then continued with treatment for an additional 20 weeks in Part B of the study. Lean subjects consumed a eucaloric diet to maintain body weight at the current value and obese subjects were prescribed a diet that reduced their daily energy intake by 500 kcal/d from the amount needed to maintain a stable weight.

At the conclusion of Part A (4 weeks' treatment), absolute weight changes across the doses studied averaged between −0.4 and −1.9 kg (Fig. 6). At the conclusion of Part B (24 weeks' treatment), absolute weight changes across the doses studied averaged between −0.7 and −7.1 kg with greatest average weight loss in the highest-dose cohort (Fig. 6). There were statistically significant dose responses for weight loss from baseline

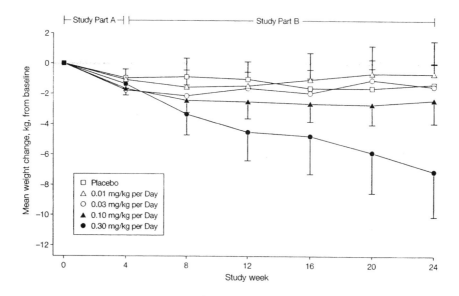

Figure 6 Pattern of weight change from baseline to week 24 in obese subjects who received recombinant methionyl human leptin (From Ref. 114). Date presented as the mean SEM. The number of subjects is not constant over the course of the study.

among those who completed 4 weeks of treatment (53 lean and 70 obese subjects, $P = .02$) and 24 weeks of treatment (47 obese subjects, $P = 0.01$). Obese subjects treated with the highest doses of rL (0.1 and 0.3 mg/kg) had lower mean energy intake than subjects treated with placebo at week 4 and at week 24 ($P = .09$ for both comparisons). Injection site reactions mild (86%) to moderate (14%) in severity were the most common adverse events are reported. None of the subjects taking rL experienced clinically significant adverse effects on major organ systems. There were no effects of rL on glycemic control or insulin action, as evidenced by serum insulin and glucose profiles obtained during oral glucose tolerance tests.

These data show that a dose-response relationship between weight loss and leptin exists both after 4 weeks of exposure to recombinant leptin in lean and obese subjects and after 24 weeks of exposure in obese subjects. Although there was considerable variability in the amount of weight lost by individual subjects, on average weight loss increased with rL dose (114). These findings demonstrate that an absolute leptin resistance does not exist in obese individuals with elevated endogenous leptin levels; however, there is relative leptin resistance with increasing adiposity. This resistance to exogenous leptin was not due to an inability of the hormone to access the brain. Fujioka et al. (115) observed that administration of recombinant methionyl human leptin resulted in greater CSF leptin concentra-

tions than in the placebo-treated controls. Although only six subjects were studied, a linear correlation between serum leptin and CSF leptin concentration was observed. The observations of Fujioka et al. (115) are consistent with data from an unusual lean patient who had a serum leptin of 700 ng/mL and a CSF value of 1.1 ng/mL. CSF leptin in this patient is predictable from the relationship between serum and CSF leptin reported by Fujioka et al. (115). It is therefore reasonable that higher doses of exogenous leptin may be required to increase the CSF leptin concentration and provide a sufficient signal for weight loss in subjects with greater adiposity (114).

In a separate study, Hukshorn et al. (116) presented data from a clinical trial designed to assess the safety of pegylated recombinant native human leptin (PEG-OB). Pegylation, the covalent linkage of proteins to amphiphilic polymers of ethylene glycol (PEG), results in increased serum half-life and reduced immunogenicity for several proteins, including leptin. Pegylated leptin was studied in 30 obese men randomized to a double-blind treatment with either subcutaneous injections of 20 mg PEG-OB, or placebo, in addition to a hypocaloric diet (500 kcal less than the daily requirement) for 12 weeks. PEG-OB was well tolerated and safe, with no adverse events observed. PEG-OB treatment produced significant suppression of appetite, as measured by eating/hunger questionnaires and a significant correlation of weight loss with percent change in serum triglycerides. No significant changes in body weight or metabolic parameters were observed, but circulating leptin levels in the actively treated group were not significantly elevated, with the exception of only two time points over the 12-week study period. The power of this study to assess changes of body weight was clearly suboptimal. Thus, it remains possible that increasing the dose and/or changing the dose schedule to achieve significantly higher circulating leptin levels in future larger trials of PEG-OB could result in significant reductions of body fat and body weight and potentially greater changes in metabolic parameters.

The results of the above studies in obese adults led Mantzoros and Flier (117) to pose several intriguing questions that need to be addressed by well-designed studies in the future. Although all leptin-deficient subjects are expected to respond dramatically to administration of low leptin doses, "leptin-resistant" obese subjects required higher doses, and their responses were highly variable. Could markers be developed to predict the response to leptin treatment? Would leptin treatment of obese subjects be more effective if the caloric restriction accompanying leptin administration had been higher? Could leptin treatment play a role in the long-term maintenance of weight loss achieved by other means? Finally, how do these initial data regarding leptin's efficacy compare with that of currently approved medications for long-term treatment of obesity? As reviewed by Mantzoros and Flier (117), administration of the highest dose of met-leptin resulted in a weight reduction to approximately 6% below the levels achieved by the placebo-treated group (114). Administration of the long-acting pegylated leptin analog decreased body weight by ~2% below the levels achieved by the placebo-treated group (116). By comparison, treatment with either orlistat or sibutramine for 24 weeks resulted in a decrease in body weight of 3–3.6% and 5–6% beyond that of the placebo-treated group, respectively (118). As for any other chronic disease, drug therapy for obesity needs to be administered continuously over a prolonged period of time, therefore, not only efficacy, but also safety, tolerability, and compliance are issues of paramount importance that need to be assessed in future long-term cost effectiveness and cost efficacy studies (117).

IV EFFECT OF LEPTIN ON OTHER PHYSIOLOGICAL PROCESSES

In addition to its role in body weight regulation, leptin has been implicated as a regulatory signal in a variety of other physiological processes. Many of these functions of leptin are mediated through the central nervous system; however, the presence of leptin receptors on numerous nonneural cells (12,26) suggests that leptin may have direct effects on these cells and tissues.

A Leptin and Metabolism

Leptin improves insulin sensitivity directly and independently of its effects on food intake and body weight. In rodents, insulin and glucose are reduced shortly after the initiation of leptin treatment, before significant reductions in body fat content are observed (32–34). With long-term leptin administration, insulin and glucose are reduced to a greater extent than in pair-fed controls (32,37). In acute infusion studies, increasing serum leptin 70-fold over basal increased whole-body glucose uptake 30% during the last 135 min of a 180-min hyperinsulinemic clamp in normal-weight rats (119). In mice, a 5-hr intravenous leptin infusion increased glucose uptake and glucose turnover and intracerebroventricular administration of leptin (5 ng/hr for 5 hr) also enhanced whole-body glucose uptake (120). This latter observation suggests that leptin influences insulin sensitivity through central mechanisms. Interestingly, leptin treatment reverses insulin resistance and diabetes in two different transgenic models of lipodystrophy through mechanisms not related to food intake (121,122).

Leptin may influence insulin action directly on target tissues but conflicting reports exist. Leptin has been reported to block insulin-stimulated phosphorylation of IRS-1 in cultured HepG2 cells (123) and inhibit glucose uptake in isolated rat adipocytes (124). However, in other studies no effect of leptin on basal or insulin-stimulated glucose uptake in rodent adipocytes and skeletal muscle, or human skeletal muscle was observed (125–127). In contrast, leptin increases basal glucose uptake in C_2C_{12} myotubes (128) and cultured human adipocytes (129). Finally, a recent report suggests that leptin activates STAT3 and MAPK in insulin target tissues within 3 min of intravenous administration (130). Future work will be necessary to determine the nature and extent of the overlap between the insulin and leptin signaling pathways in the insulin target tissues.

In the two leptin trials in humans reported to date (114,116), no effect of leptin on insulin or glucose metabolism was detected. However, preliminary reports suggest that leptin may be beneficial in lipodystrophic humans (131).

Leptin increases lipolysis in white adipose tissue both in vivo and vitro (132–134). This effect of leptin results from both centrally mediated activation of the sympathetic nervous system as well as a direct effect of leptin on adipocytes. Lipolysis induced by hyperleptinemia in rats in vivo does not result in the release of free fatty acids into the circulation (134). Evidence suggests that leptin stimulates the oxidation of fatty acids within adipocytes (135). This phenomenon has not been examined in human adipocytes to date.

B Leptin and Reproduction

Leptin functions in several different capacities during reproduction. In its role as a signal of energy stores, leptin appears to coordinate the onset of pubertal development and fertility. Leptin treatment reverses the infertilily of *ob/ob* mice (136,137) and accelerates the onset of puberty by several days in normal mice (138). Leptin prevents the starvation-induced reduction in reproductive capacity in mice by maintaining LH release and estrous cycle periodicity (96). Leptin also appears to have direct effects on ovarian steroidogenesis (139). Nocturnal leptin levels increase just prior to the nocturnal prepubertal increase in LH secretion in monkeys (140). In humans, leptin levels increase with pubertal development in both girls and boys (40–43,60) and the age of menarche in females is inversely related to serum leptin concentration (141). In boys, leptin levels rise 50% over the prepubertal baseline just before the onset of puberty (defined as the initial rise in testosterone above the limit of detection of the assay) (60). Leptin levels then decline in boys as testosterone levels rise (41–43,60). As discussed above, humans with leptin gene defects have hypothalamic hypogonadism and remain prepubertal. Gonadotropin secretion is stimulated in these patients with leptin treatment (113). Taken together, these data suggest that leptin is a coordinating signal to the central nervous system that energy stores are sufficient to support the higher energy needs associated with reproduction.

Serum leptin increases during pregnancy in both rodents (22) and humans (142–145), and this increase is not due solely to the increase in fat mass. Human placenta synthesizes leptin and appears to contribute to the rise in maternal leptin levels during pregnancy (44,145,146). Leptin does not appear to be produced by rodent placenta to any significant extent (147–149) However, murine placenta efficiently synthesizes and secretes Ob-Re, the soluble form of the leptin receptor, which acts to elevate serum leptin levels in mice (22). The role of increased leptin during pregnancy is not known. It is possible that the increase in leptin might regulate maternal-fetal energy metabolism or that leptin may act in a paracrine/autocrine manner on placental or fetal growth.

C Leptin, Bone, and Hematopoiesis

Leptin receptors are present on blast cells, promyelocytes, promonocytes, macrophages, and other bone marrow cells (150–152). Leptin stimulates proliferation of hematopoietic cell lines transfected to express leptin receptor (151–154). Leptin also stimulates proliferation of primative hematopoietic progenitors from murine bone marrow and induces granulocyte-macrophage colony formation in vitro (155). Leptin prevents the starvation-induced reduction in immune function in mice and stimulates the proliferation of naive and memory T-cells (156). Human bone marrow adipocytes differentiated in vitro synthesize and secrete leptin (157), indicating that leptin produced in the marrow could act in a paracrine fashion to regulate hematopoiesis.

In addition to effects on bone marrow, it has recently been discovered that leptin inhibits bone formation in mice (158). This effect of leptin is not mediated through a direct effect on osteoblasts or osteoclasts but by central pathways activated by leptin binding to its receptor in the hypothalamus. The significance of this finding to leptin physiology in humans has not yet been established.

V CONCLUSIONS

The discovery of leptin by Friedman's laboratory in 1994 (4) raised the hopes of millions of people that there was a simple solution to cure obesity. However, the dream of such a solution for this "complex disease" was met by a harsher reality a few months later with the first evidence of leptin resistance in human obesity (159). The fact that leptin plays a paramount role in the regulation of body weight in humans is without debate following the demonstration that mutations in the leptin gene result in early childhood obesity and that replacement of leptin to near physiologic concentrations results in dramatic weight loss in these subjects (90,113). Further, the concept of leptin resistance, defined as a pathophysiologic state where a given amount of leptin results in less than the expected biologic response, has been proven by the study of Heymsfield et al. (114). Administration of leptin, raising the plasma concentration more than 20-fold greater than the physiologic concentration, resulted in only a modest and variable weight loss in this study. Clearly, leptin resistance cannot be directly equated with insulin resistance since every patient with type 2 diabetes would have a precipitous decrease in plasma glucose concentration by raising insulin concentration more than 20-fold over its physiological levels.

That leptin can access the brain by both saturable and nonsaturable transport systems and yet patients are insensitive to supraphysiologic leptin concentrations, suggests that it is unlikely that leptin analogs of any kind, small or large molecules, would become the magic bullet many expected from the discovery of the hormone. Alternatively, leptin sensitivity enhancers that improve postleptin receptor mechanism(s) might provide the desirable therapeutic effects. It should be realized, however, that it took several decades to discover insulin sensitivity enhancers even though the extent of insulin resistance in type 2 diabetes appears to be less severe than leptin resistance in obesity. A leptin sensitivity enhancer would deceive the hypothalamus into believing that the body has a greater fat mass than it actually does. Thus, a leptin sensitivity enhancer would trigger a compensatory mechanism to lose weight. It is more difficult to predict, however, how long the hypothalamus would remain fooled by the leptin sensitivity enhancer. Because of the many overlapping pathways involved in body weight regulation, the adaptable brain might make the regrettable decision to render the entire leptin pathway ineffective. In addition, successful treatment of the obese individual without intervention in the environment, which is at least half responsible for the disease, will prove to be very difficult. Alternatively, future studies may show leptin useful in the treatment of other conditions such as insulin resistance or infertility.

ACKNOWLEDGMENTS

Work of the authors mentioned in this review has been supported by grants R01 DK45592 (J.F.C.) and R29 DK51140 (R.V.C.) from the National Institutes of Health and from the American Diabetes Association and Showalter Trust (R.V.C.).

REFERENCES

1. Kennedy GC. The role of depot fat in the hypothalamic control of food intake in the rat. Proc R Soc B 1953; 140:578–592.
2. Hervey GR. The effects of lesions in the hypothalamus in parabiotic rats. J Physiol 1959; 145:336–352.
3. Coleman DL. Obese and diabetes: two mutant genes causing diabetes-obesity syndromes in mice. Diabetologia 1978; 14:141–148.
4. Zhang Y, Proenca R, Maffei M, Barone M, Leopold L, Friedman JM. Positional cloning of the mouse obese gene and its human homologue. Nature 1994; 372:425–432.
5. Tartaglia LA, Dembski M, Weng X, Deng N, Culpepper J, Devos R, Richards GJ, Campfield LA, Clark FT, Deeds J, Muir C, Sanker S, Moriarty A, Moore KJ, Smutko JS, Mays GG, Woolf EA, Selent-Munro C, Tepper RI. Identification and expression cloning of the a leptin receptor. OB-R Cell 1995; 83:1263–1271.
6. Chen H, Charlat O, Tartaglia LA, Woolf EA, Weng X, Ellis SJ, Lakey ND, Culpepper J, Moore KJ, Breitbart RE, Duyk GM, Tepper RI, Morgenstern JP. Evidence that the diabetes gene encodes the leptin receptor: identification of a mutation in the leptin receptor gene in *db/db* mice. Cell 1996; 84:491–495.
7. Lee GH, Proenca R, Montez JM, Carroll KM, Darvishzadeh JG, Lee JI, Friedman JM. Abnormal splicing of the leptin receptor in *diabetic* mice. Nature 1996; 379:632–635.
8. Cohen SL, Halass JL, Friedman JM, Chait BT. Human leptin characterization. Nature 1996; 382:589.
9. Barr VA, Malide D, Zarnowski MJ, Taylor SI, Cushman SW. Insulin stimulates both leptin secretion and production by white adipose tissue. Endocrinology 1997; 138:4463–4472.
10. Bradley RL, Cheatham B. Regulation of ob gene expression and leptin secretion by insulin and dexamethasone in rat adipocytes. Diabetes 1999; 48:272–278.
11. Considine RV. Regulation of leptin production. Rev Endocr Metab Disord 2001; 2:357–363.
12. Tartaglia LA. The leptin receptor. J Biol Chem 1997; 272:6093–6096.
13. Vaisse C, Halaas JL, Horvath CM, Darnell JE Jr, Stoffel M, Friedman JM. Leptin activation of STAT3 in the hypothalamus of wild-type and ob/ob mice but not db/db mice. Nat Genet 1996; 14:95–97.
14. Bjorbaek C, Uotani S, Da Silva B, Flier JS. Divergent signaling capacites of the long and short isoforms of the leptin receptor. J Biol Chem 1997; 272:32686–32695.
15. Wang M-Y, Zhou YT, Newgard CB, Unger RH. A novel leptin receptor isoform in rat. FEBS Lett 1996; 392:87–90.
16. Banks WA, Kastin AJ, Huang W, Jaspan JB, Maness LM. Leptin enters the brain by a saturable system independent of insulin. Peptides 1996; 17:305–311.
17. Golden PL, Maccagnan TJ, Pardridge WM. Human blood-brain barrier leptin receptor. J Clin Invest 1997; 99:14–18.
18. Hileman SM, Tornoe J, Flier JS, Bjorbaek C. Transcellular transport of leptin by the short leptin receptor

isoform ObRa in Madin-Darby canine kidney cells. Endocrinology 2000; 141:1955–1961.

19. Sinha MK, Opentanova I, Ohannesian JP, Kolaczynski JW, Heiman ML, Hale J, Becker GW, Bowsher RR, Stephens TW, Caro JF. Evidence of free and bound leptin in human circulation. Studies in lean and obese subjects and during short-term fasting. J Clin Invest 1996; 98:1277–1282.

20. Houseknecht KL, Mantzoros CS, Kuliawat R, Hadro E, Flier JS, Kahn BB. Evidence for leptin binding to proteins in serum of rodents and humans: modulation with obesity. Diabetes 1996; 45:1638–1643.

21. Huang L, Wang Z, Li C. Modulation of circulating leptin levels by its soluble receptor. J Biol Chem 2001; 276:6343–6349.

22. Gavrilova O, Barr V, Marcus-Samuels B, Reitman M. Hyperleptinemia of pregnancy associated with the appearance of a circulating form of the leptin receptor. J Biol Chem 1997; 272:30546–30551.

23. Lewandowski K, Horn R, O'Callaghan CJ, Dunlop D, Medley GF, O'Hare P, Brabant G. Free leptin, bound leptin, and soluble leptin receptor in normal and diabetic pregnancies. J Clin Endocrinol Metab 1999; 84:300–306.

24. Moon BC, Friedman JM. The molecular basis of the obese mutation in ob^{2j} mice. Genomics 1997; 42:152–156.

25. Ghilardi N, Ziegler S, Wiestner A, Stoffel R, Heim MH, Skoda RC. Defective STAT signaling by the leptin receptor in *diabetic* mice. Proc Natl Acad Sci USA 1996; 93:6231–6235.

26. Friedman JM. Leptin, leptin receptors, and the control of body weight. Nutr Rev 1998; 56:S38–S48.

27. Phillips MS, Liu Q, Hammond HA, Dugan V, Hey PJ, Caskey CT, Hess JF. Leptin receptor missense mutation in the *fatty* Zucker rat. Nat Genet 1996; 13:18–19.

28. Chua SC Jr, White DW, Wu-Peng S, Liu SM, Okada N, Kershaw EE, Chung WK, Power-Kehoe L, Chua M, Tartaglia L, Leibel RL. Phenotype of *fatty* due to Gln269Pro mutation in the leptin receptor (lepr). Diabetes 1996; 45:1141–1143.

29. White DW, Wang DW, Chua SC Jr, Morgenstern JP, Leibel RL. Constituitive and impaired signaling of leptin receptors containing the Gln-Pro extracellular domain mutation. Proc Natl Acad Sci USA 1997; 94:10657–10662.

30. Takaya K, Ogawa Y, Hiraoka J, Hosoda K, Yamori Y, Nakao K, Koletsky RJ. Nonsense mutation of leptin receptor in the obese spontaneously hypertensive Koletsky rat. Nat Genet 1996; 14:130–131.

31. Wu-Peng S, Chua SC Jr, Okada N, Lui SM, Nicolson M, Leibel RL. Phenotype of the obese Koletsky (f) rat due to Tyr763Stop mutation in the extracellular domain of the leptin receptor (Lepr): evidence for deficient plasma to CSF transport of leptin in both the Zucker and Koletsky obese rat. Diabetes 1997; 46:513–518.

32. Pelleymounter MA, Cullen MJ, Baker MB, Hecht R, Winters D, Boone T, Collins F. Effects of the *obese* gene product on body weight regulation in ob/ob mice. Science 1995; 269:540–543.

33. Halaas JL, Gajiwala KS, Maffei M, Cohen SL, Chait BT, Rabinowitz D, Lallone RL, Burley SK, Friedman JM. Weight-reducing effects of the plasma protein encoded by the obese gene. Science 1995; 269:543–546.

34. Campfield LA, Smith FJ, Guisez Y, Devos R, Burn P. Recombinant mouse OB protein: evidence for a periperal signal linking adiposity and central neural networks. Science 1995; 269:546–549.

35. Stephens TW, Basinski M, Bristow PK, Bue-Valleskey JM, Burgett SG, Craft L, Hale J, Hoffmann J, Hsiung HM, Kriauciunas A, MacKellar W, Rosteck PR Jr, Schoner B, Smith D, Tinsley FC, Zhang XY, Heiman M. The role of neuropeptide Y in the antiobesity action of the obese gene product. Nature 1995; 377:530–532.

36. Weigle DS, Bukowski TR, Foster DC, Holderman S, Kramer JM, Lasser G, Lofton-Day CE, Prunkard DE, Raymond C, Kuijper JL. Recombinant ob protein reduces feeding and body weight in the ob/ob mouse. J Clin Invest 1995; 96:2065–2070.

37. Schwartz MW, Baskin DG, Bukowski TR, Kuijper JL, Foster D, Lasser G, Prunkard DE, Porte D Jr, Woods SC, Seeley RJ, Weigle DS. Specificity of leptin action on elevated blood glucose levels and hypothalamic neuropeptide Y gene expression in ob/ob mice. Diabetes 1996; 45:531–535.

38. Maffei M, Halaas J, Ravussin E, Pratley RE, Lee GH, Zhang Y, Fei H, Kim S, Lallone R, Ranganathan S, Kern PA, Friedman JM. Leptin levels in human and rodent: measurement of plasma leptin and ob RNA in obese and weight-reduced subjects. Nat Med 1995; 1:1155–1161.

39. Considine RV, Sinha MK, Heiman ML, Kriauciunas A, Stephens TW, Nyce MR, Ohannesian JP, Marco CC, McKee LJ, Bauer TL, Caro JF. Serum immunoreactive-leptin concentrations in normal-weight and obese humans. N Engl J Med 1996; 334:292–295.

40. Hassink SG, Sheslow DV, De Lancey E, Opentanova I, Considine RV, Caro JE. Serum leptin in children with obesity: relationship to gender and development. Pediatrics 1996; 98:201–203.

41. Garcia-Mayor RV, Andrade MA, Rios M, Lage M, Dieguez C, Casanueva FF. Serum leptin levels in normal children: relationship to age, gender, body mass index, pituitary-gonadal hormones and pubertal stage. J Clin Endocrinol Metab 1997; 82:2849–2855.

42. Blum WF, Englaro P, Hanitsch S, Juul A, Hertel NT, Muller J, Skakkebaek NE, Heiman ML, Birkett M, Attanasio AM, Kiess W, Rascher W. Plasma leptin levels in healthy children and adolescents: dependence

on body mass index, body fat mass, gender, pubertal stage, and testosterone. J Clin Endocrinol Metab 1997; 82:2904–2910.

43. Argente J, Barrios V, Chowen JA, Sinha MK, Considine RV. Leptin plasma levels in healthy Spanish children and adolescents, children with obesity, and adolescents with anorexia nervosa and bulimia nervosa. J Pediatr 1997; 131:833–838.

44. Hassink SG, deLancey E, Sheslow DV, Smith-Kirwin SM, O'Connor DM, Considine RV, Opentanova I, Dostal K, Spear ML, Leef K, Ash M, Spitzer AR, Funanage VL. Placental leptin: an important new growth factor in intrauterine and neonatal development? Pediatrics 1997; 100:e1.

45. Tome MA, Lage M, Camina JP, Garcia-Mayor RV, Dieguez C, Casanueva FF. Sex-based differences in serum leptin concentrations from umbilical cord blood at delivery. Eur J Endocrinol 1997; 137:655–658.

46. Schubring C, Kiess W, Englaro P, Rascher W, Dotsch J, Hanitsch S, Attanasio A, Blum WF. Levels of leptin in maternal serum, amniotic fluid, and arterial and venous cord blood: relation to neonatal and placental weight. J Clin Endocrinol Metab 1997; 82:1480–1483.

47. Hegele RA, Cao H, Huff MW, Anderson CM. LMNA R482Q mutation in partial lipodystrophy associated with reduced plasma leptin concentration. J Clin Endocrinol Metab 2000; 85:3089–3093.

48. Hamilton BS, Paglia D, Kwan AYM, Deitel M. Increased obese mRNA expression in omental fat cells from massively obese humans. Nat Med 1995; 1:953–956.

49. Lonnqvist F, Nordfors L, Jansson M, Thorne A, Schalling M, Arner P. Leptin secretion from adipose tissue of women. Relatioship to plasma levels and gene expression. J Clin Invest 1997; 99:2398–2404.

50. Hickey MS, Israel RG, Gardiner SN, Considine RV, McCammon MR, Tyndall GL, Houmard JA, Marks RHL, Caro JF. Gender differences in serum leptin levels in humans. Biochem Mol Med 1996; 59:1–6.

51. Rosenbaum M, Nicolson M, Hirsch J, Heymsfield SB, Gallagher D, Chu F, Leibel RL. Effects of gender, body composition, and menopause on plasma concentrations of leptin. J Clin Endocrinol Metab 1996; 81:3424–3427.

52. Rosenbaum M, Leibel RL. Role of gonadal steroids in the sexual dimorphisms in body composition and circulating concentrations of leptin. J Clin Endocrinol Metab 1999; 84:1784–1789.

53. Montague CT, Prins JB, Sanders L, Digby J, Orahilly S. Depot and sex specific differences in human leptin mRNA expression. Diabetes 1997; 46:342–347.

54. Lefebvre AM, Laville M, Vega N, Riou JP, van Gaal L, Auwerx J, Vidal H. Depot-specific differences in adipose tissue gene expression in lean and obese subjects. Diabetes 1998; 47:98–103.

55. Van Harmelen V, Reynisdotir S, Eriksson P, Thorne A, Hoffstedt J, Lonnqvist F, Arner P. Leptin secretion from subcutaneous and visceral adipose tissue of women. Diabetes 198; 47:913–917.

56. Fried SK, Kral JG. Sex differences in regional distribution of fat cell size and lipoprotein lipase activity in morbidly obese patients. Int J Obes 1987; 11:129–140.

57. Fried S, Russell CD, Grauso NL, Brolin RE. Lipoprotein lipase regulation by insulin and glucocorticoid in subcutaneous and omental adipose tissues of obese women and men. J Clin Invest 1993; 92:2191–2198.

58. Sih R, Morley JE, Kaiser FE, Perry HMIII, Patrick P, Ross C. Testosterone replacement in older hypogondal men: a 12-month randomized controlled trial. J Clin Endocrinol Metab 1997; 82:1661–1667.

59. Jockenhovel F, Blum WF, Vogel E, Englaro P, Muller-Wieland D, Reinwein D, Rascher W, Krone W. Testosterone substitution normalizes elevated serum leptin levels in hypogonadal men. J Clin Endocrinol Metab 1997; 82:2510–2513.

60. Mantzoros CS, Flier JS, Rogol AD. A longitudinal assessment of hormonal and physical alterations during normal puberty in boys. V. Rising leptin levels may signal the onset of puberty. J Clin Endocrinol Metab 1997; 82:1066–1070.

61. Elbers JM, Asscheman H, Seidell JC, Frolich M, Meinders AE, Gooren LJ. Reversal of the sex difference in serum leptin levels upon cross-sex hormone administration in transsexuals. J Clin Endocrinol Metab 1997; 82:2370–3267.

62. Casabiell X, Pineiro V, Peino R, Lage M, Camina JP, Gallego R, Vallejo LG, Dieguez C, Casanueva FF. Gender differences in both spontaneous and stimulated leptin secretion by human omental adipose tissue in vitro: dexamethasone and estradiol stimulate leptin release in women, but not in men. J Clin Endocrinol Metab 1998; 83:2149–2155.

63. Pineiro V, Casabiell X, Peino R, Lage M, Camina JP, Menendez C, Baltar J, Dieguez C, Casanueva FF. Dihydrotestosterone, stanozol, androstenedione and dehydroepiandrosterone sulphate inhibit leptin secretion in female but not male samples of omental adipose tissue in vitro: lack of effect of testosterone. J Endocrinol 1999; 160:425–432.

64. Caro JF, Sinha MK, Kolaczynski JW, Zhang PL, Considine RV. Leptin: the tale of an obesity gene. Diabetes 1996; 45:1455–1462.

65. Sinha M, Ohannesian JP, Heiman ML, Kriauciunas A, Stephens TW, Magosin S, Marco C, Caro JF. Nocturnal rise of leptin in lean, obese, and non-insulin-dependent diabetes mellitus subjects. J Clin Invest 1996; 97:1344–1347.

66. Kolaczynski JW, Considine RV, Ohannesian J, Marco C, Opentanova I, Nyce MR, Myint M, Caro JF. Responses of leptin to short-term fasting and refeeding

in humans: a link with ketogenesis but not ketones themselves. Diabetes 1996; 45:1511–1515.

67. Boden G, Chen X, Mozzoli M, Ryan I. Effect of fasting on serum leptin in normal human subjects. J Clin Endocrinol Metab 1996; 81:3419–3423.

68. Wisse BE, Campfield LA, Marliss EB, Morais JA, Tenenbaum R, Gougeon R. Effect of prolonged moderate and severe energy restriction and refeeding on plasma leptin concentrations in obese women. Am J Clin Nutr 1999; 70:321–330.

69. Schoeller DA, Cella LK, Sinha MK, Caro JF. Entrainment of the diurnal rhythm of plasma leptin to meal timing. J Clin Invest 1997; 100:1882–1887.

70. Havel PJ, Townsend R, Chaump L, Teff K. High fat meals reduce 24 h circulating leptin concentrations in women. Diabetes 1999; 48:334–341.

71. Saad MF, Khan A, Sharma A, Michael R, Road-Gabriel MG, Boyadjian R, Jinagouda SD, Steil GM, Kamdar V. Physiological insulinemia acutely modulates plasma leptin. Diabetes 1998; 47:544–549.

72. Utriainen T, Malmstrom R, Makimattila S, Yki-Jarvinen H. Supraphysiological hyperinsulinemia increases plasma leptin concentrations after 4 h in normal subjects. Diabetes 1996; 45:1364–1366.

73. Mueller WM, Gregoire FM, Stanhope KL, Mobbs CV, Mizuno TM, Warden CH, Stern JS, Havel PJ. Evidence that glucose metabolism regulates leptin secretion from cultured rat adipocytes. Endocrinology 1998; 139:551–558.

74. Mueller W, Stanhope K, Gregoire FM, Evans JL, Havel PJ. Effects of metformin and vanadium on leptin secretion from cultured rat adipocytes. Obes Res 2000; 8:530–539.

75. Rossetti L. Perspective: hexosamines and nutrient sensing. Endocrinology 2000; 141:1922–1925.

76. Wells L, Vosseller K, Hart GW. Glycosylation of nucleocytoplasmic proteins: signal transduction and O-GlcNAc. Science 2001; 291:2376–2378.

77. Wang J, Liu R, Hawkins M, Barzilai N, Rossetti L. A nutrient-sensing pathway regulates leptin gene expression in muscle and fat. Nature 1998; 393:684–688.

78. McClain DA, Alexander T, Cooksey RC, Considine RV. Hexosamines stimulate leptin production in transgenic mice. Endocrinology 2000; 141:1999–2002.

79. Considine RV, Cooksey RC, Williams LB, Fawcett RL, Zhang P, Ambrosius WT, Whitfield RM, Jones RM, Inman M, Huse J, McClain DA. Hexosamines regulate leptin production in human subcutaneous adipocytes. J Clin Endocrinol Metab 2000; 85:3551–3556.

80. Levy JR, Gyarmati J, Lesko JM, Adler RA, Stevens W. Dual regulation of leptin secretion: intracellular energy and calcium dependence of regulated pathway. Am J Physiol Endocrinol Metab 2000; 278:E892–E901.

81. Donahoo WT, Jensen DR, Yost TJ, Eckel RH. Isoproterenol and somatostatin decrease plasma leptin in

82. Pinkney JH, Coppack SW, Mohamed Ali V. Effect of isoproterenol on plasma leptin and lipolysis in humans. Clin Endocrinol (Oxf) 1998; 48:407–411.

83. Stumvoll M, Fritsche A, Tschritter O, Lehmann R, Wahl HG, Renn W, Haring H. Leptin levels in humans are acutely suppressed by isoproterenol despite acipomox-induced inhibition of lipolysis, but not by free fatty acids. Metabolism 2000; 49:335–339.

84. Slieker LJ, Sloop KW, Surface PL, Kriauciunas A, LaQuier F, Manetta J, Bue-Valleskey J, Stephens TW. Regulation of expression of ob mRNA and protein by glucocorticoids and cAMP. J Biol Chem 1996; 271:5301–5304.

85. Mantzoros CS, Qu D, Frederich RC, Susulic VS, Lowell BB, Maratos-Flier E, Flier JS. Activation of β_3-adrenergic receptors suppresses leptin expression and mediates a leptin-independent inhibition of food intake in mice. Diabetes 1996; 45:909–914.

86. Gettys TW, Harkness PJ, Watson M. The β_3-adrenergic receptor inhibits insulin-stimulated leptin secretion from isolated rat adipocytes. Endocrinology 1996; 137:4054–4057.

87. Collins S, Surwit RS. Pharmacologic manipulation of ob expression in a dietary model of obesity. J Biol Chem 1996; 271:9437–9440.

88. Kosaki A, Yamada K, Kuzuya H. Reduced expression of the leptin gene (ob) by catecholamine through a Gs protein-coupled pathway in 3T3-L1 adipocytes. Diabetes 1996; 45:1744–1749.

89. Ricci MR, Fried SK. Isoproterenol decreases leptin expression in adipose tissue of obese humans. Obes Res 1999; 7:233–240.

90. Montague CT, Farooqi IS, Whitehead JP, Soos MA, Rau H, Wareham NJ, Sewter CP, Digby JE, Mohammed SN, Hurst JA, Cheetham CH, Earley AR, Barnett AH, Prins JB, O'Rahilly S. Congenital leptin deficiency is associated with severe early-onset obesity in humans. Nature 1997; 387:903–908.

91. Rau H, Reaves BJ, O'Rahilly S, Whitehead JP. Truncated human leptin (delta133) associated with extreme obesity undergoes proteasomal degradation after defective intracellular transport. Endocrinology 1999; 140:1718–1723.

92. Strobel A, Issad T, Camoin L, Ozata M, Strosberg AD. A leptin missense mutation associated with hypogonadism and morbid obesity. Nat Genet 1998; 18:213–215.

93. Clement K, Vaisse C, Lahlou N, Cabrol S, Pelloux V, Cassuto D, Gourmelen M, Dina C, Chambaz J, Lacorte JM, Basdevant A, Bougneres P, Lebouc Y, Froguel P, Guy-Grand B. A mutation in the human leptin receptor gene causes obesity and pituitary dysfunction. Nature 1998; 392:398–401.

94. Lahlou N, Clement K, Carel JC, Vaisse C, Lotton C, Le

Bihan Y, Basdevant A, Lebouc Y, Froguel P, Roger M, Guy-Grand B. Soluble leptin receptor in serum of subjects with complete resistance to leptin: relation to fat mass. Diabetes 2000; 49:1347–1352.

95. Ahima RS, Prabakaran D, Mantzoros C, Qu D, Lowell B, Maratos-Flier E, Flier J. Role of leptin in the neuroendocrine response to fasting. Nature 1996; 382:250–252.

96. Flier JS. What's in a name? In search of leptin's physiologic role. J Clin Endocrinol Metab 1998; 83:1407–1413.

97. Wadden TA, Considine RV, Foster GD, Anderson DA, Sarwer DB, Caro JF. Short and long term changes in serum leptin in dieting obese women: Effects of caloric restriction and weight loss. J Clin Endocrinol Metab 1998; 83:214–218.

98. Kolaczynski JW, Ohannesian J, Considine RV, Marco C, Caro JF. Response of leptin to short term and prolonged overfeeding in humans. J Clin Endocrinol Metab 1996; 81:4162–4165.

99. Ravussin E, Pratley RE, Maffei M, Wang H, Friedman JM, Bennett PH, Bogardus C. Relatively low plasma leptin concentrations precede weight gain in Pima Indians. Nat Med 1997; 3:238–240.

100. Klein S, Coppack SW, Mohamed-Ali V, Landt M. Adipose tissue leptin production and plasma leptin kinetics in humans. Diabetes 1996; 45:984–987.

101. Sharma K, Considine RV, Michael R, Dunn SR, Weisberg L, Kurnik P, O'Conner J, Sinha M, Caro JF. Plasma leptin is partly cleared by the kidney and is elevated in hemodialysis patients. Kidney Int 1997; 51:1980–1985.

102. Merabet E, Dagogo-Jack S, Coyne DW, Klein S, Santiago JV, Hmiel SP, Landt M. Increased plasma leptin concentration in end-stage renal disease. J Clin Endocrinol Metab 1997; 82:847–850.

103. Banks WA, Kastin AJ, Huang W, Jaspan JB, Maness LM. Leptin enters the brain by a saturable system independent of insulin. Peptides 1996; 17:305–311.

104. Hileman SM, Tornoe J, Flier JS, Bjorbaek C. Transcellular transport of leptin by the short leptin receptor isoform ObRa in Madin-Darby canine kidney cells. Endocrinology 2000; 141:1955–1961.

105. Caro JF, Kolaczynski JW, Nyce MR, Ohannesian JP, Opentanova I, Goldman WH, Lynn RB, Zhang PL, Sinha MK, Considine RV. Decreased cerebrospinal-fluid serum leptin ratio in obesity: a possible mechanism for leptin resistance. Lancet 1996; 348:159–161.

106. Schwartz MW, Peskind E, Raskind M, Boyko EJ, Porte D Jr. Cerebrospinal fluid leptin levels: relationship to plasma levels and to adiposity in humans. Nat Med 1996; 2:589–593.

107. Van Heek M, Compton DS, France CF, Tedesco RP, Fawzi AB, Graziano MP, Sybertz EJ, Strader CD, Davis HR Jr. Diet-induced obese mice develop peripheral, but not central, resistance to leptin. J Clin Invest 1997; 99:385–390.

108. El-Haschimi K, Pierroz DD, Hileman SM, Bjorbaek C, Flier JS. Two defects contribute to hypothalamic leptin resistance in mice with diet-induced obesity. J Clin Invest 2000; 105:1827–1832.

109. Elmquist JK, Maratos-Flier E, Saper CB, Flier JS. Unraveling the central nervous system pathways underlying responses to leptin. Nat Neurosci 1998; 1:445–450.

110. Elmquist JK, Elias CR, Saper CB. From lesions to leptin: hypothalamic control of food intake and body weight. Neuron 1999; 22:221–232.

111. Chen XP, Losman JA, Rothman P. SOCS proteins, regulators of intracellular signalling. Immunity 2000; 13:287–290.

112. Bjorbaek C, Elmquist JK, Frantz JD, Shoelson SE, Flier JS. Identification of SOCS-3 as a potential mediator of central leptin resistance. Mol Cell 1998; 191:619–625.

113. Farooqi IS, Jebb SA, Langmack G, Lawrence E, Cheetham CH, Prentice AM, Hughes IA, McCamish MA, O'Rahilly S. Effects of recombinant leptin therapy in a child with congenital leptin deficiency. N Engl J Med 1999; 341:879–884.

114. Heymsfield SB, Greenberg AS, Fujioka K, Dixon RM, Kusher R, Hunt T, Lubina JA, Patane J, Self B, Hunt P, McCamish M. Recombinant leptin for weight Loss in obese and lean adults. JAMA 1999; 282:1568–1575.

115. Fujika K, Patane J, Lubina J, Lau D. Research Letter: CSF leptin levels after exogenous administration of recombinant methionyl human leptin. JAMA 1999; 282:1517–1518.

116. Hukshorn CJ, Saris WHM, Westerterp-Plantenga S, Farid AR, Smith FJ, Campfield LA. Weekly subcutaneous pegylated recombinant native human leptin (PEG-OB) administration in obese men. J Clin Endocrinol Metab 2000; 85:4003–4009.

117. Mantzoros CS, Flier JS. Editorial: Leptin as a therapeutic agent—trials and tribulations. J Clin Endocrinol Metab 2000; 85:4000–4002.

118. Bray GA, Tartaglia LA. Medicinal strategies in the treatment of obesity. Nature 2000; 404:672–677.

119. Sivitz WI, Walsh SA, Morgan DA, Thomas MJ, Haynes WG. Effects of leptin on insulin sensitivity in normal rats. Endocrinology 1997; 138:3395–3401.

120. Kamohara S, Burcelin R, Halaas JL, Friedman JM, Charron MJ. Acute stimulation of glucose metabolism in mice by leptin treatment. Nature 1997; 389:374–377.

121. Shimomura I, Hammer RE, Ikemoto S, Brown MS, Goldstein JL. Leptin reverses insulin resistance and diabetes mellitus in mice with congenital lipodystrophy. Nature 1999; 401:73–76.

122. Ebihara K, Ogawa Y, Masuzaki H, Shintani M,

Miyanaga F, Aizawa-Abe M, Hayashi T, Hosoda K, Inoue G, Yoshimasa Y, Gavrilova O, Reitman ML, Nakao K. Transgenic overexpression of leptin rescues insulin resistance and diabetes in a mouse model of lipatrophic diabetes. Diabetes 2001; 50:1440–1448.

123. Cohen B, Novick D, Rubinstein M. Modulation of insulin activities by leptin. Science 1996; 274:1185–1188.

124. Muller G, Ertl J, Gerl M, Preibisch G. Leptin impairs metabolic actions of insulin in isolated rat adipocytes. J Biol Chem 1997; 272:10585–10593.

125. Zierath JR, Frevert EU, Ryder JW, Berggren P, Kahn BB. Evidence against a direct effect of leptin on glucose transport in skeletal muscle and adipocytes. Diabetes 1998; 47:1–4.

126. Furnsinn C, Brunmair B, Furtmuller R, Roden M, Englisch R, Waldhausl W. Failure of leptin to affect basal and insulin-stimulated glucose metabolism of rat skeletal muscle in vitro. Diabetologia 1998; 41:524–529.

127. Ranganathan S, Ciaraldi TP, Henry RR, Mudaliar S, Kern PA. Lack of effect of leptin on glucose transport, lipoprotein lipase, and insulin action in adipose and muscle cells. Endocrinology 1998; 139:2509–2513.

128. Berti L, Kellerer M, Capp E, Haring HU. Leptin stimulates glucose transport and glycogen synthesis in C_2C_{12} myotubes: evidence for a PI3-kinase mediated effect. Diabetologia 1997; 40:606–609.

129. Williams LB, Ohannesian DW, Kogon BE, Jones RM, Inman M, Huse J, Considine RV. Leptin increases basal and insulin-stimulated glucose uptake into human subcutaneous adipocytes. Diabetes 1998; 47 (suppl 1):A73.

130. Kim Y-B, Uotai S, Pierroz DD, Flier JS, Kahn BB. In vivo administration of leptin activates signal transduction directly in insulin-sensitive tissues: overlapping but distinct pathways from insulin. Endocrinology 2000; 141:2328–2339.

131. Arioglu E, Simha V, Andewelt A, Ruiz E, Snell P, Depaoli A, Wagner A, Reitman M, Taylor SI, Gorden P, Garg A. Treatment of patients with lipoatrophy: efficacy of leptin treatment. 1st International Workshop on Lipoatrophic Diabetes. National Institutes of Health, Bethesda, MD, March 22–23, 2001.

132. Siegrist-Kaiser CA, Pauli V, Juge-Aubry CE, Boss O, Pernin A, Chin WW, Cusin I, Rohner-Jeanrenaud F, Burger AG, Zapf J, Meier CA. Direct effects of leptin on brown and white adipose tissue. J Clin Invest 1997; 100:2858–2864.

133. Shimabukuro M, Koyama K, Chen G, Wang MY, Trieu F, Lee Y, Newgard CB, Unger RH. Direct antidiabetic effect of leptin through triglyceride depletion of tissues. Proc Natl Acad Sci USA 1997; 94:4637–4641.

134. Fruhbeck G, Aguado M, Martinez JA. In vitro lipolytic effect of leptin on mouse adipocytes: evidence for

a possible autocrine/paracrine role of leptin. Biochem Biophys Res Commun 1997; 240:590–594.

135. Wang MY, Lee Y, Unger RH. Novel form of lipolysis induced by leptin. J Biol Chem 1999; 274:17541–17544.

136. Chehab FF, Lim ME, Lu R. Correction of the sterility defect in homozygous obese female mice by treatment with the human recombinant leptin. Nat Genet 1996; 12:318–320.

137. Barash IA, Cheung CC, Weigle DS, Ren H, Kabigting EB, Kuijper JL, Clifton DK, Steiner RA. Leptin is a metabolic signal to the reproductive system. Endocrinology 1996; 137:3144–3147.

138. Ahima RS, Dushay J, Flier SN, Prabakaran D, Flier JS. Leptin accelerates the onset of puberty in normal female mice. J Clin Invest 1997; 99:391–395.

139. Zachow RJ, Magoffin DA. Direct intraovarian effects of leptin: impairment of the synergistic action on insulin-like growth factor I on follicle stimulating hormone dependent estradiol 17 beta production by rat ovarian granulosa cells. Endocrinology 1997; 138:847–850.

140. Suter KJ, Pohl CR, Wilson ME. Circulating concentrations of nocturnal leptin, growth hormone, and insulin-like growth factor-I increase before the onset of puberty in agonadal male monkeys: potential signals for the initiation of puberty. J Clin Endocrinol Metab 2000; 85:808–814.

141. Matkovic V, Ilich JZ, Skugor M, Badenhop NE, Goel P, Clairmont A, Klisovic D, Nahhas RW, Landoll JD. Leptin is inversely related to age at menarche in human females. J Clin Endocrinol Metab 1997; 82:3239–3245.

142. Butte NF, Hopkinson JM, Nicolsol MA. Leptin in human reproduction: serum leptin levels in pregnant and lactating women. J Clin Endocrinol Metab 1997; 82:585–589.

143. Hardie L, Trayhurn P, Abramovich D, Fowler P. Circulating leptin in women: a longitudinal study in the menstrual cycle and during pregnancy. Clin Endocrinol 1997; 47:101–106.

144. Highman TJ, Friedman JE, Huston LP, Wong WW, Catalano PM. Longitudinal changes in maternal serum leptin concentrations, body composition, and resting metabolic rate in pregnancy. Am J Obstet Gynecol 1998; 178:1010–1015.

145. Masuzaki H, Ogawa Y, Sagawa N, Hosoda K, Matsumoto T, Mise H, Nishimura H, Yoshimasa Y, Tanaka I, Mori T, Nakao K. Nonadipose tissue production of leptin: leptin as a novel placenta-derived hormone in humans. Nat Med 1997; 3:1029–1033.

146. Senaris R, Garcia-Caballero T, Casabiell X, Gallego R, Castro R, Considine RV, Dieguez C, Casanueva FF. Synthesis of leptin in human placenta. Endocrinology 1997; 138:4501–4504.

147. Bi S, Gavrilova O, Gong D-W, Mason MM, Reitman M. Identification of a placental enhancer for the human leptin gene. J Biol Chem 1997; 272:30583–30588.

148. Tomimatsu T, Yamaguchi M, Murakami T, Ogura K, Sakata M, Mitsuda N, Kanzaki T, Kurachi H, Irahara M, Miyake A, Shima K, Aono T, Murata Y. Increase in mouse leptin production by adipose tissue after mid-pregnancy: gestational profile of serum leptin concentration. Biochem Biophys Res Commun 1997; 240:213–215.

149. Kawai M, Yamaguchi M, Murakami T, Shima K, Murata Y, Kishi K. The placenta is not the main source of leptin production in the pregnant rat: gestational profile of leptin in plasma and adipose tissues. Biochem Biophys Res Commun 1997; 240:798–802.

150. Cioffi JA, Shafer AW, Zupancic TJ, Smith-Gbur J, Mikhail A, Platika D, Snodgrass HR. Novel B219/OB receptor isoforms: possible role of leptin in hematopoiesis and reproduction. Nat Med 1996; 2:585–589.

151. Bennett DB, Solar GP, Yuan JQ, Mathias J, Thomas GR, Matthews W. A role for leptin and its cognate receptor in hematopoiesis. Curr Biol 1996; 6:1170–1180.

152. Gainsford T, Willson TA, Metcalf D, Handman E, McFarlane C, Ng A, Nicola NA, Alexander WS, Hilton DJ. Leptin can induce proliferation, differentiation, and functional activation of hematopoietic cells. Proc Natl Acad Sci USA 1996; 93:14564–14568.

153. Mikhail A, Beck EX, Shafer AW, Barut B, Smith-Gbur J, Zupancic TJ, Schweitzer AC, Cioffi JA, Lacaud G, Ouyang B, Keller G, Snodgrass HR. Leptin stimulates fetal and adult erythroid and myeloid development. Blood 1997; 89:1507–1512.

154. Ghilardi N, Skoda RC. The leptin receptor activates janus kinase 2 and signals for proliferation in a factor-dependent cell line. Mol Endocrinol 1997; 11:393–399.

155. Umemoto Y, Tsuji K, Yang F-C, Ebihara Y, Kaneko A, Furukawa S, Nakahata T. Leptin stimulates the proliferation of murine myelocytic and primitive hematopoietic cells. Blood 1997; 90:3438–3443.

156. Lord GM, Matarese G, Howard JK, Baker RJ, Bloom SR, Lechler RI. Leptin modulates the T-cell immune response and reverses starvation-induced immunosuppression. Nature 1998; 394:897–901.

157. Laharrague P, Larrouy D, Fontanilles A-M, Truel N, Campfield A, Tenenbaum R, Galitzky J, Corberand JX, Penicaud L, Casteilla L. High expression of leptin by human bone marrow adipocytes in primary culture. FASEB J 1998; 12:747–752.

158. Ducy P, Amling M, Takeda S, Priemel M, Schilling AF, Beil FT, Shen J, Vinson C, Rueger JM, Karsenty G. Leptin inhibits bone formation through a hypothalamic relay: a central control of bone mass. Cell 2000; 100:197–207.

159. Considine RV, Considine EL, Williams CJ, Nyce MR, Magosin SA, Bauer TL, Rosato EL, Colberg J, Caro JF. Evidence against either a premature stop codon or the absence of Ob gene mRNA in human obesity. J Clin Invest 1995; 95:2986–2988.

160. Ahima RS, Flier JS. Leptin. Annu Rev Physiol 2000; 62:413–437.

15

Drugs on the Horizon and Drugs Relegated to History

Roland T. Jung

Ninewells Hospital and Medical School, Dundee, Scotland

George A. Bray

Pennington Biomedical Research Center, Louisiana State University, Baton Rouge, Louisiana, U.S.A.

I INTRODUCTION

This chapter is a speculative resume of possible forthcoming treatments for obesity. It is based on the optimistic speculation of the two authors whose views are entirely their own. At present the obese patient has very little option for really effective, long-term, durable therapy. The best therapy at present is bariatric surgery, but even this is not necessarily durable and involves certain risk with defined mortality and significant morbidity. Surgery also does not get to the root of the problem, which is complex in the extreme. So what can the patient of the future expect from their physician in long-lasting effective therapy? Let us gaze into the crystal ball of the future derived from the latest potential of physiological and genetics research!

Twin studies suggest a heritability of fat mass 40–70% with a concordance of 0.7–0.9 between monozygotic twins compared to 0.35–0.45 between dizygotic twins (1,2). Estimates of heritability from family and adoption studies are between 0.3 and 0.4 (3). The genes for obesity exert their influence across the whole range of body weight and are consistent with a polygenic inheritance of fat mass. A human obesity gene map has been established and at present contains entries for >40 genes and 15 chromosomal regions in which studies indicate a relationship with human obesity (3).

Research in this complex area has shown new routes for the possible treatment of obesity.

II ADIPOSE SIGNALS

A Insulin and Leptin

There are two major signals of adiposity—insulin and leptin. Insulin and leptin enter the brain and reduce energy intake (4). Both hormones circulate at levels proportional to body fat content and enter the CNS in proportion to their plasma level (5,6). Both hormone receptors are expressed by areas of the brain involved in energy intake, and both reduce food intake, whereas deficiency of either alone increases food intake. Both act in the hypothalamus to stimulate energy expenditure while decreasing intake, which in turn determines body fat content. Nevertheless, both have different mechanisms to control body fat content. As weight increases, insulin secretion has to rise to compensate for the insulin resistance associated with weight gain and it is thought limits further weight gain. Failure causes type 2 (non-insulin-dependent) diabetes mellitus. Leptin secretion by adipocytes appears to involve glucose flux, possibly through the hexosamine pathway, the rate of insulin stimulated glucose utilization in adipocytes linking leptin secretion to body fat mass (7).

Leptin would appear to have a more important role than insulin in the CNS control of energy balance. The best example to illustrate this is the known leptin deficiency rodent model that results in severe obesity with hyperphagia despite high insulin levels. In contrast, obesity is not induced by severe insulin deficiency alone, as in type 1 (insulin-dependent) diabetes mellitus, as fat deposition requires insulin, and insulin is required for leptin synthesis by fat cells. The long-recognized diabetic hyperphagia is likely to be due to reduced hypothalamic signaling by insulin, leptin, or both inducing the hyperphagia. The result is that excess calories ingested cannot be stored as fat and drain out as glycosuria. Repletion of leptin in an insulin-deficient rodent prevents the development of diabetic hyperphagia, emphasizing the dominant role of leptin in controlling intake (8). Leptin's major role appears to be as a regulator of the body's response to starvation. Experiments in rats indicate that leptin acts on both fat cells and muscle. When injected into rats deprived of food, leptin had no significant effect on leptin mRNA produced by fat cells, but increased production of mRNA in muscle cells. The reason for this is speculative, but one theory is that the increase of muscle leptin mRNA is semistarvation switches the muscle cells toward fat oxidation as a source of energy rather depleting its protein and carbohydrate stores. This is suggested by recent research on the genes controlling fat oxidation where leptin increases the activity of most of these genes. However, when leptin is injected into rats fed on high-fat, high-calorie intake, leptin mRNA decreased in fat cells with little change in muscle. This appears to favor fat storage when food is plentiful. Hence, overfeeding limits the effectiveness of leptin action. This appears part of the thrifty genotype and may limit the role of leptin therapy if patients continue to overfeed or eat high-fat diets.

B Leptin Deficiency

In general, leptin levels correlate with the degree of obesity but very rare cases of leptin deficiency and massive obesity have been reported (9). Montague et al. (10) reported two cousins, both children of Pakistani origin, with undetectable levels of leptin due to a homozygous deletion of a single guanine nucleotide at codon 133, resulting in a truncated protein. The parents were heterozygous. The cousins were markedly obese, hyperphagic with no substantial impairment of energy expenditure both basal or total, had normal karyotype, had normal thyroid and normal adrenal function, were hyperinsulinemic, and had an advanced bone age

of over 3 years. Strobel et al. (11) have described a Turkish family with three siblings with leptin deficiency attributable to a missense mutation in the leptin gene. These sisters did not undergo pubertal development with hormonal features of hypogonadotropic hypogonadism. Leptin reverses the obesity and induces puberty. However, these are very rare instances, and the majority of the obese appear to have elevated leptin levels compared to the lean, suggesting that there is some resistance to leptin at the brain level (12).

C Leptin Resistance

The db/db mouse and the fa/fa rat are the archetypical leptin-resistant models due to mutant leptin receptors (9). Searches for similar genetic mutations in man, however, have been relatively fruitless except in rare circumstance. Clement et al. (13) have identified three morbidly obese sisters with very high leptin levels who are homozygous for a mutation in a splice donor site of the leptin receptor resulting in the loss of transmembrane and cytoplasmic domains because of exon skipping. These sisters were hyperphagic, had normal basal resting expenditure, and had hypogonadotropic hypogonadism with failure of pubertal development. However, unlike the above leptin-deficient patients, these sisters had mild growth retardation in early childhood with impaired basal and dynamic growth hormone secretion and decreased IGF1 and IGF-BP3 levels (see Table 1). There was also evidence of hypothalamic hypothyroidism with only mildly raised insulin levels.

Table 1 Contrast Between Leptin Deficiency and Resistance in Man

Leptin deficient	Leptin resistant
Obese + + +	Obese + + +
Hyperphagic	Hyperphagic
Energy expenditure unchanged	Energy expenditure unchanged
Normal karyotype	Normal karyotype
Normal thyroid function	Hypothalamic hypothyroidism
Normal adrenal function	
Normal cortisol levels	Normal cortisol levels
Severe hyperinsulinaemia	Mild hyperinsulinaemia
Growth advanced	Mild growth retardation
Advanced bone age	
Normal growth hormone	Impaired GH, IgF1, IgFBP3
Hypogonadotrophic hypogonadism	Hypogonadotrophic hypogonadism
Pubertal failure	Pubertal failure

The leptin-resistant, like the leptin deficient, have normal cortisol levels. Such is an extreme case of leptin resistance and both were homozygous. Their parents, although heterozygous, were not obese and had normal sexual maturation indicating that one normal allele is sufficient to control weight and neuroendocrine function. How do these rare cases support the hypothesis that human obesity may be due to reduced leptin action in the brain as the result of leptin resistance? Clearly by indicating that there must be other mechanisms that contribute to leptin resistance and genetic receptor abnormality is just one rarity. Possibly it is this area where the drugs of the future will arise to treat obesity.

D   Leptin Resistance Mechanisms

There are a number of mechanisms that may contribute to leptin resistance (4). Leptin uptake into the brain is facilitated at the endothelial cell leptin receptor level by the receptors functioning as leptin transporters (14). The cells that form the blood brain barrier produce higher levels of the mRNA that encode a shortened form of the leptin receptor called OBR-A than do any other cells in the body (review in 15). This shortened form is not tethered to the cell membrane, as it lacks the usual peptide required for tethering. This protein is essential to transport leptin. Dysfunction of this transport process might lead to obesity and is suggested as a possibility by finding of lower leptin levels in the CSF compared to blood in the obese (6,16). Another possibility is an altered leptin-receptor signal transduction. When a leptin receptor is activated, the receptor induces expression of a protein called suppressor of cytokine signaling 3 (SOCS3) that inhibits further leptin transduction. This is part of the mechanism required to halt leptin signaling when not required (14). It is possible that SOCS3 might be mediating the resistance to leptin in some obese people. If so, then SOCS3 inhibitors might reduce leptin resistance and increase the activity of endogenously produced leptin-curbing appetite. Ongoing research on the possibility of defects in OBR-A and SOCS3 as a cause of leptin resistance in human obesity are awaited with interest.

E   Recombinant Leptin Therapy

While research is proceeding in these areas, a recent trial of recombinant leptin therapy in obese man has indicated a limited outcome. Heymsfield et al. (17) reported the use of recombinant leptin for weight loss in those obese with no deficiency of leptin, i.e., the typical obese patient. A dose-reponse relationship with weight and fat

loss was observed. Weight change at 24 weeks is shown in Table 2 for each dosage used compared to placebo.

The group lost 1.3 kg on placebo while those on the highest dose of leptin (0.3 mg/kg) lost 7.1 kg. Change in fat mass accounted for most of the weight loss. Nevertheless the weight loss on lower dosages of leptin was disappointing (see Table 2). Also, the trial included small numbers, namely eight patients on the leptin and 12 on placebo at completion. The worrying feature was that the leptin level had to be raised some 19-fold above placebo (placebo 25 ng/mL vs. leptin 480 ng/mL) to achieve the weight loss observed at the highest dose. This suggests that exogenous leptin can overcome, to some extent, the functional resistance observed in obese individuals, but that to achieve this, the blood level has to be elevated to high pharmaceutical levels making it unlikely that this is a financially viable therapy for the obese. Safety profile of maintaining such high levels beyond 6 months is unknown. It also suggests that research into the areas of leptin resistance is essential if a more effective therapy is to be found.

F   Resistin

Resistin is the name recently given to a peptide produced in adipose tissue that modulates insulin resistance in vivo and in vitro (18). During treatment with thiazolidinediones such as pioglitazone or rosiglitazone, insulin resistance is reduced clinically and in experimental animals the mRNA for resistin is reduced. When this protein was identified and antibodies to it were made, a number of important findings were made. First, the peptide is made primarily by the adipocyte and is secreted into the circulation. Resistin antibodies reduce insulin resistance, and as might be expected from its name, resistin enhances insulin resistance. These studies suggest that this peptide provides the missing link between fat cells and the control of peripheral insulin

Table 2 Comparison of Weight Change in Obese Subjects Given Placebo or Variable Dosages of Recombinant Leptin Injections for 24 Weeks

Leptin dosage mg/kg per day	No. subjects	Mean weight change in kg (SD)	Mean serum leptin level (ng/mL)
Placebo	12	−1.3 (4.9)	25.0
0.01	6	−0.7 (5.4)	28.3
0.03	8	−1.4 (4.10)	115.5
0.10	13	−2.4 (5.5)	271.7
0.30	8	−7.1 (8.5)	480.3

resistance. Control of resistin may open new avenues for the treatment of obesity and diabetes mellitus (18).

G Perilipin

Hormone-sensitive lipase mediates the hydrolysis of fatty acids. Perilipin is an adipocyte protein encoded by the gene Plin. Plin-null mice have higher food intake but are the same weight as control wild-type mice with intact Plin genotype. The Plin-null mice have reduced fat depots but increased muscle mass, the latter elevating metabolic rate, which allows the higher food intake without disproportionate weight gain. The adipocytes have elevated lipolysis resistant to β-adrenergic agonist stimulation and are cold sensitive except when fed. Breeding Plin-null alleles into db/db leptin-resistant mice reverses the obesity by increasing metabolic rate. Agents that inactivate perilipin may ultimately prove to be useful as antiobesity medication (19).

III NEUROPEPTIDE MODULATORS OF ENERGY BALANCE

Upon activation of leptin receptors, a series of neuronal signals occur that ultimately alter food intake and expenditure of energy. Modulation failure of one or more of these signals may be the reason for leptin resistance and may hold the clue to future drug therapy. What are these signals? There is now a need to understand the anatomy of the process (Fig. 1). The arcuate nucleus is situated adjacent to the floor of the third ventricle occupying about half the length of the hypothalamus. This is occasionally referred to as the first order neuronal area for energy homeostasis (4). Neuropeptide Y (NPY) and Agouti-related protein (AGRP) are colocalized in the arcuate neurones, whereas two other important peptides involved in energy homeostasis, pro-opiomelanocortin (POMC) and cocaine- and amphetamine-regulated transcript (CART), are colocalized in a distinct but adjacent subset of arcuate neurones (20). A majority of NPY/AGRP and POMC/CART neurones coexpress leptin receptors and are regulated by leptin. Insulin receptors are concentrated in these areas as well.

The arcuate area innervates the so-called secondary centers of energy homeostasis—the paraventricular nucleus (PVN), zona incerta, perifornical area (PFA), and lateral hypothalamus (LH). In classical physiology, lesions in the PVN cause hyperphagia and obesity whereas bilateral lesions of the LH cause anorexia and weight loss (21).

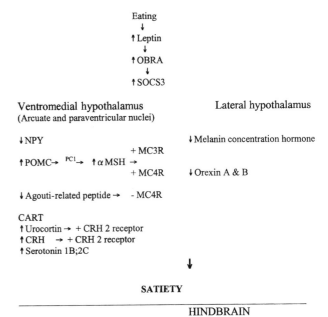

Figure 1 Effect of eating on central activity to produce satiety. OBRA = short form of leptin receptor; α-MSH = α-melanocyte stimulating hormone; SOCS3 = suppressor of cytokine signalling 3; PC1 = prohormone convertase; POMC = pro-opiomelanocortin; MC-3R,-4R = melanocortin receptor; NPY = neuropeptide Y; CRH = corticotrophin releasing hormone; CART = cocaine- and amphetamine-regulated transcript; CCK = cholecystokinin.

A Neuropeptide Y

NPY injected into the hypothalamus stimulates food intake and decreases energy expenditure (22). Ob/ob mice that lack leptin require NPY to show the full effect of the leptin deficiency because the genetic knockout of NPY reduces the hyperphagia and the obesity (23). Mice that lack NPY but otherwise are genetically normal have intact feeding responses, indicating that NPY is not the controlling anabolic force when leptin and insulin are normal (24). In other words, NPY is important during starvation but possibly not during normal nutritional periods. This has led to the reassessment of the pharmacological approach that involves NPY. NPY Y-1 receptor antagonists are being researched as a possible treatment of hypertension because NPY is a well-established vasoconstrictor and potentiates the vasoconstrictive action of noradrenaline. If the treatment with NPY Y-1 receptor antagonists results in obesity, as suggested from the NPY Y-1 knockout data, then such therapy may have limited usefulness long term. Similarly, development of obesity with NPY Y-5 receptor antagonists would also be detrimental and of limited value as a pharmacological target (22).

B POMC and Melanocortin Receptor-4

POMC is cleaved by prohormone convertase (PC1) to yield peptides (including α-melanocyte-stimulating hormone, α-MSH) that appear highly important in the feeding process (25). α-MSH binds to a family of melanocortin receptors, especially MC3-R and MC4-R (26). Synthetic agonists of these receptors suppress food intake in rodents, whereas antagonists have the opposite effect. Mice lacking MC4-R are hyperphagic, hyperinsulinemic, and severely obese (27). Mice heterozygous for the deleted MC4-R receptor allele also become obese but less so than the homozygous knockout, indicating the importance of this receptor in homeostasis. POMC deficiency and lack of MC4-R also appear to be involved in obesity in man (28). Mutations have been described in two unrelated German patients associated with isolated adrenocorticotropic hormone (ACTH) deficiency, red hair pigmentation, hyperphagia, and severe early-onset obesity (29). Another case has been reported of severe obesity associated with compound heterozygous mutations in the gene encoding PC1 (30). This patient also had impaired adrenal function, hypogonadotropic hypogonadism, and massive hyperproinsulinemia. The lack of POMC-derived ligands results in obesity primarily through a lack of α-MSH acting on the MC4-R to inhibit intake.

Another family has been described having mutations in MC4-R who are hyperphagic, tall, with severe obesity (31). MC4-R mutations have been reported in 3–5% of patients with a BMI > 40 (32). However, not all patients with MC4-R mutations are obese, and there is a considerable range of BMI. This is akin to the situation in mice where differing doses of an MC4-R knockout allele cause progressive weight gain (27). It could well be that synthetic agonists of MC4-R may prove useful in the treatment of obesity, especially in those with genetically decreased melanocortinergic activity.

C Agouti-Related Peptide and the Mahogany Gene

The agouti mouse is an autosomal-dominant model of obesity characterized by a yellow coat of fur and an obese phenotype. The obesity appears to be due to the overexpression of a protein (Agouti) produced by the Agouti gene (33). Agouti in the skin reduces MC1 receptors, lightening the coat color (28). These mice also overexpress Agouti in the hypothalamus, producing obesity by inhibiting binding of α-MSH to the melanocortin receptors (MC3-R and MC4-R). Agouti-related peptide (AGRP) found in man is homologous to the agouti peptide in mice and has a similar action in the brain. AGRP is localized to the arcuate nucleus, and is upregulated by fasting and by leptin deficiency. A single intracerebroventricular injection of AGRP increases food intake in rodents for up to 1 week (34). Compare this with NPY, whose feeding response after similar injection lasts only a few hours. It would therefore appear that lack of leptin or fasting activates the NPY/AGRP neurones in the arcuate nucleus. AGRP then blocks the action of α-MSH on MC4-R producing deactivation of MC4-R, which would normally produce satiety and decreased intake. It is possible that the development of synthetic antagonists of AGRP may have a role to play in the future treatment of the obese.

Lately another gene has been discovered that produces a peptide closely related to attractin, which itself is an immunoregulatory protein made by human T-lymphocytes. This gene has been named Mahogany because mutations darken the coat color of agouti mice, reversing the obesity in such mice (25). This suggested that the mahogany peptide was essential for agouti peptide effect on skin and on energy balance. However, the mahogany gene appears to prevent obesity in the agouti mouse by increasing energy expenditure rather than by reducing food intake. This is supported by the observation that in normal mice mutations in the mahogany gene increase both energy expenditure and energy intake (energy flux increases by 20%), weight remaining balanced. This begs the question concerning the role of mahogany in the normal situation. Does it suppress both intake and expenditure or does it act primarily on expenditure with compensatory changes occurring on the intake side? Either way there may be some mileage in the use of antagonists to mahogany gene product as long as intake can be simultaneously suppressed.

D Insulin

Insulin has been proposed as a signal for food intake (4). This hypothesis was supported by studies showing that disabling the insulin receptor in the central nervous system enhances the sensitivity to developing obesity in mice eating a high-fat diet (4). Clinical support for this idea has also come from studies blocking insulin secretion with somatostatin agonist (35,36). When children with hypothalamic obesity were treated with somatostatin agonist, the degree of reduction in weight was related to the reduction in insulin secretion as seen during an oral glucose tolerance test. In a subset of severely obese adults, monthly injections of a somatostatin agonist suppressed weight gain. These results provide a promising avenue for treatment and suggest that insulin may play a role in stimulating food intake in children and adults.

E   Secondary Centers: MCH and the Orexins

The arcuate axons innervate the secondary centers described above. Several neuropeptides synthesized in the PVN neurones reduce food intake and body weight when injected centrally. Corticotrophin-releasing hormone (CRH) produces anorexia and stimulates the sympathetic system (21). TRH and oxytocin are also anorexic. It is unlikely these agents will be of use in obesity therapy owing to predominant endocrine activities. Second-order neurones involved in satiety signaling reside within the lateral hypothalamus and perifornical area. One such peptide is melanin-concentrating hormone (MCH). MCH injected into the brains of rats increases food intake, whereas MCH knockout mice have reduced food intake and are excessively thin (37). Interestingly, the neurones making MCH project to the cortex include those regions orchestrating smell. This has led to the concept that MCH is involved in the "pizza effect" (review in 15). If a person is satiated, then MCH activity is low. However, the smell of appetizing food (e.g., the pizza) can induce a further urge to eat, and it has been proposed that the smell overrides the satiety situation by the release of MCH (15,37). Research is now under way to find a blocking agent for MCH that might be used in obesity therapy.

Two other peptides are the orexins, A and B, which increase food intake (38). The orexins are linked to arousal in animals and man, but regrettably, deletion of the orexin gene in mice induced narcolepsy, which in itself may indicate a new mode of therapy for this condition. The picture becomes even more complex when one realizes that leptin receptors have been described on the PVN and LH, indicating direct activity into the so-called secondary centers.

F   Galanin

Galanin is a peptide released from both the gastrointestinal tract and the brain. Intracerebroventricular administration or injection into the paraventricular hypothalamus or hindbrain will increase food intake, especially of fatty foods in those rodents with a fat intake preference (39). M40, a peptide antagonist to galanin, blocks the action of galanin on food intake and suggests that such antagonists may be potential therapeutic agents. Recent research has identified galaninlike peptide (GALP) in the arcuate nucleus and other hypothalamic sites (40). Fasting reduces the number of identifiable cells containing GALP mRNA in the arcuate nucleus, whereas treatment of the fasted animals with leptin produces a fourfold increase in the number of GALP mRNA cells. This indicates that GALP expression is regulated by leptin. Three G protein-linked galanin receptor subtypes have been cloned, widening the potential for selective antagonists.

G   Calcitonin Gene-Related Peptide and Amylin

Calcitonin and amylin both reduce food intake (41). Salmon calcitonin has been shown to bind irreversibly to the same receptors on which amylin acts. The suppression of food intake by salmon calcitonin is more potent and lasts longer than amylin. These findings suggest that there is another receptor system mediating suppression of food intake which can be activated by calcitonin and amylin.

H   Neuromedin U Receptor

Neuromedin U (NMU) is a peptide that is widely expressed in the gut and central nervous system. It has a variety of effects, including stimulation of smooth muscle, increasing blood pressure, and control of local blood flow. Two receptors for this peptide have been identified, one of which, neuromedin U1 receptor (NMU1R), is expressed in the ventromedial hypothalamus. Intracerebroventricular administration of NMU reduces food intake, suggesting that the central receptors for this peptide may provide another strategy for developing drugs to treat obesity (42).

IV   GASTROINTESTINAL SIGNALLING

The process of homeostasis, which also involves processes in the hindbrain for the mechanism of terminating a meal, can function in the absence of a hypothalamus or forebrain. This it does through the nucleus tractus solitarius (NTS), an area of the brainstem that integrates sensory information from the gastrointestinal tract as well as the sense of taste (4,43). Satiety signals are initiated by mechanical and chemical stimulation of the stomach and gut, neural input from the liver, and neuroendocrine hormones such as cholecystokinin (CCK) and glucagonlike peptide 1 (GLP1). MC4 R, POMC neurones, and leptin receptors are also found in the NTS, emphasizing the complexity of energy homeostasis and the extreme difficulty of finding the ideal antiobesity drug. Energy homeostasis is fundamental to survival, and the body has at its disposal backup systems in the hindbrain and forebrain. It could well be that cocktail of drugs will be required to target multiple sites if sustained weight loss is to ever achieved.

A   Cholecystokinin

The major biological functions of cholecystokinin are contraction of biliary smooth muscle, reduction in food intake, and the induction of anxiety-related behavior. Two types of CCK receptors have been identified and cloned. The CCK-A receptors are mainly located in the gastrointestinal tract but are also found in areas of the CNS. The CCK-B receptors, which are widely distributed in the brain, turned out to be identical with the gastrin receptors. Reduction of food intake is mainly mediated by type A receptors, whereas anxietylike behavior is induced by CCK-B/GRP receptors (44). There are available biologically active CCK agonists such as CCK-8S, CCK-4, cerulein, and A71378, whereas loxiglumide is a CCK antagonist (45). The literature on both the satiety effect and behavioral changes of CCK suffers from inconsistency and contradiction, making it difficult to be precise as to the role of CCK in controlling intake in man.

In rodents, the effect of CCK-8S on satiety is strongly dependent on the experimental design, with female rats less sensitive than males, and the obese less sensitive than normal-weight rats. CCK is not the most potent of the gastrointestinal released agents. The ranking order of potency on food intake inhibition has been reported as urocortin > urocortin-deamidated form >/= corticotrophin-releasing hormone (CRH) > CCK-8 > CRH6-33 > leptin (46). Adult Otsuka Long-Evans Okushima fatty (OLETF) rats lack functional CCK-A receptors and are diabetic, hyperphagic, and obese with patterns of ingestion consistent with a satiety defect secondary to CCK insensitivity (47). High-fat diets, which in normal rodents stimulates CCK release, fail to do so in this mutant strain such that gastric and duodenal fat preloads were significantly less effective in suppressing subsequent intake than were equicaloric glucose. Long-term effects of the CCK-A antagonist

loxiglumide result in weight gain, but weight is reduced by the CCK agonist cerulein in both obese and lean rodents (48). The mechanism of action has been subject to debate with some suggesting that CCK acts via the vagal system, by insulin secretion, and/or by enhancing the effect of leptin (49,50).

CCK may also be acting as a neurotransmitter or neuromodulator within two different brain regions to produce satiety. One region includes the nucleus tractus solitarius in the hindbrain and the other the medial-basal hypothalamus. In humans, two sequence changes have been noted in the gene encoding CCK in 1.9% of a cohort of 1296 individuals (44). This polymorphism showed a significantly higher percent body fat and higher levels of leptin and insulin compared to the wild (normal) type or heterozygotes. This suggests that polymorphism in the promoter region of the CCK-A receptor gene may be one of the genetic factors affecting fat deposition. Whether CCK therapy will be an effective satiety therapy in obese humans in general is certainly debatable, as is its role in those with polymorphic receptor defects where therapy would have to overcome receptor resistance.

B   Glucagonlike Peptide 1 (GLP1)

GLP1 has been found to decrease diet-induced thermogenesis in man by 47% with a decrease in carbohydrate oxidation, possibly due to delayed absorption of nutrients (51). GLP1 also decreases the desire to eat any type of food. Bombesin also released by the gut when infused in man has no significant feeding suppressive effect in obese females but did decrease intake in lean subjects (52). Whether polymorphism will be found in some obese patients for these two peptides associated with increased weight is unknown, but again the antiobesity effect is likely to be limited to such polymorphic individuals.

C   Enterostatin

A final peptide candidate in the gastrointestinal tract is enterostatin. This pentapeptide with the structure Ala-Pro-Glu-Pro-Arg is produced by cleavage of the five N-terminal amino acids from procolipase that is produced in the pancreas and secreted into the intestine. When enterostatin is injected intraperitoneally, infused into the ventricular system of the brain, or given into the stomach by gavage, it specifically reduces fat intake of animals eating a high-fat diet or when given a choice of a high-fat or low-fat diet. The receptor for this peptide is not known. In human studies it attenuates hunger ratings, but has not yet been shown to specifically reduce food intake (53).

V   FEEDING EFFICIENCY AND PARTITIONING

A   Melanocortin-3 Receptor

In the hypothalamic arcuate nucleus, leptin induces expression of POMC, which is cleaved to generate α-MSH, the principal agonist of two hypothalamic melanocortin receptor isoforms, namely MC4-R and MC3-R. As described above MC4-R regulates food intake and possibly energy expenditure, whereas MC3-R influences feed efficiency and the partitioning of fuel stores into fat. Whereas MC4-R-deficient mice are hyperphagic, hyperinsulinemic, and obese, those with MC3-R deficiency have increased body fat with a reciprocal decrease in lean mass such that body weight remains normal (54). This excessive adiposity is not due to any increase in food intake, which is actually reduced. Instead, the cause is increased feed efficiency with preferential storage of fat. This makes such MC3-R mutant mice highly susceptible to high-fat diet–induced obesity. How this is achieved has yet to be resolved for there is no alteration in resting metabolic rate or respiratory exchange ratio, just a relative physical inactivity. Consistent with the increase in fat mass, the MC3-R mutant mice are hyperleptinemic and have mild hyperinsulinemia. Mice deficient in both MC3-R and MC4-R indicate that the loss of MC3-R exacerbates the obesity associated with the MC4-R deficiency. These mutants eat excessively owing to the absence of MC4-R signaling and then store ingested calories more efficiently as fat due to the absence of MC3-R.

This animal work suggests that mutations of MC3-R in man might be part of the so-called thrifty genotype, a collection of alleles that was selected over evolution because they promote fat storage in times of plenty but do not alter fertility. Leptin and its receptors are unlikely to be candidates of the thrifty genotype as mutations would cause not only weight gain but infertility, preventing positive evolutionary selection. Central melanocortin receptors are promising targets for antiobesity therapy, MC4-R agonists decreasing food intake, and MC3-R agonists reducing fat storage with both promoting weight loss more effectively than either alone. It is of interest that a locus encoding MC3-R on human chromosome 20q has been reported to show linkage to the regulation of body mass index, subcutaneous fat mass and fasting insulin levels (55).

B   Ghrelin

Ghrelin is a peptide hormone acting primarily at the growth hormone secretagogue receptor (which releases growth hormone) in the hypothalamus and yet whose principal site of synthesis is the stomach. Ghrelin when administered peripherally to mice and rats caused both weight gain and increased fat mass by reducing fat utilization (56). Intracerebroventricular administration of ghrelin generated a dose-dependent increase in food intake and body weight. Ghrelin appears to encourage the use of carbohydrates as energy source, converting fat into adipose tissue for later use, without significantly altering energy expenditure or locomotor activity. Similar results have been observed after administration of growth hormone–releasing peptide 2 (GHRP2), a synthetic agonist of the growth hormone secretagogue receptor, indicating a possible joint mechanism. This is compatible with the need for a positive energy balance necessary to maximize the growth potential of growth hormone. Fasting increases ghrelin levels, whereas refeeding does the reverse, indicating a role for ghrelin in shifting to a more energy efficient metabolism during starvation. Sugar intake also decreases ghrelin levels. Whether manipulation of this hormone has antiobesity potential only time will tell but its action on growth hormone may be a disadvantage if IGF1 levels significantly altered.

C   Growth Hormone

Growth hormone–deficient man is associated with moderate obesity and visceral deposition of fat. Treatment of such patients with growth hormone results in weight loss in some, but this is not a consistent feature; however, most show a decrease in visceral fat with increase of lean mass, explaining the maintenance of weight in others. Trial of growth hormone therapy in obese individuals with normal growth hormone dynamics, has shown no significant total body weight loss compared to the effect of diet alone, but did produce a problem with edema and, in some, joint pains (57). Growth hormone reduces body fat preferentially with the reduction of visceral fat exceeding that of total fat. Recent trials lasting 39 weeks did not result in total body weight loss, but there were significant losses in body fat (9.2% and 3 kg) with improvements in fat-free mass. The cost of growth hormone prohibitive, and with present results it will not be a major treatment of the obese although there is a defined role in growth hormone–deficient adults (41,58,59).

VI CENTRAL NEUROTRANSMITTERS

A Dopamine

Dopamine plays a role in food intake, but the actual role is difficult to separate out from the motor impairments brought about by dopamine deficiency, which also affects feeding behavior (60). Feeding effects of dopamine vary with the brain region studied. For instance, mesolimbic dopamine pathways contibute to the rewarding aspects of consuming palatable foods (61). However, dopamine in the dorsomedial and arcuate nuclei inhibits food intake. Two dopamine receptors divided into two main groups—D1/D5, and D2/D3 and D4—have been identified as involved in altering food intake (62). Bromocriptine, a specific D2 agonist, has been reported to decrease food intake, whereas sulpiride, an antagonist of D1 receptors, can cause an increase in food intake. However, the bromocriptine data for weight loss were not significant, and this medication is no longer being evaluated as antiobesity therapy. Nevertheless, dopamine agonists used in the treatment of prolactinoma have not been conspicuous by their effect on weight in normal clinical use, although some researchers do report reduction in body fat when sufficient numbers are included in trials. This has not stopped pharmacological companies researching this area for more effective agents, and several agents are on clinical trial at present.

B Serotonin

The serotonin system has, until recently, been a primary target of pharmacological research for an antiobesity agent (e.g., dexfenfluramine and sibutramine). Such drugs increase serotonin receptor signaling and suppress food intake with the 5HT2c serotonin receptor subtype involved in the process (63). Ritanserin, a 5HT2c antagonist, blocks the satiety effect of dexfenfluramine, suggesting that such agents mediate food intake reduction through 5HT2c receptors (64). Mice with knockout of 5HT2c receptors exhibit increased food intake, and this causes a modest weight gain, indicating that normal energy homeostasis requires normal-functioning serotonin signaling (63). In contrast, the obesity of MC4-R or leptin deficiency is massive, and the latter has a profound influence on food intake with the serotonin system as shown in mice with mutant 5HT2c receptor. It is therefore debatable whether further pharmacological research into serotonin agonists is going to produce the potent antiobesity agent required.

C Antidepressants

Two antidepressants of the SSRI family, fluoxetine and sertraline, produce modest weight loss that fades out after some 20 weeks of treatment (41). The effect of fluoxetine on food intake is not inhibited by metergoline, suggesting that this effect may be by some mechanism other than serotonin. Two other drugs developed as antidepressants, mazindol and sibutramine, are inhibitors of noradrenaline uptake (mazindol) and also block reuptake of serotonin (sibutramine). This combination appears to produce better appetite-suppressant action than antidepressant activity. However, venflaxine, which blocks reuptake of both serotonin and noradrenaline, is an antidepressant but has a weak effect on food intake. This indicates that there is an interaction between serotonin and noradrenaline systems controlling food intake and mood, which is finely balanced and influenced in a different manner by drugs with various pharmacological profiles.

D GABA and Topiramate

GABA may have a role in modulating food intake. Microinjection of GABA into the medial hypothalamus increases food intake, whereas injection into the lateral hypothalamus induces satiety. Antagonists of GABA such as picrotoxin or bicuculline block the enhancement of feeding by 2-deoxyglucose (65). Topiramate, an agonist of GABA activity, is available for use in man. Topiramate is an effective anticonvulsant approved in the European Union and by the U.S. FDA for adjunctive treatment of adults and pediatric patients with refractory partial onset or generalized tonic clonic seizures (66). Topiramate appears to have a number of pharmacological properties that may contribute to its anticonvulsant activity. It blocks voltage activated sodium channels, potentiates aminobutyrate (GABA) to activate GABAA receptors, shows antagonism of glutamate at the kainite/AMPA receptor subtype, has a limited negative modulatory effect on L-type calcium channel currents, and has a weak inhibitory action on some of the isoenzymes of carbonic anhydrase (CA11 and CAIV) (66).

In genetically obese Osborne-Mendel rats, topiramate-treated rodents gained less weight with reduced body fat than did the controls. In man clinical trials have involved topiramate as adjunctive therapy to standard epileptic therapy or as monotherapy (67). Significant weight loss has been observed. Mean weight losses of 6 kg have been reported with topiramate given for

18–24 months. Weight loss appears to be dose related ranging from 1.1 kg loss on the lowest (<200 mg/day) dosage to 5.9 kg on the highest (>800 mg/day). The more obese the patient at the outset, the more weight was lost. Also, females showed greater loss than males. In the anticonvulsant trials the weight loss was considered not clinically significant, and very few had to terminate the trial for this side effect alone. Trials are now under way to study in depth the weight loss potential. Nevertheless it needs to be emphasized that topiramate has a number of significant potential side effects namely fatigue, paraesthesia, nystagmus, dizziness, impaired memory and concentration, headache, and mood problems, especially at higher dosages. Nephrolithiasis was observed in a few. Most withdrew from trials because of CNS-related events. The teratogenic potential of topiramate in humans is not known, but the fact that this drug is a weak inhibitor of carbonic anhydrase, which in general are teratogenic in rodents, might limit its use in obese potential fertile adults.

VII KETONES AND FATTY ACID SYNTHASE INHIBITION

It has been known for some time that infusion of 3-hydroxybutyrate into the brain's ventricular system will depress food intake in lean animals and enhance sympathetic activity. These effects of ketones in the CNS are in keeping with the presence of fatty acid responsive neurones in the lateral hypothalamus. Recent research on fatty acid synthase (FAS) has further elucidated the physiological role for fatty acids in the control of food intake (68). FAS catalyses the reductive synthesis of long chain fatty acids from acetyl-coenzyme A (acetyl-CoA) and malonyl-CoA (Fig. 2). When the body stores fat, FAS makes the long-chained fatty acids required. Loftus et al. (68) used a natural inhibitor of FAS, namely cerulenin, which forms a complex with FAS, but it has the drawback that its epoxide structure is

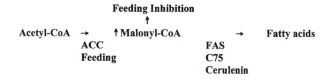

Figure 2 Feeding stimulates synthesis of acetyl-CoA carboxylase (ACC), which elevates levels of malonyl-CoA. By blocking fatty acid synthase (FAS), C75 and cerulenin prevent the removal of malonyl-CoA, keeping levels elevated and suppressing appetite.

likely to limit its utility as a drug. Epoxides are known to be unstable and reactive, so Loftus and colleagues (67) synthesized an FAS inhibitor named C75. C75 blocked FAS with the same potency of cerulenin but without the toxicity problems. Injection intraperitoneally into mice with C75 reduced FAS activity by 95% and led to an increase of 110% in the level of hepatic malonyl-CoA, the principal substrate of FAS. In mice C75 induced a dramatic but reversible decrease in appetite and weight.

C75 was found to suppress appetite with treated animals eating just 10% of their food compared to untreated littermates. The treated mice lost one third of their body weight. Surprisingly, treated mice lost 45% more weight than littermates fed the same reduced amount of food. Animals on reduced intake usually decrease their metabolic expenditure to compensate, but C75 appears to possibly prevent this. C75 is also effective when given by intracerebroventricular injection. C75 appears to inhibit NPY production, which normally would have stimulated appetite in animals with reduced intake. The effect of C75 is also leptin independent and suggests that by keeping malonyl-CoA levels high the brain centres think there is sufficient fuel when there is none. Nevertheless, NPY may not be the only candidate for the action of malonyl-CoA, for simply blocking NPY is unlikely to be responsible for the profound inhibition of food intake. Although C75 itself may never be able to be used in man as its action is severe, lesser agents based on the principle of blocking FAS may well represent a therapeutic target for the future control of appetite and body weight in man.

VIII THERMOGENESIS

A Uncoupling Proteins 1, 2, 3

The mitochondrial inner-membrane protein that uncouples proton entry from ATP synthesis in brown fat is UCP1 (69). Two homologues of UCP-1 have been identified, UCP2 and UCP3, which are 73% identical to each other and both 56% identical to UCP1 (70). UCP1 gene has been mapped to chromosome 4q31, with UCP2 and UCP3 mapped to chromosome 11q13 positioned some 150 kb of each other (71). Whereas UCP2 is expressed in most tissues, UCP3 is mainly expressed in skeletal muscle and brown fat. Brown fat is not abundant in adult humans and certainly does not have the thermogenic power in older human beings to account for the development of age-related obesity (72). Infusion of adrenaline causes a 25% increase in energy expenditure in humans, with at least 40% of this increase arising from skeletal muscle thermogenic activity (73). The mechanism of this effect on muscle is unclear as is the role of liver and white fat in thermogenic activity in adult man. An emerging view is that UCP3 may be involved in skeletal muscle thermogenesis (74). UCP3 is a transporter that shuttles anionic free fatty acids (FFA) out of mitochondria where protons are added to them and then they return to the mitochondrial matrix as neutral FFAs. This action alters the availability of FFA for fat oxidation. UCP3 is regulated by thyroid hormones, by β$_3$-adrenergic agonists, leptin, and a high-fat diet (75,76). PPAR-α and PPAR-γ are positive regulators of UCP2 ad UCP3. In man significant linkage has been reported between markers at the UCP2/UCP3 gene locus with resting metabolic rate ($P = .000002$) (77). This region is syntemic to a region in mouse chromosome 7 and has also been linked to hyperinsulinemia and obesity (78). This evidence has suggested that UCP3 may be significant therapeutic target for antiobesity drugs.

MRNA levels for both UCP2 and UCP3 in obese and lean individuals increase some 2.5-fold during fasting, which at first sight might argue against a role in adaptive thermogenesis (79). This is unlike UCP1, whose mRNA decreases with fasting. However, the role of (especially) UCP3 appears linked to fatty-acid oxidation where in the fasting state there is a need for muscle to switch on this activity to supply energy hence reducing the need for carbohydrate and protein breakdown for the same purpose. A mutation and missense polymorphisms of the UCP3 gene have been reported in severely obese humans (80). Two polymorphisms have been described in African-Americans with allele frequencies of 18% (V1021) and 10% (exon 6 splice) (74). Heterozygotes for the latter polymorphism were found to have a 50% reduction in their ability to oxidise fat. Exon-6 splice donor polymorphism is associated with the development of severe obesity in African-Americans. V1021 polymorphism was not associated with obesity. Hence an effect of exon-6 splice donor polymorphism would reduce fat oxidation promoting fat storage in keeping with the thrifty gene concept where fat would be stored in times of plenty. The mutation R143X was also found to relate to the development of early-onset severe obesity and type 2 diabetes mellitus. The control of UCP3 may therefore be an interesting target for future treatment of the obese.

Adaptive thermogenesis has other areas of interest in the development of obesity related therapy. Figure 3 shows a possible unifying model for the activation of UCP1, the uncoupling protein in brown fat proposed by Lowell and Spiegelman (70). In this model β-adrenergic

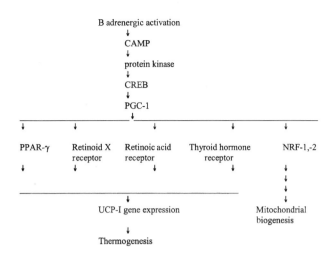

Figure 3 Adrenergic stimulation of brown fat thermogenesis. PPAR-γ = peroxisome proliferator activated receptor-γ; NRF = nuclear respiratory factors; CREB = CAMP responsive element binding protein; PKA = protein kinase A; UCP-1 = uncoupling protein 1. (From Ref. 69.).

activation stimulates generation of CAMP, which in turn activates protein kinase A (PKA). PKA then by phosphorylation of CAMP-responsive element binding protein (CREB) indirectly activates expression of peroxisome proliferator activated receptor coactivation 1 (PGC1), a coactivator of thermogenesis. PGC1 then coactivate transcription factors in the UCP1 enhancer, increasing UCP1 gene expression. Such transcription factors are PPAR-γ, retinoid X receptor, retinoic acid receptor and thyroid hormone receptor. β$_3$-adrenergic agonists have been reported to increase PGC1 mRNA levels by >50-fold, which in turn activates each of the three nuclear receptors just mentioned on the UCP1 enhancer increasing production of UCP1 (81). PGC1 also induces a new set of transcription factors called NRF1 and NRF2 associated with mitochondrial biogenesis in not only brown fat but also skeletal muscle. There is thus a mechanism by which β$_3$-agonists increase thermogenesis not only by increasing the uncoupling protein UCP1 but by causing an increase in mitochondria associated with such activated thermogenesis (70). PGC1 introduced into white fat cells induces UCPI but not UCP2 or UCP3, whereas PGC1 introduced into muscle induces UCP2 but not UCP1 or UCP3. In both fat cells and muscle, these introductions enhance both coupled and uncoupled energy expenditure. Possibly PGC1 expression may be the important developmental bifurcation between brown and white fat cells. Because of this and the analogous role of PGC1 in muscle, PGC1 has also become an interesting area of research in the development of new therapies for obesity.

B   Adrenergic Agonists

The activity of the sympathetic system has been shown to contribute to the control of the resting metabolic rate. A β_3-adrenergic gene polymorphism, a missense mutation in codon 64 (Trp^{64}ARG or W64R), has been associated with a lowered resting metabolic rate and appears to be associated with the development of obesity and type 2 diabetes mellitus (82). In female Swedish subjects the insertion of Glu instead of Gln in both alleles at codon 27 of the β_2-adrenoceptor gene was associated with a sevenfold relative risk for obesity (83). There are three α_2-adrenergic subtypes that are encoded by distinct genes located on different chromosomes with differing tissue distributions but similar pharmacological properties. The α_2-adrenergic receptors mediate part of the actions of catecholamines on the regulation of energy expenditure. A polymorphism resulting in the deletion of 3-glutamic acid repeat element appears to be important for agonist-dependent receptor desensitisation. The difference in resting metabolic rate between those with two normal long alleles and those with the abnormal two short alleles was ~5.6% or 94 kcal/d. This abnormality in the gene was discovered in 17% of a Finnish nondiabetic obese population. Research in this area might also have value in the development of obesity therapy. Nevertheless, subtype-selective pharmacological agents will need to be found before treatment options can be advanced for the early work on partial β_3/β_2 agonists which had some value as regards weight loss were associated with the side effect of tremor (84).

IX   ADRENAL HORMONOGENESIS

Adrenal glucocorticoids play an important role in the distribution of altered nutrient stores and body fat (60,85,86). Adrenal insufficiency is associated with a substantial loss in body weight and body fat (87). With excess glucocorticoids (Cushing's syndrome), excess weight develops with a central distribution of body fat. Adrenalectomy in ob/ob mice, which are deficient in leptin, or in other rodents with absent or abnormal leptin receptors, will prevent the development of obesity. Adrenalectomy in the ob/ob mice reduces hyperphagia, increases insulin sensitivity, and sympathetic activity but does not restore the hypogonadotrophic hypogonadism (87). Therefore in the rodent genetic

defects of leptin abnormality glucocorticoids are required for the phenotypic expression. Adrenalectomy is obviously not the answer in humans, but such animal work has led to further analysis of the role of glucocorticoids in the development of obesity, especially visceral obesity in man. This work has mainly centred on the cortisol-cortisone shuttle (88).

A   Cortisol-Cortisone Shuttle

Two isoenzymes of 11β-hydroxysteroid dehydrogenase (11β-HSD) catalyze the interconversion of hormonally active cortisol to inactive cortisone in man, known as type 1 and 2 (89,90). Cortisol is the principal glucocorticoid secreted from the adrenal cortex by human beings and is active as it possesses a C11 hydroxyl group, whereas cortisone with a C11 keto group is inactive. This cortisol-cortisone shuttle is an important pathway in determining corticosteroid action. Aberrant expression of the 11β-HSDs has far reaching consequences for the development of hypertension and obesity.

11β-HSD type 1 is predominantly expressed in the liver. Inhibition of this enzyme reduces to a small degree hepatic glucose output and improves insulin sensitivity (91). In knockout mice for the 11β-HSD1 gene exhibit attenuation of both fasting glucose and glucose output to food and stress compared to wild-type mice. 11β-HSD1 is also expressed in human adipose tissue, higher in omental fat than subcutaneous fat (92). In vitro 11β-HSD1 expression regulates glucocorticoid-induced adipocyte differentiation, possibly being one of the controlling factors in the development of visceral obesity (93). It has been known for decades that cortisol secretion rates are higher in obese subjects but this might not be due to increased 11β-HSD1 activity but to reduced cortisone conversion to cortisol activity increasing cortisol metabolic clearance by increasing ACTH drive (94). This reversed defect, called "apparent cortisone reductase syndrome," has also been detected in some women with polycystic ovarian syndrome (PCOS) resulting in enhanced cortisol metabolism and features due secondarily to ACTH mediated androgen excess (95,96).

Growth hormone and IGF1 inhibit 11β-HSD1 but not 11β-HSD2 expression. The increased cortisone to cortisol conversion seen in growth hormone–deficient patients (e.g., hypopituitarism) may account for some of the phenotypic features such as the visceral obesity and insulin resistance (97). 11β-HSD2 is expressed in mineralocorticoid target tissue such as kidney and salivary glands and is colocalized with the mineralocorticoid receptor in the kidney. In vitro the mineralocorticoid receptor has equal affinity for cortisol, corticosterone, and aldosterone. 11β-HSD2 by converting cortisol and corticosterone to inactive cortisone enables aldosterone to act appropriately on the mineralocorticoid receptor without interference from cortisol or corticosterone (94).

The Barker hypothesis suggests that poor nutrition in utero and in early life outside the womb programs an infant to the risk many years later of the development of cardiovascular problems, hypertension, obesity, and dyslipidemia (98). Such subjects also show altered cortisol dynamics with elevated urine cortisol as compared to those of normal birth weight and increased responsiveness to ACTH. Early work suggests that this may be related to differences in the expression of glucocorticoid receptor (personal communication, Reynolds and Walker). Clearly new medicines that act on 11β-HSD1 and target receptors may have some potential as antiobesity agents.

B DHEA

Dehydroepiandrosterone (DHEA) and its sulfated derivative are the most abundant steroid hormones secreted primarily from the adrenal cortex in man and constitute a precursor for both estrogens and testosterone. Serum levels increase markedly during adrenarche, reach peak levels in the third decade, and decline steadily and dramatically with advancing age, to 10–20% of peak values by 80 years of age (99). Although the decline in DHEA correlates with a variety of age-related changes, including reduced bone density, reduced muscle mass, increased fat mass, increased risk of atheroslerosis, and diabetes, the role that DHEA plays in these changes is still speculative (100). DHEA is also reduced in the obese person, and supplementation of the diet with DHEA in obese mice has been reported to reduce body fat (101). A recent study of modest supplementation (50 mg/day) over 6 months in obese elderly men and women (73 years average) has resulted in an average loss of 1.3 kg in total fat mass, decrease of 1.4 kg in trunk fat, and a 0.9 kg increase in lean mass, weight remaining unchanged (102). Morales et al. (103) reported that fat mass decreased with DHEA in men (−1.0 kg) but not in women (+0.5 kg). A recent structure function analysis by Lardy et al. (104) has shown that the biological effect on body fat of DHEA related steroids was greatest with the 7-oxo-DHEA derivatives. Other reports have found mixed results. Obviously this replacement might be beneficial to prevent age-related body composition adjustments but is unlikely to be a breakthrough in the treatment of the obese.

X DRUGS NO LONGER IN USE

Several groups of drugs used for treatment of obesity in the 20th century are no longer used. This paragraph will be a brief summary of these failures and the lessons, if any, that they can teach us. When measurements of metabolic rate were introduced early in the 20th century, they were rapidly applied to obesity with the hypothesis that low metabolic rate could explain the weight gain. Although oxygen uptake is higher, when the corrections were made for body weight, rather than lean body mass, overweight patients were often told that they had "low metabolism." One remedy for this was thyroid hormone, and it was one of the earliest drugs to be introduced into the treatment of obesity. We now know that obese patients do not have low metabolic rates and that, unless they are hypothyroid, there is no clinical indication for use of thyroid hormone (105). A second "thermogenic" drug arose from the observation is that workers exposed to dinitrophenol in the dye industry lost weight. Dintrophenol is an agent that uncouples oxidative phosphorylation in the mitochondrion, and on the surface might make a tempting target. Treatment with dinitrophenol produced weight loss, all right, but this treatment was associated with neuropathy and cataracts (105). However, modification of this molecule might provide some interesting compounds for further test. Hormonal injections for treatment of obesity were introduced more than 100 years ago. The most widely used in this century has been human chorionic gonadotrophin. Its wide popularity has led to a number of clinical trials that have shown it to be no better than the placebo injections (41). The final agent worthy of mention is digitalis. One of the side effects of this drug is nausea. This side effect was put to clinical use by giving digitalis leaf products to obese patients until a series of deaths associated with digitalis, diuretics, and thyroid hormone were reported.

XI CONCLUSION

Recent research has highlighted why an effective obesity agent still eludes us: namely, that the mechanism of control of intake, expenditure, and body weight is complex and polygenic. Such should be not a surprise as the survival of the human would be jeopardized by any less an effective system. It is only by understanding the rules of the system that the scientist can achieve a breakthrough in the finding of antiobesity agents. It is likely that one agent will not be the answer for everyone. Those with specific genetic faults will require correction of these either specifically or at some locus further away but downstream of their activation pathway. This may mean a package of therapy tailored to each individual's specific requirements. One the other hand, research may eventually show the final common pathway(s) which would allow pharmacological intervention with one or more agents useful for everyone with a weight problem. Nevertheless, the mass of new and varied discoveries with detection of many different genes involved does suggest that man may have to wait some decades yet before the elusive therapy is discovered. But just imagine the impact such therapy will have on the development of disease and our economies! Let it suffice to restate that it is easier for most forms of cancer to be controlled or cured at 5 years out than it is to produce substantial and maintained weight loss over the same period of time in most obese patients (106).

REFERENCES

1. Stunkard AJ, Foch TT, Hrubec Z. A twin study of human obesity. JAMA 1986; 256:51–54.

2. Borjeson M. The aetiology of obesity in children. Acta Paediatr Scand 1976; 65:279–287.

3. Perusse L, Chagnon YC, Weisnagel J, Bouchard C. The human obesity gene map: the 1998 update. Obes Res 1999; 7:111–129.

4. Schwartz MW, Woods SC, Porte D, Seeley RJ, Baskin DG. Central nervous system control of food intake. Nature 2000; 404:661–671.

5. Considine RV, Madhur K, Heiman ML, Kriaciunas A, Stephens TW, Nyce MR, Ohannesian JP, Marco CC, Mckee LJ, Bauer TL, Caro JF. Serum immunoreactive leptin concentration in normal weight and obese humans. N Engl J Med 1996; 334:292–295.

6. Schwartz MW, Peskind E, Raskind M, Boyko EJ, Porte D. Cerebrospinal fluid leptin levels; relationship to plasma levels and to adiposity in humans. Nat Med 1996; 2:589–593.

7. Wang J, Liu R, Hawkins M, Barzilia N, Possetti L. A nutrient sensing pathway regulates leptin gene expression in muscle and fat. Nature 1998; 393:684–688.

8. Sindelar DK, Havel PJ, Seeley RJ, Wilkinson CW, Woods SC, Schwartz MW. Low plasma leptin levels contribute to diabetic hyperphagia in rats. Diabetes 1999; 48:1275–1280.

9. Farooqui IS, O'Rahilly S. Recent advances in the genetics of severe childhood obesity. Arch Dis Child 2000; 83:31–34.

10. Montague CT, Farooqi IS, Whitehead JP, Soos MA, Rau H, Wareham NJ, Sewter CP, Digby JE, Mohammed SN, Hurst JA, Cheetham CH, Earley AR, Barnett AH, Prins JB, O'Rahilly S. Congential leptin deficiency is associated with severe early onset obesity in humans. Nature 1997; 387:903–908.

11. Strobel A, Issad T, Camoin L, Ozata M, Strosberg AD. A leptin missense mutation associated with hypogonadism and morbid obesity. Nat Genet 1998; 18: 213–215.

12. Van Gaal LF, Wauters MA, Mertens IL, Considine RV, De Leeuw IH. Clinical endocrinology of leptin. Int J Obes Relat Metab Disord 1999; 23(suppl 1):29–36.

13. Clement K, Vaisse C, Lahlou N, Cabrol S, Pelloux V, Cassuto D, Gourmelen M, Dina C, Chambaz J, Lacorte JM, Basdevant A, Bougneres P, Lebouc Y, Froguel P, Guy-Grand B. A mutation in the human leptin receptor gene causes obesity and pituitary dysfunction. Nature 1998; 392:398–401.

14. Bjorbaek C, Elmquist J, Frantz J, Shoelson S, Flier J. Identification of SOCS-3 as a potential mediator of central leptin resistance. Mol Cell 1998; 1:619–625.

15. Gura T. Tracing leptin's partners in regulating body weight [review]. Science 2000; 287:1738–1741.

16. Caro JF, Kolaczynski JW, Nyce MR, Ohannesian JP, Opentanova I, Goldman WH, Lynn RB, Zhang PL, Sinha MK, Considine RV. Decreased cerebrospinal fluid/serum leptin ratio in obesity: a possible mechanism for leptin resistance. Lancet 1996; 348:159–161.

17. Heymsfield SB, Greenberg AS, Fujioka K, Dixon RM, Kushner R, Hunt T, Lubina JA, Patane J, Self B, Hunt P, McCamish M. Recombinant leptin for weight loss in obese and lean adults; A randomised, controlled, dose escalation trial. JAMA 1999; 282:1568–1575.

18. Steppan CM, Bailey ST, Bhat S, Brown EJ, Banerjee RR, Wright CM, Patel HT, Ahima RS, Lazar MA. The hormone resistin links obesity to diabetes. Nature 2001; 409:307–312.

19. Martinez-Botas J, Anderson JB, Tessier D, Lapillonne A, Chang BH-J, Quast MJ, Gorenstein D, Chen K-H, Chan L. Absence of perilipin results in leanness and reverses obesity in Lepr(db/db) mice. Nat Genet 2000; 26:474–479.

20. Hahn T, Breininger J, Baskin D, Schwartz M. Co-expression of AGRP and NPY in fasting activated hypothalamic neurons. Nat Neurosci 1998; 1:271–272.

21. Bray GA, Fisler J, York DA. Neuroendocrine control of the development of obesity: understanding gained from studies of experimental animal models. Front Neuroendocrinol 1990; 11:128–181.

22. Woldbye DPD, Larsen PJ. The how and Y of eating. Nat Med 1998; 4:671–672.

23. Erickson JC, Hollopeter G, Palmiter RD. Attenuation of the obesity syndrome of ob/ob mice by the loss of neuropeptide Y. Science 1996; 274:1704–1707.

24. Erickson JC, Clegg KE, Palmiter RD. Sensitivity to

leptin and susceptibility to seizures of mice lacking neuropeptide Y. Nature 1996; 381:415–418.

25. Schwartz MW. Mahogany adds color to the evolving story of body weight regulation. Nat Med 1999; 5:374–375.

26. Cummings DE, Schwartz MW. Melanocortins and body weight: a tale of two receptors. Nat Genet 2000; 26:8–9.

27. Huszar D, Lynch CA, Fairchild-Huntress V, Dunmore JH, Fang Q, Berkmeier LR, Gu W, Kesterson RA, Boston BA, Cane RD, Smith FJ, Compfield LA, Burn P, Lee F. Targeted disruption of the melanocortin-4 receptor results in obesity in mice. Cell 1997; 88:131–141.

28. Fisher SL, Yagaloff KA, Burn P. Melanocortin-4 receptor: a novel signalling pathway involved in body weight regulation. Int J Obes Relat Metab Disord 1999; 23(suppl 1):54–58.

29. Krude H, Biebermann H, Luck W, Horn R, Brabant G, Gruters A. Severe early onset obesity, adrenal insufficiency and red hair pigmentation caused by POMC mutations in humans. Nat Genet 1998; 19: 155–157.

30. Jackson RS, Creemers JW, Ohagi S, Raffin-Sanson ML, Sanders L, Montague CT, Hutton JC, O'Rahilly S. Obesity and impaired prohormone processing associated with mutations in the human prohormone convertase I gene. Nat Genet 1997; 16:303–306.

31. Yeo GSH, Farooqi IS, Aminian S, Halsall DJ, Stanhope RG, O'Rahilly S. A frameshift mutation in MC4R associated with dominantly inherited human obesity. Nat Genet 1998; 20:111–112.

32. Hinney A, Schmidt A, Notteborm K, Heibult O, Becker I, Ziegler A, Gerber G, Sina M, Gorg T, Mayer H, Siegfried W, Fichter M, Remschoudt H, Hebebrand J. Several mutations in the melanocortin-4 receptor gene including a nonsense and a frameshift mutation associated with dominantly inherited human obesity. Nat Genet 1999; 20:111–112.

33. Bultman SJ, Michaud EJ, Woychik RP. Molecular characterisation of the mouse agouti locus. Cell 1992; 71:1195–1204.

34. Hagan M, Reisberg PA, Pritchard LM, Schwatz MW, Strack AM, Van der Ploeg LH, Woods SC, Seeley RJ. Long term orixegenic effects of AgRP (83–130) involve mechanisms other than melanocortin receptor blockade. Am J Physiol 2000; 279:R47–R52.

35. Lustig RH, Rose SR, Burgben GA, Velasquez-Mieyer P, Broome DC, Smith K, Li H, Hudson MM, Heideman RL, Kun LE. Hypothalamic obesity caused by cranial insult in children: altered glucose and insulin dynamics and reversal by a somatostatin agonist. J Pediatr 1999; 135:162–168.

36. Velasquez P, Cowan GSM, Buffington CK, Connelly BE, Spencer KA, Lustig RH. Monthly injections of long-acting octreotide promote insulin suppression and weight loss in adults with severe obesity [abstract]. Presented at Endo 2000.

37. Shimada M, Tritos N, Lowell B, Flier J, Maratos-Flier E. Mice lacking melanin concentrating hormone are hypophagic and lean. Nature 1998; 39:670–674.

38. Mondal MS, Nakazato M, Date Y, Murakami N, Hanada R, Sakata T, Matsukura M. Characterisation or orexin-A and orexin-B in the microdissected rat brain nuclei and their content in two obese rat models. Neurosci Lett 1999; 273:45–48.

39. Crawley JN. The role of galanin in feeding behaviour. Neuropeptides 1999; 33:369–375.

40. Jureus A, Cunningham MJ, McClain ME, Clifton DK, Steiner RA. Galanin-like peptide (GALP) is a target for regulation by leptin in the hypothalamus of the rat. Endocrinology 2000; 141:2703–2706.

41. Bray GA, Greenway FL. Current and potential drugs for treatment of obesity. Endocr Rev 1999; 20:705–785.

42. Howard AD, Wang R, Pong S-S, Mellin TN, Strack A, Guan X-M, Zeng Z, Williams DL Jr, Feighner SC, Nunes CN, Murphy B, Stair JN, Yu H, Hiang Q, Clements MK, Tan CP, McKee KK, Hrenluk DL, McDonald TP, Lynch KR, Evans JF, Austin CP, Caskey CT, Van der Ploeg LH, Liu Q. Identification of receptors for neuromedin U and its role in feeding. Nature 2000; 406:70–74.

43. Travers S, Norgren R. Gustatory neural processing in the hindbrain. Annu Rev Neurosci 1987; 10:595–632.

44. Funakoshi A, Miyasaka K, Matsumoto H, Yamamori S, Takiquchi S, Kataoka K, Takaka Y, Matsusue K, Kono A, Shimokata H. Gene structure of human cholecystokinin type A receptor: body fat content is related to CCK type a receptor gene promoter polymorphism. FEBS Lett 2000; 466:264–266.

45. Gouldson P, Legoux P, Carillon C, Dumont X, Le Fur G, Ferrara P, Shire D. Essential role of extracellular charged residues of the human CCK(1) receptor for interactions with SR 146131, SR 27897 and CCK-8S. Eur J Pharmacol 2000; 389:115–124.

46. Asakawa A, Inui A, Ueno N, Makino S, Fujino MA, Kasuga M. Urocortin reduces food intake and gastric emptying in lean and obese ob/ob mice. Gastroenterology 1999; 116:1287–1292.

47. Schwartz GJ, Whitney A, Skoglund C, Castonguay TW, Moran TH. Decreased responsiveness to dietary fat in Otsuka Long-Evans Tokushima fatty rats lacking CCK-A receptors. Am J Physiol 1999; 277:R1144–R1151.

48. Meereis-Schwanke K, Klonowski-Stumpe H, Erberg L, Niederau C. Long-term effects of CCK-agonist and antagonist on food intake and body weight in Zucker lean and obese rats. Peptides 1998; 19:291–299.

49. Ahren B, Holst JJ, Efendic S. Antidiabetogenic action of cholecystokinin-8 in type 2 diabetes. J Clin Endocrinol Metab 2000; 85:1043–1048.

50. Matson CA, Reid DF, Cannon TA, Ritter RC. Cholecystokinin and leptin act synergistically to reduce body weight. Am J Physiol Regul Integr Comp Physiol 2000; 278:R882–R890.

51. Flint A, Raben A, Rehfeld JF, Holst JJ, Astrup A. The effect of glucagon-like peptide-1 on energy expenditure and substrate metabolism in humans. Int J Obes Relat Metab Disord 2000; 24:288–298.

52. Lieverse RJ, Masclee AA, Jansen JB, Lam WF, Lamers C. Obese women are less sensitive for the satiety effects of bombesin than lean women. Eur J Clin Nutr 1998; 52:207–212.

53. Erlanson-Albertsson C, York D. Enterostatin–a peptide regulating fat intake [review]. Obes Res 1997; 5:360–372.

54. Chen AS, Marsh DJ, Trumbauer ME, Frazier EG, Guan X-M, Yu H, Rosenblum CI, Vongs A, Feng Y, Cao L, Metzger JM, Strack AM, Camacho RE, Mellin TN, Nunes CN, Min W, Fisher J, Gopal-Truter S, MacIntyre DE, Chen HY, Van der Ploeg LHT. Inactivation of the mouse melanocortin-3 receptor results in increased fat mass and reduced lean body mass. Nat Genet 2000; 26:97–102.

55. Lembertas AV, Perusse L, Chagnon YS, Fisler JS, Warden CH, Purcell-Huynh DA, Dianne FJ, Gagnon J, Nadeau A, Lusis AJ, Bouchard C. Identification of an obese locus on mouse chromosome 2 and evidence of linkage to fat and insulin on the human homologous region 20q. J Clin Invest 1997; 100:1240–1247.

56. Tschop M, Smiley DL, Helman ML. Ghrelin induces adiposity in rodents. Nature 2000; 407:908–913.

57. Synder DK, Clemmons DR, Underwood LE. Treatment of obese, diet-restricted subjects with growth hormone for 11 weeks: effects on anabolism, lipolysis, and body composition. J Clin Endocrinol Metab 1988; 67:54–61.

58. Johannsson G, Marin P, Lonn L, Ottosson M, Stenlof K, Bjorntorp P, Sjostrom L, Bengtsson BA. Growth hormone treatment of abdominally obese men reduces abdominal fat mass, improves glucose and lipoprotein metabolism, and reduces diastolic blood pressure. J Clin Endocrinol Metab 1997; 82:727–734.

59. Karlsson C, Stenlof K, Johannsson G, Marin P, Bjorntorp P, Bengtsson BA, Carlsson B, Carlsson LMS, Sjostrom L. Effects of growth hormone treatment on the leptin system and on energy expenditure in abdominally obese men. Eur J Endocrinol 1998; 138: 408–414.

60. Bray GA. Strategies for discovering drugs to treat obesity. In: Kopelman PG, Stock MJ, eds. Clinical Obesity Oxford: Blackwell, 1998:508–544.

61. Pothos E, Creese I, Hoebel B. Restricted eating with weight loss selectively decreases extracellular dopamine in the nucleus accumbens and alters dopamine response to amphetamine, morphine and food intake. J Neurosci 1995; 15:6640–6650.

62. Parada MA, Hernandez I, Paez X, Baptista T, De Parada MP, De Quidada M. Mechanism of the body weight increase induced by systemic sulpiride. Pharmacol Biochem Behav 1989; 33:45–50.

63. Nonogaki K, Strack A, Dallman M, Tecott I. Leptin independent hyperphagia and type 2 diabetes in mice with a mutated serotonin 5 HT_{2C} receptor gene. Nat Med 1998; 4:1152–1156.

64. Leibowitz S, Alexander J. Hypothalamic serotonin in control of eating behavior, meal size and body weight. Biol Psychiatry 1998; 44:851–864.

65. Tsujii S, Bray GA. GABA related feeding control in genetically obese rats. Brain Res 1991; 540:48–54.

66. Privitera MD. Topiramate: a new antiepileptic drug. Ann Pharmacother 1997; 31:1164–1173.

67. Shorvon SD. Safety of topiramate adverse events and relationships to dosing. Epilepsia 1996; 37(suppl 2): S18–S22.

68. Loftus TM, Jaworsky DE, Frehywot GL, Townsend CA, Ronnett GV, Lane MD, Kuhajda FP. Reduced food intake and body weight in mice treated with fatty acid synthase inhibitors. Science 2000; 288:2379–2381.

69. Nicholls DG, Locke RM. Thermogenic mechanisms in brown fat. Physiol Rev 1984; 64:1–64.

70. Lowell BB, Spiegelman BM. Towards a molecular understanding of adaptive thermogenesis. Nature 2000; 404:652–660.

71. Solanes GA, Vidal-Puig D, Grujic D, Flier JS, Lowell BB. The human uncoupling protein-3 gene: genomic structure, chromosomal localisation and genetic basis for short and long form transcripts. J Biol Chem 1997; 272:25433–25436.

72. Cunningham S, Leslie P, Hopwood D, Illingworth P, Jung RT, Nicholls DG, Peden N, Rafeal J, Rial E. The characterisation and energetic potential of brown adipose tissue in man. Clin Sci 1985; 69:343–348.

73. Simonsen L, Bulow J, Madsen J, Christensen NJ. Thermogenic response to epinephrine in the forearm and abdominal subcutaneous adipose tissue. Am J Physiol 1992; 263:E850–E855.

74. Argyropoulos G, Brown AM, Willli SM, Zhu J, He Y, Reitman M, Gevao SM, Spruill I, Garvey WT. Effects of mutations in the human uncoupling protein 3 gene on the respiratory quotient and fat oxidation in severe obesity and type 2 diabetes. J Clin Invest 1998; 102: 1345–1351.

75. Larkin S, Mull E, Miao W, Pitnner R, Abrandt K, Moore C, Young A, Denaro M, Beaumont K. Regulation of the third member of the uncoupling protein family, UCP3, by cold and thyroid hormones. Biochem Biophys Res Commun 1997; 240:222–227.

76. Matsuda J, Hosoda K, Itoh H, Son C, Doi K, Tanaka T, Fukunaga Y, Inoue G, Nishimura H, Yoshimasa Y. Cloning of rat UCP3 and UCP2 cDNAs: their gene expression in rats fed high fat diets. FEBS Lett 1997; 418:200–204.

77. Bouchard C, Perusse L, Chagnon YC, Warden C, Riquier D. Linkage between markers in the vicinity of the uncoupling protein 2 gen and resting metabolic rate in humans. Hum Mol Genet 1997; 6:1887–1889.

78. Fleury C, Neverova M, Collins S, Raimbault S, Champigny O, Levi-Meyrueis C, Bouillaud F, Seldin MF, Surwit RS, Riquier D. Uncoupling protein 2: a novel gene linked to obesity and hyperinsulinemia. Nat Genet 1997; 15:269–272.

79. Millet I, Vidal H, Andreelli F, Larrouy D, Riou JP, Ricquier D, Laville M, Langin D. Increased uncoupling protein-2 and -3 mRNA expression during fasting in obese and lean humans. J Clin Invest 1997; 100: 2665–2670.

80. Urhammer SA, Dalgaard LT, Sorensen TIA, Tybaerg-Hansen A, Echwald SM, Andersen T, Clausen JO, Pedersen O. Organisation and coding exons and mutational screening of the uncoupling protein 3 gene in subjects with juvenile onset obesity. Diabetolgia 1998; 41:241–244.

81. Boss O, Bachman E, Vidal-Puig A, Chen-Yu Z, Peroni O, Lowell BB. Role of the beta (3)-adrenergic receptor and/or a putative beta(4)-adrenergic receptor on the expression of uncoupling proteins and peroxisome-activated receptor-gamma coactivator-1. Biochem Biophys Res Commun 1999; 261:870–876.

82. Fujisawa T, Ikegami H, Kawaguchi Y, Ogihara T. Meta-analysis of the association of Trp64 arg polymorphism of beta-3 adrenergic receptor gen woth body mass. J Clin Endocrinol Metab 1998; 83:2441–2444.

83. Heinoven P, Koulu M, Pesonen U, Karvonen MK, Rissanen A, Laakso M, Valve R, Uusitupa M, Scheinin M. Identification of a three-amino acid deletion in the 2B-adrenergic receptor that is associated with reduced basal metabolic rate in obese subjects. J Clin Endocrinol Metab 1999; 84:2429–2433.

84. Connacher AA, Jung RT, Mitchell PEG. Increased weight loss in diet restricted obese subjects given BRL 26830A—a new atypical β agonist. BMJ 1988; 296: 1217–1220.

85. Bray GA, Tartaglia LA. Medicinal strategies in the treatment of obesity [review]. Nature 2000; 404:672–677.

86. Bray GA. Reciprocal relation of food intake and sympathetic activity; experimental observations and clinical implications. Int J Obes Relat Metab Dis 2000; 24(suppl 2):S8–S17.

87. Shimizu H, Ohshima K, Bray GA, Peterson M, Swerdloff RS. Adrenalectomy and castration in the genetically obese (ob/ob) mouse. Obes Res 1993; 369:215–223.

88. Stewart PM, Corrie JET, Shackleton CHL, Edwards CRW. Syndrome of apparent minerlocorticoid excess: a defect in the cortisol-cortisone shuttle. J Clin Invest 1998; 82:340–349.

89. Tannin GM, Agarwal AK, Monder C, New MI, White PC. The human gene for 11β-hydroxysteroid dehydrogenase. Structure, tissue distribution and chromosomal localisation. J Biol Chem 1991; 266:16653–16658.

90. Stewart PM, Murray BA, Mason JI. Human kidney 11β-hydroxysteroid dehydrogenase is a high affinity NAD + -dependent enzyme and differs from the cloned 'type 1' isoform. J Clin Endocrinol Metab 1994; 79: 480–484.

91. Walker BR, Connacher AA, Lindsay RM, Webb DJ, Edwards CRW. Carbenoxolone increases hepatic insulin sensitivity in man. A novel role for 11 oxo-steroid reductase in enhancing glucocorticoid receptor activation. J Clinical Endocrinol Metab 1995; 80: 3155–3159.

92. Kotelevstev YV, Holmes MC, Burchell A, Houston PM, Schmoll D, Jamieson P, Best R, Brown R, Edwards CR, Seckl JR, Mullins JJ. 11β-hydroxysteroid dehydrogenase type 1 knockout mice show attenuated glucocorticoid-inducible responses and resist hyperglycaemia on obesity or stress. Proc Natl Acad Sci USA 1997; 94:14924–14929.

93. Bujalska I, Kumar S, Stewart PM. Does central obesity reflect 'Cushing's disease' of the omentum? Lancet 1997; 349:1210–1213.

94. Stewart PM. The cortisol-cortisone shuttle: physiological and clinical implications. Topical Endocrinol 1999; 13:2–5.

95. Rodin A, Thakkar H, Taylor N, Clayton R. Hyperandrogenism in polycystic ovary syndrome; evidence of dysregulation of 11β-hydroxysteroid dehydrogenase. N Engl J Med 1994; 330:460–465.

96. Philpov G, Palermo M, Shackleton CHL. Apparent cortisone reductase deficiency. A unique form of hypercortisolism. J Clin Endocrinol Metab 1996; 81:3855–3860.

97. Weaver JU, Taylor N, Monson JP, Wood PJ, Kelly WF. Sexual dimorphism in 11β-hydroxysteroid dehydrogenase activity and its relation to fat distribution and insulin sensitivity; a study in hypopituitary subjects. Clin Endocrinol 1998; 49:13–20.

98. Barker DJ. Fetal origins of coronary heart disease. BMJ 1995; 311:171–174.

99. Belanger A, Carridas B, Dupont A, Cusan L, Diamond P, Gomez JL, Labrie F. Changes in serum concentration of conjugated and unconjugated steroids in 40–80 year old men. J Clin Endocrinol Metab 1994; 79:1310–1316.

100. Clore JN. Dehydroepiandrosterone and body fat. Obes Res 1995; 3(suppl 4):613–616.

101. Yen TT, Allan JA, Pearson DV, Acton JM, Greenberg MM. Prevention of obesity in A^{vy}/a mice be dehydroepiandrosterone. Lipids 1977; 12:409–413.

102. Villareal DT, Holloszy JO, Kohrt WM. Effects of DHEA replacement on bone mineral density and body

composition in elderly women and men. Clin Endocrinol 2000; 53:561–568.

103. Morales AJ, Haubrich RH, Hwang JY, Asakura H, Yen SS. The effect of six months treatment with a 100mg daily dose of DHEA on circulating sex steroids, body composition and muscle strength in age advanced men and women. Clin Endocrinol 1998; 49:421–432.

104. Lardy HE, Kneer N, Wei Y, Partridge B, Marwah P. Ergosteroids. II. Biologically active metabolites and synthetic derivatives of dehydroepiandrosterone. Steroids 1998; 63:158–165.

105. Bray GA. Treatment of the Obese Patient. Philadelphia: W B Saunders, 1976.

106. Council of Scientific Affairs. Treatment of obesity in adults. JAMA 1988; 260:2547–2551.

16

Drugs with Thermogenic Properties

Arne Astrup and Søren Toubro

The Royal Veterinary and Agricultural University, Frederiksberg, Denmark

I INTRODUCTION

Currently available drugs used to treat obesity exert their main action on energy balance either by reducing energy intake or by inhibiting intestinal fat absorption. However, some of the drugs that reduce food intake also possess thermogenic properties that contribute to their clinical efficacy in terms of loss of body fat and of weight maintenance. A number of other compounds possess thermogenic effects but are used for indications other than obesity. Specific thermogenic agents developed for the treatment of obesity and diabetes are in the first phases of clinical development. Compounds are reviewed in this chapter irrespective of whether they are approved for use in obesity treatment by the U.S. Food and Drug Administration (FDA), the European CPMC, or by other regulatory bodies.

II RATIONALE FOR STIMULATING ENERGY EXPENDITURE

Daily energy expenditure represents one side of the energy balance equation. Over a longer period of time, total energy expenditure should be in equilibrium with total energy intake to ensure weight stability. The inability to ensure this balance is the overall background for the prevalent weight gain in the population and the current obesity epidemic. Many efforts are exerted to produce weight loss and subsequently to maintain

energy balance with the reduced body size by adjustments of both dietary energy intake and physical exercise, but this strategy is successful only in a small proportion of obese subjects. The rapidly increasing prevalence of obesity in most countries must be due to changes in environmental factors, but there is increasing evidence that those who gain weight when exposed to these environmental factors have a genetic susceptibility. More and more genetic studies add evidence to the concept that this susceptibility is brought about by the coexistence of a cluster of certain polymorphisms at genes encoding for neurohumoral mediators, their receptors, and peripheral proteins involved in cellular substrate and energy metabolism. It is interesting that receptors and proteins important for regulation of substrate and energy metabolism, such as the β-adrenergic receptors (β_2 and β_3), and the uncoupling proteins (1–3) seem to be such susceptible genes. This knowledge, and the lack of efficacy of lifestyle changes in controlling body weight, supports the development of a pharmacological strategy to "normalize" energy and substrate metabolism as a tool to improve the results of obesity management. There is evidence to support the hypothesis that a low-energy output phenotype predisposes individuals to weight gain and obesity, the low-energy output being caused by a low resting metabolic rate (RMR), a low nonexercise activity thermogenesis (NEAT), physical inactivity, or combinations hereof (1). Increased energy metabolism and fat oxidation are therefore logical and attractive targets because they may counteract the suppression of RMR, and perhaps even diminish the hunger that accompanies weight loss, thereby allowing people to maintain food intake at more socially acceptable levels. In addition, any increase in energy expenditure is not fully counteracted by a similar increase in appetite and in energy intake (2), irrespective of whether the increased energy output is achieved through increased exercise or pharmacologically (3). Even a slight sustained increase of 2–3% in daily energy expenditure may therefore have clinical relevance, particularly in preventing the decline in RMR with weight loss, but also in decreasing the risk of weight regain following a weight loss.

Energy expenditure can be stimulated pharmacologically by interference with several steps in the regulatory system. These can be activation of the central leptin receptor, the CNS regulatory systems, peripheral efferent neurons of the sympathetic nervous system, the adrenergic receptors, the thyroid and growth hormones, or cellular mechanisms responsible for thermogenic futile mechanisms such as uncoupling proteins.

A Physiological Rationale for the Sympathoadrenal System as a Drug Target

RMR comprises 50–80% of daily energy expenditure (4). The remaining expended energy is mainly derived from the cost of physical activity and, to a lesser degree, to meal-induced thermogenesis, mental stress, cold, and thermogenic stimulants in food and beverages (nicotine, caffeine and its derivatives, polyphenols in green tea, and capsaicins in hot chilies). About 70–80% of the variance of RMR can be accounted for by differences in fat free mass, fat mass, age, and sex (4,5). However, an additional 5–8% of the variance in RMR is accounted for by family membership, which strongly supports the existence of influence by genetic factors. Some of this variance can be explained by individual differences within the normal physiological range in sympathetic tone, thyroid hormone levels, and polymorphisms in β-receptor and UCP genes (5–8). Other components of 24-hr energy expenditure are influenced by the sympathetic tone. Meal ingestion is accompanied by an increased SNS activity, and studies using β-blockade have demonstrated a facultative, β-adrenergically mediated component (9).

Physical activity also seems to be stimulated by sympathetic activity. The positive relationship between spontaneous physical activity and norepinephrine appearance rate is consistent with the idea that SNS activity is a determinant of individual differences in the level of spontaneous physical activity, i.e., how much

people move around, change position, and fidget, all of which contribute to total energy expenditure. So "fidgeters" seem either to have a constitutionally higher SNS activity (5) or to possess certain functional polymorphisms in genes controlling the activity of β-adrenoceptors and uncoupling proteins (7,8).

The contribution of the sympathoadrenal system to 24-hr energy expenditure has been addressed using measurements in whole-body calorimeters. Administration of the β-antagonist propranolol causes a 2–4% decrease in 24-hr energy expenditure, suggesting that a total blockade of the β-mediated pathways of the sympathoadrenal system may suppress 24-hr EE by 4–6%, equivalent to 50–150 kcal/d (5). This is consistent with observations from meta-analyses of clinical trials showing that treatment with β-adrenoceptor antagonists produces weight gain (10). SNS activity also influences the substrate oxidized, and norepinephrine increases intracellular lipolysis and NEFA uptake in the muscle (11), which seem to be impaired in some obese subjects (12). The stimulatory effect of β-adrenergic agonists on fat oxidation is well established. β-Antagonists accordingly have the opposite effect; that is, they decrease energy expenditure and the relative rate of fat oxidation. The effect of substrate utilization may be attributed, in part, to the important β-adrenergic stimulatory effect on lipolysis.

B Role of Low-Energy Expenditure in the Development of Obesity

Several studies support the idea that a low RMR is associated with weight gain. A low metabolic rate has been shown to precede body weight gain in infants, children, and in adult Pima Indians and Caucasians (5). Based on the assumption that formerly obese, weight-reduced subjects exhibit the metabolic characteristics that predisposed them to obesity, several studies have compared metabolic rates in formerly obese subjects to those of weight-matched controls who have never been obese. A meta-analysis of 12 such studies corroborates the prospective data by demonstrating a 3–5% lower mean RMR in the formerly obese subjects (13). Moreover, these data indicate that a low RMR is more frequent among formerly obese subjects than among never-obese control subjects. Studies of the contribution of the sympathoadrenal activity to this trait have yielded conflicting results, probably because comparisons of lean and obese subjects provide only very limited information about the role of the SNS in the aetiology of obesity (5). Furthermore, they do not discern between the causes and the consequences of weight gain. However, longitudinal studies both in Pima Indians and in Caucasians have shown a relationship between low urinary norepinephrine excretion and weight gain, and a relationship between low urinary epinephrine excretion and the development of central obesity (5). These results strongly suggest that a low SNS activity is also a risk factor for weight gain in humans. SNS activity increases in response to weight gain, thereby attenuating the original impairment (see Macdonald and Ravussin, this book).

III THYROID HORMONES AND DERIVATES

Thyroid hormones are the physiological controllers of basal metabolism. Hypothyroid and hyperthyroid states are associated with predicted changes in energy expenditure and in body weight and composition. Mean body weight and fat mass are normally decreased by 15% in hyperthyroidism, and hypothyroid patients weigh 15–30% more than in their euthyroid states. These pertur-

bations in thyroid hormone metabolism are good examples of primary changes in energy expenditure that are not fully compensated for by corrective adjustments in energy intake. Normal physiological variations in T_3 concentrations have also been shown to be responsible for differences between individuals in daily energy expenditure by up to 150 kcal/d (6). An increase of this magnitude is an attractive goal for the treatment of obesity. The short-term thermogenic effect of thyroid hormone involves a direct interaction between T_2 and mitochondrial enzymes with an onset after 6 hr and lasting for 2 days, whereas the long-term effects are mediated by T_3 through nuclear receptors (TR_α and TR_β) (14). The long-term effects require binding to the regulatory regions of the genes. Effects are seen after 30 hr and last up to 60 days (14). Thyroid hormones produce actions as a result of interactions with several genes controlling energy metabolism, and many of these effects result in increased energy production and utilization of fat as substrate. One of the important effects of T_3 is upregulation of the uncoupling proteins (Fig. 1), which subsequently leads to heat dissipation without

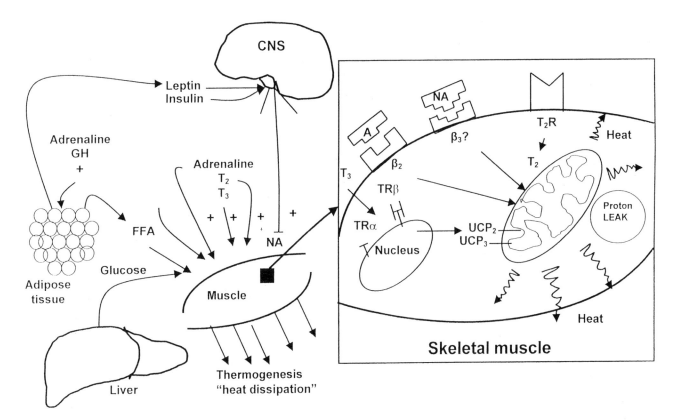

Figure 1 Where can thermogenesis be stimulated pharmacologically in humans? Model of the effector side of decreased metabolic efficiency in humans. Thyroid hormones, growth hormones, circulating catecholamines, and sympathetic nerves stimulate thermogenesis, fat oxidation, and uncoupling in skeletal muscle and liver.

synthesis of ATP. In hypothyroidism UPC$_3$ levels are decreased threefold and they are increased sixfold in hyperthyroidism, but the expression of the UCP$_3$ gene is also influenced by energy balance, leptin, and β$_3$-adrenoceptors. Although obesity is not normally characterized by a subnormal T$_3$, the receptors responsible for the T$_3$ actions remain attractive targets for enhancing energy expenditure.

A Clinical Trials with Thyroid Hormone Therapy in Euthyroid Obese Subjects

Thyroid hormones have been used to treat obesity for more than a century (15). Initially thyroid extracts were used, but after the identification of T$_4$, and later T$_3$, several studies of the specific actions of these components were conducted in the 1960s and '70s. Desiccated thyroid extract, T$_4$, and T$_3$, have all been used in clinical trials, but the design of many of these studies was not optimal, and the outcome was therefore variable. More recent trials using T$_3$ in controlled designs generally support that T$_3$ is effective in producing substantial weight loss in obese euthyroid subjects (for complete review see 15), most of the studies used high doses of T$_3$ varying from 0.15 to 2.00 mg/day (16). High doses of T$_3$ caused several side effects, serious cardiac problems, and muscle weakness, all of which can probably be attributed to excessive loss of lean body tissue (16–20). Recent studies using T$_3$ treatment following a very low calorie diet where endogenous T$_3$ levels are suppressed, have failed to find excessive urinary nitrogen loss or changes in leucine or lysine kinetics (21–23). Although there is a widespread use of T$_3$ supplementation among overweight and obese subjects, this is not endorsed by the existing data on efficacy and safety. Clinical trials with current state of the art design and methodology are required (14,15), but recent experimental evidence shows that even mild hyperthyroidism has adverse effects (24).

B Selective Thyroid Receptor Analogs

Selective agonists at the TR$_β$ have been developed and have been shown in animal models to have fewer side effects than T$_3$ (25). In comparison with T$_3$, one of these agonists, GC-1 [3,5-dimethyl-4-(4′-hydroy-3′-isopropylbenzyl)-phenoxy acid], has more marked lipid-lowering acetic acid], has more marked lipid-lowering effect, does not increase heart rate and has less positive inotropic effect (26). Ribeiro et al. (27) have shown that TR$_α$ is essential for thyroid hormone to restore the levels of a factor in the norepinephrine signalling pathway,

downstream of the adrenergic receptors, that is limiting for the norepinephrine action in hypothyroidism. This effect is seen in several tissues and could be a way to increase thermogenesis. Compounds taking advantage of the fact that thyroid-induced thermogenesis is thyroid hormone receptor isoform-specific may be promising for the treatment of obesity and the metabolic syndrome, but no human data are yet in the public domain.

IV CONTROLLED UNCOUPLERS

A 2,4-Dinitrophenol

Mitochondria are the cellular organelles that convert food energy to carbon dioxide, water, and ATP, and they are fundamental in mediating effects on energy dissipation. Mitochondria are responsible for 90% of cellular oxygen consumption and the majority of ATP production. However, not all of the available energy is coupled to ATP synthesis. Much is lost by uncoupled reactions when protons move from the cytosol back into the mitochondrial matrix via pathways which circumvent the ATP synthase and other uses of the electrochemical gradient (28). Proton cycling has been estimated to account for 20–25% of resting metabolic rate, and there is very good evidence to support that drugs can further stimulate it. 2,4-Dinitrophenol (DNP) is an artificial uncoupler that acts as a protonophore because it can cross membranes protonated, lose its proton, and return as the anion, then reprotonate and repeat the cycle. By this mechanism DNP increases the basal proton conductance of mitochondria and uncouples. DNP was introduced as a drug in the 1930s and was used with enormous success for weight loss purposes. The ability of DNP to produce effective weight loss without dieting led to widespread use, but several problems occurred due to its low therapeutic index (28). Owing to a steep dose dependence of metabolic rate, a number of people were literally "cooked to death" in the 1930s because of accidental or deliberate overdose (29). Reports of cataracts and deaths from overdose led to its withdrawal from the market by the FDA in 1938 (28). Currently, pharmaceutical companies are developing derivatives of DNP with a less steep dose response relationship, and with a built-in inhibition that limits the uncoupling process.

B Uncoupling Proteins

Uncoupling protein UCP$_2$ and UCP$_3$ are proteins that can uncouple ATP production from mitochondrial respiration, thereby dissipating energy as heat and reducing energy metabolism efficiency (28,30). In rodents, brown adipose tissue (BAT) functions to dissipate energy in the form of heat through the action of UCP_1. Heat production by brown adipocytes results from a controlled uncoupling of oxidative phosphorylation by an UCP_1-mediated proton conductance pathway in the inner mitochondrial membrane. In animal models the β_3-receptor stimulates lipolysis in WAT and BAT, and in BAT both activates UCP and upregulates the UCP gene, both of which result in a further increase in energy expenditure. BAT is abundant in rodents but has no functional role in adult humans (31), and the β_3-receptor is a questionable drug target (see Sec. V.E). In humans, however, the major site of catecholamine induced thermogenesis is skeletal muscle, which can account for 50–60% of the whole-body response (32).

In contrast to UCP_1, which is only present in brown adipose tissue, UCP_2 has a wide tissue distribution, whereas UCP_3 is expressed predominantly in skeletal muscle. Linkage and association studies have provided some evidence of a role for UCPs in modulating metabolic rate in human studies. Until recently, the cellular thermogenic mechanisms were unknown, but the discovery of both UCP_2 and UCP_3 expressed in skeletal muscle offers a plausible mechanism for heat dissipation (33). Treatment with thyroid hormone increases expression of the UCP_2 and UCP_3 genes. Other regulators of UCP_2 and UCP_3 gene expression are β_3-adrenergic agonists and glucocorticoids. The UCP_3 and UCP_2 genes are located adjacent to each other in a region implicated in linkage studies as contributing to obesity (34,35), and a polymorphism in the gene encoding for both UCP_2 and UCP_3 has been associated with reduced RMR and fat oxidation (7,8,34). However, it is still controversial whether UCP_2 and UCP_3 are real uncoupling proteins, but they may yet be found to catalyse an uncoupling similar to that of UCP_1, which is induced by unidentified agonists. Indeed, recent studies suggest that both UCP_2 and UCP_3 are functional (36). Other promising drug targets for uncoupling are the adenine nucleotide transporters responsible for uncoupling by free fatty acids and AMP (28).

V THERMOGENIC PROPERTIES OF ENHANCERS OF SYMPATHETIC ACTIVITY

A Leptin

Animals and humans that have a genetic deficiency of the adipocyte-derived hormone leptin, or of its receptor, exhibit extreme obesity (37). Leptin acts on the hypothalamus to suppress appetite and increase energy expenditure, and the negative energy balance produced by exogenous administration of leptin in deficient animals is partly mediated by increased SNS outflow to several organs, including BAT. Accordingly, rodents with defective leptin biosynthesis or receptor function (*ob/ob* mouse, *db/db* mouse, or *fa/fa* rat) exhibit severely reduced SNS activity, gain weight rapidly, and become obese. Leptin deficiency is extremely rare in humans and has been identified as a cause of obesity in only ~10 patients. By contrast, serum concentrations of leptin increase with body fat in all the obese persons who do not have this mutation in the gene encoding for leptin. The high leptin levels in obese individuals suggest leptin insensitivity and pose questions about the potential for leptin in the treatment of simple obesity. However, observational studies in humans suggests that leptin, in humans as in animals, stimulates SNS and energy expenditure (38,39). Recombinant leptin has indeed proved to be very effective in two children with leptin deficiency, although the investigators did not detect any stimulatory impact of leptin on energy expenditure, which could easily have been blurred by the pronounced concomitant decrease in body weight (40). However, physical activity level index increased from 1.6 to 1.9 after 12 months of treatment, which is most probably due to movement being less restrained with less adiposity and is thus not a direct effect of leptin. In normal-weight subjects and in leptin-intact obese subjects, injections of recombinant leptin produced only a modest reduction in weight and fat loss over 24 weeks (41). Moreover, a recent study of Hukshorn et al. did not find any effect of subcutaneous pegylated recombinant native human leptin treatment on body fat, energy expenditure, or substrate utilization in obese men (42). Leptin and analogs are therefore not very promising thermogenic agents for the treatment of simple obesity.

B Ephedrine/Caffeine

Numerous studies have shown that ephedrine (E) as monotheraphy decreases body fat in obese subjects by a combined action of suppression of appetite and stimulation of energy expenditure (43). Adenosine antagonists such as caffeine (C) potentiate the thermogenic and clinical effects. Dose-response studies found that the combination of ephedrine 20 mg and caffeine 200 mg produced the best synergistic effect on thermogenesis (44). Ephedrine is both an indirect sympathomimetic, causing release of norepinephrine from the sympathetic nerve endings (32), and a direct agonist on β-receptors.

Experimental human studies suggest that not only β_1 and β_2, but also β_3 are involved in its peripheral thermogenic effect (45).

Combinations of E + C have been shown to be effective for treatment of obesity for up to 50 weeks (Fig. 2). In a study including 180 obese patients it was found that E + C (20 mg/200 mg TID) produced a larger weight loss than placebo, caffein, or ephedrine, in combination with a hypoenergetic diet over 24 weeks (46). After 24 weeks the placebo group had lost 13.2 kg, and E + C further increased the weight loss by 3.4 kg to a total loss of 16.6 kg. Also, more patients in the E + C group than in the placebo group lost >5% and 10% of the initial body weight. Breum et al. tested E + C against dexfenfluramine in a double-blind placebo-controlled trial, and found E + C produced a greater weight loss than dexfenfluramine in subjects with a BMI of >30 kg/m² (47). The reductions in pulse rate and blood pressure were similar with the two treatments. E + C has also been evaluated for prevention of weight gain after smoking cessation. The double-blind placebo-controlled trial included 225 subjects, and after 12 weeks weight gain was less in the E + C group than in placebo group (48). However, after 1 year there was no difference in the proportion of subjects not smoking.

Molnar et al. reported a 20-week, randomized double-blind placebo-controlled trial of E + C in adolescents aged 16 years and Tanner stage III–V, and found that E + C produced more substantial weight loss than placebo (14.4% vs. 2.2%) (49). Subjects dropped out only in the placebo group, and adverse effects were mild and not different from placebo after 4 weeks.

1   Cardiovascular Effects of E + C

Notably, E + C increases blood pressure and heart rate slightly with the first exposure (44). However, during chronic treatment tachyphylaxis develops to the cardiovascular effects of the compound, but not to the anorectic and thermogenic (46). In the largest trial of E + C, only a slight increase in blood pressure and heart rate could be detected when the treatment was initiated, but after 12 weeks dietary treatment the reductions in blood pressure were similar in the E + C group to those in the placebo group (46). A hypothetical cardiovascular safety concern could be raised by the combination of E + C and exercise. However, Stich et al. studied the metabolic and hemodynamic responses to submaximal exercise before and after 3 days of E + C treatment in obese patients and found no indications of an enhanced exer-

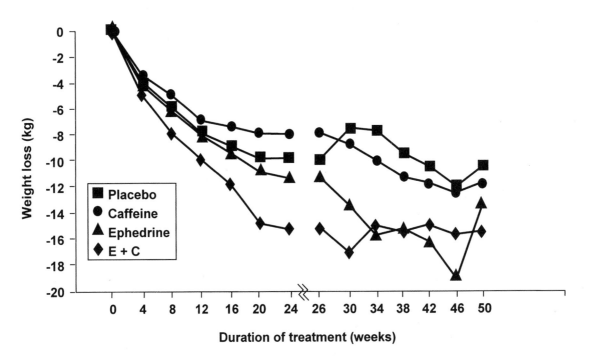

Figure 2 Effect of a combination of 20 mg ephedrine and 200 mg caffeine TTD as adjuvant to a hypocaloric diet on weight loss and weight maintenance for 1 year. The first 24 months involved a randomized, double-blind, placebo-controlled study, whereas all groups received E + C from week 26 to 50. (From Refs. 46 and 56.)

cise induced increase in blood pressure and heart rate as compared with placebo (50). With more extensive measurement of cardiovascular function by thoracic impedance, automatic sphygmomanometry, and continuous electrocardiographic recording, Waluga et al. concluded that E + C had no undesirable effects on cardiovascular function in obese subjects (51). E + C has also been tested in overweight subjects with controlled hypertension (52). Treatment with E + C produced a larger weight loss than placebo, and reduced systolic blood pressure 5.5 mm Hg more than placebo, and the antihypertensive effect of β-blockers was not reduced by E + C (52).

E + C does not seem to have any long-term effect on glucose and lipid metabolism apart from the beneficial changes in risk factors secondary to weight loss. Buemann et al. reported that E + C prevented the decline in HDL cholesterol associated with weight loss, and it increased the ratio of HDL cholesterol to total cholesterol, whereas no effect on fasting glucose metabolism was observed (53).

How much of the fat loss produced by E + C can be attributed to the thermogenic action of the compound? Measurements of 24-hr energy expenditure in whole-body calorimeters, combined with measurements of body composition, during 8 weeks of treatment with a hypocaloric diet and either E + C or placebo found that 25% of the additional fat loss seen in the intervention group could be explained by an enhanced fat oxidation and thermogenic effect of E + C (54). Similar results have been found in nonhuman primates, where E + C caused fat loss and increased sleeping energy expenditure by 20–25% (55).

The clinical studies of E + C clearly show that the compound is effective in the treatment of obesity for up to 1 year (56). However, owing to the limited number of patients treated in the trials the total evidence does not meet the efficacy and safety requirements of the American FDA or the European CPMC for licensing E + C as a prescription compound. Unfortunately, the pharmaceutical industry does not invest in such a compound, which is difficult to protect. A recent systematic review concluded that the risks of E + C are outweighed by the benefits of achieving and maintaining a healthy weight (43).

Various herbal combinations of E + C based on Ma Huang, guarana, and aspirin are sold OTC in United States, and the total sales reached ~$950 million in 1999. The pharmacokinetics of these herbal preparations may be variable, and they contain many other ingredients such as minerals and herbs that might alter or interact with E or C (43). As concluded by Greenway:

"These herbal products containing ephedrine and caffeine should be tested in controlled clinical trials to confirm their presumed efficacy and safety which cannot truly be extrapolated from the peer-reviewed scientific literature using pharmaceutical grade caffeine and ephedrine in isolation" (43).

C Thermogenic Properties of Sibutramine

Sibutramine is a serotonin and norepinephrine reuptake inhibitor, and it causes weight loss in laboratory animals through effects on both food intake and metabolic rate (57). Controlled trials conducted in obese patients have consistently shown dose-related weight loss, and optimal weight loss at 10 mg and 15 mg sibutramine (58). Typically, weight loss was 3–5 kg greater than placebo at 24 weeks, and the loss was sustained for 2 years. The STORM trial demonstrates that sibutramine is also more effective in maintaining 2-year weight loss than placebo (59). Sibutramine causes dose-dependent inhibition of daily food intake in rats owing to the enhancement of satiety, whereas eating patterns and other behaviors remain similar to those exhibited by control animals. Sibutramine also stimulates thermogenesis in rats, producing sustained (> 6 hr) elevation of energy expenditure of up to 30% (57). The thermogenic effect of sibutramine results from central stimulation of efferent sympathetic activity because it is inhibited by ganglionic blockade and by high doses of nonselective β-adrenergic antagonists. Sibutramine also decreases food intake in humans by increasing meal induced satiety (60,61).

The thermogenic properties of sibutramine were tested in a number of acute tests and in one long-term trial using indirect calorimetry. Seagle et al. evaluated the thermogenic response to sibutramine in 44 obese women on a hypocaloric diet and receiving either placebo, 10 mg or 30 mg sibutramine for 8 weeks (62). There was no difference in the thermogenic response to sibutramine and placebo measured 3 hr after acute dosing. However, the active metabolite of sibutramine does not peak in plasma before 3–3.5 hr after oral intake, and it is possible that Seagle et al. missed the thermogenic effect by too early termination of the measurements. Having taken the pharmacokinetic profile of sibutramine and its active metabolites into consideration, Hansen et al. found that sibutramine increased basal metabolic rate, the thermic effect of meals and core temperature more than placebo in normal weight males (63). The increased energy expenditure was covered by higher levels of both glucose and fat utilization and was linked to activation of sympathoadrenal activity.

The contribution of the thermogenic effect of sibutramine to weight loss was examined in two trials. Hansen et al. studied the chronic effect of sibutramine in 32 obese subjects randomized to 8 weeks of treatment with either 15 mg of sibutramine daily or placebo in a double-blind design (61). Twenty-four hour energy expenditure was measured before the start and on the last day of treatment. Weight loss was 2.4 kg in the sibutramine group versus 0.3 kg in the placebo group ($P < .001$). Despite larger loss of both fat-free mass and fat mass in the sibutramine treated group, 24-hr EE did not decrease more than in the placebo group (-2.6% vs. -2.5%, NS). As expected, the reduction in body weight during the 8 weeks was associated with a decrease in 24-hr EE ($r = .42$, $P < .01$). When the body weight changes were taken into account, 24-hr EE decreased less in the sibutramine than in the placebo group (0.8% vs. 3.8%, $P < .02$). In a trial by Walsh et al., 19 obese females were instructed to consume a hypocaloric diet for 12 weeks and, in a double-blind design, received 15 mg sibutramine or placebo daily. RMR was measured before and after 12 weeks of treatment (64). After RMR was adjusted for weight loss, there was a tendency toward sibutramine blunting the decline in RMR, although this was not statistically significant. No change in thermogenic response to an infusion of epinephrine was found after chronic treatment with sibutramine.

These studies demonstrate that sibutramine possesses mild thermogenic properties in humans, sufficient to prevent the decline in 24-hr EE that normally occurs in obese subjects during energy restriction and weight loss. It can be estimated that the thermogenic effect of sibutramine could account for $\sim 23\%$ of the fat loss induced during 8 weeks of treatment (64). Future studies should carefully consider the pharmacokinetics of sibutramine and its active metabolites, and study designs should possess sufficient statistical power to detect differences in 24-hr EE of the order of 2–4% (65).

D β₂-Adrenoceptor Agonists

The β_2-adrenoceptor is involved in several regulatory systems, such as vasodilatation and bronchodilatation, but also in lipolysis in adipose tissue and skeletal muscle metabolism (glucose uptake, thermogenesis, and muscle anabolism). Genetic studies have addressed the importance of this receptor subtype for body weight regulation and obesity by looking at a common polymorphism (Gln27Glu) in the gene encoding for the receptor. The amino acid substitution has been shown to have a functional impact on the biological response to receptor stimulation, and the genetic studies suggest that those

bearing the Glu allele are more likely to be obese if they have a sedentary lifestyle (66,67). The sedentary behavior may actually be linked to the effect of the polymorphism. Larsen et al. found that individuals with the Gln/Gln genotype had a 7% higher daily spontaneous physical activity than those bearing the Glu allele (68).

β_2-Agonists, such as terbutaline and salbutamole, are used in the treatment of asthma, but they have been shown to be thermogenic, to increase insulin-mediated glucose disposal, and to increase the ratio of T_3 to T_4 (69). In a 6-week crossover trial, Acheson et al. studied the impact of treatment with terbutaline versus placebo in healthy volunteers (70). They found that terbutaline increased fat oxidation and T_3/T_4 ratio and decreased nitrogen excretion. These results support that β_2-adrenoceptor stimulation in man produces repartitioning with reduction of fat mass and increase in the lean tissue mass. The clinical value for obesity treatment is limited due to the effect on heart rate, tremor, and the uterus.

E β₃-Adrenoceptor Agonists

Sympathomimetic agents are widely used in the treatment of obesity due to their appetite suppressant activity and thermogenic effect (e.g., ephedrine, sibutramine). However, the use of unselective β-adrenoceptor stimulants is associated with adverse effects such as palpitations, tremor, and insomnia attributable to β_1 and β_2 stimulation. A unique β-adrenergic receptor subtype, termed β_3 has been identified. This receptor is pharmacologically distinct from the classical β_1 and β_2 receptors. In animal models, the β_3-receptor stimulates lipolysis in white adipose tissue and BAT, and in BAT it both activates UCP_1 and up-regulates the UCP_1 gene, both of which result in a further increase in energy expenditure (71). BAT is abundant in rodents and in neonatal humans, where it is important for thermoregulation, but it also appears that chronic β_3-adrenergic stimulation in white adipose tissue increases the expression of UCP_2 and UCP_3, and a "reawakening" of dormant brown adipocytes. In humans, the presence of β_3-adrenergic receptor mRNA has been demonstrated in brown and white adipose tissue, gallbladder, colon, stomach, small intestine, prostate gland (72,73), and more recently also in human brain, gastrocnemius muscle, and right atrium (74,75). A functional role for the β_3-receptor in adipocyte lipolysis has been suggested by studies in isolated human omental and subcutaneous fat cells (76–78), and in in vivo microdialysis studies with such agonists (78–80). However, these drugs are not available for use in humans, usually because of additional β_{1+2} antagonism (e.g., CGP 12177), so their thermogenic efficacy is unknown. Indirect studies, using combinations of different sympathomimetics and blockers to dissect out the contribution of the β_3-receptor to human thermogenesis have yielded inconsistent results (81–83).

Shortly after their discovery in the early 1980s β_3-agonists were found to possess potent antiobesity and antidiabetic properties in rodents. Despite these promising qualities, several pharmaceutical problems and theoretical concerns have slowed the development of these products as therapeutic agents in humans during the last 20 years. Initial problems were due to disregarded differences between rodent and human β_3-receptors and to the difficulty in finding a compound with sufficient bioavailability whilst being highly selective and a full agonist at the human receptor (84). Most of these problems were solved with the cloning of the human β_3-receptor, which has made it possible to develop novel compounds directly and specifically aimed at the human receptor. A few companies have been successful in developing compounds fulfilling these criteria, compounds that also have the bioavailability necessary to increase systemic levels sufficiently to produce an optimal biological stimulation of the human β_3-receptor.

1 From Rodent to Human Agonist

Examples of the first generation of β_3-agonists are ZD7114, ZD2079, and CL316243, compounds that proved to have no thermogenic effect in human clinical trials (85–88). Despite the failure of the first generation compounds in man, their proven acute effects on metabolic rate and insulin action suggest that the β_3-adrenoceptor is a valid target. It might be argued that the acute effects of BRL-26830, BRL-35135, and ZD-2079 after first exposure in man were due to stimulation of β_2- or even β_1-adrenoceptors. Indeed, 60% of the thermogenic effect of BRL-35135 was resistant to blockade with the β_1/β_2-adrenoceptor antagonist nadolol, but the remaining activity appears nevertheless to be mediated by the β_3-adrenoceptor (89). In humans, treatment with CL 316,243 for 8 weeks, in spite of limited bioavailability, induced marked plasma concentration-dependent increases in insulin sensitivity, lipolysis, and fat oxidation in lean volunteers, without causing β_1- or β_2-mediated side effects (86). However, the compound had no effect on 24-hr energy expenditure. This finding may be explained by a low intrinsic activity at the human β_3-receptor (84).

L-796568 (Merck) is a newly developed β_3-adrenergic receptor agonist with high affinity (EC_{50} = 3.6 nM) and efficacy (94% of maximal cAMP accumulation by iso-

prenaline) for the human β_3-adrenoceptor (90). L-796568 is a weak partial agonist at the human β_1 and β_2 receptor, with EC_{50}s of 4.8 and 2.4 µM, respectively, and efficacy of 25% of isoprenaline activity (91). The first study conducted was a randomized, placebo-controlled trial in which the obese patients were exposed acutely to either 250 mg or 1000 mg L-796568, or placebo (91). During the 4-hr postdose period energy expenditure increased after the 1000 mg dose ($\sim$ 8%), and this was accompanied by an increase in plasma glycerol and free fatty acid concentrations. Systolic blood pressure also increased by 12 mm Hg with 1000 mg, but no changes occurred in heart rate, diastolic blood pressure, core temperature, plasma catecholamine, or potassium. This is the first study to demonstrate such an effect of β_3-adrenergic receptor agonists in humans, without significant evidence for β_2-adrenergic receptor involvement. In the second study, the effect of 28 days daily oral dosing with 375 mg L-796568 on 24-hr EE, substrate oxidations, and body composition was studied in 20 obese subjects (92). Twenty-four-hour EE change from baseline did not differ between L-796568 and placebo ($+92 \pm 586$ vs. $+86 \pm 512$ kJ/24 hr). Likewise, no effect could be found on body weight and composition, 24-hr RQ_{np}, or glucose tolerance, but triacylglycerides were decreased by L-796568. However, fat loss was correlated with plasma L-796568 concentration in the L-796568 group ($r = -.69$, $P < .03$).

Other human β_3-agonists are in preclinical development. A single dose of LY-377604 (Lilly), which has been reported as having $> 20\%$ oral bioavailability, increased metabolic rate by 17.5% at the highest dose used (120 mg) in normal-weight and obese subjects (93). This compound did not move on to clinical tests because of toxicological problems. A compound from Takeda (AJ-9677) may go into clinical trials soon. AJ-9677 is structurally similar to the first generation compounds BRL-37344 (active metabolite of BRL-35135) and, although its selectivity is 100-fold, it retains some β_1- and β_2-adrenoceptor agonist activity (84). It remains to be to be seen whether it overcomes the efficacy and selectivity problems of the first generation of compounds.

2 The Future of β_3-Receptor as a Drug Target

BAT is abundant in rodents and in neonatal humans, where it is important for thermoregulation, but no functional BAT remains in adult humans (31). However, recent morphological and functional studies in humans have found small pockets of BAT dispersed in white adipose tissue. The observation that patients with the catecholamine-secreting adrenal tumor pheochromocytoma display an increase in metabolic rate and weight loss in conjunction with the appearance of BAT, demonstrates the potential for recruitment and activation of BAT in adult humans and other primates (94) under certain circumstances. But why does the highly selective β_3-agonist L-796568 possess pronounced lipolytic and thermogenic efficacy following the first exposure in humans, but no efficacy after 28 days of chronic treatment? (Fig. 3). Clearly, the plasma concentrations achieved during the chronic study were 20- to 30-fold higher than the EC_{50} for stimulation of the human β_3-adrenoceptor (92). It cannot entirely be ruled out that the thermogenic effect observed in the acute dosing study was mediated by β_{1+2} receptors, and tachyphylaxis to this effect developed during chronic treatment. In this scenario, there were insufficient β_3-adrenoceptors in the adult human to achieve a measurable thermogenic effect. It is also likely that recruitment of BAT needs an initial sustained β_1 stimulation as described in rodents. This prerequisite may explain why an enhanced thermogenic response to β-adrenergic stimulation can be achieved in humans during chronic β_{1-3} stimulation (95).

The initial reports that the Trp64Arg polymorphism in the β_3-adrenoceptor gene was associated with increased body weight, clinical features of insulin resistance, and early development of type 2 diabetes in several populations, provided some support for the theory that the receptor is of physiological importance also in humans. However, two different meta-analyses based on the same studies have provided conflicting conclusions about whether this polymorphism is associated with BMI (96,97).

In conclusion, based on studies of the latest highly selective and potent agonists, the human β_3-adrenoceptor does not seem to be a promising drug target for antiobesity compounds.

VI   OTHER THERMOGENIC COMPOUNDS

Hormones such as testosterone and growth hormone have been used to treat obesity, and it is likely that both have thermogenic effects (15). Growth hormone increases lean body mass and reduces body fat through stimulation of thermogenesis and fat oxidation (98,99).

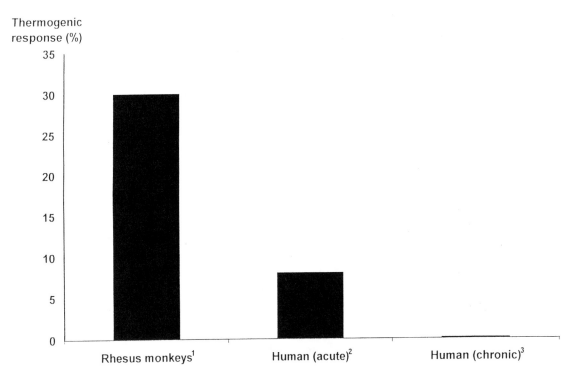

Figure 3   Thermogenic effects of the highly selective human β_3-adrenergic receptor agonist L-796,568 (L-755,507) in rhesus monkeys, and in humans following acute and chronic exposure. Thermogenic response is expressed as increased above resting metabolic rate (%). [1]The thermogenic response in rhesus monkeys after acute intravenous bolus administration of 0.1 mg/kg (93). [2]After oral intake of 100 mg (90). [3]Change in placebo-subtracted 24-hr energy expenditure after 28 days of daily treatment with 375 mg L-796,568 in 20 obese subjects (91).

However, owing to serious side effects its use is restricted to growth hormone–deficient patients. A number of thermogenic compounds with other modes of action are currently being tested in animal studies, and some in human Phase I studies. These include derivatives of thyroid hormone, $PPAR_\gamma$ coactivator, PCC-1 (30), new uncouplers related to dinitrophenol, capsacain from hot chilies (100), and polyphenols from green tea (101,102). None of them had gone into clinical trials as of mid-2002.

ACKNOWLEDGMENTS

Supported by grants from Desirée and Niels Yde's Foundation, Denmark.

REFERENCES

1. Astrup A. Macronutrient balances and obesity: the role of diet and physical activity. Public Health Nutr 1980; 2:314–347.
2. Bray GA. The MONA LISA hypothesis: most obesities known are low in sympathetic activity. In: Oomura Y, Inoue S, Shimazu T, eds. Progress in Obesity Research London: John Libbey, 1990:61–74.
3. Grujic D, Susulic VS, Harper M-E, Himms-Hagen J, Cunningham BA, Corkey BA, Lowell BB. β_3-Adrenergic receptors on white and brown adipocytes mediate β_3-selective agonist-induced effects on energy expenditure, insulin secretion, and food intake. J Biol Chem 1997; 28:17686–17693.
4. Ravussin E, Lillioja S, Anderson TE, Christin L, Bogardus C. Determinants of 24-hour energy expenditure in man. J Clin Invest 1986; 78:1568–1578.
5. Snitker S, Macdonald I, Ravussin E, Astrup A. The sympathetic nervous system and obesity: role in etiology and treatment. Obes Rev 2000; 1:5–15.
6. Toubro S, Sørensen TIA, Rønn B, Christensen NJ, Astrup A. Twenty-four-hour energy expenditure: the role of body composition, thyroid status, sympathetic activity and family membership. J Clin Endocrinol Metab 1996; 81:2670–2674.
7. Astrup A, Toubro S, Dalgaard LT, Urhammer SA, Sørensen TIA, Pedersen O. Impact of the v/v 55 polymorphism of the uncoupling protein 2 gene on 24-hour energy expenditure. Int J Obes 1999; 23:1030–1034.
8. Bnemann B, Schierning B, Toubro S, Bibby BM, Sørensen T, Dalgaard L, Pedersen O, Astrup A. The association between the VAL/ALA-55 polymorphism of the uncoupling protein 2 gene and exercise efficiency. Int J Obes 2001; 25:467–471.
9. Astrup A, Simonsen L, Bülow J, Madsen J, Christensen NJ. Epinephrine mediates facultative carbohydrate-induced thermogenesis in human skeletal muscle. Am J Physiol 1989; 257:E340–E345.
10. Sharma AM, Pischon T, Hardt S, Kunz I, Luft FC. β_3-Adrenergic receptor blockers and weight gain. A systematic analysis. Hypertension 2001; 37:250–254.
11. Snitker S, Tataranni PA, Ravussin E. Respiratory quotient is inversely associated with muscle sympathetic nerve activity. J Clin Endocrinol Metab 1998; 83:3977–3979.
12. Ranneries C, Bülow J, Buemann B, Christensen NJ, Madsen J, Astrup A. Fat metabolism in formerly obese women: effect of exercise on substrate oxidation and adipose tissue lipolysis. Am J Physiol (Endocrinol Metab) 1998; 274:155–161.
13. Astrup A, Gøtzsche PC, van de Werken K, Ranneries C, Toubro S, Raben A, Buemann B. Meta-analysis of resting metabolic rate in formerly obese subjects. Am J Clin Nutr 1999; 69:1117–1122.
14. Krotkiewski M. Thyroid hormones and treatment of obesity. Int J Obes 2000; 24(suppl 2):S116–S119.
15. Bray GA, Greenway FL. Current and potential drugs for treatment of obesity. Endocr Rev 1999; 20:805–875.
16. Hollingsworth DR, Amatruda TT, Schei R. Quantitative and qualitative effects of L-triiodothyronine in massive obesity. Metabolism 1970; 19:934–945.
17. Moore R, Grant AN, Howard AN, Mills IH. Treatment of obesity with triiodothyronine and a very-low calorie liquid formula diet. Lancet 1980; 1:233–226.
18. Koppeschaar HPF, Meinders AE, Schwarz F. Metabolic responses in grossly obese subjects treated with a very-low-calorie diet with and without triiodothyronine treatment. Int J Obes 1983; 7:133–141.
19. Burman KD, Wartofsky L, Dinterman RE, Kesler P, Wannemacher RW. The effect of T3 and reverse T3 administration on muscle protein catbolism during fasting as measured by 3-methylhistindine excretion. Metabolism 1979; 28:805–813.
20. Abraham RR, Densen JW, Davies P, Davie MWJ, Wynn V. The effects of triiodothyronine on energy expenditure, nitrogen balance and rates of weight and fat loss in obese patients during prolongued caloric restriction. Int J Obes 1985; 9:433–442.
21. Byerley LO, Heber D. Metabolic effects of triiodothyronine replacement during fasting in obese subjects. J Clin Endocrinol Metab 1996; 81:968–976.
22. Nair KS, Halliday D, Ford GC, Garrow JS. Effect of triiodothyronine on leucine kinetics, metabolic rate, glucose concentration and insulin secretion rate during two weeks fasting in obese women. Int J Obes 1989; 13:487–496.
23. Wilson JH, Lamberts SW. The effect of triiodothyronine on weight loss and nitrogen balance of obese patients on a very-low calorie liquid-formula diet. Int J Obes 1981; 5:279–282.
24. Lovejoy JC, Smith SR, Bray GA, DeLany JP, Rood JC, Gouvier D, Windhauser M, Ryan DH, Macchiavelli R,

Tulley R. A paradigm of experimentally induced mild hyperthyroidism: effects on nitrogen balance, body composition, and energy expenditure in healthy young men. J Clin Endocrinol Metab 1997; 82:765–770.

25. Trost SU, Swanson E, Gloss B, Wang-Iverson DB, Zhang H, Voldarsky T, Grover GJ, Baxter JD, Chiellin G, Scanlan TS, Dillman WH. The thyroid hormone receptor-beta-selective agonis GC-1 differentially affects plasma lipids and cardiac activity. Endocrinology 2000; 141:3055–3056.

26. Wagner RL, Huber BR, Shiau AK, Kelly A, Cunha S, Lima T, Scanlan TS, Apriletti JW, Baxter JD, West BL, Fletterick RJ. Hormone selectivity in thyroid hormone receptors. Mol Endocrinol 2001; 15:398–410.

27. Ribeiro MO, Carvalho SD, Schultz JJ, Chiellini G, Scanlan TS, Bianco AC, Brent GA. Thyroid hormones–sympathetic interaction and adaptive thermogenesis are thyroid hormone receptor isoform-specific. J Clin Invest 2001; 108:97–105.

28. Harper JA, Dickinson K, Brand MD. Mitochondrial uncoupling as a target for drug development for the treatment of obesity. Obes Rev 2001; 2:255–265.

29. Tainter ML, Cutting WC, Stickton AB. Use of dinitrophenol in nutritional disorders: a critical survey of clinical results. Am J Public Health 1934; 24:1045–1053.

30. Lowell BB, Spiegelman BM. Towards a molecular understanding of adaptive thermogenesis. Nature 2000; 404:652–677.

31. Astrup A. Thermogenesis in human brown adipose tissue and skeletal muscle induced by sympathomimetic stimulation. Acta Endocrinol Scand 1986; 112:1–32.

32. Astrup A, Bülow J, Madsen J, Christensen NJ. Contribution of brown adipose tissue and skeletal muscle to thermogenesis induced by ephedrine in man. Am J Physiol 1985; 248:E507–E515.

33. Simoneau JA, Kelley DE, Neverova M, Warden CH. Over-expression of muscle uncoupling protein protein 2 content in human obesity associates with reduced skeletal muscle lipid utilization. FASEB J 1998; 12:1739–1745.

34. Agryropoulos G, Brown AM, Willi SM, Zhu J, He Y, Reitman M. Effects of mutations in the human uncoupling protein 3 gene on the respiratory quotient and fat oxidation in severe obesity and type 2 diabetes. J Clin Invest 1998; 102:1345–1351.

35. Esterbauer H, Schneitler C, Oberkofler H, Ebenbichler C, Paulweber B, Sandhofer F, Ladurner G, Hell E, Strosberg AD, Patsch JR, Krempler F, Patsch W. A common polymorphism in promoter of UCP2 is associated with decreased risk of obesity in middle-aged humans. Nature Genetics 2001; 28:178–183.

36. Schrauwen P, Troost FJ, Xia J, Ravussin E, Saris WHM. Skeletal muscle UCP2 and UCP3 expression in trained and untrained male subjects. Int J Obes 1999; 23:966–972.

37. Montague CT, Farooqu IS, Whitehead J-P. Congential leptin deficiency is associated with severe early-onset obesity in humans. Nature 1997; 387:903–908.

38. Salbe AD, Nicolson M, Ravussin E. Total energy expenditure and the level of physical activity co-relates with plasma leptin concentrations in five-year-old children. J Clin Invest 1997; 99:592–595.

39. Verdich C, Toubro S, Buemann B, Holst JJ, Bülow J, Simonsen L, Søndergaard SB, Christensen NJ, Astrup A. Leptin levels are associated with fat oxidation and dietary-induced weight loss in obesity. Obes Res 2001; 9:452–61.

40. Farooqi IS, Jebb SA, Langmack G, Lawrence E, Cheetham CH, Prentice AM, Hughes IA, McCamish MA, O'Rahilly S. Effects of recombinant leptin therapy in a child with congenital leptin deficiency. N Engl J Med 1999; 341:879–884.

41. Heymsfield SB, Greenberg AS, Fujioka K, Dixon RM, Kushner R, Hunt T, Lubina JA, Patane J, Self B, Hunt P, McCamish M. Recombinant leptin for weight loss in obese and lean adults. JAMA 1999; 282:1568–1575.

42. Hukshorn CJ, Saris WH, Westerterp-Plantenga MS, Farid AR, Smith FJ, Campfield LA. Weekly subcutaneous pegylated recombinant native human leptin (PEG-OB) administration in obese men. J Clin Endocrinol Metab 2000; 85:4003–4009.

43. Greenway FL. The safety and efficacy of pharmaceutical and herbal caffeine and ephedrine use as a weight loss agent. Obes Rev 2001; 2:199–211.

44. Astrup A, Toubro S. Thermogenic, metabolic and cardiovascular responses to ephedrine and caffeine in man. Int J Obes 1993; 17:S41–S43.

45. Liu Y-L, Toubro S, Astrup A, Stock MJ. Contribution of β3-adrenoceptor activation to ephedrine-induced thermogenesis in humans. Int J Obes 1995; 19:678–685.

46. Astrup A, Breum L, Toubro S, Hein P, Quaade F. The effect and safety of an ephedrine/caffeine compound compared to ephedrine, caffeine and placebo in obese subjects on an energy restricted diet. A double blind trial. Int J Obes 1992; 16:269–277.

47. Breum L, Pedersen JK, Ahlstrom F, Frimodt-Moller J. Comparison of an ephedrine/caffeine combination and dexfenfluramine in the treatment of obesity. A double-blind multi-centre trial in general practice. Int J Obes 1994; 18:99–103.

48. Norregaard J, Jorgensen S, Mikkelsen KL, Tonnesen P, Iversen E, Sorensen T, Soeberg B, Jakobsen HB. The effect of ephedrine plus caffeine on smoking cessation and postcessation weight gain. Clin Pharmacol Ther 1996; 60(6):679–686.

49. Molnar D. Effects of ephedrine and aminophylline on resting energy expenditure in obese adolescents. Int J Obes Metab Disord 2000; 24:1573–1578.

50. Stich V, Hainer V, Kunesova M. Effect of ephedrine/caffeine mixture on metabolic response to exercise in obese subjects. Int J Obes 1993; 17:31.

51. Waluga M, Janusz M, Karpel E, Hartleb M, Nowak A.

Cardiovascular effects of ephedrine, caffeine and yohimbine measured by thoracic electrical bioimpedance in obese women. Clin Physiol 1998; 18:69–76.

52. Svendsen TL, Ingerslev J, Mork A. Is Letigen contraindicated in hypertension? A double-blind, placebo controlled multipractice study of Letigen administered to normotensive and adequately treated patients with hypersensitivity. Ugeskr Laeger 1998; 160:4073–4075.

53. Buemann B, Astrup A, Marckmann P, Christensen NJ. The effect of ephedrine + caffeine on plasma lipids and lipoproteins during a 4.2-MJ/d diet. Int J Obes 1994; 18:329–332.

54. Astrup A, Buemann B, Christensen NJ, Toubro S, Thorbek G, Victor OJ, Quaade F. The effect of ephedrine/caffeine mixture on energy expenditure and body composition in obese women. Metabolism 1992; 41:686–688.

55. Ramsey JJ, Colman RJ, Swick AG, Kemnitz JW. Energy expenditure, body composition, and glucose metabolism in lean and obese rhesus monkeys treated with ephedrine and caffeine. Am J Clin Nutr 1998; 68:42–51.

56. Toubro S, Astrup A, Breum L, Quaade F. Safety and efficacy of long-term treatment with ephedrine, caffeine and an ephedrine/caffeine mixture. Int J Obes 1993; 17:S69–S72.

57. Stock MJ. Sibutramine: a review of the pharmacology of a novel anti-obesity agent. Int J Obes 1997; 21:25–29.

58. Bray GA, Ryan DH, Gordon D, Heidingsfelder S, Cerise F, Wilson K. A double-blind randomized placebo-controlled trial of sibutramine. Obes Res 1996; 4:263–270.

59. James WPT, Astrup A, Finer N, Hilsted J, Kopelman P, Rössner S, Saris WHM, Van Gaal LF. Effect of sibutramine on weight maintenance after weight loss: a randomised trial. Lancet 2000; 356:2119–2125.

60. Rolls BJ, Thorwart ML, Shide DJ, Ulbrecht JS. Sibutramine reduces food intake in non-dieting women with obesity. Obes Res 1998; 6:1–11.

61. Hansen DL, Toubro S, Stock MJ, Macdonald IA, Astrup A. The effect of sibutramine on energy expenditure and appetite during chronic treatment without dietary restriction. Int J Obes 1999; 23:1016–1024.

62. Seagle HM, Bessesen DH, Hill JO. Effects of sibutramine on resting metabolic rate and weight loss in overweight women. Obes Res 1998; 6:115–121.

63. Hansen DL, Toubro S, Stock MJ, Macdonald IA, Astrup A. Thermogenic effects of sibutramine in humans. Am J Clin Nutr 1998; 68:1180–1186.

64. Walsh KM, Leen E, Lean MEJ. The effect of sibutramine on resting energy expenditure and adrenaline-induced thermogenesis in obese females. Int J Obes 1999; 23:1009–1015.

65. Danforth E. Sibutramine and thermogenesis in humans. Int J Obes 1999; 23:1007–1008.

66. Meirhaeghe A, Helbecque N, Cottel D, Amouyel P. Beta2-adrenoceptor gene polymorphism, body weight, and physical activity. Lancet 1999; 353:896.

67. Large V, Hellstrom L, Reynisdottir S, Lonnqvist F, Eriksson P, Lannfelt L, Arner P. Human beta-2 adrenoceptor gene polymorphisms are highly frequent in obesity and associate with altered adipocyte beta-2 adrenoceptor function. J Clin Invest 1997; 100:3005–3013.

68. Larsen TM, Buemann B, Toubro S, Astrup A. β_2-Receptor polymorphism Gln27Glu associated with 24 hr spontaneous physical activity. Int J Obes 2001; 25(suppl 2):S13.

69. Scheidegger K, O'Connell M, Robbins DC, Danforth EJ. Effects of chronic beta-receptor stimulation on sympathetic nervous system activity, energy expenditure, and thyroid hormones. J Clin Endocrinol Metab 1984; 58:895–903.

70. Acheson KJ, Tavussin E, Schoeller DA, Christin L, Bourquin L, Baertschi P, Danforth E Jr, Jecquier E. Two-week stimulation or blockade of the sympathetic nervous system in man: influence on body weight, body composition, and twenty-four hour energy expenditure. Metabolism 1988; 37:91–98.

71. Van Baak MA. The peripheral sympathetic nervous system in human obesity. Obes Rev 2001; 2:3–14.

72. Krief S, Lönnqvist F, Raimbault S, Baude B, Van Spronsen A, Arner P, Strosberg AD, Ricquier D, Emorine LJ. Tissue distribution of β_3-adrenergic receptor mRNA in man. J Clin Invest 1993; 91:344–349.

73. Berkowitz DE, Nardone NA, Smiley RM, Price DT, Kreutter DK, Fremeau RT, Schwin DA. Distribution of β_3-adrenoceptor mRNA in human tissues. Eur J Pharmacol 1995; 289:223–228.

74. Rodriguez M, Carillon C, Coquerel A, Le Fur G, Ferrara P, Caput D, Shire D. Evidence for the presence of beta$_3$-adrenergic receptor mRNA in the human brain. Brain Res Mol Brain Res 1995; 29:369–375.

75. Chamberlain PD, Jennings KH, Paul F, Cordell J, Berry A, Holmes SD, Park J, Chambers J, Sennitt MV, Stock MJ, Cawthorne MA, Young PW, Murphy GJ. The tissue distribution of the human β-adrenoceptors studied using a monoclonal antibody: direct evidence of the β_3-adrenoceptor in human adipose tissue, atrium and skeletal muscle. Int J Obes 1999; 23:1057–1065.

76. Lönnqvist F, Krief S, Strosberg AD, Nyberg B, Emorine LJ, Arner P. Evidence for a functional β_3-adrenoceptor in man. Br J Pharmacol 1993; 110:929–936.

77. Hoffstedt J, Shimizu M, Sjöstedt S, Lönnqvist F. Determination of β_3-adrenoceptor mediated lipolysis in human fat cells. Obes Res 1995; 3:447–457.

78. Enocksson S, Shimizu M, Lönnqvist F, Nordenström J, Arner P. Demonstration of an in vivo functional β_3-adrenoceptor in man. J Clin Invest 1995; 95:2239–2245.

79. Barbe P, Millet L, Galitzky J, Lafontan M, Berlan M. In situ assessment of the role of the β_1-, β_2 and β_3-

adrenoceptors in the control of lipolysis and nutritive blood flow in human subcutaneous adipose tissue. Br J Pharmacol 1996; 117:907–913.

80. Tavernier G, Barbe P, Galitzky J, Berlan M, Caput D, Lafontan M, Langin D. Expression of β_3-adrenoceptor with low lipolytic action in human subcutaneous white adipocytes. J Lipid Res 1996; 37:87–97.

81. Wheeldon NM, McDevitt DG, Lipworth BJ. Do β_3-adrenoceptors mediate metabolic responses to isoprenaline. Q J Med 1993; 86:595–600.

82. Blaak EE, Saris WHM, Van Baak MA. Adrenoceptor subtypes mediating catecholamine-induced thermogenesis in man. Int J Obes 1993; 17(suppl 3):S78–S81.

83. Schiffelers SLH, Blaak EE, Saris WHM, Van Baak MA. In vivo β_3-adrenergic stimulation of human thermogenesis and lipid use. Clin Pharmacol Ther 2000; 67:558–566.

84. Arch JRS, Wilson S. Prospects for β_3-adrenoceptor agonists in the treatment of obesity and diabetes. Int J Obes 1996; 20:191–199.

85. Weyer C, Gautier JF, Danforth E Jr. Development of beta 3-adrenoceptor agonists for the treatment of obesity and diabetes—an update. Diabetes Metab 1999; 25:11–21.

86. Weyer C, Tataranni PA, Snitker S, Danforth E Jr, Ravussin E. Increase in insulin action and fat oxidation after treatment with CL-316,243, a highly selectiv beta 3-adrenoceptor agonist in humans. Diabetes 1998; 47:1555–1561.

87. Buemann B, Toubro S, Astrup A. Effects of the two β_3-agonists, XD7114 and ZD2079, on 24-hour energy expenditure and respiratory quotient in obese subjects. Int J Obes 2000; 24:1553–1560.

88. Melnyk A, Zingaretti MC, Ceresi E, De Matteis R, Cancello R, Cinti S, Himms-Hagen J. Transformation of some unilocular (UL) into multilocular (ML) adipocytes in white adipose tissue (WAT) of CL 316,243(CL)-treated rats. Obes Res 1999; 7:74.

89. Wheeldon NM, McDevitt DG, McFarlane LC, Lipworth BJ. β-Adrenoceptor subtypes mediating the metabolic effects of BRL 35135 in man. Clin Sci 1994; 86:331–337.

90. Mathvink RJ, Tolman JS, Chitty D, Candelore MR, Cascieri MA, Colwell LF. Discovery of a potent, orally bioavailable β_3 adrenergic receptor agonist, (R)-N-[4-[2-[[2-hydroxy-2-(3-piridinyl)ethyl]amino]ethyl]-phenyl]-4-[4-[4-(trifluoromethyl)phenyl]thiazol-2-yl]benzenesulfonamide. J Med Chem 2000; 43:3832–3836.

91. Van Baak MA, Hul GBJ, Toubro S, Astrup A, Gottesdiener KM, DeSmet M, Saris WHM. Acute effect

of L-796568, a β_3-adrenergic receptor agonist, on energy expenditure in obese men. Clin Pharmacol Ther 2002; 71:272–279.

92. Larsen TM, Toubro S, Van Baak MA, Gottesdiener KM, Larson P, Saris WHM, Astrup A. The effect of 28 days treatment with L-796568, a novel β_3-adrenoceptor agonist, on energy expenditure and body composition in obese men. Am J Clin Nut 2002; 76:780–788.

93. Harada H, Kato S, Kawashima H, Furutani Y. A new β_3-adrenergic agonist: synthesis and biological activity of indole derivatives. 214th Meeting of the American Chemical Society, Las Vegas, Medi 208, 1997.

94. Fisher MH, Amend AM, Bach TJ, Barker JM, Brady EJ, Candelore MR. A selective human β_3 adrenergic receptor agonist increases metabolic rate in rhesus monkeys. J Clin Invest 1998; 101:2387–2393.

95. Astrup A, Lundsgaard C, Madsen J, Christensen NJ. Enhanced thermogenic responsiveness during chronic ephedrine treatment in man. Am J Clin Nutr 1985; 42:83–94.

96. Fujisawa T, Ikegami H, Kawaguchi Y, Ogihara T. Meta-analysis of the association of Trp[64]Arg polymorphism of β_3-adrenergic receptor gene with body mass index. J Clin Endocrinol Metab 1998; 83:2441–2444.

97. Allison DB, Heo M, Faith MS, Pietrobelli. Meta-analysis of the association of the Trp[64]Arg polymorphism in the beta3 adrenergic receptor with body mass index. Int J Obes 1998; 22:559–566.

98. Karlsson C, Stenlof K, Johannsson G, Marin P, Bjorntorp P, Bengtsson BA, Carlsson B, Carlsson LM, Sjostrom L. Effects of growth hormone treatment on the leptin system and on energy expenditure in abdominally obese men. Eur J Endocrinol 1998; 138:408–414.

99. Møller N, Jørgensen JO, Møller N, Christiansen JS, Weeke J. Growth hormone enhances effects of endurance training on oxidative muscle metabolism in elderly women. Am J Physiol 2000; 279:E989–E996.

100. Yoshioka M, St-Pierre S, Suzuki M, Tremblay A. Effects of red pepper added to high-fat and high-carbohydrate meals on energy metabolism and substrate utilization in Japanese women. Br J Nutr 1998; 80:503–510.

101. Dulloo AG, Duret C, Rohrer D, Girardier L, Mensi N, Fathi M, Chantre P, Vandermander J. Efficacy of a green tea extract rich in catechin polyphenols and caffeine in increasing 24-h energy expenditure and fat oxidation in humans. Am J Clin Nutr 1999; 70:1040–1045.

102. Astrup A. Thermogenic drugs as a strategy for treatment of obesity. Endocrine 2000; 13:207–212.

17

Herbal and Alternative Approaches to Obesity

Frank L. Greenway

Pennington Biomedical Research Center, Louisiana State University, Baton Rouge, Louisiana, U.S.A.

David Heber

David Geffen School of Medicine at UCLA and UCLA Center for Human Nutrition, Los Angeles, California, U.S.A.

I INTRODUCTION

The use of herbal and alternative medicines has increased in the last decade in the United States and is now the subject of clinical and basic science investigations supported by the NIH Office of Dietary Supplements Research and the National Center for Complementary and Alternative Medicine. The Dietary Supplements Health Education Act of 1994 enables manufacturers to market these approaches without proving efficacy or safety. The FDA has limited resources for this purpose and relies on adverse effects reporting to monitor safety, but this method has significant drawbacks in terms of scientifically examining the causative relationship of a particular herbal or alternative approach to a reported side effect.

The most widely used herbal approaches for weight loss comprise dietary supplements that contain ephedra alkaloids (sometimes called ma huang). These are widely promoted and used in the United States as a means of losing weight at least in part by purportedly increasing energy expenditure. In light of recently reported adverse events related to use of these products, the U.S. Food and Drug Administration (FDA) has proposed limits on the dose and duration of use of such supplements. The FDA requested an independent review of reports of adverse events related to the use of supplements that contained ephedra alkaloids to assess causation and to estimate the level of risk the use of these supplements poses to consumers, and this report was published in the New England Journal of Medicine and widely publicized (1). A total of 140 reports of adverse events related to the use of dietary supplements containing ephedra alkaloids that were submitted to the FDA between June 1, 1997, and March 31, 1999, were reviewed. A standardized rating system for assessing causation was applied to each adverse event. Thirty-one percent of cases were judged by the authors to be related to the use of supplements containing ephedra alkaloids, and 31% were deemed to be possibly related to the use of supplements. Among the adverse events that were deemed definitely, probably, or possibly related to the use of supplements containing ephedra alkaloids, 47% involved cardiovascular symptoms and 18% involved the central nervous system. Hypertension was the single most frequent adverse effect (17 reports), followed by palpitations, tachycardia, or both (13); stroke (10); and seizures (7). Ten events were associated with deaths, and 13 associated events resulted in permanent disability, representing 26% of the definite, probable, and possible cases. These reports, while possibly associating the use of herbal dietary supplements containing ephedra with side effects, do not in any way prove a causative relationship between herbal use and these problems.

On the other hand, controlled studies of supplements containing ephedra provide considerable evidence reviewed below of efficacy in weight loss and weight maintenance. There is also a biological rationale for combining ephedra and caffeine to obtain enhanced efficacy as reviewed below. This widely used combination and other putative thermogenic aids are discussed, including green tea catechins and capsaicin from chili peppers.

There are biological rationales for the actions of the different alternative medical and herbal approaches to weight loss discussed in detail below. First, thermogenic aids such as ephedra and caffeine, synephrine, tea catechins, and chili pepper capsaicin are directed at increasing fat burning or metabolism during dieting. Many individuals attempting to lose weight believe that their metabolism is abnormally slow. The adaptive decrease in metabolism which occurs in response to caloric restriction is 10–15% of resting metabolic rate. The popularity of stimulants suggests that they have some effects on weight loss reviewed below, and there is some evidence that these agents can affect metabolism. Second, the same principles have been applied to the development of topical fat reduction creams. Second, a number of supplements and herbs claim to result in nutrient partitioning so that ingested calories will be directed to muscle rather than fat. This diverse group includes an herb (*Garcinia cambogia*), a lipid that is the product of bacterial metabolism (conjugated linoleic acid), a mineral (chromium), a hormone precursor (dehydroepiandrosterone), and an amino acid metabolite (beta-hydroxymethylbutyrate). Third, a number of approaches attempt to influence food intake and satiety through effects on noradrenergic, serotoninergic, or dopaminergic mechanisms including tyrosine, phenylalanine, and 5-hydroxytryptophan (5HT). Fourth, a series of approaches attempt to physically affect gastric satiety by filling the stomach. Fiber swells after ingestion and has been found to result in increased satiety. A binding resin (chitosan) has the ability to precipitate fat in the laboratory and is touted for its ability to bind fat in the intestines so that it is not absorbed. However, there has been some success noted with the use of a gastric pacemaker or detection of stomach fullness through a waist cord. Finally, psychophysiological approaches including hypnosis and aromatherapy have been evaluated. For the most part, the discussion has been restricted to methods of weight reduction for which some clinical or basic research could be found. However, there may be other methods including traditional herbal medicines from other cultures which remain to be discovered and studied in the future.

Clearly, one attraction of alternative obesity treatments to consumers is the lack of any required professional assistance with these approaches. For those obese individuals who cannot afford to see a physician, these approaches often represent a more accessible solution. For many others, these approaches represent alternatives to failed attempts at weight loss using more conventional approaches. These consumers are often discouraged by previous failures, and are likely to combine approaches or use these supplements at doses higher than recommended doses.

II HERBAL THERMOGENIC AIDS

A Herbal Caffeine and Ephedrine

Selling caffeine and ephedrine in herbal form for weight loss is now a large industry. Caffeine in the herbal products is the same chemical contained in pharmaceutical caffeine. Herbal ephedra has four isomers, but the pharmaceutical grade product contains the most potent of these (2). Therefore, the herbal form of ephedrine should be even safer than equivalent doses of the pharmaceutical grade product, because it contains less of the most potent isomer.

In 1972, Dr. Erikson, a general practitioner in Elsinore, Denmark, noted unintentional weight loss when he prescribed a compound containing ephedrine, caffeine, and phenobarbital to patients he was treating for asthma. As he pursued his observation, rumor spread from his patients to the rest of the country. By 1977, over 70,000 patients were taking the "Elsinore Pill," and one Danish pharmaceutical house was producing 1 million tablets a week.

During the time that the Elsinore Pill was used for the treatment of obesity, there were more skin rashes, some serious, reported. These were most likely due to the phenobarbital in the Elsinore Pill. In 1977, the Danish Institute of Health issued a warning to doctors not to prescribe the compound because of increased incidence of skin rashes, and Dr. Erikson was harshly criticized in the public and scientific press.

The Elsinore Pill without phenobarbital was compared to the appetite suppressant diethylpropion and to a placebo in 132 subjects in a 12-week double-blind trial. Diethylpropion 25 mg TID and the Elsinore Pill without phenobarbital (caffeine 100mg and ephedrine 40 mg TID) gave 8.4 kg and 8.1 kg weight loss, respectively, which were not different from each other, but greater than the placebo weight loss of 4.1 kg ($P < .01$). Tremor and agitation were more frequent on the Elsinore Pill but were transient, and the withdrawal for side effects was equal in the diethylpropion and Elsinore Pill groups. There was no increase in blood pressure, pulse rate, or laboratory parameters. The authors concluded that ephedrine and caffeine had the advantage over diethylpropion because of its lower cost with equivalent safety and efficacy (3).

Other early studies of ephedrine and caffeine also used commercial asthma preparations. Theophylline and caffeine are both methylxanthines and have the same pharmacologic actions. One milligram of theophylline is equivalent to 2 mg of caffeine (4). Miller used the "Do-Do" pill manufactured by Ciba-Geigy in the United Kingdom containing 22 mg ephedrine, 30 mg caffeine, and 50 mg theophylline per pill. Each pill, therefore, contained the equivalent of 22 mg ephedrine and 130 mg caffeine (5). Ephedrine with theophylline was the primary treatment for asthma in the 1960s and '70s, and ephedrine is still sold in the United States without a prescription for the treatment of asthma (6). Ephedrine with caffeine is still the most widely sold prescription weight loss medication in Denmark and held 80% of the market share even when dexfenfluramine was available.

Caffeine has been studied separately in animals and humans since it can increase sympathetic nervous system activity, and obesity has been associated with low sympathetic activity (7). In genetically obese mice without endogenous leptin production (ob/ob mice) caffeine decreased body fat and improved sympathetic activity suggesting a possible role in the treatment of human obesity (8). Caffeine in an oral dose of 250 mg increased free fatty acids and glucose but not cortisol levels in obese and lean humans compared to a water placebo with each subject acting as his own control (9). Oxygen consumption, fat oxidation, and serum free fatty acids were increased in six normal subjects given caffeine 8 mg/kg orally compared to 0.5 g glucose. Oxygen consumption and fat oxidation were also increased in seven normal and six obese subjects after 4 mg/kg of caffeinated coffee compared to a decaffeinated control after fasting and after a mixed meal (10).

Six obese, six lean, and four postobese women were evaluated after 4 mg/kg oral caffeine. Caffeine levels were higher in the lean than in the obese and postobese, and the rise in oxygen consumption and free fatty acids was lower in the postobese than in the obese and lean. These changes were felt to be due to differences in lipolysis (11). Caffeine 100 mg was shown to increase resting oxygen consumption 3–4% in nine lean and nine postobese subjects. Caffeine 100 mg also improved the defective diet induced thermogenesis over 150 min that was present in the postobese. Five lean and six post-

obese subjects were given 100 mg caffeine every 2 hr for 6 hr. Daily energy expenditure increased 150 kcal/d in the lean and 79 kcal/d in the postobese (12). Ten lean and 10 obese women were evaluated for 24 hr in a metabolic chamber on two occasions, one with 4 mg/kg caffeine five times a day and the other with placebo. Caffeine increased energy expenditure and lipid oxidation, but less in the obese than in the lean (13). The response of serum catecholamines to 4 mg/kg caffeine was evaluated in 12 prepubertal lean, 15 prepubertal obese, 12 pubertal lean, and 24 pubertal obese subjects. The rise in serum catecholamines was less in the pubertal obese group (14). Caffeine administration significantly elevated systolic blood pressure 4.5–6.6 mmHg, but there was no change in diastolic blood pressure or pulse rate. Subjects reported no symptoms or side effects. The caffeine-induced increase in thermogenesis is dissipated through an increase in skin temperature (15). The increase in resting metabolic rate induced by 4 mg/kg caffeine predicts the amount of weight lost in response to a diet and exercise program (16). The volume of distribution of caffeine was found to be proportional to body weight, with caffeine having the same clearance in the obese as in the lean (17). Therefore, for metabolic studies one might justify a loading dose, but for chronic treatment no change in dosage is necessary for the obese (18,19). Therefore, the scientific evidence in animals and humans supports a potential role for caffeine in weight reduction through increases in oxygen consumption and fat oxidation.

Several epidemiologic studies have addressed the safety of caffeine. The positive correlation found between heavy coffee drinking and elevated cholesterol is felt to be due to factors other than caffeine in coffee, since caffeine consumption in the form of tea or cola has no effect on cholesterol (20,21). Heavy caffeine use is associated with hypertension and snoring. Heavy caffeine use is also associated with cigarette smoking. Since cigarette smoking is associated with hypertension and snoring, it may be the smoking that is responsible for the association with these conditions rather than the caffeine. (22,23). When consumed on a chronic basis, caffeine consumption has been correlated with a decreased risk of hospitalization for coronary heart disease (24). It has also been associated with lower blood pressure (25,26). Therefore, caffeine consumption on a chronic basis appears to reduce the risk of cardiovascular disease, the opposite suggested by caffeine's acute cardiovascular response. A clinical trial with 288 healthy subjects evaluated the effects of a single 200 mg/d dose of caffeine compared to placebo. Caffeine gave a 2.2 mmHg in diastolic blood pressure which was felt to be clinically insignificant. There was no change in pulse rate or systolic blood pressure (27).

Although the intake of >2 cups of coffee per day is associated with osteoporosis, this association has only been demonstrated in women between 50 and 98 years of age and only when they consume < 1 glass of milk per day, far below the intake recommended by nutritional guidelines (28). As noted before, coffee contains more than caffeine, and any negative effect on bone could as easily be related to one of the other components of coffee.

Caffeine has a long history of safe use in food and has been used in headache preparations, to treat fatigue, intracranial hypertension, and respiratory distress in the neonate (29,30). The FDA approves caffeine for sale without a prescription for use as a stimulant by persons 12 years of age or older at a dose up to 200 mg every 3 hr (1600 mg/d) and as an ingredient in pain medications, which gives further support to its safety.

Ephedrine was proposed as a potential treatment for obesity on the basis of a study comparing it to tri-iodothyronine in six animal models of obesity and in lean controls. Tri-iodothyronine increased both oxygen consumption and food intake, causing death in genetically obese animals. Ephedrine elevated oxygen consumption without increasing food intake while causing weight and fat loss (31). There were no deaths in the ephedrine group. Two other animal models of obesity were treated with ephedrine. Increased energy expenditure, decreased food intake, and fat loss were demonstrated (32,33). In an effort to discover a potential drug to treat obesity, 33 compounds known to stimulate oxygen consumption were screened in several animal models of obesity. In general, these compounds gave selective fat loss without loss of body protein by increasing energy expenditure without increasing food intake. Ephedrine was one of the two most efficient compounds, and this led to its proposed use in the treatment of obesity (34,35).

Ephedrine stimulates brown adipose tissue thermogenesis through the activation of beta-receptors. It has been estimated that 40% of the acute rise in oxygen consumption in response to ephedrine is due to activation of the beta-3-adrenergic receptor (36). The isomer of ephedrine in pharmaceutical preparations is the most active of the four existing isomers (37). Propranalol prevents the weight loss induced in ob/ob mice by ephedrine (38), demonstrating its action through the beta receptors. Aspirin has been shown to increase ephedrine-induced thermogenesis. Mice made obese by MSG and treated with aspirin had no change in their energy expenditure, body fat, or body weight. Mice made obese with MSG and treated with ephedrine increased their energy expenditure by 9%, reduced their body fat by 50%, and reduced their body weight by 18%. The combination of aspirin and ephedrine increased energy expenditure by 18%, reduced body fat by 75%, and reversed the obesity in these animals (39).

Ephedrine was studied in humans in 1974 but was felt to give side effects in doses adequate to suppress appetite (40). Ephedrine 20 mg TID increased oxygen consumption at baseline by 1.3 L over 3 hr. Stimulation of oxygen consumption increased to 7 L over 3 hr at week 4 and 12 of treatment accompanied by weight losses of 2.5 kg and 5.5 kg, respectively (41). Chronic treatment with ephedrine increased metabolic rate by 10% and increased fat oxidation as well (42). A 3-month trial comparing ephedrine 25 mg TID (13 subjects) and 50 mg TID (17 subjects) with placebo (16 subjects) showed similar weight losses in all groups with significantly more side effects (blood pressure elevation, pulse elevation, agitation, insommia, headache, weakness, palpitations, giddiness, euphoria, tremor, and diarrhea) in the ephedrine 50 mg TID group compared to placebo (43). There was more weight loss in the ephedrine groups, however, at the end of months 1 and 2, a difference that was lost by the end of month 3 (44). A second trial compared ephedrine 50 mg TID with placebo over 8 weeks in 10 low-energy adapted women who had already lost weight. The study used a crossover design. Weight loss was greater during the 2-month period on ephedrine (2.4 kg) than on placebo (0.6 kg). Side effects were uncommon: agitation (two subjects), insomnia (three subjects), giddiness (two subjects), and palpitations (two subjects), and none required withdrawal of medication (45). Ephedrine has also been evaluated in conjunction with a very low calorie diet. Ephedrine decreased urinary nitrogen and blunted the fall in resting metabolic rate (46). The rise in oxygen consumption to ephedrine 1 mg/kg was increased by 5 weeks of exercise training 1 hr/d on a bicycle at a heart rate of 140–160 beats per minute (BPM) (47).

Attempts have been made to explore the mechanisms by which ephedrine exerts its effects in humans. Although ephedrine stimulates brown adipose tissue in rodents, ephedrine-induced thermogenesis in humans takes place primarily in skeletal muscle, since humans have little brown adipose tissue (48). Ephedrine has also been shown to decrease gastric emptying which may contribute to its effect on food intake (49). As one might expect from a compound that stimulates beta-1, beta-2, and beta-3 receptors, intravenous ephedrine acutely increases oxygen consumption, serum glucose, insulin, and c-peptide (50). Beta-1 receptors stimulate heart rate, and beta-2 receptors increase glucose in addition to stimulating oxygen consumption along with the beta-3 receptors. Post-prandial thermogenesis measured for 160 min following a liquid meal was greater in 10 obese women to an acute dose of ephedrine 30 mg and aspirin 300 mg than to an acute dose of ephedrine 30 mg alone. Aspirin did not have this additional effect on thermogenesis in 10 lean women (51). Ephedrine and aspirin normalized the postprandial thermogenesis in obese women to levels equal to the lean (52). Side effects with ephedrine were agitation, insomnia, headache, weakness, palpitations, giddiness, tremor, and constipation, but were only seen with the 50 mg TID dose and dissipated with time. No significant changes were seen in pulse or blood pressure (53). Ephedrine has been reported to cause urinary difficulty in subjects with prostatic hypertrophy and can exacerbate angle closure glaucoma (54).

Ephedra and methylxanthines have been demonstrated to be synergistic in animals. Caffeine or theophylline given alone to mice with MSG-induced obesity caused no change in weight, fat, or energy expenditure. Ephedrine decreased weight by 14%, decreased fat by 42%, and increased energy expenditure by 10%. When caffeine or theophylline was added to ephedrine, weight decreased by 25%, fat decreased by 75%, energy expenditure increased by 20%, and body composition was normalized to that of lean control animals (55). Caffeine with ephedrine and theophylline also normalized obesity in Zucker fatty (fa/fa) rats by decreasing food intake by 40% and increasing energy expenditure from 25% to 33% (56). Oxygen consumption was increased by 32% with ephedrine, 48% with caffeine, and 47% with caffeine and ephedrine in the LA-corpulent rat, another rodent obesity model. These rats lost three times more weight with caffeine and ephedrine in combination than with ephedrine alone (57). Not only can rodent obesity be effectively treated with ephedrine and methylxanthines, but caffeine, ephedrine, and theophylline also prevent obesity in fa/fa rats by normalizing energetic efficiency to that of lean animals (58). Caffeine and ephedrine gave fat loss in both lean and obese monkeys, but weight loss and decreased food intake was only seen in obese animals. Nocturnal energy expenditure increased by 21% and 24% in the lean and obese monkeys, respectively. There was no change in the glucose tolerance test, but leptin levels decreased (59).

Genetically obese mice (ob/ob and db/db) and mice with MSG-induced obesity have low adipsin levels that precede the obesity, and the obesity in these animals is associated with low levels of sympathetic activity. Since caffeine and ephedrine correct both the obesity

and the adipsin levels, it was postulated that adipsin is under sympathetic control (60). Since it was later demonstrated that BRL 26830A, a selective beta-3-adrenergic stimulator, depressed adipsin levels, it was suggested that adipsin was inversely related to body fat (61). It now appears that adipsin levels are controlled by food intake, since both ephedrine with caffeine and food restriction increase adipsin levels (62). The mechanism by which methylxanthinines potentiate ephedrine-induced thermogenesis was assumed to be inhibition of the adenosine receptor, a known effect of methylxanthines. Using an in vitro assay of brown fat cell respiration, it was shown that the adenosine receptor plays only a minor role, and most of the methylxanthine effect is due to phosphodiesterase inhibition (63). Ephedrine and theophylline also increase hepatic lipase activity, the enzyme that degrades atherogenic intermediate density lipoproteins (64), which should theoretically help to prevent from atherosclerotic vascular disease.

Herbal forms of caffeine and ephedrine have also been evaluated in rodents. Bofu-tsusho-san containing ephedra and a phosphodiesterase inhibitor when fed to mice with MSG-induced obesity decreased both fat and body weight by activating brown fat thermogenesis (65). Oolong tea prevented the obesity and fatty liver induced by a high-fat diet, stimulated noradrenaline-induced lipolysis, stimulated hormone sensitive lipase, and inhibited pancreatic lipase activity in rodents (66). This effect was attributed to caffeine, but more recent studies demonstrate that green tea contains not only caffeine, but also catechin polyphenols that inhibit catechol-O-methyl transferase, the enzyme that breaks down norepinephrine. Just as caffeine and ephedrine are synergistic in their effect on the respiration of brown fat cells in vitro, so are the catechins in green tea synergistic with caffeine, ephedrine and the combination of caffeine with ephedrine (67).

Ephedrine 40 mg and caffeine 100 mg given TID in combination increased metabolism, but thyroid hormone did not seem to be responsible for this increase. Diet, diethylpropion, and the Elsinore Pill all significantly decreased levels of T_3 by a mean of 9% during weight loss (68). Extrapolating from animal studies, the increase in energy expenditure was postulated to come from stimulation of brown adipose tissue. Further studies with ephedrine demonstrated that, at maximum, 15% of the increase in human thermogenesis could come from brown adipose tissue, the majority being due to thermogenesis in muscle (48).

Do-Do pills, a nonprescription asthma medication containing 22 mg ephedrine, 30 mg caffeine, and 50 mg theophylline made by Ciba-Geigy was twice as effective in raising resting metabolic rate in lean and postobese subjects as ephedrine alone. Although there was no change in 24-hr energy expenditure in lean subjects measured in a metabolic chamber, the postobese increased their energy expenditure by 8%. The ephedrine-methylxanthine combination normalized the defective thermogenic response to a meal in the postobese (69).

Since aspirin and methylxanthines both potentiate ephedrine-induced thermogenesis, aspirin 100 mg with ephedrine 50 mg and caffeine 50 mg was given TID for 8 weeks in a double-blind clinical trial. Weight loss was faster in the aspirin-ephedrine-caffeine group than placebo, and there were no significant differences in pulse rate, blood pressure, fasting glucose, or symptoms (70). In an effort to evaluate the best combination of caffeine and ephedrine, single doses of ephedrine (10 mg and 20 mg) and caffeine (100 mg and 200 mg) were compared with three combinations of caffeine with ephedrine (10 mg/200 mg, 20 mg/100 mg, and 20 mg/200 mg). Ephedrine 20 mg with caffeine 200 mg gave increases in oxygen consumption that were greater than the sum of the increase seen with ephedrine 20 mg and caffeine 200 mg separately. The other two doses of caffeine and ephedrine were equivalent to the additive effect of their component doses of caffeine and ephedrine separately on oxygen consumption. The acute dose of caffeine and ephedrine elevated systolic blood pressure 9 mm Hg and pulse rate 7 BPM. Plasma glucose, insulin, and c-peptide were also elevated (71). This acute effect of caffeine and ephedrine in raising blood pressure, pulse, and glucose is lost with chronic treatment (66).

A combination of 20 mg ephedrine with 200 mg caffeine given TID was studied in 180 obese subjects randomized to ephedrine 20 mg TID, caffeine 200 mg TID, ephedrine 20 mg with caffeine 200 mg TID, or placebo for a 24-week double-blind trial. Weight loss with caffeine and ephedrine was greater than placebo from 8 weeks to the end of the trial. Ephedrine alone and caffeine alone were not different than placebo. The caffeine with ephedrine group lost 17.5% of their body weight in the 24-week trial. Side effects of tremor, insomnia, and dizziness reached the levels of placebo by 8 weeks, and blood pressure fell similarly in all four groups. Heart rate rose in a statistically significant manner in the ephedrine group compared to placebo, but fell below the baseline value in the caffeine and ephedrine group (72). Two weeks after cessation of the 24-week trial, headache and tiredness were more frequent in the group that had taken caffeine with ephedrine. At the end of the 2-week washout period, all subjects were given the opportunity to participate in an additional 24-week open-label trial using caffeine

with ephedrine. Those subjects remaining on caffeine with ephedrine maintained their weight loss to the end of trial at week 50 (73). Seventy-five percent of the weight loss was explained by anorexia, and 25% was explained by increased thermogenesis (74). Since acute treatment with caffeine 200 mg and ephedrine 20 mg TID had cardiovascular and metabolic effects, the chronic effects were evaluated in the 24-week trial. By week 12 the blood pressure had dropped 4–11 mm Hg below baseline and remained similar to the placebo group. The pulse rate dropped 1–2 BPM from baseline during the trial, and reductions in plasma glucose, cholesterol, and triglycerides were not different between the groups at the end of the 24-week double-blind trial (75). These findings were confirmed in an 8-week trial using ephedrine 50 mg, caffeine 50 mg, and aspirin 110 mg given TID that was double blinded and placebo controlled. There was no significant change in heart rate, blood pressure, blood glucose, insulin, cholesterol, or side effects relative to placebo, but weight loss was greater in the ephedrine, caffeine, and aspirin group (76).

The effect of caffeine 200 mg with ephedrine 20 mg TID on body composition has been studied using bio-impedance analysis. At the end of 8 weeks, weight loss was not different, but the group on caffeine and ephedrine lost 4.5 kg more fat and 2.5 kg less lean tissue than the placebo group, a significant difference. As one might expect, the fall in energy expenditure was 13% in the placebo group and only 8% in the group treated with caffeine and ephedrine (77). Treatment with caffeine and ephedrine over 8 weeks also prevented the expected drop in HDL cholesterol. Since HDL cholesterol protects from atherogenesis, this finding suggests that caffeine and ephedrine may have the potential to reduce atherosclerotic cardiovascular disease. The placebo group experienced the drop in HDL cholesterol routinely reported with diet-induced weight loss (78).

Ephedrine with or without a methylxanthine was evaluated in adolescents. The effect of ephedrine in stimulating thermogenesis was lost after 1 week of treatment, but was restored by combining it with aminophylline for 1 week (79). This would explain why the trials with ephedrine alone give more weight loss than placebo early in trial that decreases with time unless combined with a methylxanthine. The same group reported a 20-week, double-blind, placebo-controlled and randomized clinical trial of caffeine and ephedrine in 32 adolescents age of 16 ± 1 years and Tanner stage III–V (80). Subjects < 80 kg were given 1 tablet containing 100 mg caffeine and 10 mg ephedrine TID, and subjects > 80 kg were given 2 pills TID. The loss of initial body weight was 14.4% and 2.2% in the caffeine with ephedrine and placebo groups, respectively ($P <$ .01). All three dropouts were in the placebo group, and adverse events were described as negligible. After the first 4 weeks the adverse events in the caffeine group were not different than placebo.

Caffeine with ephedrine give weight losses in the range of 15–20% of initial body weight in 6 months—a weight loss comparable to what was seen with phentermine/fenfluramine (81). Caffeine 200 mg with ephedrine 20 mg TID was compared to dexfenfluramine 15 mg BID in a double-blind trial. In subjects with a BMI > 30 kg/m^2, the weight loss was greater with caffeine and ephedrine treatment. Blood pressure declined significantly in both groups (7.8/4.6 mmHg in the dexfenfluramine group and 10.6/3.5 mmHg in the caffeine and ephedrine group), but the differences were not significantly different from each other. Pulse rate declined 1.1 to 2.7 BPM and was not different between the groups. The subjects treated with dexfenfluramine had more gastrointestinal symptoms (diarrhea, dry mouth, and thirst), and the subjects treated with caffeine and ephedrine had more symptoms of central nervous system stimulation (tremor, insomnia, agitation). Symptoms in both groups declined by the end of the first month of the 15-week trial (82).

Although dexfenfluramine is no longer available owing to cardiac valvular toxicity, caffeine and ephedrine are available without prescription. The cardiac valvular problems associated with fenfluramine and dexfenfluramine are felt to be related to serotonin and have not been associated with caffeine and ephedrine, which have a noradrenergic mechanism of action. Fenfluramine with phentermine, fenfluramine, with mazindol, and caffeine with ephedrine and mazindol alone were compared in their ability to reduce weight, cardiovascular risk, and LDL cholesterol. Caffeine with ephedrine was found to be the most cost-effective treatment (83).

Ephedrine 25 mg and caffeine 200 mg TID for 10 days had no effect on resting cardiovascular function measured by thoracic bioimpedance, automatic sphygmomanometry, or continuous electrocardiographic recording. During cycle ergometer exercise, there was a small increase in the cardiac ejection fraction. Based on these results, the authors concluded that, in the doses studied, caffeine and ephedrine had no undesirable effects on cardiovascular function in the obese (84). The efficacy of caffeine and ephedrine in the treatment of human obesity is summarized in Table 1.

The safety of caffeine and ephedrine in human obesity studies are summarized in Table 2, which compiles the incidence of side effects in the various trials of caffeine and ephedrine, expressing them as a percentage of the total number of subjects studied. Since one trial compared caffeine and ephedrine to diethylpropion and another to dexfenfluramine, some comparison to the safety of these compounds can also be made (see Table 2).

Another way to evaluate the safety of caffeine and ephedrine is to compare the dropouts in caffeine with ephedrine groups to placebo groups or to groups of compounds with which caffeine with ephedrine have been compared in obesity studies (see Table 3). The raw dropout rates, however, do not reflect the reasons for the dropouts. Safety can also be evaluated by comparing the dropouts for adverse events in the caffeine with ephedrine groups to the dropouts for adverse event in the placebo groups or other compounds with which caffeine with ephedrine have been compared (see Table 4).

Caffeine and ephedrine are unique in that the side effects return to placebo levels by 8 weeks and remain at placebo levels at least to 24 weeks despite subjects remaining on the compounds (72) (Fig. 1). Therefore, the incidence of adverse events may overestimate their true clinical significance in obesity studies, since obesity is a chronic disease and one for which chronic treatment is appropriate. Catechins in green tea (see below) are synergistic with caffeine in stimulating thermogenesis in man. No adverse effects were detectable, even with acute dosing of caffeine with catechins in a study performed in a metabolic chamber (85). Caffeine 200 mg and ephedrine 20 mg TID have been tested for the prevention of weight gain after smoking cessation. Two-thirds of 225 subjects were randomized to receive caffeine and ephedrine for 12 weeks, and the rest were randomized to placebo. All subjects were off medication by week 39, and at 1-year weight loss and the percent not smoking were similar in the two groups. At 12 weeks, however, weight gain was less in the caffeine and ephedrine group (86).

Concerns have been raised regarding the safety of caffeine and ephedrine use in subjects with controlled hypertension. One hundred thirty-six overweight normotensive or drug-controlled hypertensive subjects randomized to five groups. After 6 weeks of treatment, systolic blood pressure was reduced 5.5 mmHg more in controlled hypertensive subjects treated with caffeine 200 mg and ephedrine 20 mg TID than placebo in subjects treated with medication other than beta-blockers. The antihypertensive effect of beta-blocker medication was not reduced by caffeine and ephedrine. Normotensive patients treated with caffeine and ephedrine had a 4.4/3.9 mmHg greater drop in blood pressure

Table 1 Efficacy of Caffeine and Ephedrine

Ref.	Start D/P	End D/P	Dose (E/C)	Length	kg lost D/P	% wt lost D/P	Comments
(3)	49/33	42/31	80/300 mg/d	12 wk	8.1/4.1	8.3/4.5	Diethylpropion and E/C gave equal wt loss
(69)	16	16	22/130 mg/d	1 d	0[a]	0	E/C normalized TEF of postobese to lean level
(70)	29	11/13	150/150 mg/d	8 wk	2.2/0.7	—[b]	E/C with aspirin 330 mg/d
(71)	6	6	20/200 mg/d	1 d	0	0	E/C dose synergistic
(72)	45/45	35/35	60/600 mg/d	24 wk	16.6/13.2	17.5/13.6	E or C alone and placebo gave equal wt loss; C/E maintained wt loss for 24 wk on open-label C/E
(77)	7/7	6/6	60/600 mg/d	8 wk	10.1/8.4	—	C/E gave more fat loss and less lean tissue loss than placebo
(78)	20/20	16/16	60/600 mg/d	8 wk	9.07.6	9.6/8.2	C/E gave no drop in HDL
(79)	8	8	75/880 mg/d	1 d	0	0	Ephedrine loses its effect without methylxanthine in adolescents
(82)	50/53	38/43	60/600 mg/d	15 wk	9.0/7.0	9.7/7.8	P = dexfenfluramine 30 mg/d in this study
(89)	20	20	75/600 mg/d	24 wk	—	8.6	C/E was most cost-effective obesity treatment in the trial
(84)	9/9	9/9	50/400 mg/d	10 d	0	0	C/E gave no cardiovascular toxicity at 10 d
(80)	16/16	16/13	30/300 and 60/600 mg/d	20 wk	7.9/0.5	14.4/2.2	C/E toxicity negligible and equal to placebo by 4 weeks in adolescents

The table lists the human caffeine (C) and ephedrine (E) studies by number in the reference list. The number of subjects that started and finished the studies in the drug (D) and placebo (P) groups are listed. The study length is given, and the weight lost in kilograms and/or percent initial body weight lost is also given. The comment section lists special aspects of the various studies.
[a] 10 = 0.
[b] — = no data.

than those treated with placebo. The mean loss of weight of 4 kg was significant for all groups (87).

Caffeine was combined with phenylpropanolamine in the past to treat obesity (88). Since caffeine is not synergistic or even additive to phenylpropanolamine in stimulating weight loss, and can give central nervous system stimulation, it was removed from phenylpropanolamine products sold for weight loss (89). This is in contradistinction to caffeine and ephedrine that do give more weight loss when combined than either compound induces alone. The addition of caffeine to ephedrine in a 6-month trial blocked the rise in pulse rate seen with ephedrine alone (72). Energy expenditure with mention of caffeine has been reviewed (90), and nonprescription appetite suppressants including caffeine have also been reviewed (91).

Ephedrine has been proposed as an adjunct to cognitive restructuring (92). Ephedrine has been considered in reviews relative to nonprescription weight loss sup-

plements (93), obesity management (94), energy balance (95), and obesity treatment (96).

Caffeine and ephedrine have been included in recent reviews of obesity medication (97–102). Thermogenic approaches to treat obesity have been reviewed (103). More specifically, caffeine and ephedrine relative to obesity treatment have also been reviewed (104–107). In a letter to the editor of the journal in which the clinical trial was published, the authors reported that ephedrine alone, on reanalysis, actually gave more weight loss than placebo, but less than ephedrine and caffeine, in the 24-week trial of caffeine, ephedrine, caffeine with ephedrine, and placebo (108). Caffeine and ephedrine have also been used to induce weight loss prior to comparing different weight maintenance diets (109).

Ephedrine products are sold without a prescription for the treatment of asthma and have a recommended dosage up to 150 mg/d. Caffeine sold without a prescription has a recommended dose up to 1600 mg/d. The

Table 2 Adverse Effects

Symptom	C&E	No.	Pl	No.	DEP	No.	Dex	No.
Agitation (jitteriness, anxiety)	5.9%	(15/256)	0%	(0/143)	8%	(4/50)	0%	(0/53)
Dizziness	3.5%	(9/256)	2.1%	(3/143)	0%	(0/50)	7.5%	(4/53)
Headache	1.6%	(4/256)	0%	(0/143)	0%	(0/50)	5.7%	(3/53)
Tremor	9.4%	(24/256)	4.2%	(6/143)	4%	(2/50)	0%	(0/53)
Depression (fatigue)	0.8%	(2/256)	0%	(0/143)	0%	(0/50)	5.7%	(3/53)
Insomnia	12.5%	(32/257)	6.3%	(9/143)	10%	(5/50)	1.9%	(1/53)
Postural hypotension	0.8%	(2/256)	0.7%	(1/143)	0%	(0/50)	0%	(0/53)
Nausea	4.7%	(12/256)	3.5%	(5/143)	0%	(0/50)	11.3%	(6/53)
Thirst	0.4%	(1/256)	0%	(0/143)	0%	(0/50)	9.4%	(5/53)
Paresthesias	0%	(0/256)	0%	(0/143)	0%	(0/50)	5.7%	(3/53)
Diarrhea	0%	(0/256)	0%	(0/143)	0%	(0/50)	11.3%	(6/53)
Arrhythmia	5.5%	(14/256)	2.1%	(3/143)	0%	(0/50)	1.9%	(1/53)
Constipation	1.2%	(3/256)	1.4%	(2/143)	2%	(1/50)	3.8%	(2/53)
Urinary problems	0.4%	(1/256)	0.7%	(1/143)	2%	(1/50)	0%	(0/53)
Dry mouth	1.6%	(4/256)	0%	(0/143)	0%	(0/50)	1.9%	(1/53)
Heart rate	0.8%	(2/256)	0%	(0/143)	0%	(0/50)	0%	(0/53)
BP elevated	0.4%	(1/256)	0.7%	(1/143)	0%	(0/50)	0%	(0/53)
Glucose	0%	(0/256)	0%	(0/143)	0%	(0/50)	0%	(0/53)
Other	4.9%	(10/256)	6.3%	(9/143)	0%	(0/50)	0%	(0/53)

Adverse events reported in trials of caffeine and ephedrine are listed as a percent incidence with the number of subjects experiencing the symptoms and the total number of subjects in the trials in parentheses. One trial compared caffeine (C) and ephedrine (E) to diethylpropion (DEP) 25 mg TID in 50 subjects and another trial compared caffeine and ephedrine to dexfenfluramine (Dex) 15 mg BID in 53 subjects. Pl, placebo.

popular herbal products containing caffeine and ephedrine and taken for weight loss have dosage recommendations up to 100 mg/d of ephedrine equivalent as ephedra. The caffeine content of these herbal products containing caffeine and ephedrine varies, but is < 600 mg/d. The most popular and widely sold herbal product

containing caffeine and ephedra has only 240 mg/d of caffeine, < 3 cups of coffee. Pharmaceutical grade products have greater potency than the herbal products containing caffeine and ephedrine in equivalent doses because the herbal products contain some of the less active isomers of ephedra. The peer-reviewed literature

Table 3 Subjects Withdrawn from the Caffeine and Ephedrine Trials

Ref.	C&E	Placebo	DEP	Dexfen
(3)	0	4	4	—
(72)	10	10	—	—
(77)	1	1	—	—
(78)	4	4	—	—
(82)	10	—	—	7
(80)	0	3	—	—
—	11.3%	11.2%	8%	13.2%
	(29/256)	(16/143)	(4/50)	(7/53)

All subjects who withdrew from the studies of caffeine (C) and ephedrine (E) are listed. Each study is identified by reference list number. The bottom row on the table expresses the dropout incidence in percent followed by the number of subjects who dropped out and the total number of subjects in the trials. There was one trial in which caffeine and ephedrine were compared to 50 subjects on diethylpropion (DEP) 25 mg TID and one trial in which caffeine and ephedrine were compared to 53 subjects on dexfenfluramine (Dexfen) 15 mg.

Table 4 Adverse Events Responsible for Withdrawal Listed for Subjects Participating in Caffeine and Ephedrine Trials

Adverse event	C&E	Placebo	Dexfen[a]
HTN[b]	1	2	0
Arrhythmia	2	0	0
Agitation	1	0	0
Vomiting	2	0	0
Insomnia	3	0	0
Headache	0	0	1
Diarrhea	0	0	1
Totals	3.3%	1.6%	3.8%
	(8/241)	(2/127)	(2/53)

This table lists the reasons given for study withdrawal in subjects dropping out for adverse events during the caffeine (C) and ephedrine (E) trials. The bottom row lists the incidence of dropouts for adverse events described in the trials followed by the number withdrawing and the number in the trials.

[a] Dexfenfluramine.
[b] Hypertension.

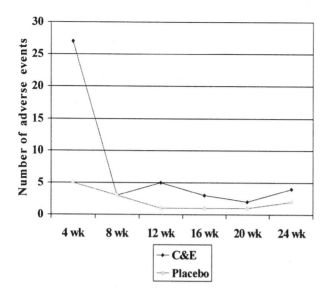

Figure 1 Incidence of adverse events with caffeine and ephedrine compared to placebo at monthly intervals during a 6-month trial (68). The incidence of adverse events (dizziness, tremor, headache, depressed mood, anxiety, euphoria, insomnia, postural hypotension, palpitation, and tachycardia) were mild and transient and reached the placebo level at 8 weeks where they remained for the rest of the trial.

documents central nervous system stimulation, an increase in pulse, an increase in blood pressure, and an increase in glucose when caffeine and ephedrine are given acutely either separately or together. These side effects disappear with chronic treatment and are no longer present after 4–12 weeks, depending on the trial. A 24-week trial of caffeine and ephedrine found a decrease in pulse and blood pressure. The pulse rate in that trial was no different from placebo in the caffeine and ephedrine group, but was significantly higher than placebo in the ephedrine group. There were no differences between the caffeine with ephedrine group and the placebo group relative to serum glucose, serum cholesterol, or symptoms of stimulation.

Ephedrine and caffeine have each been sold for years without a prescription for the treatment of asthma and to combat drowsiness, respectively. Toxicity has not been a concern, even with recommended doses higher than that used in herbal products containing caffeine and ephedrine for weight loss. Overweight and obesity are common problems affecting more than half of the population, yet obesity is stigmatized by society. Therefore, it is not surprising that an effective weight loss product containing compounds with a long history of safe nonprescription use would be embraced enthusias-

tically by the public. When large numbers of the public use any product, adverse events can be associated with the use of the product, but establishing that there is a cause-and-effect relationship of these adverse events to the product should be required prior to the withdrawal, prohibition, or licensing of such products.

B   Green Tea Catechins

Green tea prepared by heating or steaming the leaves of *Camelia sinensis* is widely consumed on a regular basis throughout Asia. However, the most widely consumed tea is black tea consumed by > 80% of the world's population. Black tea is made by allowing the green tea leaves to auto-oxidize enzymatically, leading to the conversion of a large percentage of green tea catechins to theaflavins. The catechins are a family of compounds including epigallocatechin gallate, considered to be the most potent antioxidant in the family of compounds. Drinking 1 cup of tea per day has been reported to decrease the odds ratio of suffering a myocardial ifarction to 0.56 compared to non tea drinkers (110). These compounds are flavonoids in the class of polyphenols and have many activities including inhibition of the catechol-O-methyl transferase (COMT) enzyme, which degrades norepinephrine (111). The catechins appear to be able to enhance sympathetic nervous system activity at the level of the fat cell adrenoreceptor. In vitro, a green tea extract containing both catechins and caffeine was more potent in stimulating brown adipose tissue thermogenesis than equimolar concentrations of caffeine alone (112). The use of ephedrine to release norepinephrine increased the thermogenic effect noted with green tea catechins. Oolong tea or placebo was orally administered to mice over a 10-week period during high-fat feeding. Mean food consumption was not different between the groups, but oolong tea prevented the obesity and fatty liver induced by the high-fat diet. Noradrenaline-induced lipolysis was shown to increase and pancreatic lipase activity to be inhibited by the oolong tea (113). Since caffeine occurs naturally in green tea extract, it has been difficult to separate the effects of green tea from caffeine in humans. However, a recent study by Dulloo et al. (67) gave subjects green tea extract capsules TID providing a total of 150 mg caffeine and 375 mg total catechins, of which 270 mg was epigallocatechin gallate. Subjects spent three 24-hr periods in an energy chamber during which they received the above green tea extract, 150 mg of caffeine or placebo. Twenty-four-hour urinary excretion of norepinephrine but not epinephrine increased in the 24 hr when green tea was administered compared to the caffeine or placebo treatment periods. Energy expenditure was higher by 4.5% in the green tea period compared to placebo and 3.2% higher than when the same dose of caffeine was given alone. In addition, fat oxidation was increased. The net effect attributable to green tea could be estimated at 328 kJ/d, or ~ 80 kcal/d. Clearly, it is difficult to demonstrate the effects of green tea catechins alone, but there is the possibility of a synergistic interaction with ephedrine independent of the caffeine content of green tea which should be evaluated.

C Synephrine from Citrus Aurantium

Bitter Orange (*Citrus aurantium*) contains small amounts of alkaloids such as synephrine and octopamine, which are direct and indirect sympathomimetic agonists. These substances occur in minute concentrations in orange juice on the order of parts per million. In one placebo-controlled study (114), 23 subjects with body mass index > 25 kg/m2 were randomly assigned to receive a maltose placebo, nothing or 975 mg *Citrus aurantium* extract with 528 mg of caffeine and 900 mg St. John's wort daily. Subjects in the treated group lost 1.4 kg more weight than those in the placebo groups and also lost a significant amount of body fat (2.9%), while there was no fat loss in the placebo groups. It is claimed that these alkaloids act in a similar but milder fashion than the ephedra alkaloids, but this has not been carefully studied in a bioequivalence trial.

D Capsaicin from Chili Peppers

Capsaicin from chili peppers and red peppers have been shown to stimulate fat oxidation and thermogenesis (115,116). The exact mechanism for this effect is not known, but the constituents appear to activate neural signals that result in vasodilatation and endorphin release. There are also reports of modest weight loss in subjects consuming chili peppers regularly.

III FAT METABOLISM AND NUTRIENT PARTITIONING

A Conjugated Linoleic Acid

The *cis*-9,*trans*-11 isomer of conjugated linoleic acid (117) is formed naturally in the rumen of cattle (118), and supplementation of cattle feed with linoleic or linolenic acids increases the amount of conjugated linoleic acid in milk (119). Synthetic conjugated linoleic acid is a mixture of the *cis*-9,*trans*-11 isomer and *trans*-10,*cis*-12 isomer (120). The 9–11 isomer is thought to be responsible for the anticancer activity of conjugated linoleic acid (121) while the 10–12 isomer is thought to be responsible for the body compositional changes observed in animals (122,123).

Mice fed a diet supplemented with 0.5% conjugated linoleic acid at constant calories develop 60% less body fat than animals fed a control diet (124). This decrease in body fat is most likely due to a combination of reduced fat deposition, increased lipolysis, and increased fat oxidation. These findings were confirmed by West et al. (125), who demonstrated that conjugated linoleic acid reduced energy intake, growth rate, carcass lipid, and carcass protein in mice. Metabolic rate was increased and nocturnal respiratory quotient was decreased in these mice. On a high-fat diet, however, DeLany et al. (126) showed that conjugated linoleic acid decreased body fat without suppressing energy intake in mice. In this study, there was a marked decrease in body fat, and increase in body protein and without changes in food intake. Rats also respond to conjugated linoleic acid with a decrease in body fat (127).

Conjugated linoleic acid induces apoptosis of adipocytes and results in a form of lipodystrophy in which there is a decrease in white adipose tissue with the development of insulin resistance and enlargement of the liver (128). The mechanism is far from certain, however. Satory and Smith (129) postulate a reduction in fat accumulation in growing animals by inhibition of stromal vascular preadiposite hyperplasia. Azain et al. (130) found a reduction in fat cell size rather than a change in fat cell number. Initial studies in humans to treat obesity, presented in abstract form, suggest a lack of efficacy and increases in insulin resistance in animals raises safety concerns as well.

B *Garcinia cambogia* (Hydroxycitric Acid)

Garcinia cambogia contains hydroxycitric acid (HCA), which is extracted from the rind of the brindall berry. HCA is one of 16 isomers of citric acid and the only one that inhibits citrate lyase, the enzyme that catalyzes the first step in fatty acid synthesis outside the mitochondrion. HCA was studied by Roche Pharmaceuticals in the 1970s in rodents. Those studies, using the sodium salt of HCA, demonstrated weight reduction in three rodent models of obesity—the mature rat, the goldthioglucose-induced obese mouse, and the ventromedial hypothalamic lesioned obese rat. Food intake, body weight gain, and body lipid content were all reduced with no change in body protein (131). Three clinical trials have evaluated the efficacy and safety of HCA.

The first trial evaluated a product containing both HCA *Garcinia cambogia* and chromium picolinate. This single-arm open-label trial of 8 weeks in 77 adults, 500 mg *Garcinia cambogia* extract was combined with 100 μg of chromium picolinate taken TID. A 5.5% weight loss was seen in women, and 4.9% weight loss in men (132). HCA is also sold as an herbal supplement containing the calcium salt for which the dose is 3 g/d as a treatment for obesity. Two human clinical trials have evaluated the safety and efficacy of this marketed product. The first trial used 10 males acting as their own controls in a crossover trial evaluating energy expenditure and substrate oxidation. There was no difference in respiratory quotient, energy expenditure, glucose, insulin, glucagon, lactate, or beta-hydroxybutyrate at rest or during exercise (133). The second trial randomized 135 obese adults using a double-blind placebo-controlled design. HCA 1500 mg/d was administered daily for 12 weeks, and both groups were given a low-fat, high-fiber diet. In this trial, there was no significant difference in the weight loss observed in both groups (3.2 ± 3.3 for HCA group vs. 4.1 ± 3.9 kg for placebo, $P = .14$) (134). It is unclear whether the insolubility of the calcium salt or a species difference between rodents and humans are responsible for the lack of efficacy in humans. Further trials with measures of bioavailability are needed to resolve this issue, but the currently available HCA herbal dietary supplements appear to have no effect in human obesity.

C Dehydroepiandrosterone

Dehydroepiandrosterone (DHEA) and its sulfate are the most abundant circulating steroids in humans They originate in the adrenal gland and gonads, and are weak androgens. However, they can be converted into estrogens by enzymes found in many tissues. In lower animals, DHEA acts as an antiobesity agent (135) in amounts manyfold greater than those naturally produced in these animals. The mechanism of this effect has not been established. DHEA has been tested for the treatment of obesity in humans, and has been sold as a dietary supplement for weight loss. The reduction of endogenous DHEA production with aging and with malnutrition or illness, has suggested that DHEA may be more effective in elderly obese subjects. However, the evidence of any efficacy is minimal.

Abramsson and Hackl (136) treated obese women with 200 mg DHEA enanthate per day. Half of the women lost >1 kg/month, and these women were older with lower levels of urinary ketosteroids (136). Nestler

et al. (137) treated normal men with DHEA 1600 mg/d orally for 1 month. The percent body fat decreased 31% by skinfold measures without weight change (137). Mortola and Yen (138) performed a similar study in older women without a change in body weight or body fat by underwater weighing. Usiskin et al. (139) tried to repeat the study in men performed by Nestler et al. (137) using the more sensitive method of underwater weighing. They could not confirm a loss of fat and weight did not change. Welle et al. (140) also treated men with DHEA 1600 mg for one month without a change in body weight or indices of lean body mass.

Since DHEA is known to decrease through life, Morales et al. (141) treated aging humans with 50 mg DHEA per day for 6 months. There was no change in body fat. The same group treated aging humans for 1 year with DHEA 100 mg/d and placebo for 6 months, each in a crossover design. DHEA supplementation restored youthful levels of the hormone. Body fat by DEXA decreased by 1 kg in men during the DHEA treatment, but not in women. Women gained 1.4 kg of body mass, but men did not (142). Taken in total, these studies suggest that the effect of DHEA on body fat or body weight in humans is minimal if it exists at all.

D Chromium Picolinate

Chromium picolinate is a dietary supplement that has gained popularity for both weightlifters and people desiring weight loss (143). The concept is that it enhances the effectiveness of insulin, and has been called "glucose-tolerance factor." Page et al. (144) reported an increased percentage of muscle and a decreased percentage of fat in swine supplemented with chromium picolinate during growth from 55 kg to 119 kg, a phase of growth called finishing (144). These findings were confirmed by Mooney and Cromwell as well as by Lindeman et al. who also demonstrated an increased litter size in reproducing sows (145–147). Boleman et al. demonstrated that the chromium picolinate effect on body composition was limited to supplementation during the finishing phase of growth and was not seen when the chromium picolinate supplementation was given throughout growth from 19 kg to 106 kg (148). Myers et al. could not confirm the effects of chromium picolinate on body composition, but gave the supplementation throughout growth from 20 kg to 90 kg (149). Evock-Clover et al., who supplemented with chromium picolinate during growth from 30 kg to 60 kg, demonstrated a lowering of glucose and insulin concentrations, but failed to find an effect on body composition (150).

Bunting et al., studying cattle, demonstrated an increased rate of glucose clearance with chromium picolinate supplementation (151).

Although the animal literature is encouraging, the studies in humans have not confirmed the experience in swine. Hasten et al. studied the effect of 200 µg/d of chromium as chromium picolinate compared to placebo and administered to students of both sexes beginning a 12-week weight training class using a randomized double-blind design. Although there was an increase in circumferences and a decrease in skinfolds in all groups, the only significant difference seen was a greater increase in body weight in the females supplemented with chromium picolinate compared to the other three groups (152). These findings were confirmed by Grant et al., who studied 43 obese women using 400 µg/d of chromium. Women taking chromium picolinate gained weight unless engaged in exercise, which lowered weight and the insulin response to glucose (153).

Clancy et al. (154) performed a double-blind placebo-controlled study in football players attending a 9-week spring training. There was no effect of 200 µg/d of chromium as picolinate on strength or body composition, but the group taking chromium picolinate had urinary chromium that was five times higher than the placebo group. Trent and Thieding-Cancel studied obese U.S. Navy personnel (>22% fat for men and >30% fat for women by skinfolds) in a double-blind placebo-controlled protocol utilizing 400 µg/d of chromium picolinate. The 95 out of 212 military personnel who completed the 16-week study lost a small amount of weight and body fat, but no effect of chromium picolinate was demonstrated (155).

Lukaski et al. compared chromium chloride and chromium picolinate to placebo in an 8-week double-blind study in 36 men on a weight program. Serum and urine chromium increased equally in both chromium-supplemented groups, but the transferrin saturation decreased more in the chromium picolinate group than in the chromium chloride or the placebo groups. There was no effect of chromium supplementation on strength or body composition by DEXA (156). Bahadori et al. compared 200 µg/d of chromium picolinate with 200 µg/ d of chromium as yeast in 36 obese subjects during an 8-week very low calorie diet (VLCD) and an 18-week follow-up. Chromium picolinate, but not chromium as yeast, increased lean body mass without altering weight loss (157).

Pasman et al. compared 200 µg/d chromium picolinate to fiber, caffeine, and 50 g carbohydrate in 33 obese subjects during a 16-month weight loss study, the first 2 months of which included a VLCD. Chromium had no effect on body composition (158). Walker et al. compared 200 µg of chromium picolinate with placebo in 20 wrestlers over 14 weeks. There was no effect of chromium on body composition or performance (159). Campbell et al. evaluated the effect of chromium picolinate 200 µg/d in 18 men between 56 and 69 years of age during a resistance-training program (160). Chromium had no effect on body composition or strength.

Although chromium picolinate, 200 and 400 µg/d, has no effect upon body composition in humans, it has a significant effect on lipids, blood pressure, and glucose tolerance. Press et al. found that chromium picolinate 200 µg/d reduced LDL cholesterol and apolipoprotein B, and increased apolipoprotein A-1 in 28 subjects in a double-blind, placebo controlled, crossover trial (161). Lee and Reasner demonstrated a significant 17% drop of triglycerides in 30 non-insulin-dependent diabetic subjects using a similar design (162). Chromium ameliorates sucrose-induced blood pressure elevations in hypertensive rats and improves insulin sensitivity in man (163,164). The extent to which this is due to urinary losses of chromium and depletion of chromium stores in diabetic patients has not been evaluated. Chromium also reduces glycohemoglobin in diabetic subjects (165).

The toxicity of chromium, and chromium picolinate in particular, has been questioned. Evans and Bowman compared the effect of chromium chloride, chromium nicotinate, and chromium picolinate on insulin, glucose, and leucine internalization in cultured cells. Increased internalization was specific to chromium picolinate, since the other chromium salts and zinc picolinate did not have an effect. This was attributed to the demonstrated effect of chromium picolinate on the membrane fluidity in synthetic microsomal membranes (166). Chromium picolinate has been shown to produce chromosomal damage in Chinese hamster ovary cells, an effect attributed to the picolinate (167). Although not demonstrated, it has been postulated that with the use of dietary supplements of chromium picolinate over extended periods, levels could become high enough to damage DNA in humans (168).

Toxicology testing in animals, however, suggests that chromium supplements have a wide margin of safety (169). Chromium's effect upon insulin resistance is mediated through the oligopeptide chromodulin, which binds chromium. The chromium-chromodulin complex binds the insulin receptor and activates tyrosine kinase (170). Regardless of other beneficial uses, chromium picolinate does not alter body composition in humans, and as such is not helpful for the treatment of obesity.

Double-Blind, Placebo-Controlled Chromium Picolinate Studies on Body Composition in Humans

Ref.	Year	Duration	Dose	No. drug and placebo	Comments
(10)	1994	12 weeks	200 μg/d	30 and 29	Weight training. Females on Cr gained weight.
(11)	1997	9 weeks	400 μg/d	22 and 21	Obese women gained weight on Cr.
(12)	1994	9 weeks	200 μg/d	19 and 19	Football players. Cr—no change in body composition.
(13)	1995	16 weeks	400 μg/d	106 and 106	Obese Navy personnel. Cr—no change in body composition.
(14)	1996	8 weeks	200 μg/d	18 and 18	Cr—no effect on strength or body composition in men.
(15)	1997	26 weeks	200 μg/d	18 and 18	Cr picolinate not as yeast increased lean mass after VLCD.
(16)	1997	16 months	200 μg/d	11 and 22	Obese. Cr—no effect on body composition.
(17)	1998	14 weeks	200 μg/d	10 and 10	Cr—no effect of body composition or performance.
(18)	1999	13 weeks	200 μg/d	9 and 9	Men 56–69 yo. Cr—no effect on body composition or strength.

E Beta-Hydroxy-Beta-Methylbutyrate

Beta-hydroxy-beta-methylbutyrate (HMB) is a metabolite of leucine that is sold as a supplement to burn fat and build both strength and muscle tissue. Nissen et al. reported that HMB supplementation at 1.5–3 g/d reduced muscle catabolism and increased fat-free mass during a weightlifting program of 2–6 weeks' duration (171). These effects were not seen, however, in trained athletes (172). Although supplementation with HMB has been shown to be safe in studies lasting 3–8 weeks, it has not yet been tested for efficacy in the treatment of obesity (173).

F Topical Fat Reduction

The goal of local fat reduction is the cosmetic benefit to individuals who are dissatisfied with the distribution of their fat tissue. The primary cosmetic concerns with fat topography has come from women who have a concentration of fat in the thigh area with a dimply appearance that has been termed cellulite (174). The actual cause of the dimpling is an increased growth of fibrous boundaries in the subcutaneous fat tissue occurring in the third and fourth decades of life. This is usually associated with childbearing and postpregnancy weight gain, but can also occur in women with a primarily gynoid fat distribution in the second decade of life. The cosmetic goal of reducing and smoothing thigh fat can be approached with topical treatment, which will be discussed here, and liposuction, which, being a cosmetic surgical procedure, is beyond the scope of this chapter.

The lipolytic threshold in various fat tissues is determined by the balance of stimulatory and inhibitory GTP-binding proteins (G proteins) on the cell surface influencing the activity of adenylate cyclase. Women have more alpha-2 receptors in the thigh area with inhibitory effects on the lipolytic beta-2 receptors due to their higher levels of circulating estrogen. Adenosine receptors are also inhibitory G protein receptors, and phosphodiesterase, by degrading adenylate cyclase, also plays an inhibitory role in the lipolytic process (175–179).

Local application of substances to the fat cells that stimulate the lipolytic process have the potential to reduce the size of the treated fat cells. Using one thigh as a control, isoproterenol injections (a beta receptor stimulator), forskolin ointment (a direct stimulator of adenylate cyclase), yohimbine ointment (an alpha-2 receptor inhibitor), and aminophylline (an inhibitor of phosphodiesterase and the adenosine receptor) gave more girth loss from the treated than the control thigh. Treatments were given once daily, 5 days a week, for 1 month (180).

A 6-week study with 10% aminophylline ointment in 23 subjects, a 5-week study with 2% aminophylline cream in 11 subjects, and a 5-week study with 0.5% aminophylline cream in 12 subjects confirmed these findings. None of the creams were more effective than the 0.5% aminophylline, which had more than a 3 cm difference between the treated and untreated thighs (181). Another study, by Collis et al., however, was unable to reproduce these results in a 12-week study of aminophylline cream using a similar design (182).

An oral product containing gingko biloba, sweet clover, seaweed, grapeseed oil, lecithins, and evening promrose oil has been marketed orally for the treatment of cellulite. In a 2-month placebo-controlled trial, there was no reduction in body weight, fat content, thigh circumference, hip circumference, or dimply appearance of the fat (183).

IV AMINO ACIDS AND NEUROTRANSMITTER MODULATION

A 5-Hydroxytryptophan

Changes in plasma amino acid levels can modify food intake by affecting the brain availability of neurotransmitter precursors (184,185). Both theoretical and experimental data support a role for serotonin in the central nervous system regulation of satiety. Wurtman has suggested that serotonin may also play a role in the selection of carbohydrate-rich foods contributing to so-called carbohydrate craving (186). Blundell and Leshem (187) reported in 1975 that food intake could be reduced in hyperphagic rats through the parenteral administration of 5-hydroxytryptophan (5HTP), the metabolic precursor of serotonin. 5HTP is used based on the rationale that at high brain tryptophan concentrations conversion of tryptophan to serotonin is limited by reduced activity of 5-tryptophan hydroxylase, the enzyme that forms 5HTP from 1-tryptophan (188). Osborne-Mendel rats have reduced activity of 5-tryptophan hydroxylase (189) and a genetic predisposition to obesity.

There have been two studies in humans from the same group evaluating the effects of 5HTP on weight loss (190,191). In 19 obese women in a randomized, controlled double-blind crossover study comparing 5HTP and placebo without diet instruction, a small but significant difference in weight loss was noted over 5 weeks between subjects treated with 5HTP at a dose of 8 mg/kg/d and placebo. In a second study, 20 of 28 subjects completed a 12-week study in which there was no dietary instruction in the first 6 weeks and a 1200-calorie diet in the second 6 weeks. Subjects on 5HTP lost ~5% of starting weight in the trial, more than was observed in subjects treated with placebo with 2 kg additional lost in the first 6 weeks and 3 kg additional lost in the next 6 weeks. The high dropout rate and small size of this trial support preliminary data that 5HTP is effective, but further studies must be done to establish this as a reasonable adjunct to weight loss therapies.

B L-Tyrosine

L-tyrosine administration to rats increases the rate at which brain neurons synthesize and release catecholamine neurotransmitters (192). If a similar mechanism was operative in humans, then L-tyrosine could be used to increase catecholamine synthesis and affect satiety. Administration of 100 mg/kg/d of tyrosine led to increased CSF tyrosine concentrations in nine patients with Parkinson's disease changing from 3.5 ± 1.9 to 5.9 ± 3.4 µg/mL (192). In mice undergoing caloric restriction to 40% of usual intake, there was impairment of cognitive functions evaluated in a maze not seen at 60% of usual intakes. However, when 100 mg/kg/d tyrosine was injected into the mice, no decrease in cognitive function was seen at 40% of usual intake (193). While there are no studies of weight loss in humans taking tyrosine, these observations suggest that this might be useful in restoring normal well-being during dietary restriction.

Not withstanding these observations suggesting a benefit of 1-tyrosine supplementation, the enzyme tyrosine hydroxylase has been thought to be the rate-limiting step in the synthesis of norepinephrine, not the availability of the substrate L-tyrosine. Hull and Maher have suggested that this relationship might change in the presence of drugs that release catecholamines. The anorectic activity of phenlypropanolamine, ephedrine, and amphetamine are increased in food deprived rats from 37–50% by L-tyrosine supplementation in a dose-dependent manner (25–400 mg/kg). This enhanced anorectic activity is mediated by catecholamines and was not seen with direct-acting beta agonists (194). Hull and Maher also demonstrated that the effect of tyrosine to enhance the anorectic effect of drugs that release catecholamines was limited to the central nervous system. The peripheral actions of these drugs such as blood pressure elevation were not enhanced by tyrosine supplementation (195,196). Although these studies suggest a role for tyrosine supplementation in enhancing the anorectic effect of centrally acting anorectic medications that release catecholamines without increasing side effects, evaluation of this possibility in humans has not been reported.

V FIBERS

A Soluble and Insoluble Dietary Fibers

It has been suggested that the increase in obesity in Western countries since 1900 may be related to changes in dietary fiber. The fiber associated with starchy foods has decreased while the fiber associated with fruits and vegetables has increased (197). Efforts to evaluate the association of dietary fiber with body weight regulation began in the 1980s. Guar gum, a water-soluble fiber, was shown to reduce hunger and weight more effectively than water-insoluble bran fiber in the absence of a prescribed diet (198).

Glucomannan, another water-soluble fiber supplemented at 20 g/d over 8 weeks gave a 5.5-lb weight loss with no prescribed diet (199). These results were confirmed in a 2-month study using the same fiber with a calorie-restricted diet (200). In a 2-week trial 45 subjects on psyllium, a third water-soluble fiber, were compared to 40 subjects on bran, a water-insoluble fiber, and a control without a specific diet. There was no difference in weight, but hunger was reduced in both fiber groups (201).

In an effort to further define the physiology of fiber, 31 normal-weight males and 19 overweight males were given a 5.2- or 0.2-g fiber preload. The high fiber preload increased fullness in both normal and overweight subjects, but only overweight decreased food intake at the subsequent meal (202). Another study confirmed fiber's ability to decrease appetite (203). The relationship between appetite and fiber was further defined by a study using two doses of water-soluble fiber. During 1 week of supplementation (40 g/d) without calorie restriction, food intake was reduced without change in appetite. During 1 week of supplementation (20 g/d) with calorie restriction, hunger was suppressed without a change in food intake (204).

Baron et al. compared two 1000 kcal/d diets in 135 subjects, one low in carbohydrate and fiber, the other higher in both these components. In contrast to subsequent studies, there was significantly more weight loss (5.0 vs. 3.7 kg) over 3 months on the lower-fiber diet (205). In a trial of 52 overweight subjects randomized to 7 g of fiber per day or a placebo with a calorie-restricted diet for 6 months. The fiber-supplemented group lost more weight (5.5 vs. 3.0 kg) and had less hunger (206).

Solum et al. randomized 60 overweight women to dietary fiber tablets or placebo and a weight-reducing diet for 12 weeks. The group on fiber lost more (8.5 vs. 6.7 kg) than those on placebo (207). An 8-week study compared fiber tablets (5 g/d) with placebo on a calorie-restricted diet in 60 obese females. The fiber group lost significantly more weight (7.0 vs. 6.0 kg). This finding was confirmed in a second study of 45 obese females. The group on 7 g fiber per day lost more weight than the placebo (6.2 vs. 4.1 kg) (208).

Owing to its safety, dietary fiber supplementation has been evaluated in obese children. There was no difference between a 15 g/d supplement and control during a 4-week trial (209). Longer-term trials in adults were conducted as well. Ninety obese females were randomly assigned to a 6- to 7-g/d dietary supplement or placebo and a 1200- to 1600-kcal/d diet in 1-year double-blind trial. The fiber group lost 3.8 kg (4.9% of initial body weight) compared to 2.8 kg (3.6%), a statistically significant difference (210).

Fiber, 30 g/d, has been supplemented in a VLCD in a 4-week crossover trial. Weight loss was not different, but hunger was less during the supplementation with fiber (211). In a 2-month trial of a VLCD followed by a 12-month maintenance phase with 20 obese subjects and 11 obese controls, there was no difference in weight loss between the group supplemented with 20 g guar gum per day compared to placebo (212).

The relationship between obesity and fiber has also been evaluated epidemiologically. Using food frequency questionnaires, obese men and women had significantly more fat and less fiber in their diets than lean men and women (213). These findings were confirmed using 3-day food diaries. Total fiber intake was higher in the lean than the obese group and the grams of fiber per 1000 kcal was inversely related to BMI (214).

In summary, the bulk of evidence suggests that dietary fiber decreases food intake, decreases hunger and water-soluble fiber may be more efficient than water insoluble fiber. Dietary fiber supplements (5–40 g/d) lead to small (1–3 kg) weight losses greater than placebo. Although the weight loss obtained with dietary fiber is less than the 5% of initial body weight felt to confer clinically significant health benefits, the safety of dietary fiber and its other potential benefits on cardiovascular risk factors recommend it for inclusion in weight reduction diets.

B Chitosan

Chitosan is acetylated chitin from the exoskeletons of crustaceans such as shrimp. The product has a molecular weight of >1 million daltons, and is designed to bind to intestinal lipids including cholesterol and triglycerides. Originally developed as a lipid binding resin in the 1970s based on its properties as a charged nonabsorbable carbohydrate, chitosan has received a great deal of attention as a potential weight loss aid working through a "fat blocker" mechanism. In public demonstrations, chitosan is mixed with corn oil in a glass, and the precipitation of the oil and clarification of the solution is emphasized as a mechanism that would result in fat malabsorption and weight loss in humans. This promises individuals that they can eat the fatty foods they desire without gaining weight.

Mice fed a high-fat diet with 3–15% chitosan for 9 weeks had less weight gain, hyperlipidemia, fatty liver, and higher fecal fat excretion than high-fat-diet-fed controls. These changes were shown to be the result of chitosan binding of dietary fat rather than through the inhibition of fat digestion (215).

Two double-blind clinical trials have been performed to evaluate the effect of chitosan 1200–1600 mg orally BID. One trial included 51 obese women who were treated for 8 weeks without any reduction in weight

Controlled Studies of Dietary Fiber for the Treatment of Obesity

Ref.	Number Fiber (Control)	Time	Weight loss Fiber (control)	Water-soluble	Water-insoluble	Diet	Hunger	Comment
(201)	95 (23)	2 wk	4.6 vs. 4.2 kg (NS)	Psyllium (45)	Bran (40)	No	Less	20 g fiber/d
(199)	10 (10)	8 wk	5.5 vs. − 1.5	Glucomannan 3 g/d		No		3 g fiber/d
(198)	5 (5)	1 meal	NS	Guar 20 g/d		No	Less	Blood sugar 10% less
(205)	169 (66)	3 mo	3.7 vs. 5.0 kg			Yes		20 vs. 27 g fiber/d
(207)	30 (30)	3 mo	8.5 vs. 6.7 kg	10%	90%	Yes		6 g fiber/d
(208)	30 (30)	2 mo	7.0 vs. 6.0 kg	10%	90%	Yes		5 g fiber/d
	45	3 mo	6.2 vs. 4.1 kg	10%	90%	Yes		7 g fiber/d
(209)	9 (9)	8 wk	NS	10%	90%	Yes		Children 15 g fiber/d
(210)	45 (45)	52 wk	3.8 vs. 2.8 kg	10%	90%	Yes		6–7 g fiber/d
(211)	22 (22)	4 wk	NS			VLCD	Less	
(206)	26 (26)	6 mo	5.5 vs. 3.0	10%	90%	Yes	Less	7 g fiber/d
(200)	15 (15)	2 mo		Glucomannan		Yes	Less	
(158)	20 (11)	14 mo	NS	Guar gum 20 g/d		VLCD		20 g fiber/d

(216). The second trial included 34 overweight men and women who were treated for 28 days without any weight reduction relative to control (217). There were no serious adverse events or changes in safety laboratory in either trial, and no changes in fat-soluble vitamins or iron metabolism were seen. It would appear that chitosan has the potential for weight reduction by binding dietary fat, but is not effective in the doses presently used in humans.

VI PHYSICAL AGENTS

A Jaw Wiring

Jaw wiring has been used for the treatment of obesity since the 1970s. Rogers et al. wired the jaws of 17 subjects with resistant obesity. The mean weight loss was 25.3 kg in 6 months, which is comparable to obesity surgery over the same period of time. The majority of the subjects regained weight after the wires were removed (218). Kark and Burke, who wired the jaws of nine subjects for 6–8 months, confirmed this observation. Their subjects lost 28.8 kg making gastric bypass surgery less difficult (219).

Castelnuovo-Tedesco et al. attempted jaw wiring in 14 self-referred obese women who were immature and had passive-dependent or passive-aggressive personalities. Only one-third completed the 6-month study, and most of those regained weight (220). Ross et al. confirmed that psychologically frail subjects do not tolerate this procedure well, and demonstrated that one could predict success of the jaw wiring with a phychological questionnaire (221). They also demonstrated that subjects with panic or fear did not tolerate jaw wiring well (222).

Garrow demonstrated that weight is almost inevitably regained when the jaw wires are removed by following a group of nine subjects who lost 30.3 kg in 9 months of jaw wiring (223). Discouraged by these results, 10 subjects with jaw wiring were compared to 10 subjects treated with milk-based liquid diets. The group with jaw wiring lost twice the amount of weight as the group on the milk-based diets, demonstrating that compliance was enhanced by jaw wiring (224). Pacy et al. confirmed these results by comparing diet advice to jaw wiring in 17 obese individuals followed for more than a year. The dietary advice group lost 17 kg compared to 33 kg in the jaw-wiring group (225).

Ramsey-Stewart and Martin treated 10 subjects with jaw wiring who lost an average 85% of their excess body weight in 16–40 weeks. Five of these subjects then underwent gastric reduction surgery and continued to lose further weight. Four of the five subjects who did not have surgery regained their weight, and only one subject maintained a significant weight loss after removal of the jaw wires. These authors concluded that jaw wiring has no place as a stand-alone treatment for obesity. It can, however, be useful for inducing a rapid weight loss safely, if it is sustained by an effective weight maintenance strategy (226).

B Gastric Balloon

Gastric balloons have been associated with weight loss in uncontrolled studies. In a trial with 60 morbidly obese subjects, an average of 21 kg was lost in a mean of 39 weeks. The procedure was not benign, however. There were two gastric ulcers and three cases of ileus, one of which required operative intervention (227). A second study in 60 subjects using a 550-mL pear-shaped balloon gave an 11% weight loss in 16 weeks without significant adverse events (228). Another study gave an average weight loss of 16 kg (229). Two subjects lost 18 kg and 15.5 kg in 6 and 5 months, respectively, prior to an elective surgery (230).

Both failure and complications tempered this initial enthusiasm. A trial in five adolescents with morbid obesity using a 500- to 700-mL balloon failed to give weight loss (231). A 3-month trial of a gastric balloon in 40 subjects resulted in a gastric ulcer, a spontaneous anal extrusion, and a duodenal ulcer (232). A gastric balloon caused severe abdominal cramps during pregnancy, almost necessitating a cesarean section (233), and a woman experienced a small bowel obstruction from migration of the balloon into the pyloric channel that required percutaneous deflation to avoid laparotomy (234).

Several controlled trials were conducted to resolve the issues surrounding the safety and efficacy of gastric balloons. One study inserted the Garren-Edwards gastric bubble into 34 subjects and performed a sham insertion in 25. All subjects participated in diet, behavior modification, and exercise. Weight loss at 3 months was not different in the two groups (18.7 lb vs. 17.2 lb) (235). In a second study, a balloon was passed into the stomachs of 10 obese subjects. The balloon was inflated with 400 mL for 1 month and deflated for 1 month. Inflation resulted in slower gastric emptying and one gastric ulcer. Significant weight loss occurred during the second and third weeks of inflation, but the difference was small and did not continue into the fourth week (236).

A larger gastric balloon, the 500-mL Ballobes, was inserted into obese subjects who qualified for obesity surgery. These subjects lost an average of 38 kg in the first 17 weeks and 12 kg in the second 18 weeks. The weight loss in the four groups—sham-sham, sham-balloon, balloon-sham, and balloon-balloon—were not different, and there were three gastric erosions and one gastric ulcer (237). Another study evaluated a 300-mL silicone rubber balloon. Eighty-six subjects were treated for 6 months in four groups–balloon only,

balloon and 1000 kcal/d diet, 1000 kcal/d diet only, and no treatment. The balloon-only group lost 3.2 kg, balloon and diet group lost 5.1 kg, but the diet-only group lost the most weight, 6.9 kg. Gastroscopy revealed three ulcers and two erosions. Subjects with smaller gastric volumes lost more weight (238).

Another evaluation of the gastric balloon divided 40 subjects into four groups of 10—gastric balloon and 1500 kcal/d diet, gastric balloon and intensive diet therapy, sham and 1500-kcal/d diet, and sham with intensive diet therapy. The two groups with the gastric balloon lost more weight at 6 months when the balloons were removed, and this significant difference was still present at 19 months. This study is exceptional in that it is the only one that supports the use of the gastric balloon (239).

Bariatric surgery has been the accepted invasive method of treating obesity. For this reason the 57 subjects with the Garren-Edwards gastric bubble were compared to 77 subjects undergoing bariatric surgery. Bariatric surgery gave more effective weight loss at 12 months, and the yearly cost for uncomplicated cases was comparable (240).

In the face of questions regarding the efficacy of the gastric bubble, more attention was focused on possible mechanisms by which it might be made more effective. Subjects with the 500-mL Ballobes balloon had less hunger in the 2–3 days following the insertion, but hunger returned to baseline at 2 months (241). The effect of inflating a gastric balloon with 200 mL and 500 mL in dogs demonstrated that food intake was suppressed only with the larger inflation volume (242).

Rats with a gastric balloon had a transient decrease in food intake and body weight at 3 days that was gone by 18 days compared to sham controls. This transient weight loss was not seen in capsaicin-treated rats, suggesting that vagal afferents are essential for the gastric balloon to cause weight loss (243). Inflating a gastric balloon was shown to decrease hunger in humans, an effect that was enhanced by infusing CCK-8 (244). Infusion of CCK-8 decreased food intake in subjects who were obese from hypothalamic injury and in obese subjects with normal brains. Placement of a gastric balloon did not enhance this effect on food intake (245).

Further evaluation of gastric distension in humans, revealed that hunger is reduced by 30% in the first week following balloon insertion, but hunger returns to baseline by 12 weeks (246). A 4-month study randomized 20 obese and 20 normal subjects to a low-calorie diet with or without a 500-mL gastric balloon. There was weight loss and gastric slowing irrespective of the presence or absence of a gastric balloon in both groups (247). Weight loss has been shown to decrease gastric capacity suggesting that alterations in stomach size impact the effect of the gastric balloon on hunger (248).

In summary, the gastric balloon has a minor and transient effect in suppressing hunger and food intake. It is not a cost-effective treatment for obesity in humans.

C Gastric Pacing

The concept of gastric stimulation electrically, also called gastric pacing, is to induce a neural feedback satiety signal so as to reduce food intake. This concept has been tested in animals by Cigaina et al., who induced antegrade and retrograde gastric peristalsis in three pigs with a bipolar pacing electrode on the serosal surface of the antrum (249). Using chronic gastric antral pacing with different gastric pacing parameters resulted in a decrease in food intake with weight loss in three pigs and an increase in food intake with weight gain in three pigs compared to three control animals over a period of 90 days (250). Therefore, gastric pacing can clearly have effects on weight gain.

This method was also tested by the same investigators in a 23-year-old Caucasian female weighing 149 kg with a BMI of 52.5 kg/m^2 who was treated with antral gastric pacing for weight loss (251). She was given no instructions other than to avoid sweet drinks. At ~1 year, she had lost 51 kg, >50% of her excess body weight (weight above a BMI of 25 kg/m2). The only reported side effects were an increase from 0.8 to 2.0 formed stools per day, and the conversion of preoperative gallbladder sludge to a gallstone. Gastroscopy and a gastrograffin meal revealed impaired gastric peristalsis. Not only was gastric emptying impaired, but the increased stool frequency also suggested accelerated intestinal transit.

The experience with gastric pacing in humans for the treatment of obesity was reviewed in 1999 (252). In 1995 and 1996, platinum electrodes were placed at laparotomy on the lesser curvature of the anterior gastric antrum in four subjects with a BMI >40 kg/m^2. Pacing parameters were: 24 hr/d, 180–400 msec pulse width, and 40–100 Hz (2 sec on and 3 sec off) with a burst amplitude of 2–8.5 mA. Two patients had monopolar electrodes, and two had bipolar electrodes. Subjects were only instructed not to drink sweet liquids. One patient with monopolar pacing lost 3% of her excess body weight in 31 months, and the other gained 16% of her excess body weight in 24 months. One patient with the bipolar electrode lost 38% of her excess body weight in 34 months, and the other lost 83% of her excess body weight in 40 months.

Ten similar patients were implanted with bipolar electrodes for gastric pacing in 1998. Three had the pacemaker placed near the fundus and 7 had the pacemaker placed near the antrum. At 6–12 months of follow-up (mean 8.5 months), the three subjects with the electrode placement near the fundus lost 13.7% of their excess body weight while the seven subjects with the electrode placement near the antrum lost 26.7% of their excess body weight. A clinical trial is now in progress testing the safety and efficacy of antral bipolar pacing for the treatment of obesity.

D Waist Cord

The waist cord was first tried as a method of maintaining a weight loss induced by jaw wiring (223). Jaw wiring can induce a 40-kg weight loss in ~9 months, a weight loss comparable to obesity surgery. The length of time that the jaw wires stay in place is 9 months and is limited by dental considerations. Following the removal of jaw wires, weight is almost inevitably regained. Nine subjects with an average weight of 115 kg had jaw wiring for an average of 8.1 months losing an average of 30.3 kg. During the 10 months following removal of the jaw wires, these subjects regained 17.8 kg. Another seven subjects with an average weight of 107 kg had jaw wiring for an average of 9.3 months and lost an average of 38.1 kg. When these seven subjects had the jaw wires removed, a 2-mm nylon cord was placed around their waists and left permanently in place. The group with the waist cord regained only 5.6 kg in an average of 7.8 months compared to 15 kg in the control group. The difference between the two groups was statistically significant ($P < .05$) (223).

Simpson et al. (253) compared two groups of obese subjects for weight loss and weight maintenance, one with a waist cord that was progressively tightened as weight was lost, and the other group without a waist cord. Both groups were treated with 4-week periods of very low calorie dieting alternating with 4-week periods of 1200 kcal/d high-fiber dieting. At 18–20 weeks the two groups lost 7.7 and 7.8 kg, respectively, which was not significantly different. At the end of the 48-week study 14 of 27 subjects remained in the waist cord group and seven of 19 remained in the group without a waist cord. The group with a waist cord lost 16 kg and regained 1.2 kg compared with a regain of 6.6 kg in the group not treated with a waist cord ($P < .01$). This suggests that a waist cord can be a useful tool for weight maintenance, but does not improve weight loss.

Garrow (254) subjected a series of 38 subjects to jaw wiring for weight loss. Twenty-six of these 38 subjects tolerated the jaw wiring and completed the weight loss phase losing 43 kg and had a waist cord applied. The waist cord was removed in 12 subjects for pregnancy, abdominal operations, or personal reasons. The 14 subjects continuing to wear the waist cord maintained a 33-kg weight loss at 3 years of follow-up, 77% of the weight loss achieved with jaw wiring (254).

Garrow also described three subjects who achieved a weight loss of 41.7 kg by conventional dieting followed by the application of a waist cord (255). These three subjects maintained a 33-kg weight loss at 21 months of follow-up, 79% of the weight lost with dieting. This suggests that the maintenance of large weight losses using the waist cord are achievable with diet induced weight loss. The waist cord is believed to provide a feedback signal whenever weight gain occurs triggering behaviors designed to result in prevention of weight gain (256).

A new design for the fastener of the waist cord was proposed in which the patient could adjust the tightness within limits. This new design also allowed for the cord to be tightened during weight loss (257). Although this new design was claimed to be better tolerated and successful clinically, trials with this new design have not been published.

VII PSYCHOPHYSIOLOGICAL APPROACHES

A Hypnosis

Hypnosis consists of relaxing subjects so that they are prone to carry out posthypnotic suggestions. The majority of the psychiatric literature suggests that this methodology is only useful in a subset of patients suggestible enough to be hypnotized. Hypnosis was evaluated by Kirsch et al. in a meta-analysis of 18 studies in which cognitive behavior therapy was compared with and without hypnosis (258). Kirsch concluded that, averaged across posttreatment and follow-up periods, the hypnosis groups lost 11.3 lb compared to 6.0 lb in the nonhypnosis groups. At the last assessment period the weight loss in the hypnosis group was 14.8 lb compared to 6.0 lb in the nonhypnosis group, suggesting that the benefits of hypnosis increased with time (259). Allison and Faith, on the other hand, performed a meta-analysis on the same studies and found that by eliminating one questionable study the statistical significance between the hypnosis and nonhypnosis groups was no longer present (260). These studies suggest that hypnosis is only useful in some subjects and on balance is not better than cognitive behavioral therapy.

Since these meta-analyses were done, Johnson and Karkut reported a lack of difference in weight loss between hypnosis with and without aversive therapy (261). Johnson reported an uncontrolled study describ-

ing weight loss with hypnotherapy (262). Stradling et al. treated obese subjects with sleep apnea using hypnotherapy compared to dietary advice. Weight loss was equal at 3 months, but the hypnotherapy group maintained a significant 3.8 kg weight loss at 18 months that was not present in the dietary group (263).

With the exception of a report citing adverse reactions to hypnotherapy in developing adolescents, hypnotherapy for obesity appears to be a safe treatment (264). Schoenberger, in a review of the literature on hypnosis as an adjunct to cognitive-behavioral psychotherapy, states that although the studies cite benefits, the numbers are relatively small and many have methodologic limitations suggesting the need for well-designed randomized clinical trials (265). Therefore, although promising, the place of hypnotherapy in the treatment of obesity remains unresolved.

B Aromatherapy

The lay literature has suggested aromatherapy may be effective in the treatment of obesity. We could find only one controlled trial to assess this approach. This was an 8-week treatment program in which one group had 25 selected foods paired with noxious odors each week while the control group had air paired with these foods. The 14 subjects in the group given noxious odors lost significantly more weight (4.7 lb) compared to the air group (3.6 lb). Weight returned to baseline in both groups 8 weeks after treatment, suggesting that aromatherapy has limited potential to treat obesity, which is a chronic disease (266).

C Acupuncture

Acupuncture has been suggested as a treatment for obesity. Using acupuncture points that stimulate the auricular branch of the vagus nerve in the ear, appetite suppression has been postulated. There have been three controlled trials to evaluate this claim. Mok et al. randomized 24 overweight subjects in a single-blind trial to acupuncture needles placed for 9 weeks in active or inactive auricular sites. These needles were stimulated before eating. The treatment was safe, but there was no difference in weight loss between the groups. A simultaneous trial was run in six guinea pigs with no change in weight (267).

Richards and Marley randomized 60 overweight subjects in a 4-week trial to a transcutaneous nerve stimulator device placed on the auricular branch of the vagus nerve in the ear or on the thumb as a control. Appetite was suppressed in a higher percentage of the active (ear) group ($P < .05$), and there was greater weight loss in the active group (2.98 kg vs. 0.62 kg, $P < .05$) (268).

Allison et al. randomized 96 obese subjects to an acupressure device that was massaged before each meal for 12 weeks. The active device fit into the ear like a hearing aid, putting pressure on the auricular branch of the vagus nerve. The inactive device was placed on the wrist. The treatment was safe, but there was no significant difference in weight loss, fat loss, or blood pressure between the groups (269).

Two of three human studies using acupuncture with good clinical trial designs and one animal study gave no significant weight loss. The one positive study used a transcutaneous nerve stimulation approach. In this study there was less than a 2.5 kg difference between the active and inactive groups. Although there were no adverse events in these studies, the efficacy of using stimulation of the auricular branch of the vagus nerve for weight loss appears to be marginal.

VIII EFFICACY AND SAFETY ASSESSMENT

While many of the studies presented above are not conclusive, and others are incomplete or poorly controlled, there are some general conclusions which can be drawn as to the safety and efficacy of the herbal and alternative approaches reviewed above.

One of the key problems in this assessment is that only those agents found to be effective have had adequate clinical studies performed to begin to look at safety. Even in these cases, it may be that adverse effects reports will be obtained in the field. It is sometimes difficult to assess whether the effects are caused by the agent being used. This problem will require careful documentation, but this work is only likely to be done with the most effective agents that become widely used.

IX CONCLUSION

The opportunities for additional research in this area are plentiful. Unfortunately, there has been relatively limited funding by comparison to funding for research on pharmaceuticals. However, botanical dietary supplements often contain complex mixtures of phytochemicals that have additive or synergistic interactions. For example, the tea catechins include a group of related compounds with effects demonstrable beyond those seen with epigallocatechin gallate (EGCG), the most potent catechin. The metabolism of families of related compounds may be different from the metabolism of purified crystallized compounds. Herbal medicines in some cases may be simply less purified forms of single active ingredients, but in other cases represent unique formulations of multiple related compounds that may have superior safety and efficacy compared to single ingredients.

Herbal/alternative approach	Evidence of efficacy	Evidence of safety
Caffeine and ephedra	Good—clinical trial	Good
Green tea catechins	Good—metabolic study	Excellent
Synephrine	Modest—clinical trial	Excellent
Capsaicin	Good—clinical trial	Excellent
Conjugated linoleic acid	Weak—clinical trial	Questionable
Garcinia cambogia	Poor—clinical trial	Excellent
Dehydroepiandrosterone	Minimal, if any—clinical trial	Questionable
Chromium picolinate	Ineffective	Good
Beta-hydroxy-beta-methylbutyrate	Ineffective for weight loss	Good
Topical fat reduction	Cosmetic only	Excellent
5-Hydroxytryptophan	Modest—clinical trial	Excellent
L-Tyrosine	None	Excellent
Dietary fiber	Modest—clinical trial	Excellent
Chitosan	Ineffective—clinical trial	Excellent
Jaw wiring	Effective	Dental problems
Gastric balloon	Ineffective	Unsafe
Gastric pacing	Questionable	Safe
Waist cord	Effective maintenance	Safe
Hypnosis	Ineffective	Safe
Aromatherapy	Ineffective	Safe
Acupuncture	Ineffective	Safe

Obesity is a global epidemic, and traditional herbal medicines may have more acceptance than prescription drugs in many cultures with emerging epidemics of obesity. A large number of ethnobotanical studies have found herbal treatments for diabetes, and similar surveys, termed bioprospecting, for obesity treatments may be productive.

Unfortunately, there have been a number of instances where unscrupulous profiteers have plundered the resources of the obese public with nothing to show for it. While Americans spend some $30 billion per year on weight loss aids, our regulatory and monitoring capability as a society are woefully inadequate. Without adequate resources, the FDA has resorted to "guilt by association" adverse events reporting which often results in the loss of potentially helpful therapies without adequate investigation of the real causes of the adverse events being reported. Scientific investigations of herbal and alternative therapies represent a potentially important source for new discoveries in obesity treatment and prevention. Cooperative interactions in research between the Office of Dietary Supplements, the National Center for Complementary and Alternative Medicine, and the FDA could lead to major advance in research on the efficacy and safety of the most promising of these alternative approaches.

REFERENCES

1. Haller CA, Benowitz NL. Adverse cardiovascular and central nervous system events associated with dietary supplements containing ephedra alkaloids. N Engl J Med 2000; 343:1833–1838.

2. Vansal SS, Feller DR. Direct effects of ephedrine isomers on human beta-adrenergic receptor subtypes. Biochem Pharmacol 1999; 58:807–810.

3. Malchow-Moller A, Larsen S, Hey H, Stokholm KH, Juhl E, Quaade F. Ephedrine as an anorectic: the story of the "Elsinore pill". Int J Obes 1981; 5:183–187.

4. Goodman L, Gilman A. The Pharmacological Basis of Therapeutics, 7 ed. New York: Macmillan, 1985.

5. Miller DS. A controlled trial using ephedrine in the treatment of obesity [letter]. Int J Obes 1986; 10:159–160.

6. Drug Topics Red Book Montvale, NJ: Medical Economics Company, 2000.

7. Macdonald IA. Advances in our understanding of the role of the sympathetic nervous system in obesity. Int J Obes Relat Metab Disord 1995; 19(suppl 7):S2–S7.

8. Chen MD, Lin WH, Song YM, Lin PY, Ho LT. Effect of caffeine on the levels of brain serotonin and catecholamine in the genetically obese mice. Chung Hua I Hsueh Tsa Chih (Taipei) 1994; 53:257–261.

9. Oberman Z, Herzberg M, Jaskolka H, Harell A, Hoerer E, Laurian L. Changes in plasma cortisol, glucose and free fatty acids after caffeine ingestion in obese women. Isr J Med Sci 1975; 11:33–36.

10. Acheson KJ, Zahorska-Markiewicz B, Pittet P, Anantharaman K, Jequier E. Caffeine and coffee: their influence on metabolic rate and substrate utilization in normal weight and obese individuals. Am J Clin Nutr 1980; 33:989–997.

11. Jung RT, Shetty PS, James WP, Barrand MA, Callingham BA. Caffeine: its effect on catecholamines and metabolism in lean and obese humans. Clin Sci 1981; 60:527–535.

12. Dulloo AG, Geissler CA, Horton T, Collins A, Miller DS. Normal caffeine consumption: influence on thermogenesis and daily energy expenditure in lean and postobese human volunteers. Am J Clin Nutr 1989; 49:44–50.

13. Bracco D, Ferrarra JM, Arnaud MJ, Jequier E, Schutz Y. Effects of caffeine on energy metabolism, heart rate, and methylxanthine metabolism in lean and obese women. Am J Physiol 1995; 269:E671–E678.

14. Bondi M, Grugni G, Velardo A, et al. Adrenomedullary response to caffeine in prepubertal and pubertal obese subjects. Int J Obes Relat Metab Disord 1999; 23:992–996.

15. Tagliabue A, Terracina D, Cena H, Turconi G, Lanzola E, Montomoli C. Coffee induced thermogenesis and skin temperature. Int J Obes Relat Metab Disord 1994; 18:537–541.

16. Yoshida T, Sakane N, Umekawa T, Kondo M. Relationship between basal metabolic rate, thermogenic response to caffeine, and body weight loss following combined low calorie and exercise treatment in obese women. Int J Obes Relat Metab Disord 1994; 18:345–350.

17. Abernethy DR, Todd EL, Schwartz JB. Caffeine disposition in obesity. Br J Clin Pharmacol 1985; 20:61–66.

18. Cheymol G. Clinical pharmacokinetics of drugs in obesity. An update. Clin Pharmacokinet 1993; 25:103–114.

19. Caraco Y, Zylber-Katz E, Berry EM, Levy M. Caffeine pharmacokinetics in obesity and following significant weight reduction. Int J Obes Relat Metab Disord 1995; 19:234–239.

20. Haffner SM, Knapp JA, Stern MP, Hazuda HP, Rosenthal M, Franco LJ. Coffee consumption, diet, and lipids. Am J Epidemiol 1985; 122:1–12.

21. La Vecchia C, Franceschi S, Decarli A, Pampallona S, Tognoni G. Risk factors for myocardial infarction in young women. Am J Epidemiol 1987; 125:832–843.

22. Toner JM, Close CF, Ramsay LE. Factors related to treatment resistance in hypertension. Q J Med 1990; 77:1195–1204.

23. Ohayon MM, Guilleminault C, Priest RG, Caulet M. Snoring and breathing pauses during sleep: telephone interview survey of a United Kingdom population sample [see comments]. BMI 1997; 314:860–863.

24. Gartside PS, Glueck CJ. Relationship of dietary intake to hospital admission for coronary heart and vascular disease: the NHANES II national probability study. J Am Coll Nutr 1993; 12:676–684.

25. Stamler J, Caggiula A, Grandits GA, Kjelsberg M, Cutler JA. Relationship to blood pressure of combinations of dietary macronutrients. Findings of the Multiple Risk Factor Intervention Trial (MRFIT). Circulation 1996; 94:2417–2423.

26. Wakabayashi K, Kono S, Shinchi K, et al. Habitual coffee consumption and blood pressure: a study of self-defense officials in Japan. Eur J Epidemiol 1998; 14:669–673.

27. Noble R. A controlled clinical trial of the cardiovascular and psychological effects of phenylpropanolamine and caffeine. Drug Intell Clin Pharm 1988; 22:296–299.

28. Barrett-Connor E, Chang JC, Edelstein SL. Coffee-associated osteoporosis offset by daily milk consumption. The Rancho Bernardo Study. JAMA 1994; 271:280–283.

29. Sawynok J. Pharmacological rationale for the clinical use of caffeine. Drugs 1995; 49:37–50.

30. Ramadan NM. Headache caused by raised intracranial pressure and intracranial hypotension. Curr Opin Neurol 1996; 9:214–218.

31. Massoudi M, Miller DS. Ephedrine, a thermogenic and potential slimming drug. Proc Nutr Soc 1977; 36:135A.

32. Yen TT, McKee MM, Bemis KG. Ephedrine reduces weight of viable yellow obese mice (Avy/a). Life Sci 1981; 28:119–128.

33. Wilson S, Arch JR, Thurlby PL. Genetically obese C57BL/6 ob/ob mice respond normally to sympathomimetic compounds. Life Sci 1984; 35:1301–1309.

34. Massoudi M, Evans E, Miller DS. Thermogenic drugs for the treatment of obesity: screening using obese rats and mice. Ann Nutr Metab 1983; 27:26–37.

35. Dulloo AG, Miller DS. Thermogenic drugs for the treatment of obesity: sympathetic stimulants in animal models. Br J Nutr 1984; 52:179–196.

36. Liu YL, Toubro S, Astrup A, Stock MJ. Contribution of beta 3-adrenoceptor activation to ephedrine-induced thermogenesis in humans. Int J Obes Relat Metab Disord 1995; 19:678–685.

37. Bukowiecki L, Jahjah L, Follea N. Ephedrine, a potential slimming drug, directly stimulates thermogenesis in brown adipocytes via beta-adrenoreceptors. Int J Obes 1982; 6:343–350.

38. Bailey CJ, Thornburn CC, Flatt PR. Effects of ephedrine and atenolol on the development of obesity and diabetes in ob/ob mice. Gen Pharmacol 1986; 17:243–246.

39. Dulloo AG, Miller DS. Aspirin as a promoter of ephedrine-induced thermogenesis: potential use in the treatment of obesity. Am J Clin Nutr 1987; 45:564–569.

40. Sapeika N. Drugs in obesity. S Afr Med J 1974; 48:2027–2030.

41. Astrup A, Lundsgaard C, Madsen J, Christensen NJ. Enhanced thermogenic responsiveness during chronic ephedrine treatment in man. Am J Clin Nutr 1985; 42:83–94.

42. Astrup A, Madsen J, Holst JJ, Christensen NJ. The effect of chronic ephedrine treatment on substrate utilization, the sympathoadrenal activity, and energy expenditure during glucose-induced thermogenesis in man. Metabolism 1986; 35:260–265.

43. Pasquali R, Baraldi G, Cesari MP, et al. A controlled trial using ephedrine in the treatment of obesity. Int J Obes 1985; 9:93–98.

44. Pasquali R, Cesari MP, Besteghi L, Melchionda N, Balestra V. Thermogenic agents in the treatment of human obesity: preliminary results. Int J Obes 1987; 11:23–26.

45. Pasquali R, Cesari MP, Melchionda N, Stefanini C, Raitano A, Labo G. Does ephedrine promote weight loss in low-energy-adapted obese women? Int J Obes 1987; 11:163–168.

46. Pasquali R, Casimirri F, Melchionda N, et al. Effects of chronic administration of ephedrine during very-low-calorie diets on energy expenditure, protein metabolism and hormone levels in obese subjects. Clin Sci (Colch) 1992; 82:85–92.

47. Nielsen B, Astrup A, Samuelsen P, Wengholt H, Christensen NJ. Effect of physical training on thermogenic responses to cold and ephedrine in obesity. Int J Obes Relat Metab Disord 1993; 17:383–390.

48. Astrup A. Thermogenesis in human brown adipose tissue and skeletal muscle induced by sympathomimetic stimulation. Acta Endocrinol Suppl 1986; 278:1–32.

49. Jonderko K, Kucio C. Effect of anti-obesity drugs promoting energy expenditure, yohimbine and ephedrine, on gastric emptying in obese patients. Aliment Pharmacol Ther 1991; 5:413–418.

50. Jaedig S, Henningsen NC. Increased metabolic rate in obese women after ingestion of potassium, magnesium- and phosphate-enriched orange juice or injection of ephedrine. Int J Obes 1991; 15:429–436.

51. Horton TJ, Geissler CA. Aspirin potentiates the effect of ephedrine on the thermogenic response to a meal in obese but not lean women. Int J Obes 1991; 15:359–366.

52. Geissler CA. Effects of weight loss, ephedrine and aspirin on energy expenditure in obese women. Int J Obes Relat Metab Disord 1993; 17(suppl 1):S45–S48.

53. Pasquali R, Casimirri F. Clinical aspects of ephedrine in the treatment of obesity. Int J Obes Relat Metab Disord 1993; 17(suppl 1):S65–S68.

54. Dvorak R, Starling RD, Calles-Escandon J, Sims EA, Poehlman ET. Drug therapy for obesity in the elderly. Drugs Aging 1997; 11:338–351.

55. Dulloo AG, Miller DS. The thermogenic properties of ephedrine/methylxanthine mixtures: animal studies. Am J Clin Nutr 1986; 43:388–394.

56. Dulloo AG, Miller DS. Reversal of obesity in the genetically obese fa/fa Zucker rat with an ephedrine/methylxanthines thermogenic mixture. J Nutr 1987; 117:383–389.

57. Tulp OL, Buck CL. Caffeine and ephedrine stimulated thermogenesis in LA-corpulent rats. Comp Biochem Physiol C 1986; 85:17–19.

58. Dulloo AG, Miller DS. Prevention of genetic fa/fa obesity with an ephedrine-methylxanthines thermogenic mixture. Am J Physiol 1987; 252:R507–R513.

59. Ramsey JJ, Colman RJ, Swick AG, Kemnitz JW. Energy expenditure, body composition, and glucose metabolism in lean and obese rhesus monkeys treated with ephedrine and caffeine. Am J Clin Nutr 1998; 68:42–51.

60. Lowell BB, Napolitano A, Usher P, et al. Reduced adipsin expression in murine obesity: effect of age and treatment with the sympathomimetic-thermogenic drug mixture ephedrine and caffeine. Endocrinology 1990; 126:1514–1520.

61. Napolitano A, Lowell BB, Flier JS. Alterations in sympathetic nervous system activity do not regulate adipsin gene expression in mice. Int J Obes 1991; 15:227–235.

62. Spurlock ME, Hahn KJ, Miner JL. Regulation of adipsin and body composition in the monosodium glutamate (MSG)-treated mouse. Physiol Behav 1996; 60:1217–1221.

63. Dulloo AG, Seydoux J, Girardier L. Potentiation of the thermogenic antiobesity effects of ephedrine by dietary methylxanthines: adenosine antagonism or phosphodiesterase inhibition? Metabolism 1992; 41:1233–1241.

64. Malecka-Tendera E. Effect of ephedrine and theophylline on weight loss, resting energy expenditure and lipoprotein lipase activity in obese over-fed rats. Int J Obes Relat Metab Disord 1993; 17:343–347.

65. Yoshida T, Sakane N, Wakabayashi Y, Umekawa T, Kondo M. Thermogenic, anti-obesity effects of bofutsusho-san in MSG-obese mice. Int J Obes Relat Metab Disord 1995; 19:717–722.

66. Han LK, Takaku T, Li J, Kimura Y, Okuda H. Anti-obesity action of oolong tea. Int J Obes Relat Metab Disord 1999; 23:98–105.

67. Dulloo AG, Seydoux J, Girardier L, Chantre P, Vandermander J. Green tea and thermogenesis: interactions between catechin-polyphenols, caffeine and sympathetic activity. Int J Obes Relat Metab Disord 2000; 24:252–258.

68. Stokholm KH, Hansen MS. Lowering of serum total T3 during a conventional slimming regime. Int J Obes 1983; 7:195–199.

69. Dulloo AG, Miller DS. The thermogenic properties of ephedrine/methylxanthine mixtures: human studies. Int J Obes 1986; 10:467–481.

70. Krieger DR, Daly PA, Dulloo AG, Ransil BJ, Young JB, Landsberg L. Ephedrine, caffeine and aspirin promote weight loss in obese subjects. Trans Assoc Am Physicians 1990; 103:307–312.

71. Astrup A, Toubro S, Cannon S, Hein P, Madsen J. Thermogenic synergism between ephedrine and caffeine in healthy volunteers: a double-blind, placebo-controlled study. Metabolism 1991; 40:323–329.

72. Astrup A, Breum L, Toubro S, Hein P, Quaade F. The effect and safety of an ephedrine/caffeine compound compared to ephedrine, caffeine and placebo in obese subjects on an energy restricted diet. A double blind trial. Int J Obes Relat Metab Disord 1992; 16:269–277.

73. Toubro S, Astrup A, Breum L, Quaade F. The acute and chronic effects of ephedrine/caffeine mixtures on energy expenditure and glucose metabolism in humans. Int J Obes Relat Metab Disord 1993; 17(suppl 3):S73–S77; discussion S82.

74. Astrup A, Toubro S, Christensen NJ, Quaade F. Pharmacology of thermogenic drugs. Am J Clin Nutr 1992; 55:246S–248S.

75. Astrup A, Toubro S. Thermogenic, metabolic, and cardiovascular responses to ephedrine and caffeine in man. Int J Obes Relat Metab Disord 1993; 17(suppl 1):S41–S43.

76. Daly PA, Krieger DR, Dulloo AG, Young JB, Landsberg L. Ephedrine, caffeine and aspirin: safety and efficacy for treatment of human obesity. Int J Obes Relat Metab Disord 1993; 17(suppl 1):S73–S78.

77. Astrup A, Buemann B, Christensen NJ, et al. The effect of ephedrine/caffeine mixture on energy expenditure and body composition in obese women. Metabolism 1992; 41:686–688.

78. Buemann B, Marckmann P, Christensen NJ, Astrup A. The effect of ephedrine plus caffeine on plasma lipids and lipoproteins during a 4.2 mJ/day diet. Int J Obes Relat Metab Disord 1994; 18:329–332.

79. Molnar D. Effects of ephedrine and aminophylline on resting energy expenditure in obese adolescents. Int J Obes Relat Metab Disord 1993; 17(suppl 1):S49–S52.

80. Molnar D, Torok K, Erhardt E, Jeges S. Safety and efficacy of treatment with an ephedrine/caffeine mixture. The first double-blind placebo-controlled pilot study in adolescents. Int J Obes Relat Metab Disord 2000; 24:1573–1578.

81. Atkinson RL, Blank RC, Loper JF, Schumacher D, Lutes RA. Combined drug treatment of obesity. Obes Res 1995; 3(suppl 4):497S–500S.

82. Breum L, Pedersen JK, Ahlstrom F, Frimodt-Moller J. Comparison of an ephedrine/caffeine combination and dexfenfluramine in the treatment of obesity. A double-blind multi-centre trial in general practice. Int J Obes Relat Metab Disord 1994; 18:99–103.

83. Greenway FL, Ryan DH, Bray GA, Rood JC, Tucker EW, Smith SR. Pharmaceutical cost savings of treating obesity with weight loss medications. Obes Res 1999; 7:523–531.

84. Waluga M, Janusz M, Karpel E, Hartleb M, Nowak A. Cardiovascular effects of ephedrine, caffeine and yohimbine measured by thoracic electrical bioimpedance in obese women. Clin Physiol 1998; 18:69–76.

85. Dulloo AG, Duret C, Rohrer D, et al. Efficacy of a

green tea extract rich in catechin polyphenols and caffeine in increasing 24-h energy expenditure and fat oxidation in humans. Am J Clin Nutr 1999; 70:1040–1045.

86. Norregaard J, Jorgensen S, Mikkelsen KL, et al. The effect of ephedrine plus caffeine on smoking cessation and postcessation weight gain. Clin Pharmacol Ther 1996; 60:679–686.

87. Svendsen TL, Ingerslev J, Mork A. Is Letigen contra-indicated in hypertension? A double-blind, placebo controlled multipractice study of Letigen administered to normotensive and adequately treated patients with hypersensitivity. Ugeskr Laeger 1998; 160:4073–4075.

88. Altschuler S, Conte A, Sebok M, Marlin RL, Winick C. Three controlled trials of weight loss with phenylpro-panolamine. Int J Obes 1982; 6:549–556.

89. Greenway FL. Clinical studies with phenylpropanol-amine: a metaanalysis. Am J Clin Nutr 1992; 55:203S–205S.

90. Jequier E. Energy utilization in human obesity. Ann NY Acad Sci 1987; 499:73–83.

91. Drew R. Nonprescription appetite suppressants. N C Med J 1983; 44:573–574.

92. Zgourides GD, Warren R, Englert ME. Ephedrine-induced thermogenesis as an adjunct to cognitive restructuring and covert conditioning: a proposal for treatment of obese individuals. Percept Mot Skills 1989; 69:563–572.

93. Egger G, Cameron-Smith D, Stanton R. The effective-ness of popular, non-prescription weight loss supple-ments [see comments]. Med J Aust 1999; 171:604–608.

94. Poston WS 2d, Foreyt JP, Borrell L, Haddock CK. Challenges in obesity management [see comments]. South Med J 1998; 91:710–720.

95. Doucet E, Tremblay A. Food intake, energy balance and body weight control. Eur J Clin Nutr 1997; 51:846–855.

96. Dulloo AG, Stock MJ. Ephedrine in the treatment of obesity [editorial]. Int J Obes Relat Metab Disord 1993; 17(suppl 1):S1–S2.

97. Ryan DH. Medicating the obese patient. Endocrinol Metab Clin North Am 1996; 25:989–1004.

98. Davis R, Faulds D. Dexfenfluramine. An updated review of its therapeutic use in the management of obesity. Drugs 1996; 52:696–724.

99. Finer N. Present and future pharmacological ap-proaches. Br Med Bull 1997; 53:409–432.

100. Carek PJ, Dickerson LM. Current concepts in the pharmacological management of obesity. Drugs 1999; 57:883–904.

101. Bray GA, Greenway FL. Current and potential drugs for treatment of obesity. Endocr Rev 1999; 20:805–875.

102. Bray GA. Drug treatment of obesity. Baillieres Best Pract Res Clin Endocrinol Metab 1999; 13:131–148.

103. Astrup A, Lundsgaard C. What do pharmacological approaches to obesity management offer? Linking pharmacological mechanisms of obesity management agents to clinical practice. Exp Clin Endocrinol Diabe-tes 1998; 106:29–34.

104. Astrup AV. Treatment of obesity with thermogenic agents [editorial]. Nutrition 1989; 5:70.

105. Dulloo AG, Miller DS. Ephedrine, caffeine and aspirin: "over-the-counter" drugs that interact to stimulate thermogenesis in the obese. Nutrition 1989; 5:7–9.

106. Dullo AG. Ephedrine, xanthines and prostaglandin-inhibitors: actions and interactions in the stimulation of thermogenesis. Int J Obes Relat Metab Disord 1993; 17(suppl 1):S35–S40.

107. Astrup A, Breum L, Toubro S. Pharmacological and clinical studies of ephedrine and other thermogenic agonists. Obes Res 1995; 3(suppl 4):537S–540S.

108. Astrup A, Breum L, Toubro S, Hein P, Quaade F. Ephedrine and weight loss. Int J Obes Relat Metab Disord 1992; 16:715.

109. Toubro S, Astrup A. Randomised comparison of diets for maintaining obese subjects' weight after major weight loss: ad lib, low fat, high carbohydrate diet v fixed energy intake. Bmj 1997; 314:29–34.

110. Sesso HD, Gaziano JM, Buring JE, Hennekens CH. Coffee and tea intake and the risk of myocardial infarction. Am J Epidemiol 1999; 149:162–167.

111. Borchardt RT, Huber JA. Catechol O-methyltransfer-ase. 5. Structure-activity relationships for inhibition by flavonoids. J Med Chem 1975; 18:120–122.

112. Dulloo AG, Seydoux J, Giradier L. Tealine and ther-mogenesis: interactions between polyphenols, caffeine and sympathetic activity. Int J Obes Relat Metab Disord 1996; 20(suppl 4):71.

113. Han LK, Takaku T, Li J, Kimura Y, Okuda H. Anti-obesity action of oolong tea. Int J Obes Relat Metab Disord 1999; 23:98–105.

114. Colker C, Kalman D, Torina G, Perlis T, Street C. Effects of citrus aurantium extract, caffeine and St. John's wort on body fat loss, lipid levels and mood state in overweight healthy adults. Curr Ther Res 1999; 60:145–153.

115. Henry CJ, Emery B. Effect of spiced food on metabolic rate. Hum Nutr Clin Nutr 1986; 40:165–168.

116. Yoshioka M, St-Pierre S, Suzuki M, Tremblay A. Effects of red pepper added to high-fat and high-carbohydrate meals on energy metabolism and sub-strate utilization in Japanese women. Br J Nutr 1998; 80:503–510.

117. Choi Y, Kim YC, Han YB, Park Y, Pariza MW, Ntambi JM. The *trans*-10,*cis*-12 isomer of conjugated linoleic acid downregulates stearoyl-CoA desaturase 1 gene expression in 3T3-L1 adipocytes. J Nutr 2000; 130:1920–1924.

118. Griinari JM, Corl BA, Lacy SH, Chouinard PY, Nur-mela KV, Bauman DE. Conjugated linoleic acid is synthesized endogenously in lactating dairy cows by delta(9)-desaturase. J Nutr 2000; 130:2285–2291.

119. Dhiman TR, Satter LD, Pariza MW, Galli MP, Albright K, Tolosa MX. Conjugated linoleic acid (CLA) content of milk from cows offered diets rich in linoleic and linolenic acid. J Dairy Sci 2000; 83:1016–1027.

120. Kritchevsky D. Antimutagenic and some other effects of conjugated linoleic acid. Br J Nutr 2000; 83:459–465.

121. MacDonald HB. Conjugated linoleic acid and disease prevention: a review of current knowledge. J Am Coll Nutr 2000; 19:111S–118S.

122. Pariza MW, Park Y, Cook ME. Conjugated linoleic acid and the control of cancer and obesity. Toxicol Sci 1999; 52:107–110.

123. Park Y, Storkson JM, Albright KJ, Liu W, Pariza MW. Evidence that the trans-10,cis-12 isomer of conjugated linoleic acid induces body composition changes in mice. Lipids 1999; 34:235–241.

124. Park Y, Albright KJ, Liu W, Storkson JM, Cook ME, Pariza MW. Effect of conjugated linoleic acid on body composition in mice. Lipids 1997; 32:853–858.

125. West DB, Delany JP, Camet PM, Blohm F, Truett AA, Scimeca J. Effects of conjugated linoleic acid on body fat and energy metabolism in the mouse. Am J Physiol 1998; 275:R667–R672.

126. DeLany JP, Blohm F, Truett AA, Scimeca JA, West DB. Conjugated linoleic acid rapidly reduces body fat content in mice without affecting energy intake. Am J Physiol 1999; 276:R1172–R1179.

127. Yamasaki M, Mansho K, Mishima H, et al. Dietary effect of conjugated linoleic acid on lipid levels in white adipose tissue of Sprague-Dawley rats. Biosci Biotechnol Biochem 1999; 63:1104–1106.

128. Tsuboyama-Kasaoka N, Takahashi M, Tanemura K, et al. Conjugated linoleic acid supplementation reduces adipose tissue by apoptosis and develops lipodystrophy in mice. Diabetes 2000; 49:1534–1542.

129. Satory DL, Smith SB. Conjugated linoleic acid inhibits proliferation but stimulates lipid filling of murine 3T3-L1 preadipocytes. J Nutr 1999; 129:92–97.

130. Azain MJ, Hausman DB, Sisk MB, Flatt WP, Jewell DE. Dietary conjugated linoleic acid reduces rat adipose tissue cell size rather than cell number. J Nutr 2000; 130:1548–1554.

131. Sullivan C, Triscari J. Metabolic regulation as a control for lipid disorders. I. Influence of (−)-hydroxycitrate on experimentally induced obesity in the rodent. Am J Clin Nutr 1977; 30:767–776.

132. Badmaev V, Majeed M. Open field, physician-controlled clinical evaluation of botanical weight loss formula citrin. Nutracon 1995: nutraceuticals, dietary supplements and functional foods. Las Vegas, July 11–13, 1995.

133. Kriketos AD, Thompson HR, Greene H, Hill JO. Hydroxycitric acid does not affect energy expenditure and substrate oxidation in adult males in a post-absorptive state. Int J Obes Relat Metab Disord 1999; 23:867–873.

134. Heymsfield SB, Allison DB, Vasselli JR, Pietrobelli A, Greenfield D, Nunez C. Garcinia cambogia (hydroxycitric acid) as a potential antiobesity agent: a randomized controlled trial. JAMA 1998; 280:1596–1600.

135. Clore JN. Dehydroepiandrosterone and body fat. Obes Res 1995; 3(suppl 4):613S–616S.

136. Abrahamsson L, Hackl H. Catabolic effects and the influence on hormonal variables under treatment with Gynodian-Depot or dehydroepiandrosterone (DHEA) oenanthate. Maturitas 1981; 3:225–234.

137. Nestler JE, Barlascini CO, Clore JN, Blackard WG. Dehydroepiandrosterone reduces serum low density lipoprotein levels and body fat but does not alter insulin sensitivity in normal men. J Clin Endocrinol Metab 1988; 66:57–61.

138. Mortola JF, Yen SS. The effects of oral dehydroepiandrosterone on endocrine-metabolic parameters in postmenopausal women. J Clin Endocrinol Metab 1990; 71:696–704.

139. Usiskin KS, Butterworth S, Clore JN, et al. Lack of effect of dehydroepiandrosterone in obese men. Int J Obes 1990; 14:457–463.

140. Welle S, Jozefowicz R, Statt M. Failure of dehydroepiandrosterone to influence energy and protein metabolism in humans. J Clin Endocrinol Metab 1990; 71:1259–1264.

141. Morales AJ, Nolan JJ, Nelson JC, Yen SS. Effects of replacement dose of dehydroepiandrosterone in men and women of advancing age. J Clin Endocrinol Metab 1994; 78:1360–1367.

142. Morales AJ, Haubrich RH, Hwang JY, Asakura H, Yen SS. The effect of six months treatment with a 100 mg daily dose of dehydroepiandrosterone (DHEA) on circulating sex steroids, body composition and muscle strength in age-advanced men and women. Clin Endocrinol (Oxf) 1998; 49:421–432.

143. Porter DJ, Raymond LW, Anastasio GD. Chromium: friend or foe? Arch Fam Med 1999; 8:386–390.

144. Page TG, Southern LL, Ward TL, Thompson DL Jr. Effect of chromium picolinate on growth and serum and carcass traits of growing-finishing pigs. J Anim Sci 1993; 71:656–662.

145. Mooney KW, Cromwell GL. Efficacy of chromium picolinate and chromium chloride as potential carcass modifiers in swine. J Anim Sci 1997; 75:2661–2671.

146. Mooney KW, Cromwell GL. Effects of dietary chromium picolinate supplementation on growth, carcass characteristics, and accretion rates of carcass tissues in growing-finishing swine. J Anim Sci 1995; 73:3351–3357.

147. Lindemann MD, Wood CM, Harper AF, Kornegay ET, Anderson RA. Dietary chromium picolinate additions improve gain: feed and carcass characteristics in growing-finishing pigs and increase litter size in reproducing sows. J Anim Sci 1995; 73:457–465.

148. Boleman SL, Boleman SJ, Bidner TD, et al. Effect of

chromium picolinate on growth, body composition, and tissue accretion in pigs. J Anim Sci 1995; 73:2033–2042.

149. Myers MJ, Farrell DE, Evock-Clover CM, Cope CV, Henderson M, Steele NC. Effect of recombinant growth hormone and chromium picolinate on cytokine production and growth performance in swine. Pathobiology 1995; 63:283–287.

150. Evock-Clover CM, Polansky MM, Anderson RA, Steele NC. Dietary chromium supplementation with or without somatotropin treatment alters serum hormones and metabolites in growing pigs without affecting growth performance. J Nutr 1993; 123:1504–1512.

151. Bunting LD, Fernandez JM, Thompson DL Jr, Southern LL. Influence of chromium picolinate on glucose usage and metabolic criteria in growing Holstein calves. J Anim Sci 1994; 72:1591–1599.

152. Hasten DL, Rome EP, Franks BD, Hegsted M. Effect of chromium picolinate on beginning weight training students. Int J Sport Nutr 1992; 2:343–350.

153. Grant KE, Chandler RM, Castle AL, Ivy JL. Chromium and exercise training: effect on obese women. Med Sci Sports Exerc 1997; 29:992–998.

154. Clancy SP, Clarkson PM, DeCheke ME, et al. Effects of chromium picolinate supplementation on body composition, strength, and urinary chromium loss in football players. Int J Sport Nutr 1994; 4:142–153.

155. Trent LK, Thieding-Cancel D. Effects of chromium picolinate on body composition. J Sports Med Phys Fitness 1995; 35:273–280.

156. Lukaski HC, Bolonchuk WW, Siders WA, Milne DB. Chromium supplementation and resistance training: effects on body composition, strength, and trace element status of men [see comments]. Am J Clin Nutr 1996; 63:954–965.

157. Bahadori B, Wallner S, Schneider H, Wascher TC, Toplak H. Effect of chromium yeast and chromium picolinate on body composition of obese, non-diabetic patients during and after a formula diet. Acta Med Austriaca 1997; 24:185–187.

158. Pasman WJ, Westerterp-Plantenga MS, Saris WH. The effectiveness of long-term supplementation of carbohydrate, chromium, fibre and caffeine on weight maintenance. Int J Obes Relat Metab Disord 1997; 21:1143–1151.

159. Walker LS, Bemben MG, Bemben DA, Knehans AW. Chromium picolinate effects on body composition and muscular performance in wrestlers. Med Sci Sports Exerc 1998; 30:1730–1737.

160. Campbell WW, Joseph LJ, Davey SL, Cyr-Campbell D, Anderson RA, Evans WJ. Effects of resistance training and chromium picolinate on body composition and skeletal muscle in older men. J Appl Physiol 1999; 86:29–39.

161. Press RI, Geller J, Evans GW. The effect of chromium picolinate on serum cholesterol and apolipoprotein fractions in human subjects [see comments]. West J Med 1990; 152:41–45.

162. Lee NA, Reasner CA. Beneficial effect of chromium supplementation on serum triglyceride levels in NIDDM. Diabetes Care 1994; 17:1449–1452.

163. Preuss HG, Grojec PL, Lieberman S, Anderson RA. Effects of different chromium compounds on blood pressure and lipid peroxidation in spontaneously hypertensive rats. Clin Nephrol 1997; 47:325–330.

164. Anderson RA. Nutritional factors influencing the glucose/insulin system: chromium. J Am Coll Nutr 1997; 16:404–410.

165. Anderson RA, Cheng N, Bryden NA, Polansky MM, Chi J, Feng J. Elevated intakes of supplemental chromium improve glucose and insulin variables in individuals with type 2 diabetes. Diabetes 1997; 46:1786–1791.

166. Evans GW, Bowman TD. Chromium picolinate increases membrane fluidity and rate of insulin internalization. J Inorg Biochem 1992; 46:243–250.

167. Stearns DM, Wise JP Sr, Patierno SR, Wetterhahn KE. Chromium (III) picolinate produces chromosome damage in Chinese hamster ovary cells. FASEB J 1995; 9:1643–1648.

168. Stearns DM, Belbruno JJ, Wetterhahn KE. A prediction of chromium (III) accumulation in humans from chromium dietary supplements. FASEB J 1995; 9:1650–1657.

169. Anderson RA, Bryden NA, Polansky MM. Lack of toxicity of chromium chloride and chromium picolinate in rats. J Am Coll Nutr 1997; 16:273–279.

170. Vincent JB. The biochemistry of chromium. J Nutr 2000; 130:715–718.

171. Nissen S, Sharp R, Ray M, et al. Effect of leucine metabolite beta-hydroxy-beta-methylbutyrate on muscle metabolism during resistance-exercise training. J Appl Physiol 1996; 81:2095–2104.

172. Kreider RB, Ferreira M, Wilson M, Almada AL. Effects of calcium beta-hydroxy-beta-methylbutyrate (HMB) supplementation during resistance-training on markers of catabolism, body composition and strength. Int J Sports Med 1999; 20:503–509.

173. Nissen S, Sharp RL, Panton L, Vukovich M, Trappe S, Fuller JC. Beta-hydroxy-beta-methylbutyrate (HMB) supplementation in humans is safe and may decrease cardiovascular risk factors. J Nutr 2000; 130:1937–1945.

174. Ronsard N. Cellulite: Those Lumps, Bumps, and Bulges You Couldn't Lose Before. New York: Beauty and Health Publishing Co., 1973.

175. Arner P. Adrenergic receptor function in fat cells. Am J Clin Nutr 1992; 55:228S–236S.

176. Arner P, Hellstrom L, Wahrenberg H, Bronnegard M. Beta-adrenoceptor expression in human fat cells from different regions. J Clin Invest 1990; 86:1595–1600.

177. Lafontan M, Berlan M. Fat cell adrenergic receptors and the control of white and brown fat cell function. J Lipid Res 1993; 34:1057–1091.

178. Presta E, Leibel RL, Hirsch J. Regional changes in adrenergic receptor status during hypocaloric intake do not predict changes in adipocyte size or body shape. Metabolism 1990; 39:307–315.

179. Vernon RG. Effects of diet on lipolysis and its regulation. Proc Nutr Soc 1992; 51:397–408.

180. Greenway FL, Bray GA. Regional fat loss from the thigh in obese women after adrenergic modulation. Clin Ther 1987; 9:663–669.

181. Greenway FL, Bray GA, Heber D. Topical fat reduction. Obes Res 1995; 3(suppl 4):561S–568S.

182. Collis N, Elliot LA, Sharpe C, Sharpe DT. Cellulite treatment: a myth or reality: a prospective randomized, controlled trial of two therapies, endermologie and aminophylline cream. Plast Reconstr Surg 1999; 104:1110–1114; discussion 1115–1117.

183. Lis-Balchin M. Parallel placebo-controlled clinical study of a mixture of herbs sold as a remedy for cellulite. Phytother Res 1999; 13:627–629.

184. Mellinkoff S. Digestive system. Ann Rev Physiol 1957; 19:175–204.

185. Fernstrom JD. Role of precursor availability in control of monoamine biosynthesis in brain. Physiol Rev 1983; 63:484–546.

186. Wurtman J, Wurtman R, Growdon JPH, Lipscomb M, Zeisel S. Carbohydrate-craving in obese people: suppression by treatments affecting serotoninergic neurotransmission. Int J Eat Disord 1981; 1:2–15.

187. Blundell JE, Leshem MB. The effect of 5-hydroxytryptophan on food intake and on the anorexic action of amphetamine and fenfluramine. J Pharm Pharmacol 1975; 27:31–37.

188. Birdsall TC. 5-Hydroxytryptophan: a clinically-effective serotonin precursor. Altern Med Rev 1998; 3:271–280.

189. Weekley LB, Maher RW, Kimbrough TD. Alterations of tryptophan metabolism in a rat strain (Osborne-Mendel) predisposed to obesity. Comp Biochem Physiol A 1982; 72:747–752.

190. Ceci F, Cangiano C, Cairella M, et al. The effects of oral 5-hydroxytryptophan administration on feeding behavior in obese adult female subjects. J Neural Transm 1989; 76:109–117.

191. Cangiano C, Ceci F, Cascino A, et al. Eating behavior and adherence to dietary prescriptions in obese adult subjects treated with 5-hydroxytryptophan. Am J Clin Nutr 1992; 56:863–867.

192. Growdon JH, Melamed E, Logue M, Hefti F, Wurtman RJ. Effects of oral L-tyrosine administration on CSF tyrosine and homovanillic acid levels in patients with Parkinson's disease. Life Sci 1982; 30:827–832.

193. Avraham Y, Bonne O, Berry EM. Behavioral and neurochemical alterations caused by diet restriction—the effect of tyrosine administration in mice. Brain Res 1996; 732:133–144.

194. Hull KM, Maher TJ. L-tyrosine potentiates the anorexia induced by mixed-acting sympathomimetic drugs in hyperphagic rats. J Pharmacol Exp Ther 1990; 255:403–409.

195. Hull KM, Maher TJ. L-tyrosine fails to potentiate several peripheral actions of the sympathomimetics. Pharmacol Biochem Behav 1991; 39:755–759.

196. Hull KM, Maher TJ. Effects of L-tyrosine on mixed-acting sympathomimetic-induced pressor actions. Pharmacol Biochem Behav 1992; 43:1047–1052.

197. Van Itallie TB. Dietary fiber and obesity. Am J Clin Nutr 1978; 31:S43–S52.

198. Krotkiewski M. Effect of guar gum on body-weight, hunger ratings and metabolism in obese subjects. Br J Nutr 1984; 52:97–105.

199. Walsh DE, Yaghoubian V, Behforooz A. Effect of glucomannan on obese patients: a clinical study. Int J Obes 1984; 8:289–293.

200. Cairella M, Marchini G. Evaluation of the action of glucomannan on metabolic parameters and on the sensation of satiation in overweight and obese patients. Clin Ter 1995; 146:269–274.

201. Hylander B, Rossner S. Effects of dietary fiber intake before meals on weight loss and hunger in a weight-reducing club. Acta Med Scand 1983; 213:217–220.

202. Porikos K, Hagamen S. Is fiber satiating? Effects of a high fiber preload on subsequent food intake of normal-weight and obese young men. Appetite 1986; 7:153–162.

203. Witkowska A, Borawska MH. The role of dietary fiber and its preparations in the protection and treatment of overweight. Pol Merkuriusz Lek 1999; 6:224–226.

204. Pasman WJ, Saris WH, Wauters MA, Westerterp-Plantenga MS. Effect of one week of fibre supplementation on hunger and satiety ratings and energy intake. Appetite 1997; 29:77–87.

205. Baron JA, Schori A, Crow B, Carter R, Mann JI. A randomized controlled trial of low carbohydrate and low fat/high fiber diets for weight loss. Am J Public Health 1986; 76:1293–1296.

206. Rigaud D, Ryttig KR, Angel LA, Apfelbaum M. Overweight treated with energy restriction and a dietary fibre supplement: a 6-month randomized, double-blind, placebo-controlled trial. Int J Obes 1990; 14:763–769.

207. Solum TT, Ryttig KR, Solum E, Larsen S. The influence of a high-fibre diet on body weight, serum lipids and blood pressure in slightly overweight persons. A randomized, double-blind, placebo-controlled investigation with diet and fibre tablets (DumoVital). Int J Obes 1987; 11:67–71.

208. Rossner S, von Zweigbergk D, Ohlin A, Ryttig K. Weight reduction with dietary fibre supplements. Results of two double-blind randomized studies. Acta Med Scand 1987; 222:83–88.

209. Gropper SS, Acosta PB. The therapeutic effect of fiber in treating obesity. J Am Coll Nutr 1987; 6: 533–535.

210. Ryttig KR, Tellnes G, Haegh L, Boe E, Fagerthun H. A dietary fibre supplement and weight maintenance after weight reduction: a randomized, double-blind, placebo-controlled long-term trial. Int J Obes 1989; 13:165–171.

211. Quaade F, Vrist E, Astrup A. Dietary fiber added to a very-low caloric diet reduces hunger and alleviates constipation. Ugeskr Laeger 1990; 152:95–98.

212. Pasman WJ, Westerterp-Plantenga MS, Muls E, Vansant G, Van Ree J, Saris WH. The effectiveness of long-term fibre supplementation on weight maintenance in weight-reduced women. Int J Obes Relat Metab Disord 1997; 21:548–555.

213. Miller WC, Niederpruem MG, Wallace JP, Lindeman AK. Dietary fat, sugar, and fiber predict body fat content. J Am Diet Assoc 1994; 94:612–615.

214. Alfieri MA, Pomerleau J, Grace DM, Anderson L. Fiber intake of normal weight, moderately obese and severely obese subjects. Obes Res 1995; 3:541–547.

215. Han LK, Kimura Y, Okuda H. Reduction in fat storage during chitin-chitosan treatment in mice fed a high-fat diet. Int J Obes Relat Metab Disord 1999; 23:174–179.

216. Wuolijoki E, Hirvela T, Ylitalo P. Decrease in serum LDL cholesterol with microcrystalline chitosan. Methods Find Exp Clin Pharmacol 1999; 21:357–361.

217. Pittler MH, Abbot NC, Harkness EF, Ernst E. Randomized, double-blind trial of chitosan for body weight reduction. Eur J Clin Nutr 1999; 53:379–381.

218. Rodgers S, Burnet R, Goss A, et al. Jaw wiring in treatment of obesity. Lancet 1977; 1:1221–1222.

219. Kark AE, Burke M. Gastric reduction for morbid obesity: technique and indications. Br J Surg 1979; 66:756–761.

220. Castelnuovo-Tedesco P, Buchanan DC, Hall HD. Jaw-wiring for obesity. Gen Hosp Psychiatry 1980; 2:156–159.

221. Ross MW, Kalucy RS, Morton JE. Locus of control in obesity: predictors of success in a jaw-wiring programme. Br J Med Psychol 1983; 56:49–56.

222. Ross MW, Goss AN, Kalucy RS. The relationship of panic-fear to anxiety and tension in jaw wiring for obesity. Br J Med Psychol 1984; 57:67–69.

223. Garrow JS, Gardiner GT. Maintenance of weight loss in obese patients after jaw wiring. BMJ (Clin Res Ed) 1981; 282:858–860.

224. Garrow JS, Webster JD, Pearson M, Pacy PJ, Harpin G. Inpatient-outpatient randomized comparison of Cambridge diet versus milk diet in 17 obese women over 24 weeks. Int J Obes 1989; 13:521–529.

225. Pacy PJ, Webster JD, Pearson M, Garrow JS. A cross-sectional cost/benefit audit in a hospital obesity clinic. Hum Nutr Appl Nutr 1987; 41:38–46.

226. Ramsey-Stewart G, Martin L. Jaw wiring in the treatment of morbid obesity. Aust N Z J Surg 1985; 55:163–167.

227. Mathus-Vliegen EM, Tytgat GN. Intragastric balloons for morbid obesity: results, patient tolerance and balloon life span. Br J Surg 1990; 77:76–79.

228. Marshall JB, Schreiber H, Kolozsi W, et al. A prospective, multi-center clinical trial of the Taylor intragastric balloon for the treatment of morbid obesity. Am J Gastroenterol 1990; 85:833–837.

229. Sniegocki G. Comparison of the treatment of obesity by surgical methods and gastric balloon. Wiad Lek 1990; 43:268–274.

230. De Waele B, Reynaert H, Urbain D, Willems G. Intragastric balloons for preoperative weight reduction. Obes Surg 2000; 10:58–60.

231. Vandenplas Y, Bollen P, De Langhe K, Vandemaele K, De Schepper J. Intragastric balloons in adolescents with morbid obesity. Eur J Gastroenterol Hepatol 1999; 11:243–245.

232. Perez-Cuadrado Martinez E, Silva Gonzalez C, Vazquez Dourado R, et al. Complications of the intragastric balloon prosthesis. Rev Esp Enferm Dig 1993; 84:291–295.

233. Butterwegge M, Gethmann U, Ohlenroth G. Ileus in pregnancy induced by a gastric balloon. Zentralbl Gynakol 1993; 115:238–240.

234. Mirich DR, Gray RR, Haber GB. Percutaneous deflation of a gastric balloon: technical note. Cardiovasc Intervent Radiol 1989; 12:164–165.

235. Hogan RB, Johnston JH, Long BW, et al. A double-blind, randomized, sham-controlled trial of the gastric bubble for obesity. Gastrointest Endosc 1989; 35:381–385.

236. Geliebter A, Melton PM, Gage D, McCray RS, Hashim SA. Gastric balloon to treat obesity: a double-blind study in nondieting subjects. Am J Clin Nutr 1990; 51:584–588.

237. Mathus-Vliegen EM, Tytgat GN, Veldhuyzen-Offermans EA. Intragastric balloon in the treatment of super-morbid obesity. Double-blind, sham-controlled, crossover evaluation of 500-milliliter balloon. Gastroenterology 1990; 99:362–369.

238. Geliebter A, Melton PM, McCray RS, et al. Clinical trial of silicone-rubber gastric balloon to treat obesity. Int J Obes 1991; 15:259–266.

239. Krakamp B, Leidig P, Gehmlich D, Paul A. Stomach volume reduction balloon for weight loss: what is the justification for this controversial method? Zentralbl Chir 1997; 122:349–356.

240. Kirby DF, Wade JB, Mills PR, et al. A prospective assessment of the Garren-Edwards gastric bubble and bariatric surgery in the treatment of morbid obesity. Am Surg 1990; 56:575–580.

241. Pasquali R, Besteghi L, Casimirri F, et al. Mechanisms of action of the intragastric balloon in obesity: effects on hunger and satiety. Appetite 1990; 15:3–11.

242. Durrans D, Taylor TV, Holt S. Intragastric device for weight loss. Effect on energy intake in dogs. Dig Dis Sci 1991; 36:893–896.

243. Northway MG, Geisinger KR, Gilliam JH, MacLean DB. Weight loss induced by gastric implant in rats. Effects of capsaicin sensory denervation. Dig Dis Sci 1992; 37:1051–1056.

244. Melton PM, Kissileff HR, Pi-Sunyer FX. Cholecystokinin (CCK-8) affects gastric pressure and ratings of hunger and fullness in women. Am J Physiol 1992; 263:R452–R456.

245. Boosalis MG, Gemayel N, Lee A, Bray GA, Laine L, Cohen H. Cholecystokinin and satiety: effect of hypothalamic obesity and gastric bubble insertion. Am J Physiol 1992; 262:R241–R244.

246. Rigaud D, Trostler N, Rozen R, Vallot T, Apfelbaum M. Gastric distension, hunger and energy intake after balloon implantation in severe obesity. Int J Obes Relat Metab Disord 1995; 19:489–495.

247. Tosetti C, Corinaldesi R, Stanghellini V, et al. Gastric emptying of solids in morbid obesity. Int J Obes Relat Metab Disord 1996; 20:200–205.

248. Geliebter A, Schachter S, Lohmann-Walter C, Feldman H, Hashim SA. Reduced stomach capacity in obese subjects after dieting. Am J Clin Nutr 1996; 63:170–173.

249. Cigaina V, Pinato G, Rigo V, et al. Gastric peristalsis control by mono situ electrical stimulation: a preliminary study. Obes Surg 1996; 6:247–249.

250. Cigaina V, Saggioro A, Rigo V, Pinato G, Ischai S. Long-term effects of gastric pacing to reduce feed intake in swine. Obes Surg 1996; 6:250–253.

251. Cigaina V. The long-term effects of gastric pacing on an obese young woman. Obes Surg 1996; 6:312–313.

252. Cigaina V. Gastric myo-electrical pacing as therapy for morbid obesity: preliminary results. Obes Surg 1999; 9:333–334.

253. Simpson GK, Farquhar DL, Carr P, et al. Intermittent protein-sparing fasting with abdominal belting. Int J Obes 1986; 10:247–254.

254. Garrow JS. Morbid obesity: medical or surgical treatment? The case for medical treatment. Int J Obes 1987; 11:1–4.

255. Garrow JS. Treatment of morbid obesity by nonsurgical means: diet, drugs, behavior modification, exercise. Gastroenterol Clin North Am 1987; 16:443–449.

256. Garrow JS. Is it possible to prevent obesity? Infusionstherapie 1990; 17:28–31.

257. Garrow JS. The management of obesity. Another view. Int J Obes Relat Metab Disord 1992; 16(suppl 2):S59–S63.

258. Kirsch I, Montgomery G, Sapirstein G. Hypnosis as an adjunct to cognitive-behavioral psychotherapy: a meta-analysis. J Consult Clin Psychol 1995; 63:214–220.

259. Kirsch I. Hypnotic enhancement of cognitive-behavioral weight loss treatments—another meta-reanalysis. J Consult Clin Psychol 1996; 64:517–519.

260. Allison DB, Faith MS. Hypnosis as an adjunct to cognitive-behavioral psychotherapy for obesity: a meta-analytic reappraisal. J Consult Clin Psychol 1996; 64:513–516.

261. Johnson DL, Karkut RT. Participation in multicomponent hypnosis treatment programs for women's weight loss with and without overt aversion. Psychol Rep 1996; 79:659–668.

262. Johnson DL. Weight loss for women: studies of smokers and nonsmokers using hypnosis and multicomponent treatments with and without overt aversion. Psychol Rep 1997; 80:931–933.

263. Stradling J, Roberts D, Wilson A, Lovelock F. Controlled trial of hypnotherapy for weight loss in patients with obstructive sleep apnoea. Int J Obes Relat Metab Disord 1998; 22:278–281.

264. Haber CH, Nitkin R, Shenker IR. Adverse reactions to hypnotherapy in obese adolescents: a developmental viewpoint. Psychiatr Q 1979; 51:55–63.

265. Schoenberger NE. Research on hypnosis as an adjunct to cognitive-behavioral psychotherapy. Int J Clin Exp Hypn 2000; 48:154–169.

266. Cole AD, Bond NW. Olfactory aversion conditioning and overeating: a review and some data. Percept Mot Skills 1983; 57:667–678.

267. Mok MS, Parker LN, Voina S, Bray GA. Treatment of obesity by acupuncture. Am J Clin Nutr 1976; 29:832–835.

268. Richards D, Marley J. Stimulation of auricular acupuncture points in weight loss. Aust Fam Physician 1998; 27(suppl 2):S73–S77.

269. Allison DB, Kreibich K, Heshka S, Heymsfield SB. A randomised placebo-controlled clinical trial of an acupressure device for weight loss. Int J Obes Relat Metab Disord 1995; 19:653–658.

18

Surgical Treatment of Obesity: An Overview and Results from the SOS Study

Lars Sjöström

Sahlgrenska University and Sahlgrenska University Hospital, Göteborg, Sweden

I INTRODUCTION

Previous chapters and many separate publications (1–4) have shown that conventional as well as pharmacological treatment of obesity is associated with poor long-term results. Recent publications from the intervention study Swedish Obese Subjects (SOS) have shown that conventional treatment results are particularly poor in settings not specialized in the treatment of overweight and obesity (5–8). Drug treatment of obesity results in 8–10% weight loss under conditions when placebo gives 4–6% weight loss (9). Although this is encouraging, much more efficient drugs are needed in the future. All these circumstances have constituted incentives for surgeons to develop techniques resulting in malabsorptive or restrictive effects on food intake. Several techniques achieve weight loss through both of these mechanisms and most likely also by changing the gastrointestinal signaling systems by which energy expenditure and/or appetite regulation may be modulated.

Literally dozens of surgical antiobesity techniques have been described. This chapter will focus more on results than surgical methodology. For technical procedures and unusual methods the reader is referred to textbooks of obesity surgery (10). Obviously inefficient techniques, such as the gastric bubble (11), will not be reviewed. The outcome of the eight techniques having been most commonly used over the last 30 years will be examined, and studies comparing conventional and

surgical treatment will be reviewed. The overall aim of the chapter is to illustrate that bariatric surgery is safe and so far more long-term efficient than any other technique available for the treatment of obesity. Some parts of this chapter overlap with sections written for other books or journals (7,8).

II INDICATIONS FOR SURGICAL TREATMENT OF OBESITY

Obesity is associated with increased morbidity (12) and mortality (13) and with a poor health related quality of life (14,15). Since conventional treatment results are poor (1–4), surgical procedures may be indicated in many cases. At the 1991 consensus conference, NIH recommended that obesity surgery should be restricted to individuals with BMI $\geq 40 \, \text{kg/m}^2$ with a lower cut off for subjects with pronounced metabolic complications (16). At that time, the SOS project had already used the BMI cutoff $38 \, \text{kg/m}^2$ for women and $34 \, \text{kg/m}^2$ for men for 4 years. Today it is obvious that a cut off of $40 \, \text{kg/m}^2$ leaves a large fraction of the obese population virtually without efficient treatment and often in very bad shape in spite of the fact that new antiobesity drugs have been added to the therapeutic arsenal.

In a preliminary report, Näslund (17) has analyzed effects and complications in surgically treated SOS patients with BMI < 40 and BMI $\geq 40 \, \text{kg/m}^2$. In absolute terms, weight loss was larger in the heavier, while this was not the case in relative terms. The frequency of complications was similar in the two groups, and, from a risk factor point of view, the two groups benefited similarly from the surgical treatment.

The surgical mortality rate has rapidly decreased since the late 1970s, when it ranged from 2% to 5%. In the SOS study, which included patients between August 1987 and January 2001, the postoperative mortality has been 0.25% (five cases in 2010 operated) (7). Most of these patients have been operated with open surgery. With the advent of laparoscopic techniques, the complication rate and operative mortality are expected to be further decreased. This favorable development makes it warranted to lower the recommended BMI cutoff for surgical treatment, particularly since surgery is the only documented long-term efficient treatment available. Unfortunately, the guidelines for surgical obesity treatment have not been updated. This author would like to suggest a BMI of 34 kg/m^2 as a lower cutoff for surgical treatment of obesity. If concomitant risk factors are present even lower cutoffs may be considered.

It has often been suggested that documented failure to respond to conventional treatment should be a requirement for surgical treatment. This may be correct in principle but meaningless in practice because virtually all patients being considered for surgical treatment have a history of repeated conventional treatment failures. In the SOS study, males (n = 975) and females (n = 1330) had made on average 7.6 and 18.2 serious attempts to reduce weight, respectively, when included in the study (18). The best attempt had resulted in mean weight loss of 17.7 kg in men and 20.3 kg in women. However, the best weight losses were maintained for only 7 and 10 months, respectively (18). Therefore, the treating physician must consider, on a case-by-case basis, if it is in the interest of the patient or an expression of prejudice against the obese to require one more treatment failure.

Treating severely obese children with conventional methods is at least as difficult as treating adult obesity. The experience of bariatric obesity in children is very limited. In one study, 22 superobese children, aged 8–18 years, were operated with vertical banded gastroplasty, gastric bypass, or biliopancreatic diversion (19). No acute complication occurred, and effects on BMI and sleep apnea were excellent. In obese children with the Prader-Willi syndrome, biliopancreatic diversion has resulted in conflicting results (20,21). More explorative studies are needed until guidelines for bariatric surgery in children can be established.

Numerous attempts have been made to select patients for weight loss programs based on anthropometric, biochemical, or psychological variables. The larger the body weight at baseline, the larger the absolute weight loss after conventional treatment—but the faster also the relapse (22). In other respects, no unequivocal predictors of weight loss or maintenance are available, at least not with respect to surgical treatment (for review see 23). Therefore, the current recommendation must be to select patients based on general exclusion criteria for surgery and to remain skeptical about selection criteria of unproven value. In research settings, it may rather be warranted to collect as many baseline variables as possible on patients in the effort to try to understand how future patients should be optimally selected in an ethically correct way. After all, the aim of obesity surgery is not to be able to publish extraordinary results from low risk individuals but to help as many obese patients as possible while keeping complications at acceptable levels.

III METHODS

The intestinal operations are illustrated in Figure 1, gastric operations in Figure 2, and the combined gastric and intestinal operations in Figure 3.

A Intestinal Operations

The *jejunocolic shunt* (Fig. 1A) was first described by Payne in 1963 (24). The jejunum was divided 37–75 cm from the ligament of Trietz. The proximal segment was connected end-to-side to transverse colon while the distal segment of the divided jejunum was closed. The

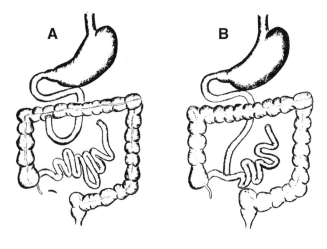

Figure 1 Intestinal operations for weight control. (A) Jejunocolic shunt. (B) Jejunoileal bypass (JIB). Copyright Sofia Karlsson and Lars Sjöström.

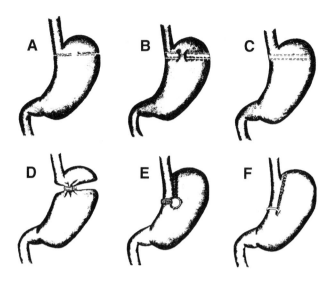

Figure 2 Gastric operations for weight control. (A) Horizontal gastroplasty. (B) Horizontal gastroplasty with gastrogastrostomy. (C) Gomez horizontal gastroplasty. (D) Gastric banding. (E) Vertical banded gastroplasty (VBG). (F) Silastic ring VBG. Copyright Sofia Karlsson and Lars Sjöström.

operation resulted in large weight reductions and dramatic improvement of blood lipids. However, the technique was soon abandoned owing to severe diarrhea and hepatic failure.

Thirteen years later Payne's group (25) described the end-to-side jejunoileal bypass (JIB) (Fig. 1B). The jejunum was divided 35–37.5 cm from the ligament of Trietz. The proximal end was anastomosed to ileum 10–12 cm from the ileocecal valve. The distal part of the divided jejunum was closed. Several variants of JIB have been described (26–28).

B   Gastric Operations

Horizontal gastroplasties were introduced by Pace et al. in 1979 (29). After having removed three central staples, a double staple row was applied horizontally across the upper part of the stomach resulting in a ≤50-mL pouch with a 9-mm central opening (Fig. 2A). The stoma between the pouch and remaining stomach was rapidly dilated, and thus the long-term results were poor. Attempts were undertaken to circumvent this problem by means of an intact staple row plus a gastrogastrostomy (30,31) (Fig. 3B) or by placing a reinforced stoma at the major curvature (Gomez horizontal gastroplasty) (32) (Fig. 3C).

A *gastric banding (GB)* operation was first undertaken by Wilkinson in 1976 (33), but the technique was not published until 8 years later (34,35). A band (usually silicon) is strapped around the upper part of the stomach, resulting in a small pouch (20–25 mL) (Fig. 2D). This was the original gastric banding.

A *variable gastric banding* is achieved by placing a balloon on the gastric side of the band. The balloon is connected with a subcutaneous reservoir or port sup-

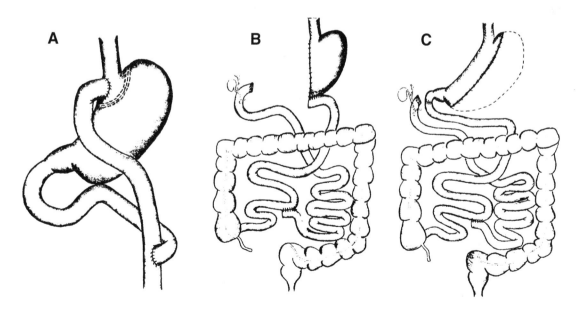

Figure 3 Combined intestinal and gastric operations for weight control. (A) Roux-en-Y gastric bypass (GBP). (B) Biliopancreatic diversion (BPD). (C) Biliopancreatic diversion with duodenal switch (BPD/DS). Copyright Sofia Karlsson and Lars Sjöström.

plied with a self-healing membrane. By percutaneous puncture of the reservoir, fluid can be added or removed from the system, thereby changing the size of the stoma. At least two different techniques have been developed— the American "adjustable silicone gastric banding" (ASGB) (36), and the European "Swedish adjustable gastric banding" (SAGB) (37).

Variable banding with the *band positioned at the gastroesophageal junction* (cardia) has been reported (38). Weight loss seems to be as good as after ordinary banding, and the operation is simpler to perform. Gastric erosions have been observed in 1–2% of patients operated with banding at cardia (39,40). Randomized comparisons between ordinary banding and high banding have not been performed.

The *vertical banded gastroplasty (VBG)* was introduced by Mason in 1980 and published 2 years later (41,42). After pressing the anterior and posterior wall of the stomach together, a hole is punched through both walls by means of a so-called EEA stapler (end-to-end anastomosis) and at the same time the walls are stapled together (Fig. 2E). Thus, a channel through the stomach, with no contact with its interior, is created. The front and back walls are then stapled together with four rows of staples from the punched channel to the angle of His. Finally, a polypropylene strip (1.5 cm wide) is brought through the punched hole and around the lesser curvature and sutured to itself so that its circumference is 5.0 cm (Fig. 2E). A circumference of 4.5 cm creates more vomiting and an increased frequency of staple row insufficiency while 5.5 cm has a lower weight-reducing effect than 5 cm (42).

A variant on Mason's VBG operation is the *silastic ring VBG* (43,44). With this technique no hole is punched, but a thin silicon tubing is threaded onto a suture circumscribing the outlet of the vertical pouch. Only the suture (not the tubing) is penetrating the ventricle between the staple rows (Fig. 2F).

C   Combined Gastric and Intestinal Operations

The *gastric bypass technique (GBP)* was developed by Mason in the 1960s (45,46) and has subsequently been refined through several steps (47–52) so that the GBP of today is usually characterized by a pouch along the lesser curvature and a so called Roux-en-Y arrangement of the jejunum (Fig. 3A) (51). Thus, the jejunum is divided 45 cm from the ligament of Trietz, and the distal segment is brought up retrocolically and antegastrically for the lesser curvature gastrojejunal anastomosis to the pouch. Finally, the proximal segment of the divided jejunum is used for an end to side jejunojejunostomy 35–60 cm from the pouch (Fig. 3A).

The *biliopancreatic diversion (BPD)* was constructed by Scopinaro to overcome the serious side effects of JIB related to bacterial overgrowth in its blind loop (53,54). Seventy-five percent of the distal stomach is removed, and the remaining proximal stomach as well as the duodenal stump is closed (Fig. 3B). The ileum is divided 250 cm from the ileocecal valve, and the distal segment (alimentary limb) is anastomosed to the remaining stomach. The proximal segment of the divided ileum (the biliopancreatic limb) is anastomosed to the side of the terminal ileum 50 cm from the ileocecal valve. Thus, the digestion of food by means of juices from the upper intestinal tract can occur only in the most distal 50 cm of ileum.

The *distal gastric bypass Roux-en-Y (DGBP), or long-limb gastric bypass*, is a mixture of GBP and BPD (55). It can be described as a GBP with a distal enteroentero anastomosis or as a BPD without gastrectomy.

GBP, BPD, and DGBP are associated with risk for marginal ulcerations in the gastroenteric anastomosis (56). To avoid this problem and to preserve a normal pyloric function the *biliopancreatic diversion with duodenal switch (BPD/DS)*, also called *distal gastric bypass with duodenal switch*, was introduced by Hess in 1988 (57–59) (Fig. 3C). The duodenum is first exposed and divided 4 cm distal to pylorus. The distal segment of the duodenum (with papilla Vateri) is closed. Then a retro-colic end-to-end anastomosis is performed between the proximal duodenum and the alimentary enteric limb obtained in the same way as in the BPD operations. The stomach is sectioned vertically to yield a pouch (140 ± 40 cc) along the lesser curvature from cardia to pylorus. Finally the biliopancreatic limb is anastomosed to the ileum ~100 cm from the ileocecal valve.

D   Laparoscopic Procedures

Banding operations by means of laparoscopic techniques were first undertaken in 1993 by Fried and Peskova (60) and by Balachew et al. (61). Later, several reports on laparoscopic procedures for nonadjustable (62) and adjustable (63–66) banding have appeared. Interestingly, the necessary abdominal insufflation during laparoscopy disturbs the hemodynamic (67) and respiratory (68) functions less in obese than in lean individuals. This may indicate that the insufflation adds only marginally to a preexisting adaptation to an increased abdominal pressure due to intraabdominal fat (69).

Hans Lönroth was the pioneer in the development of laparoscopic techniques for *VBG* [first operation October 1993 (70)] and *gastric bypass* (71). Studies based on 1040 (72) and 275 (73) laparoscopically performed GBP operations were later published by other investigators.

Recently a laparoscopical procedure for *BPD/DS* (74) and a hand-assisted laparoscopic technique via a Hand-Port introduced through an 8-cm right subcostal incision (75) have also been described.

IV RESULTS OF BARIATRIC TECHNIQUES

This section is mainly based on publications comparing different bariatric techniques, but, when comparisons are lacking, results of individual techniques will also be described. Table 1 shows available comparisons and illustrates the development of bariatric surgery over the last 30 years.

A Jejunocolic Shunt Versus Other Techniques

No comparisons between the jejunocolic shunt and other techniques are available. Even if blood lipids improved markedly, side effects in the form of electrolyte disturbances and hepatic failure were so serious that the technique was abandoned after a few years (24,76,77).

B Jejunoileal Bypass (JIB) Versus Other Techniques

1 JIB Versus Gastric Bypass (GBP)

Two randomized (48,78) and two prospective nonrandomized (47,79) comparisons were published between 1977 and 1981 (Table 1). In the study of Griffen (48), 32 patients were randomized to GBP and 27 patients to JIB. On average, body weight was 152 kg and age 33 years. The 1-year follow up was 68%. Weight loss was similar in GBP (51 kg) and JIB (58 kg) patients (NS). Although early side effects were more common in GBP-treated patients, late complications were much more common in JIB patients. At operation all patients within both groups had some degree of liver steatosis. Some patients accepted a liver biopsy after 1 year. Among 12 GBP patients two were unchanged while 10 were improved with respect to steatosis. In contrast 12 of 15 JIB patients had deteriorated in their steatosis while the remaining three were unchanged. One JIB patient died in liver coma, and in another the shunt had to be taken down owing to threatening liver insufficiency.

The study of Buckwalter (78) was planned as a 2-year randomized study, but at the time of the publication only 12 patients had been followed for 1 year. Weight loss was 31.5 kg in the JIB group and 43.0 kg in the GBP group.

Although difficult to evaluate for several reasons, the two nonrandomized studies (47,79) with a total of 506 starting patients followed for up to 3 years are consistent with the Griffen (48) study: similar weight reductions with GBP and JIB but more complications with JIB. Both techniques result in reduced serum levels of triglycerides and cholesterol, the latter being more reduced by JIB (79).

2 JIB Versus Gomez Horizontal Gastroplasty (GHGP)

Only one nonrandomized comparison is available (80) (Table 1). JIB resulted in a larger weight loss than GHGP (33% vs. 16% after 2 years) but also in more complications. However, this study adds a temporal aspect to Griffen's (48) data on liver steatosis. A nonspecified number of JIB patients demonstrated deterioration in liver steatosis after 9 months, improvement after 18 months, and normalization after 30 months (80). It is not clear to this author to what extent the same patients were examined on the three occasions.

3 Prospective Noncomparative Studies on JIB

In total, some 40 noncomparative JIB studies have been published. At the 1991 NIH consensus conference on surgical treatment of obesity, O'Leary (81) summed up the JIB literature as follows: (1) excellent weight loss; (2) patients usually satisfied, and psychosocial adjustments are satisfactory; (3) perioperative mortality can be limited to 0.5% and wound infections to 3%; (4) all patients develop diarrhea; (5) electrolyte disturbances can be controlled; (6) 50% of the patients develop some kind of late metabolic complications; and (7) liver insufficiency, kidney stones, autoimmune arthritis, or skin diseases are seen among 20% of JIB-operated individuals, and these complications can appear late, often > 10 years after the operation. The NIH consensus conference advised against using JIB (16).

C Gastric Bypass (GBP) Versus Other Techniques

1 GBP Versus Horizontal Gastroplasties (HGP)

GBP has been compared with HGP in randomized studies with follow-up periods ranging from 1 to 3 years (30,31,82–87) and in nonrandomized studies with 1–2 years of follow-up (88,89). These studies were published between 1981 and 1990 (Table 1).

Hall's study is the largest (n = 204) and among the longest (3 years) (87). The median baseline weight was 112 kg, and after 3 years the weight loss was 39 kg in the GPB group and 17 kg in the HGP group. Similar results have been observed in two other 2- to 3-year studies: 38.4 versus 24.7 kg (85,86), and 44.2 versus 32.3 kg (84).

Table 1 Evolution of Surgery for Weight Control as Reflected in Comparative Prospective Studies

References Year/(No.)	Random yes/no matched	Years of follow-up	Conventional treatment	Intestinal operations (JIB)	Combined intestinal and gastric operations			Gastric operations			
					GBP	BPD	BPD/DS	HGP	VBG	Banding	Adjustable banding
1977 (47)	No	1		O	O						
1977 (48)	Yes	1		O	O						
1977 (78)	Yes	1		O	O						
1979 (145,146)	Yes	3	X	O							
1981 (79)	No	1		O	O						
1981 (82)	Yes	1			O			O			
1981 (83)	Yes	2			O			O			
1982 (80)	No	2.5		O				O			
1982 (30)	Yes	1.5			O			O			
1982 (88)	No	2			O			O			
1983 (84)	Yes	3			O			O			
1984 (89)	No	1			O			O		O	
1984 (90)	No	1			O			O–O[a]			
1984 (147)	Yes	2	X		O			O			
1986 (52)	No	2			O			O			
1986 (85)	Yes	2			O			O			
1986 (31)	Yes	2			O			O	O		
1987 (86)	Yes	3			O				O		
1987 (93)	Yes	3			O–O[b]						
1987 (91)	Yes	4			O				O		
1987 (95)	No	5	X		O						
1987 (107)	Yes	1			O			O	O		
1988 (148)	Yes	5			O			O	O		
1989 (93,96)	No	2–4			O–O[c]				O–O[c]		
1990 (87)	Yes	3			O–O[d]			O	O		
1992 (55)	Yes	4				O–O[e]					
1993 (129)	No	3			O				O		
1993 (94)	Yes	3			O				O		
1995 (92)	Yes	5			O				O		
1995 (149)	No	2–6	X		O						

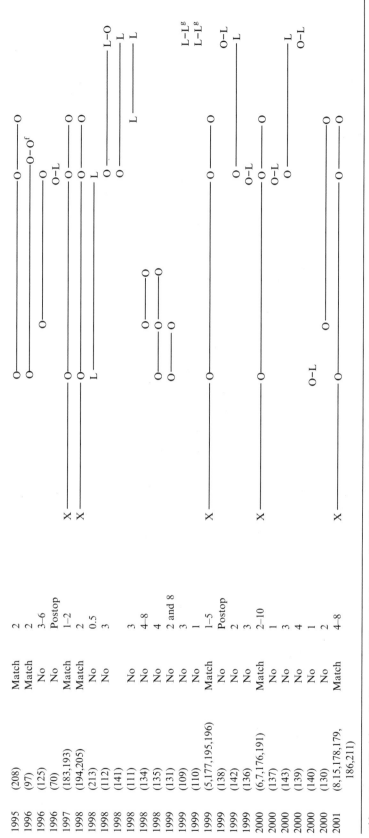

Abbreviations: JIB, jejuno-ileal bypass; GBP, gastric bypass; BPD, biliopancreatic diversion; BPD/DS, biliopancreatic diversion with duodenal switch; HGP, horizontal gastroplasties; VBG, vertical banded gastroplasty; O = open surgery; L = laparoscopic surgery; X = nonsurgical treatment.

[a] 1984, Sugerman (90), three different horizontal gastroplasties.
[b] 1987, Gleysteen (91) reinforced vs. nonreinforced stoma.
[c] 1989, Sugerman (93,96) sugar eaters vs. non sugar eaters.
[d] 1992, Brolin (55), normal vs. long-limb GBP.
[e] 1993, Clare (129), normal vs. equal-limb PPD.
[f] 1996, Lindroos (97), VBG and banding groups are pooled.
[g] 1999, Miller (109), and 1999, Berrevoet (110): American (36) vs. Swedish (37) adjustable band.

Results from the shorter and nonrandomized studies are in line with the 3-year studies.

In most studies, HGP has required a higher frequency of reoperations than GBP. Sugerman (90) reported that 39 out of 122 HGP patients required 43 revisions. On 10 occasions the HGP was converted into a GBP. The repaired HGPs resulted in many complications but not in improved weight loss. Compared to primary GBP operations, the conversions from HGP to GBP resulted in more complications but in similar weight loss.

In a detailed report, Näslund (31) showed that dilatation of stoma as well as pouch was associated with a reduction of weight loss in HGP but not in GBP. Similarly, Gleysteen (91) followed randomized GBP patients over 4 years without finding a difference in weight loss between patients with and without a reinforced gastrojejunostomy. Other mechanisms than pouch size and stoma diameter may thus be of importance for weight loss after GBP (see Sec. IV.C.5).

2   GBP Versus VBG

One randomized 5-year study (92), three randomized 3-year studies (87,93,94), and matched (SOS) or non-randomized 8-year (6), 5-year (95), and 2-year (5,52) studies have been published between 1986 and 2000 (Table 1). In none of the studies was VBG superior or equal to GBP as far as weight loss was considered. The percentage weight losses (as roughly calculated on means) in GBP and VBG groups were 24% versus 16% (6) (8-year), 34% versus 28% (87) (3-year, silastic ring VGB), 32% versus 20% (93) (3-year), 35% versus 30% (52) (2.5-year), and 32% versus 22% (5) (2-year). Howard (92) (5 years) and MacLean (94) (3 years) did not report weight losses. Howard reported the percentage of subjects losing >75% of excess weight at 1 year (18% in VBG, 60% in GBP) and the percent sustaining an excess weight loss of 50% (0% in VBG, 100% in GBP). MacLean defined a satisfactory result as BMI < 35. This was achieved among 83% of GBP patients with isolated pouch, in 58% of patients with ordinary GBP, and in 43% of those with VBG. In earlier studies, complications seem to have been more common in the GBP groups.

In his randomized 3-year report from 1987 (93) cited above, Sugerman also reported that VBG resulted in larger weight losses among "non-sweet eaters" than among "sweet eaters." In a nonrandomized study from 1989, non-sweet eaters were selectively operated with VBG while sweet eaters were subjected to GBP (96). Compared to the randomized VBG patients from 1987, the non sweet eaters with VBG (1989) achieved a larger weight reduction while there was no difference in weight loss between GBP patients from 1987 and 1989. From these results, Sugerman concluded that sweet eaters should be operated with GBP rather than VBG. In the SOS study, a careful assessment of food intake before and after gastroplasty (VBG and Banding) has not been able to verify a relationship between sugar intake and weight loss (97). More studies are needed to elucidate this question.

3   GBP Versus Banding

No randomized studies are available. In the SOS study, GBP is clearly superior to banding at both 2 (5) and 8 years follow-up (6). One single nonrandomized and small study has found a larger 1-year weight loss after banding (50 kg) than GBP (34 kg) (89).

4   GBP Versus Long-Limb Gastric Bypass

Brolin compared the outcome in 22 patients operated with traditional GBP (75-cm defunctionalized jejunum) with results from 23 patients treated with distal GBP (150-cm defunctionalized) in a randomized study (55). At baseline, BMI was 63 and 62 kg/m^2, respectively, and the mean follow-up was 43 months. After 2 years, the excess weight lost was 50% in GBP and 64% in the long-limb GBP ($P = .02$). After 4 years, only 33% of originally randomized patients were available for examination, and the weight loss was by then not significantly different between the two groups (63.5 vs. 72.1 kg, respectively, NS). Side effects were comparatively low and similar in the two groups. Brolin concluded that long-limb GBP is an appropriate method in the super-obese.

5   Mechanisms Behind the Superiority of GBP

The mechanisms behind the superior results with GBP as compared to gastroplasties are not known. That GBP is both a restrictive and a malabsorptive procedure is often suggested as an explanation. Dumping problems after intake of sweet food has been brought forward as an explanation for reduced energy intake. However, Lindroos reported similar energy intake at 6, 12, and 24 months after GBP and gastroplasty operations but larger weight loss in GBP patients (97). Flancbaum (98) found an energy expenditure higher than predicted in GBP individuals. GLP-1 (glucagonlike peptide 1, enteroglucagon) is elevated after gastric bypass (99), and it has been suggested that GLP-1 release from terminal ileum is increased after operations causing a food bypass of the pyloric muscle (100). GLP-1 may have multiple peripheral and central effects on the energy balance (100,101), and therefore an increased GLP-1 release may at least partly explain the larger weight loss after GBP. Cholecystokinin has anorectic effects but is not changed after GBP (99).

Grehlin is a novel gastrointestinal peptide, secreted mainly from gastric mucosa (102). It acts both as a growth hormone secretagogue (103) and as a stimulator of NPY release (104). Grehlin administration causes obesity in rodents by decreasing energy expenditure and increasing food intake (105). However, grehlin concentrations are low in human obesity (106), indicating a downregulation secondary to long-lasting positive energy balance or increased energy stores. Whether GBP changes the grehlin regulation in a direction causing larger weight losses than seen after gastroplasties remains to be examined.

D   VBG Versus Other Techniques

1   VBG Versus Horizontal Gastroplasty (HGP)

In an elegant study, Andersen et al. pretreated 74 patients (median body weight 125.1 kg) with a very low calorie diet (VLCD) resulting in 25-kg weight loss (107). Forty-five patients with sufficient weight loss according to predetermined criteria were then randomized to either VBG or HGP. Twelve months after surgery, VBG patients were reduced on average another 9.7 kg while HGP patients had increased with 1.0 kg ($P < .0005$). VLCD plus surgery had resulted in 48.5- and 32.6-kg weight loss, respectively (107). The study convincingly shows that VBG is superior to HGP.

2   VBG Versus Banding

No randomized studies comparing VBG and banding are available. From the SOS study, 2-year (5) and 8-year (6) follow-ups have been reported. In the 2-year report, results from 191 banding patients were compared with results from 534 VBG patients. At 8 years, the corresponding numbers of patients were 86 and 227. Body weights of banding and VBG patients were 120.2 and 120.6, respectively, at baseline, 94.6 and 93.0 at 2 years, and 101.6 and 101.5 kg at 8 years. Thus, the initial weight loss as well as the subsequent modest relapse was very similar with the two techniques, but banding was associated with a higher frequency of reoperations (17).

E   Banding with Variable Bands

As described earlier, one American (ASGB) (36) and one Swedish (SAGB) (37,108) band are in use. The two

devices seem to result in similar weight losses (109,110), although the SAGB band seems to be associated with less complications (110). Compared to laparoscopic nonadjustable banding, laparoscopic adjustable banding results in similar postoperative morbidity and weight loss but in less vomiting and food intolerance (111). In one large, nonrandomized study, results from 350 laparoscopic adjustable bandings undertaken from 1993 to 1997 were compared with the outcome of 200 open adjustable bandings and 210 open VBGs undertaken between 1991 and 1993 (112). The weight loss was similar in all three groups. In a 4-year follow-up of 50 patients treated with the SAGB technique, the weight loss was reported to be remarkable at 54 kg with amazingly few complications (113).

Although most reports on laparoscopic variable banding are positive, some authors are critical (114, 115) and report a high frequency of anatomical and functional complications with the ASGB (116) as well as the SAGB (117) technique.

F   Biliopancreatic Diversion (BPD)

Scopinaro reported on 1968 BPD operated cases in 1996 (118) and on 2241 BPD in 1998 (119). In the latter report, the operative mortality was low (0.5%), and the excess body weight loss was 75%. The follow-up ranged from 1 year to 21 years. Anemia during iron and folate therapy was < 5%, stomal ulcer during H_2-blocker therapy was 3.2%, and protein malnutrition was 3%. While protein malabsorption figures are similar in smaller study groups, higher frequencies of stomal ulcers ($\approx 10\%$) have been reported (120–122). In these reports, weight loss was excellent: BMI was decreased from 48 to 33, 51 to 29, and 49 to 29, respectively, after 2–3 years.

Scopinaro's group has reported on 239 pregnancies occurring in 129 of 1136 women who had undergone BPD (123). Of the 129 women, 35 had been infertile before BPD. Three babies died postpartum, and some were born preterm or were small for gestational age. The results were not contrasted against normal weighing or superobese reference mothers. The general impression from the publication is, however, that infertility and pregnancy risks were reduced by BPD and that the pregnancies usually resulted in healthy babies. In a more recent report, Scopinaro's group found that binge eating disappeared almost completely after PBD while night eating was not influenced (124).

In a nonrandomized study, Chapin et al. described results from 12 BPD and 10 VBG operations (125). The weight losses were 75 and 55 kg, respectively. Urinary calcium excretion and serum concentrations of calcium and vitamin D were lower in the BPD patients, while serum parathyroid hormone, serum alkaline phosphatase, and the urinary hydroxyproline/creatine ratio were higher in BPD. The laboratory data indicated that following BPD, secondary hyperparathyroidism attributed to hypocalcemia resulted from malabsorption of vitamin D although concurrent calcium malabsorption was not excluded.

Chapin's study illustrates the importance of supplementation with fat-soluble vitamins, B$_{12}$, folate, and calcium, a fact that has always been stressed by Scopinaro. Brolin examined supplementation habits among 109 surgeons performing BPD and gastric bypass operations (126). He found that most surgeons give multivitamin, iron, and B$_{12}$ supplementation after both types of operations. BPD patients also obtain calcium and fat-soluble vitamins to a great extent (63–97% of patients), and 21% obtain protein supplementation. Brolin concluded that most surgeons protect patients from developing severe metabolic deficiencies after BPD and gastric bypass. Occasional case reports on night blindness with optic neuropathy (127) and severe corneoconjunctival xerosis (128) after BPD emphasize the importance of lifelong supplementary treatment.

1 BPD Versus BPD Modification

In an attempt to improve the postoperative nutritional state after BPD, 106 patients had a BPD with a division of the small intestine at its midpoint to create equal biliopancreatic and alimentary limbs rather than a 250-cm alimentary limb as recommended by Scopinaro (129). The results were compared with traditional PBD ad modum Scopinaro. After 36 months, patients with equal limb BPD had lost 71% of their excess weight while the ordinary BPD had lost 77%. With the modification hypoproteinemia was reduced from 8% to 2%, and iron deficiency anemia from 20% to 10%. If these nutritional improvements can be verified in controlled studies, the modification might be warranted to consider in spite of the slightly smaller weight loss.

2 BPD Versus Gastric Banding

In a retrospective, nonradomized comparison of BPD (n = 142) and banding (n = 93), performed with open surgery, the excess weight lost was 60% and 48%, respectively (130). Early complications were common (15%) after BPD and uncommon after banding (1%). Late mortality was restricted to the BPD group (3.5%), while late complications were evenly distributed over the groups. Malnutrition was most common after BPD and outlet stenosis after banding. Removal of band

was necessary in 17% of the patients operated with banding.

3 BPD Versus Long-Limb Gastric Bypass

In a nonrandomized small study, 11 patients treated with BPD were compared with 19 patients obtaining long limb Roux-en-Y GBP (131). The median follow-up time was 96 and 24 months, respectively. From the latest available observation, BMI was reduced from 64 to 37 kg/m^2 in the BPD group and from 67 to 42 in the long-limb GBP group. Early complications seemed to occur at approximately the same rate in both groups (BPD, n = 2, 18%; GBP, n = 5, 26%). Serious late complications were not observed in the GBP group, but two cases of metabolic bone disease and one death due to liver failure occurred in the BPD group. It should be observed, however, that both groups were small and that the median observation time was four times longer in the BPD group.

G Biliopancreatic Diversion with Duodenal Switch (BPD/DS)

Hess, who introduced BPD/DS, has published a noncomparative study on his BPD/DS operations in 440 subjects with an average body weight of 183 kg (41% with BMI > 50) (132). The patients lost 80% of the initial excess weight after 2 years and 70% after 8 years. Complications were seen in 9% of the patients including two patients dying postoperatively. No marginal ulcers and no cases of the dumping syndrome were observed. Seventeen revisions were performed to correct excessive weight loss and low protein levels.

In contrast to Hess, Baltasar et al. found BPD/DS (n = 60, 2.5 years) to be an unsafe operation with unacceptably high operative (n = 2) and late (n = 2) mortality (133). The two late fatalities were due to liver failure and malnutrition, respectively. The mean percent excess weight lost was 86%. Eleven patients had minor liver abnormalities, and one had severe diarrhea for more than a year.

1 BPD/DS Versus BPD

Marceau et al. reported on a nonrandomized 4-to-8-year comparison between 252 patients operated with BPD and 465 treated with biliopancreatic diversion with duodenal switch (BPD/DS) (134). PBD/DS was associated with greater weight loss (46 vs. 36 kg), fewer side effects (diarrhea, vomiting, bone pain), less abnormal lab values (serum calcium, parathyroid hormone, ferritin, and vitamin A), and a lower annual revision rate due to severe malabsorption 0.1% vs. 1.7%). Rabkin reported 4-year BMI reductions that were similar after gastric bypass (from 49 to 30, n = 138), BPD (from 45 to 29, n = 32), and BPD/DS (from 49 to 31, n = 105) (135). Unfortunately, side effects of all three operations were not compared in Rabkin's study.

H   Open Versus Laparoscopic Techniques

Open and laparoscopic VBG have been compared in several studies (70,136,137), and in all studies the weight loss was similar with the two techniques. Laparoscopically operated patients had less postoperative pain, a faster mobilization, an improved respiratory status, and a shorter hospital stay. Comparisons of open versus laparoscopic adjustable banding (138,139), open versus laparoscopic GBP (140), and open VBG versus laparoscopic adjustable banding (141–143) have resulted in similar conclusions.

Large (n = 1040, 500, and 275), noncomparative studies of laparoscopically performed GBP also suggest that rapid mobilization and excellent weight loss can be achieved (72,73,144). In a smaller study (n = 40) on laparoscopically performed BPD/DS, the median post-operative hospital stay was 4 days (range 3–210 days) (74).

V   SURGICALLY VERSUS CONVENTIONALLY ACHIEVED WEIGHT LOSS

Three studies compared surgical treatment with dietary treatment undertaken by more or less specialized obesity clinics (145–149), and one study compared surgical treatment with treatment delivered by general practitioners at 480 primary heath care centers in Sweden (150). Results from the latter study, Swedish Obese Subjects (SOS), will be discussed separately in Section VII of this chapter. Pories' study on nonoperated and GBP-operated diabetic obese individuals (151) will be discussed in Section VI.

A   Jejunoileal Bypass Versus Diet

In the Danish Obesity Project (145,146), 202 patients were randomized in the proportions 2:1 to jejunoileal bypass or diet treatment. Six patients never came to treatment. The remaining 130 surgically treated and 66 diet-treated patients were followed for 2–3 years. After 2 years, the weight loss was 42.9 kg in the surgically treated group and 5.9 kg in the diet group. The quality of life as well as blood pressure was markedly improved in the surgical group. However, the surgical group had a large number of complications, some of which were serious.

B   Horizontal Gastroplasty Versus VLCD Followed by Diet

In another early Danish study, 60 patients were randomized to horizontal gastroplasty or VLCD followed by traditional dieting. A 2-year (147) and a 5-year (148) report have appeared. Unfortunately, <50% of the patients had in fact been followed for 2 and 5 years, respectively, when the reports were written. At 2 years, the weight loss was 30.6 kg in the gastroplasty group and 8.2 kg in the VLCD/diet group. Weight losses are not reported at 5 years. Instead, a "cumulated success rate" defined as >10 kg maintained weight loss was given. This success rate was 16% in the patients operated with horizontal gastroplasty and 3% in the VLCD/diet group. As discussed above, and further emphasized by this Danish study, horizontal gastroplasties are not any longer used owing to poor long-term results.

C   Gastric Bypass Versus VLCD and Diet

In a prospective, nonrandomized, nonmatched study, Martin compared gastric bypass (n = 201) with VLCD followed by diet (n = 161) (149). After VLCD, the diet group was offered one counseling session per week for 18 months and then annual follow-ups. The follow-up ranged from 2 to 6 years. At 6 years, the follow up rate was 34.5% in the GBP group and 19.7% in the VLCD/diet group. In the GBP group, BMI dropped from 49.3 to a minimum of 31.8 after 2 years. At 6 years BMI was 33.7 kg/m^2. In the VLCD/diet group, the corresponding figures were 41.2, 32.1, and 38.5 kg/m^2. As compared to VLCD/diet treatment, GBP thus resulted in twice-as-large BMI drops and in much smaller relapses.

VI   IMPROVEMENTS OF RISK FACTORS, MORBIDITY, AND MORTALITY

Improvements of risk factors and morbidity after surgically induced weight loss will mainly be covered when reviewing the results from the SOS study in Section VII. Here, only the most important results from other studies will be summarized.

Several reports on the surgical treatment of obesity have demonstrated improvements of blood pressure (152–159), blood lipids (152–157,160–163), diabetes/ fasting glucose (152–155,157,161,164–169), sleep apnea (152,153,156,157,170), and various symptoms (152, 156). With few exceptions, these studies are based on within-group comparisons over comparatively short periods of time. In lack of obese control groups with little or no weight change reflecting the natural history of obesity, amelioration of risk factors cannot be properly evaluated in obese study groups with weight loss. Thus, impacts of weight loss on the incidence of various conditions cannot be examined without obese control groups, and the evaluation of recoveries from disease conditions will be uncertain. In addition, risk factor improvements seen after 6–24 months may disappear after more prolonged periods of follow-up, despite the fact that weight loss is maintained, as discussed in Section VII. Thus, even the most encouraging short-term within-group improvements of risk factors must be interpreted with great caution.

Walter Pories was the first to notice the favorable effect of gastric bypass on established type 2 diabetes (169). Subsequently, he has documented this effect not only in several long-term (10 years and more) within group reports (166–168) but also in a retrospective study examining 154 obese type 2 diabetics operated with gastric bypass and 78 obese diabetics not being operated (controls) (151). At baseline the two groups were comparable with respect to age, sex, BMI, and occurrence of hypertension. The follow-up was 9 years in the surgically treated group and 6.2 years in the control group. Although the retrospective design, different follow-up times, and the comparatively small study groups make the evaluation difficult, it is remarkable that the annual mortality rate was 4.5% in the control group but only 1% in the surgically treated group (151). The improvement in mortality rate was mainly explained by a decreased number of cardiovascular deaths.

Several authors, including Pories, have suggested that the improved diabetic state after gastric bypass is not only due to the reduced body weight but also to a changed gastrointestinal signaling system (100,171, 172). However, the exact non-weight-loss mechanisms remain to be established. It should be noted that although the metabolic clearance rate of glucose improves after gastric bypass, it is not completely normalized (173). After massive weight losses achieved by means of VBG, the normal insulin oscillatory secretion is not restored in previously type 2 diabetic obese subjects (174).

VII   SWEDISH OBESE SUBJECTS

A   SOS Aims

The main goal of SOS is to examine if large and long-term intentional weight loss will reduce the elevated morbidity and mortality of obese subjects. Several secondary aims, related to the genetics of obesity, quality of life, and health economics, have also been defined (150).

B   Study Design

SOS originally consisted of one registry study and one intervention study (150). One randomized reference study and one genetic sib pair study were added later.

In the registry study, 6322 obese men (BMI $\geq$ 34) and women (BMI $\geq$ 38) in the age interval 37–60 years were health examined by physicians at 480 of the existing 700 primary health care centers in Sweden. From the registry, patients were recruited into the intervention study consisting of one surgically treated group (n = 2010) and one matched control group (n = 2038) treated conventionally at the 480 primary health care centers. The surgically treated patients obtained (variable) banding (Fig. 2D), VBG (Fig. 2E) or gastric bypass (Fig. 3A) at one of the 28 participating surgical departments. The obese controls received the customary obesity treatment of the center at which they were registered. Up to 1998, no antiobesity drugs were approved in Sweden. Given the poor long-term results at specialized obesity units after traditional obesity management (1–4), poor weight loss was anticipated following the nonsurgical treatment in SOS. Thus these patients were expected to constitute a control group, which on average would not experience intentional weight loss.

Patients were entered into the registry and intervention studies between September 1, 1987, and January 31, 2001. After having reached the goal 2000 patients per intervention arm, the inclusions into the registry and intervention studies have now ceased. All patients in the intervention study will be followed for 20 years.

SOS is a matched and not a randomized study since, in 1987, ethical approval for randomization was not obtained owing to the high operative mortality (1–5%) observed in most surgical study groups from the 1970s and '80s. Thus, patients are choosing for themselves if they want surgical or conventional treatment. When a surgical patient has been accepted according to a number of inclusion and exclusion criteria, a matching program, taking 18 different matching variables into account, selects the optimal control among eligible individuals in the registry study (150). The selection is based on an algorithm moving the mean values of the matching variables of the control group towards the current mean values of the surgically treated patients. Thus a group match rather than an individual match is undertaken. The participating centers can not influence the matching program.

A surgically treated patient and the control selected together with him or her start the intervention on the operation day of the surgically treated individual. Both patients are examined just before inclusion and then after 0.5, 1, 2, 3, 4, 6, 8, 10, 15, and 20 years. For special reasons, 28 surgically treated patients obtained two controls each. Centralized biochemistry is obtained at 0, 2, 10, 15, and 20 years. All visits are automatically booked by a computer at the SOS secretariat and all centers obtain the necessary forms, test tubes, etc., for a given patient visit some weeks before the booked appointment. If information is not coming back as expected from patients or centers, the program is automatically sending out reminders or is asking the staff of the secretariat to solve the problem by phone.

Over the years, several interim reports with different number of patients have been published from the ongoing SOS-study. In this review, reference is given to published reports rather than to available patients after completion of inclusion unless stated otherwise.

C Matching and Follow-Up

The matching program resulted in two similar groups. For instance, within the surgically treated group and the obese control group the fraction of women was 70.3% and 70.3%, age was 47 ± 6 and 48 ± 6 years, body weight was 118.7 ± 15.6 and 116.9 ± 16.6 kg, and height 1.69 ± 0.09 and 1.69 ± 0.09 m, respectively.

The matching is based on data from the registry study. The waiting time between registry examination and inclusion into the intervention was on average 9 months. During this period the surgical group increased in weight while the conventionally treated controls reduced their weight without any interference from the investigators. Therefore, body weight and several risk factors were higher in the surgically treated group at the baseline examination of the SOS intervention study.

The 10-year compliance rate is currently 74.3% in both study groups. All deceased individuals are so far included among the non-compliant individuals since the safety monitoring committee has not yet released mortality data. Considering that most antiobesity trials have 30–50% dropout after 2 years, the 26% dropout rate (including mortality) in SOS after 10 years is very encouraging. We believe that the high follow-up rate is explained in part by the centralized scheduling and monitoring system, which includes frequent and timely reminders. When participating centers of a study are responsible for the scheduling of reexaminations, the follow-up rates are much lower. For instance, in the North American NBSR registry of surgically treated obese patients, the 1-, 2-, and 3-year follow-up rates were 90% (6064/6764), 46% (2737/5977), and 23% (1124/4890), respectively (175).

D Weight Loss in SOS

In one 2-year report on 767 surgically treated patients and 712 obese controls, the weight loss was 28 ± 15 kg (mean ± SD) and 0.5 ± 8.9 kg, respectively (5). The percentage reductions after gastric bypass, VBG, and banding were 33 ± 10%, 23 ± 10%, and 21 ± 12%, respectively. Similar 2-year changes in body weight were recently reported for 1210 surgically treated and 1099 control subjects of SOS (176).

In other publications, 4-year (177), 6-year (178,179), and 8-year (6) follow-ups of weight loss have been reported. Figure 4 gives the weight changes over 10 years. As expected from the literature, GBP resulted in larger weight losses than banding and VBG at all time points between 6 months and 10 years. With all three surgical techniques the lowest weight was observed after 1 year. Between 1 and 8 years a moderate relapse occurred while body weight appeared to be stable between 8 and 10 years. In contrast, virtually no weight change was observed in the obese, conventionally treated control group (Fig 4). Two years after inclusion, the average weight change was −22.9% in the surgically treated groups taken together (n = 1592 completers) while the weight change was −0.2% in the obese control group (n = 1431 completers) (P < .001 for difference in change between groups). Corresponding figures after 10 years (n = 263 + 263 completers by 2001) were −16.7% and +1.1% (P < .001).

Thus conventional, nonpharmacological treatment is, on the average, almost meaningless when undertaken by GPs at nonspecialized treatment units. This implies personal tragedies for millions of obese individuals around the world who do not have access to specialized treatment and immense consequences from a public health point of view. It should be noted, however, that the treatment offered to the control group by general physicians may have prevented further weight gain since the self-reported gain prior to the registry examination was 13–21 kg per decade, depending on gender and age (18).

The energy intake before and during weight loss was studied over the first 2 years after inclusion by means of a validated dietary questionnaire (180,181) in 365 patient operated with VBG or banding and in 34 patients operated with gastric bypass (97). Although the weight loss was 38.6 kg in the gastric bypass group but only 26.7 kg in the combined VBG and banding group, the energy intake before and after surgery did not differ between the groups (Fig. 5). As discussed above (Sec. IV.C.), this

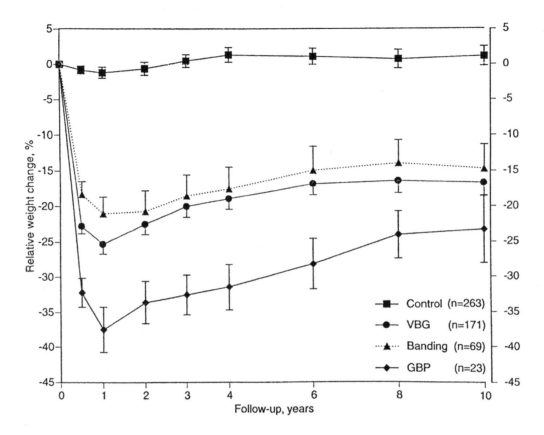

Figure 4 Weight change (95% CI) in 263 obese controls and 263 surgically treated patients over 10 years of follow-up in the SOS intervention study. Analysis based on completer population. Each one of the surgical groups had a significantly ($P < .01$) larger weight reduction than the controls.

finding suggests that gastric bypass is associated with increased energy expenditure, perhaps due to an increased secretion of GLP-1 or a decreased grehlin secretion.

E   Surgical Complications in SOS

Five postoperative deaths in 2010 operated patients have occurred in the SOS study (0.25%, Jan. 31, 2001). Three of these fatal cases were due to leakage that was detected too late. One death was caused by a technical mistake during a laparoscopic operation and one by a postoperative myocardial infarction.

Peri- and postoperative complications have been calculated on 1164 patients followed for 4 years (17 and unpublished observations). During the primary stay at the hospital the following complications occurred: bleeding 0.5%; embolus and/or thrombosis 0.8%; wound complications 1.8%; deep infections (leakage, abscess) 2.1%; pulmonary 6.1%; other complications 4.8%. The number of complications was 193 and the number of patients with complications 151

(13%). In 26 patients (2.2%) the postoperative complications were serious enough to cause a reoperation.

Over 4 years, 12% of the 1164 patients were reoperated, usually owing to poor weight loss but in some cases due to vomiting or other side effects. Usually banding and VBG were converted to gastric bypass but in some cases the original operation was repaired.

Over the 4 years a number of other operations were undertaken in both groups. In the control group, 10.1 operations per 100 person-years were undertaken while the corresponding figure in the surgical group was 15.2. Operations due to ventral hernia, gallbladder disease, intestinal obstruction, and surplus of skin were more common in the surgical group while, on the average, operations due to malignancy, gynecological disorders, and all other reasons taken together were more common in the control group.

F   Risk Factors at Baseline in SOS

In an early cross-sectional analysis of 450 men and 556 women from the registry study of SOS it was shown that

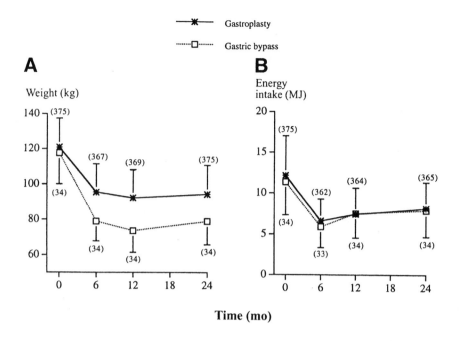

Figure 5 Weight loss (panel A) and energy intake (panel B) over 2 years in SOS patients operated by means of gastroplasty and gastric bypass. The gastroplasty operations were banding and VBG pooled. Mean ± SD. Values in parentheses indicate number of patients at each examination. Energy intake, estimated with validated technique (180,181), did not differ between groups at any time point. Body weights were significantly lower in gastric bypass patients at all time points after surgery ($P < .0001$), whereas body weight before surgery did not differ significantly between groups. (From Ref. 97.)

as compared to randomly selected controls most cardiovascular risk factors were elevated in the obese (Table 2) (150). The exception was total cholesterol, which was similar in obese and non-obese males and lower in obese women as compared to reference women.

Later, risk factors have also been analyzed in relation to body composition in 1083 men and 1367 women from the SOS registry study (182). This analysis revealed one body compartment, risk factor pattern, and one subcutaneous adipose tissue distribution, risk factor pattern. Within the first pattern, risk factors were positively and strongly related to the visceral adipose tissue mass and, more weakly, to the subcutaneous adipose tissue mass. Some risk factors, such as glucose and triglycerides in men and insulin in women, were negatively related to lean body mass. In addition, the

Table 2 BMI and Risk Factors in 50-Year-Old Men and Women from SOS and in 50-Year-Old Randomly Selected Reference Subjects[a]

	SOS males	Ref. males	$P <$	SOS females	Ref. females	$P <$
N	102	220		121	398	
Age (years)	48–52	50		48–52	50	
BMI	37.3 ± 3.9	24.0		41.4 ± 4.4	24.8	
Systolic, mmHg	146 ± 16	137 ± 22	.001	147 ± 18	140 ± 22	.01
Diastolic, mmHg	94 ± 9	90 ± 14	.01	89 ± 9	85 ± 11	.001
Blood glucose mmol/L	5.9 ± 2.0	4.7 ± 1.3	.001	5.5 ± 1.6	4.2 ± 0.9	.001
Insulin, mU/L	31 ± 25	9.6 ± 8.0	.001	22 ± 12	14 ± 5	.001
Triglycerides, mmol/L	2.7 ± 2.0	1.3 ± 0.8	.001	2.0 ± 1.0	1.3 ± 0.6	.001
HDL chol, mmol/L	1.2 ± 0.4	1.6 ± 0.4	.001	1.4 ± 0.4	–	
Total chol, mmol/L	6.2 ± 1.2	6.4 ± 1.3	n.s.	6.1 ± 1.1	7.2 ± 1.1	.001

[a] Risk factor levels for other age groups, see Ref. 150.
Source: Ref. 150.

subcutaneous adipose tissue distribution was related to risk factors when both taking and not taking the body compartments into account statistically. A preponderance of subcutaneous adipose tissue in the upper part of the trunk, as indicated by the neck circumference, was positively related to risk factors while the thigh circumference was negatively related to risk factors. These two risk factor patterns have also been observed longitudinally; i.e, changes in risk factors and changes in body composition and adipose tissue distribution are related (183) in the same way as in the cross-sectional observations (182).

G Risk Factor Changes in SOS

In a 2-year report of 282 men and 560 women, pooled from the surgically treated group and the control group, risk factor changes were examined as a function of weight change (183). A 10-kg weight loss was enough to introduce clinically significant reductions in all tra-

ditional risk factors except total cholesterol (Fig. 6). Although it is known that total cholesterol is reduced short term (1–6 months) by moderate weight losses (9,184), Figure 6 illustrates that 30–40 kg of maintained weight loss is required to preserve the reduction in total serum cholesterol after 2 years.

In another 2-year report, on 767 surgically treated patients and 712 controls, the weight loss of the surgical group resulted in dramatic reductions in the incidence of hypertension, diabetes, hyperinsulinemia, hypertriglyceridemia, and low HDL cholesterol (5) (Fig. 7). In the case of diabetes, a 32-fold risk reduction was observed while the incidences of other risk conditions were reduced 2.6- to 10-fold. In analogy with Figure 6, weight loss had no effect on the incidence of hypercholesterolemia (Fig. 7). To illustrate the amount of weight loss necessary to prevent the development of diabetes, the surgically treated group and the control group were pooled and the diabetes incidence plotted by decile of weight change (185). As can be seen in Figure 8, weight

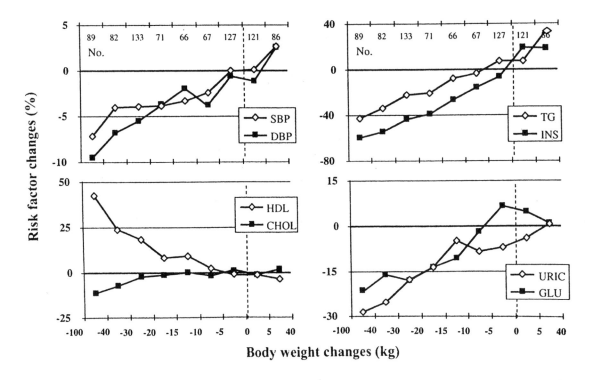

Figure 6 Adjusted risk factor changes (%) in relation to body weight changes (kg) over 2 years in 842 obese men and women pooled from the surgically treated group and the obese control group of the SOS intervention study. The percent change of each risk factor was adjusted for the basal value of that risk factor, initial body weight, sex, age, and height. The number of subjects in each weight-changing class is shown at the top of the figure (as No.). SBP and DBP, systolic and diastolic blood pressure; HDL, serum HDL cholesterol; CHOL, serum total cholesterol; TG, serum triglycerides; INS, serum insulin; URIC, serum uric acid; GLU, blood glucose. All serum samples collected after an overnight fast. (From Ref. 183.)

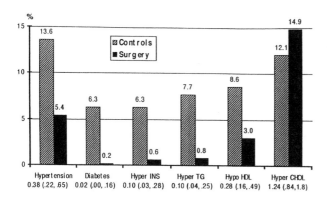

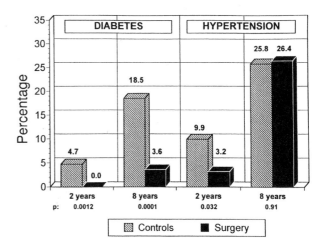

Figure 7 Two-year unadjusted incidence of indicated conditions in 712 obese controls (striped bars) and in 767 surgically treated completers (solid bars) from the SOS intervention study. Below bars, odds ratios (95% CI) adjusted for baseline values of age, sex, weight, smoking, and perceived health. $P < .001$ for all differences between groups except for hypercholesterolemia. Abbreviations as in Figure 6. (From Ref. 5.)

Figure 9 Two-year and 8-year unadjusted incidence of diabetes and hypertension in 232 obese controls (striped bars) and 251 surgically treated patients (solid bars) from the SOS intervention study. Calculations based on completer population. Almost identical odds ratios were obtained with and without adjustments in completer and intent-to-treat populations (not shown). (From Ref. 6.)

changes close to zero were associated with a 2-year diabetes incidence of 7–9%. A mean weight loss of 7% was still associated with a 2-year diabetes incidence of 3% while no new cases of diabetes were seen for mean weight losses of 12% or larger.

In the 8-year follow-up (6), the incidence of diabetes was still five times lower in the surgical group than in the control group (Fig. 9). However, there was no difference

between the two groups with respect to the 8-year incidence of hypertension (Fig. 9). This was the case with or without multiple adjustments in the completer population as well as in the intent-to-treat population (6). In a follow-up study, the final blood pressure has been shown to be closely related to recent weight changes and the length of the follow-up but more weakly associated with initial weight and the initial weight loss (186).

Table 3 sums up unpublished results from 263 surgically and 263 conventionally treated subjects followed for 10 years. The mean changes of systolic blood pressure, glucose, insulin, TG, HDL cholesterol, and uric acid were significantly more favorable in the surgically treated group than the control group, while no effects were observed with respect to diastolic blood pressure and total cholesterol. Surgery significantly decreased the incidence (of new cases) of diabetes, hypertriglyceridemia, and hyperuricemia while it increased the recovery from hypertension, diabetes, hypertriglyceridemia, and hyperuricemia.

Thus, surgically induced weight loss seems to have favorable effects on already established hypertension, diabetes, hypertriglyceridemia, and hyperuricemia, and it reduces the development of new cases of diabetes, hypertriglyceridemia, and hyperuricemia. However, these 10-year data need to be validated when more patients are available. The need for obesity treatment

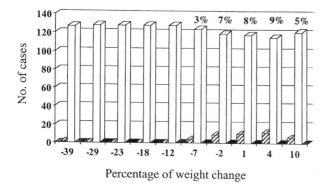

Figure 8 Two-year incidence of diabetes by decile of percent weight change in the SOS intervention study. Pooled data from 1281 obese controls and surgically treated subjects not having diabetes at baseline. Striped bars indicate new cases of diabetes. At bottom, the average percent weight change within each decile. At top, the 2-year incidence of diabetes within each weight change decile. (From Refs. 5 and 185.)

Table 3 Summary of Unpublished Observations on SOS 10-Year Data Regarding Significant and Favorable Differences (+) or Lack of Such Differences (−) Between Surgically Treated Subjects and Obese Controls

	Mean change of value[a]	Incidence	Recovery
Syst. BP	+		
Diast. BP	−		
Hypertension		−	+
Glucose	+		
Insulin	+		
Diabetes		+	+
TG	+	+	+
HDL-cholest.	+	−	(−)[b]
Total cholesterol	−	−	−
Uric acid	+	+	+

[a] "Mean change of value" refers to continuous variables such as blood pressure and biochemical risk factors independent of medication. Incidence and recovery calculations are based on medication and cut-offs of continuous variables.
[b] Sign within parentheses indicates power problems due to too few cases at baseline.

in the case of obesity plus diabetes has recently been the subject of a Lancet review (187).

H Hard End Points

SOS will not be able to report on total mortality until 2004–2006. Reports on myocardial infarction and stroke will probably not be available until 2010.

While short-term weight losses improve all cardiovascular risk factors (Fig. 6) (9,184), several observational epidemiological studies have shown an association between weight loss and increased total as well as cardiovascular mortality, even in those being obese at baseline (188). This discrepancy has usually been explained by the inability of observational studies to separate intentional from unintentional weight loss. Williamson has provided some evidence for this in women (189) but not in men (190). The 8-year (6) and 10-year observations discussed above suggest another possibility: in the long term, some risk factors, such as hypercholesterolemia (and hypertension?), may relapse in spite of maintained weight loss.

A third explanation for increased mortality after weight loss may be that unknown or nontraditional risk factors deteriorate during weight loss. Recently, 10-year data from SOS have demonstrated that homocysteine increases with increasing weight loss, independent of the weight loss method (surgery or conventional), even when adjusting for changes in folate and B_{12} (191).

Homocysteine levels have been shown to be related to cardiovascular mortality (192). Since homocysteine and folate are negatively related and since folate intake is reduced during caloric restriction, our observations suggest that all weight-reducing treatment, surgical or not, should be accompanied by substitution with multivitamin pills, folic acid, and possibly B_{12} in order to counteract an increased incidence of cardiovascular disease due to hyperhomocysteinemia.

Taken together, the pattern of known and unknown risk factor responses after long-term, maintained weight loss may well determine the incidence of hard end points such as total mortality, myocardial infarction, and stroke. Since the net effect of known risk factor changes are difficult to estimate and since unknown risk factors are always likely to exist, the importance of controlled obesity interventions is obvious.

I Effects on the Cardiovascular System

In subsample of the SOS study, cardiac and vascular structure and function was examined at baseline and after 1–4 years of follow-up. At baseline a surgically treated group (n = 41) and an obese control group (n = 31) were compared with a lean reference group (n = 43) (193,194). Compared to lean subjects, the systolic and diastolic blood pressure, left ventricular mass, and relative wall thickness were increased in the obese, while the systolic function (measured as left ventricular ejection fraction) and the diastolic function (estimated from the E/A ratio, i.e., the flow rate over the mitral valve early in diastole divided by the flow rate late in diastole during the artrial contraction) were impaired. After 1 year, all these variables had improved in the surgically treated group but not in the obese control group. When pooling the two obese groups and plotting left ventricular mass or E/A ratio as a function of quintiles of weight change a "dose" dependency was revealed; i.e., the larger the weight reduction, the larger the reduction in left ventricular mass (Fig. 10) and the more pronounced the improvement in diastolic function (Fig. 11). Unchanged weight was in fact associated with a measurable deterioration in diastolic function over 1 year.

In other small subgroups from SOS, heart rate variability from 24-hr Holter EKG recordings and 24-hr catecholamine secretion were examined (195). Compared to lean subjects, our examination indicated an increased sympathetic activity and a withdrawal of vagal activity at baseline. Both these disturbances were normalized in the surgically treated group but not in the control group after 1 year of treatment.

The intima-media thickness of the carotid bulb was examined by means of ultrasonography at baseline and

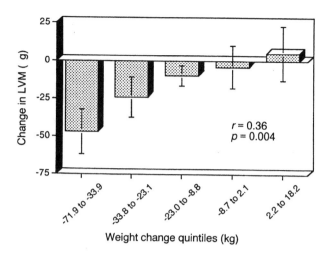

Figure 10 Changes in left ventricular mass (g) as a function of 1-year weight change quintiles (kg) in the SOS intervention study. Mean ± SEM. Pooled echocardiographic data of 38 surgically treated patients and 25 obese controls. Correlation for trend based on individual observations (n = 63). (From Ref. 193.)

after 4 years in the SOS intervention study (196). A randomly selected lean reference group matched for gender, age, and height was examined at baseline and after 3 years. As shown in Figure 12, the annual progression rate was almost three times higher in the obese control group (n = 9) as compared to lean reference subjects ($P < .05$). In the surgically treated group, the progression rate was normalized. Although results from this small study group need to be confirmed in larger trials, this study offers the first data on hard end points after intentional weight loss.

We have also shown that the pulse pressure increases more slowly in the surgically treated group than in the obese control group after a mean follow-up of 5.5 years (186). In gastric bypass individuals the pulse pressure is in fact decreasing. These observations are of interest since it has been shown that, at a given systolic blood pressure, a high pulse pressure is associated with increased arterial stiffness (197), increased intima-media thickness (198), and increased cardiovascular mortality (199). Thus, pulse pressure changes (186) as well as ultrasonographic measurements (196) indicate that surgical treatment is slowing down the increased atherosclerotic process in the obese.

Finally, questionnaire data from 1210 surgically treated patients and 1099 obese SOS controls examined at baseline and after 2 years were analyzed with respect

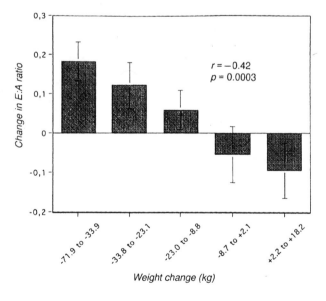

Figure 11 Changes in diastolic function, as indicated by the E/A ratio, in relation to 1-year weight change quintiles (kg) in the SOS intervention study. Mean ± SEM. Pooled transmitral Doppler data of 41 surgically treated patients and 30 obese controls. Correlation for trend based on individual observations (n = 71). For explanation of E/A ratio, see text. (From Ref. 194.)

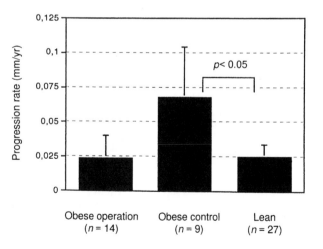

Figure 12 Annual progression rate of intima-media thickness in the carotid artery bulb in surgically treated obese (n = 14), obese controls (n = 9), and lean controls (n = 27) matched for gender, age, and height. Mean ± SEM. Progression rate measured ultrasonographically over 4 years in the two obese groups and over 3 years in the lean reference group. The weight change was −22 ± 10 kg in the operated group and 0 ± 13 kg in the obese control group. (From Ref. 196.)

to various cardiovascular symptoms (176). At baseline the two groups were comparable in most respects. After 2 years, dyspnea and chest discomfort were reduced in a much larger fraction of surgically treated as compared to controls. For instance, 87% of the surgically treated reported baseline dyspnea when climbing two flights of stairs, while only 19% experienced such dyspnea at the 2-year follow-up. In the obese control group the corresponding figures were 69% and 57%, respectively ($P < .001$ for difference in change between groups).

Physical inactivity was observed in 46% of the surgically treated before weight reduction but only in 17% after 2 years. Corresponding figures in the obese control group were 33% and 29%, respectively ($P < .001$) (176). Thus, not only does physical inactivity contribute to the development of obesity, but obesity favors physical inactivity. This cycle is broken by surgical treatment.

J Effects on Sleep Apnea

Sleep apnea was examined in patients from the SOS register study (1324 SOS men and 1711 SOS women) by means of a questionnaire (200,201). A high likelihood for sleep apnea was observed in 26% of obese men and in 9% of obese women. Sleep apnea was associated with WHO grade 4 daytime dyspnea, admission to hospital with chest pain, myocardial infarction, and elevations of blood pressure, insulin, triglycerides, and uric acid when adjusting for body fat, adipose tissue distribution, and other potential confounders (200). In addition, sleep apnea was also associated with increased psychosocial morbidity before and after these adjustments (201).

Sleep apnea has also been investigated in the SOS intervention study (176). A high likelihood for sleep apnea was observed in 23% of 1210 surgically treated cases at baseline but only in 8% 2 years postsurgery. In the control group (n = 1099), the corresponding figures were 22% and 20%, respectively ($P < .001$ for difference in change between groups) (176). Finally, a small experimental study in obese SOS patients demonstrated an association among sleep apnea, elevated catecholamine secretion, and elevated energy expenditure, particularly during sleep (202). Affected individuals were improved by means of nighttime treatment with continuous positive airway pressure (202).

K Quality of Life in SOS Subjects Before and After Weight Loss

Cross-sectional information from 800 obese men and 943 women of the SOS registry study demonstrated that obese patients have a much worse health-related quality of life (HRQL) than age-matched reference subjects (14). In fact, HRQL in the obese was as bad as, or even worse than, in patients with severe rheumatoid arthritis, generalized malignant melanoma, or spinal cord injuries. The measurement were performed with generic scales such as General Health Rating Index, Hospital Anxiety and Depression Scale, Mood Adjective Checklist, and Sickness Impact Profile in original or short form (14,203) and with more obesity-specific instruments such as OP measuring obesity-related psychosocial problems (14) and Stunkard's Three-Factor Eating Questionnaire (TFEQ) (204). All scales have been validated under Swedish conditions.

In 2- (205) and 4-year (15) reports, results from all measuring instruments improved dose-dependently; i.e., the larger the weight loss, the more improvement of HRQL. However, different instruments resulted in different effect sizes as illustrated by Figure 13, showing 4-year results in surgically treated patients divided by weight loss ≥25% and <25% and in the obese, weight-stable controls. In subjects with weight loss ≥25%, large effects (>0.8 SRM) were seen for obesity-related measures reflecting eating patterns and psychosocial problems and for general health and functional health domains such as ambulation, recreation, passtimes, and social interaction. Moderate effect sizes (0.5 < SRM < 0.8) were observed for depressive symptoms (HAD-D), self-esteem (SE), and overall mood (MACL), while the effect on anxiety symptoms (HAD-A) were minor (Fig 13). In the obese control group only trivial effects were seen.

Stunkard's original findings based on the TFEQ (204) (cognitive restraint, disinhibition, hunger) could not be replicated among 4377 obese SOS patients with respect to convergent and discriminative validity of the factors. Using multitrait/multi-item analysis and factor analysis, a short revised 18-item instrument has been constructed, representing the derived factors of Cognitive Restrain, Uncontrolled Eating, and Emotional Eating (206).

In summary, HRQL is very poor in obese subjects. Large (>25%) and moderate (10–25%) weight losses maintained over 4 years improve virtually all aspects of HRQL.

L Economical Consequences of Obesity and Weight Loss in SOS

In cross-sectional studies of SOS patients, it was shown that sick leave was twice as high and disability pension twice as frequent than in the general Swedish population independent of age and gender (207–209). The annual indirect costs (sick leave plus disability pension) attrib-

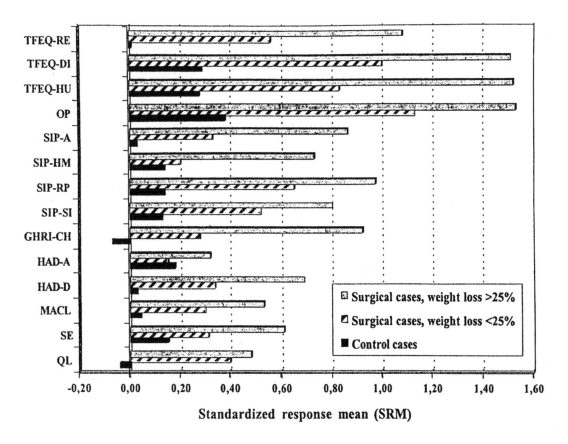

Figure 13 Treatment effects on health-related quality of life (HRQL) in surgically treated patients and controls after 4 years in the SOS intervention study. HRQL change scores from baseline to 4-year follow-up are transformed to standardized response means (SRM). SRM (214) is calculated as score mean change of a test divided by the standard deviation of change. *Abbreviations*: TFEQ, Three-Factor Eating Questionnaire; RE, restrained eating; DI, disinhibition; HU, hunger; OP, obesity-related psychosocial problems; SIP, sickness impact profile; A, ambulation; HM, home management; RP, recreation and pastime; SI, social interaction; GHRI, General Health Rating Index; CH, current health; HAD, Hospital Anxiety and Depression Scale; A, anxiety symptoms; D, depression symptoms; MACL, Mood Adjective Checklist; SE, self-esteem. (From Ref. 15.)

utable to obesity were estimated at $6 billion SEK in Sweden or $1 million U.S. per 10,000 inhabitants per year.

The number of lost days due to sick leave and disability pension the year before inclusion into the SOS intervention was almost identical in the surgically treated group and the obese control group (104 and 107 days, respectively) (177). The year after inclusion, the number of lost days was higher in the surgically treated group but, 2–4 years after inclusion, the lost days were lower in the surgically treated group (Fig. 14). This was particularly evident in those individuals above the median age (46.7 years, not shown) (177).

The total direct costs attributable to obesity in Sweden and their changes after weight loss are currently examined in the SOS project. So far, we have no data from the general population (but a 30,000 sample has

just been collected) to use as reference for obese SOS individuals with respect to costs for hospital care. However, we do know that surgical obesity treatment is associated with higher hospital costs ($10,200) than conventional treatment ($2800) over 6 years (179). When adjusting for the surgical intervention as such ($4300) in the surgical group and conditions common after bariatric surgery in both groups ($2800 in surgically treated, $400 in controls) the remaining costs were not different in the two groups. This study (179) indicates that the lag time between weight loss and improvement of hard endpoints requiring hospitalization is longer than 6 years. It is still an open question if surgical treatment will result in smaller hospitalization costs than conventional care of the obese in a 10-to-20 year perspective.

At baseline, the fraction of individuals on medication for various conditions was usually higher in obese

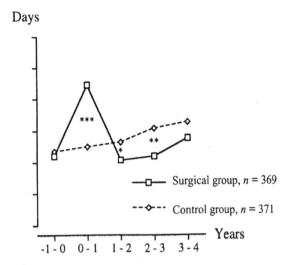

Figure 14 Days of sick leave plus disability pension per year in 369 surgically treated and 371 obese controls the year before inclusion and over 4 years after inclusion into the SOS intervention study. All data adjusted for age, gender, and several predictive variables. During years 1–4, the number of days is also adjusted for days of sick leave plus disability pension the year before inclusion. Significant differences between groups indicated as $*P < .05$, $**P < .01$, $***P < .001$. (From Ref. 177.)

subjects of the SOS intervention study (Int) than in lean randomly selected individuals of the SOS reference study (Ref) (178). The fraction on medication for the following conditions was significantly different between groups: diabetes (Int 6.1%, Ref 0.7%), CVD (Int 27.8%, Ref 8.2), pain (Int 10.8%, Ref 4.1%), while medication for the following conditions were not significantly different: asthma (Int 5.2%, ref 2.3%), psychiatric disorders (Int. 7.2%, Ref 4.6%) anemia (Int 1.3%, Ref 1.6%) gastrointestinal disorders (Int 4.4%, Ref 3.5%), all others (Int 20.5%, Ref 23.6%).

Among those SOS intervention patients on medication at baseline, the fraction on medication dropped significantly more over 6 years in the surgically treated group than in the control group (178). In contrast, surgery did not significantly prevent the start of medication among those who had no medication at baseline. While the average cost per individual over 6 years was lower in the surgically than the conventionally treated control group regarding medication for diabetes and CVD, the costs were higher for anemia and gastrointestinal disorders. The total annual cost for all medication averaged over 6 years was not significantly different between surgically treated individuals (1386 Swedish crowns/year) and control individuals (1261/year).

In a separate study on CVD and diabetes medication, we found that a weight loss ≥10% was necessary to reduce the costs of medication among subjects with such treatment at baseline while a ≥15% weight loss was required to prevent the initiation of a new treatment against the two conditions (210,211). Overall, the annual average cost over 6 years for medication against diabetes and CVD increased by 463 SEK (96%) in subjects with weight loss <5%, and decreased by 39 SEK (8%) with weight loss ≥15% (210,211).

Modern economists are often using estimates of patients' willingness to pay for a given treatment as an expression for degree of urgency. We measured the willingness to pay for an efficient obesity treatment at baseline and found it to be twice as high as the monthly salary of the participants (212). After inclusion, the willingness to pay for an efficient treatment increased markedly in the surgically treated group (to be published).

Taken together, the direct plus indirect costs of surgical obesity treatment seem to be only marginally higher than conventional treatment over 6 years. Taking the reduced risk factors and the improved quality of life into account, the surgical approach seems worthwhile in spite of the fact that it is yet too early to judge its effects on hard endpoints and their associated costs.

VIII SURGICAL METHODS OF CHOICE

The previous discussion has emphasized that gastric bypass (GBP) and jejunoileal bypass (JIB) are resulting in similar weight loss. However, late side effects are more common and much more serious after JIB operations (81). Most experts as well as NIH (16) are therefore discouraging the use of JIB.

GBP results in larger weight loss than vertical banded gastroplasty (VBG) and gastric banding. The two latter techniques give similar weight reductions. Banding is associated with more reoperations than GBP and VBG. GBP is technically more demanding than VBG and banding, and it results in iron and B_{12} insufficiency that must be substituted. It is not known whether GBP will cause negative calcium balance or other malabsorptive problems in a 10-to-30 year perspective. Such hypothetical problems are less likely with VBG and banding since these methods do not change the normal passage of food through the gastrointestinal tract. Finally, patients subjected to GBP cannot easily have their stomach examined endoscopically, which makes malignancy examination more complicated.

Taken together, these circumstances suggest that GBP should be reserved for individuals with a considerable degree of obesity (BMI $\geq$ 40 kg/m^2) while VBG according to the SOS experience can be used with BMIs as low as 34kg/m^2. Banding in its original form as well as all forms of horizontal gastroplasties should not be used owing the high rate of reoperations. It should be noticed, however, that banding and VBG results in similar weight loss over 10 years. Variable banding has not been evaluated in randomized studies but seems to have a place in the obesity therapy, particularly when used with laparoscopic techniques.

The biliopancreatic diversion generates impressive weight reductions, but it is also associated with malabsorption of protein, fat-soluble vitamins, and calcium. Hence treatment with this technique should be reserved for the heaviest (BMI > 45 kg/m^2) and should only be undertaken in experienced surgical departments (rather than by individual surgeons) prepared to take a lifelong responsibility for the patients. The experience with biliopancreatic diversion with duodenal switch is still limited. However, it seems as if this technique is at least as efficient as the original biliopancreatic diversion and associated with less frequent and milder side effects. Although less efficient, the long-loop gastric bypass may be considered as an alternative to biliopancreatic diversions with or without duodenal switch owing to its lower frequency of serious adverse effects.

Randomized multicenter studies comparing gastric bypass, long-loop gastric bypass, biliopancreatic diversion, and biliopancreatic diversion with duodenal switch are urgently needed. While randomized studies were fairly common in the early days of bariatric surgery, no such studies seem to have been published since 1995 (Table 1).

Compared to open surgery, the advantages of the laparoscopic bariatric surgical procedures are so convincing that the aim should be to use the laparoscopic procedures almost universally in the future. Such a change will require elaborate educational activities within all surgical departments and perhaps also a new generation of surgeons. However, if the choice is between open surgery and no bariatric surgery at all, open surgery is still clearly recommended in most morbidly obese patients.

IX   OVERALL CONCLUSIONS

The prevalence of obesity is high and increasing, and obesity is associated with a dramatically increased morbidity and mortality. Nonpharmacological conventional treatment at specialized obesity units may achieve, on average, a 5% weight loss over 2–5 years

of follow-up. This is not enough to keep the risk factors down long term. Nonpharmacological, conventional obesity treatment at primary health care centers is not, on average, associated with any weight loss in the short or the long term. Unfortunately, most obese patients worldwide have no access to specialized obesity treatment. Treatment with currently available antiobesity drugs results, on average, in 8–10% weight reduction over 2 years, compared to 4–6% in the placebo groups. This is encouraging, but more efficient drugs are clearly needed. So far no randomized drug trials with durations longer than 2 years have been published.

The obese type 2 diabetic patient deserves extra attention. It is more difficult to achieve conventional or pharmacologically induced weight loss in diabetic obese patients. Moreover, even when weight loss is achieved, almost all patients relapse within a few years. Treatment with sulfonylureas or insulin causes weight increase. Thus, obesity not only causes diabetes but is also a complication of its treatment. This vicious spiral must be broken.

Surgery is the only treatment of obesity resulting, on average, in >15% documented weight loss over 10 years. This treatment has dramatic positive effects on most but not on all cardiovascular risk factors over a 10-year period. It has excellent effects on established diabetes, and it prevents the development of new cases of diabetes. Large weight reductions achieved by surgery also improve left ventricular structure and function and slow down the atherosclerotic process as estimated from intima-media measurements. Finally, quality of life is markedly improved. Since all these positive effects are well documented and since long-term direct and indirect costs for bariatric surgery treatment seem to be only moderately higher than for conventional obesity treatment, surgical treatment must become attainable for many more obese individuals.

In reality, however, primary health care centers will continue to assure the worldwide basis for obesity treatment also in the future. It can only be hoped that better programs and more efficient antiobesity drugs will improve treatments at these centers within the next 10 years. There is an urgent need for one specialized obesity center per ~500,000 inhabitants. At these centers, internists, surgeons, nurses, and dietitians would need to work full time with obese patients referred to them by general practitioners. The demand for such treatment is almost unlimited. Obese patients in a region with 500,000 inhabitants will generate at least 20,000–30,000 visits annually.

While waiting for more efficient antiobesity drugs, the surgical treatment of obesity must become more universally available. This author estimates that the real need is for at least 500–1000 operations annually per 500,000 inhabitants in most Western countries even if the current demand for operations is at a lower level. All obese patients with BMI $\geq$40 kg/m^2 need to be considered for bariatric surgery. However, a very large number of individuals with BMIs as low as 34 kg/m^2 will also benefit from surgical treatment. Finally, in the case of obese, diabetic patients, the question must now be raised, if it can be considered *lege artis* not to offer surgical treatment for their obesity and associated metabolic disorders.

REFERENCES

1. Stunkard AJ, McLaren-Hume M. The results of treatment for obesity. Arch Intern Med 1959; 79:103.
2. Sohar E, Sneh E. Follow-up of obese patients: 14 years after a successful reducing diet. Am J Clin Nutr 1973; 26:845–848.
3. Safer DJ. Diet, behavior modification, and exercise: a review of obesity treatments from a long-term perspective. South Med J 1991; 84:1470–1474.
4. Glenny AM, O'Meara S, Melville A, Sheldon TA, Wilson C. The treatment and prevention of obesity: a systematic review of the literature. Int J Obes Relat Metab Disord 1997; 21:715–737.
5. Sjöström CD, Lissner L, Wedel H, Sjöström L. Reduction in incidence of diabetes, hypertension and lipid disturbances after intentional weight loss induced by bariatric surgery: the SOS Intervention Study. Obes Res 1999; 7:477–484.
6. Sjöström CD, Peltonen M, Wedel H, Sjöström L. Differentiated long-term effects of intentional weight loss on diabetes and hypertension. Hypertension 2000; 36:20–25.
7. Sjöström L. Surgical intervention as a strategy for treatment of obesity. Endocrine 2000; 13:213–230.
8. Sjöström L. Swedish Obese Subjects, SOS. In: Björntorpp, ed. International Textbook of Obesity. Chichester: John Wiley & Sons, 2001:519–533.
9. Sjöström L, Rissanen A, Andersen T, Boldrin M, Golay A, Koppeschaar HP, Krempf M. Randomised placebo-controlled trial of orlistat for weight loss and prevention of weight regain in obese patients. European Multicentre Orlistat Study Group [see also editorial]. Lancet 1998; 352:167–172.
10. Deitel M. Surgery for the Morbidly Obese Patient. Philadelphia: Lea & Febiger, 1989.
11. Hogan RB, Johnston JH, Long BW, Sones JQ, Hinton LA, Bunge J, Corrigan SA. A double-blind, randomized, sham-controlled trial of the gastric bubble for obesity. Gastrointest Endosc 1989; 35:381–385.
12. Sjöström L. Morbidity of severely obese subjects. Am J Clin Nutr 1992; 55(suppl):508S–515S.
13. Sjöström L. Mortality of severly obese subjects. Am J Clin Nutr 1992; 55(suppl):516S–523S.
14. Sullivan M, Karlsson J, Sjöström L, Backman L, Bengtsson C, Bouchard C, Dahlgren S, Jonsson E, Larsson B, Lindstedt S. Swedish obese subjects (SOS)—an intervention study of obesity. Baseline evaluation of health and psychosocial functioning in the first 1743 subjects examined. Int J Obes Relat Metab Disrd 1993; 17:503–512.
15. Sullivan M, Karlsson J, Sjöström L, Taft C. Why quality-of-life measures should be used in the treatment of patients with obesity. In: Björntorpp, ed. International Textbook of Obesity Chichester: John Wiley and Sons, 2001:485–510.
16. NIH. Gastrointestinal surgery for severe obesity: National Institutes of Health Consensus Development conference Statement, March 25–27, 1991. Am J Clin Nutr 1992; 55(suppl):615–619.
17. Näslund I. Effects and side-effects of obesity surgery in patients with BMI below and above 40 in the SOS study. Int J Obes 1998; 22(suppl 3):S52.
18. Lissner L, Sjostrom L, Bengtsson C, Bouchard C, Larsson B. The natural history of obesity in an obese population and associations with metabolic aberrations. Int J Obes Relat Metab Disord 1994; 18:441–447.
19. Breaux CW. Obesity Surgery in Children. Obes Surg 1995; 5:279–284.
20. Antal S, Levin H. Biliopancreatic diversion in Prader-Willi syndrome associated with obesity. Obes Surg 1996; 6:58–62.
21. Grugni G, Guzzaloni G, Morabito F. Failure of biliopancreatic diversion in Prader-Willi syndrome. Obes Surg 2000; 10:179–181; discussion 182.
22. Krotkiewski M, Sjöström L, Björntorp P, Carlgren G, Garellick G, Smith U. Adipose tissue cellularity in relation to prognosis for weight reduction. Int J Obes Relat Metab Disord 1977; 1:395–416.
23. Kral J. Surgical treatment of obesity. In: Kopelman PG, Stock MJ, eds. Clinical Obesity. Oxford: Blackwell Science, 1998:545–563.
24. Payne JH, DeWind LT, Commons RR. Metabolic observations in patients with jejunocolic shunts. Am J Surg 1963; 106:273–289.
25. DeWind LT, Payne JH. Intestinal bypass surgery for morbid obesity. Long-term results. JAMA 1976; 236:2298–2301.
26. Scott HW Jr, Dean RH, Shull HJ, Gluck F. Results of jejunoileal bypass in two hundred patients with morbid obesity. Surg Gynecol Obstet 1977; 145:661–673.
27. Palmer JA. The present status of surgical procedures for obesity. In: DM, ed. Nutrition in Clinical Surgery. Baltimore: Williams & Williams, 1980:281–292.
28. Eriksson F. Biliointestinal bypass. Int J Obes 1981; 5:437–447.

29. Pace WG, Martin EW Jr, Tetirick T, Fabri PJ, Carey LC. Gastric partitioning for morbid obesity. Ann Surg 1979; 190:392–400.

30. Pories WJ, Flickinger EG, Meelheim D, Van Rij AM, Thomas FT. The effectiveness of gastric bypass over gastric partition in morbid obesity: consequence of distal gastric and duodenal exclusion. Ann Surg 1982; 196: 389–399.

31. Näslund I. The size of the gastric outlet and the outcome of surgery for obesity. Acta Chir Scand 1986; 152:205–210.

32. Gomez CA. Gastroplasty in morbid obesity. Surg Clin North Am 1979; 59:1113–1120.

33. Kuzmark LI. Gastric banding. In: Deitel M, ed. Surgery for the Morbidly Obese Patient. Philadelphia: Lea & Febiger, 1989:226.

34. Bö O, Modalsli O. Gastric banding, a surgical method of treating morbid obesity: preliminary report. Int J Obes 1983; 7:493–499.

35. Solhaug JH. Gastric banding: a new method in the treatment of morbid obesity. Curr Surg 1983; 40:424–428.

36. Kuzmark LI. A review of seven years' experience with silicon gastric banding. Obes Surg 1991; 1:403–408.

37. Forsell P, Hallberg D, Hellers G. Gastric banding for morbid obesity: initial experience with a new adjustable band. Obes Surg 1993; 3:369–374.

38. Hallerbäck BJ. Laparoscopy in the gastroesophageal junction. Int Surg 1995; 80:307–310.

39. Hallerbäck B, Glise H, Johansson B, Johnson E. Laparoscopic surgery for morbid obesity. Eur J Surg Suppl 1998; 582:128–131.

40. Dargent J. Laparoscopic adjustable gastric banding: lessons from the first 500 patients in a single institution. Obes Surg 1999; 9:446–452.

41. Mason EE. Vertical banded gastroplasty for obesity. Arch Surg 1982; 117:701–706.

42. Mason EE. Morbid obesity: use of vertical banded gastroplasty. Surg Clin North Am 1987; 67:521–537.

43. Eckhout GV, Willbanks OL, Moore JT. Vertical ring gastroplasty for morbid obesity. Five year experience with 1,463 patients. Am J Surg 1986; 152:713–716.

44. Fobi MA, Lee H. SILASTIC ring vertical banded gastric bypass for the treatment of obesity: two years of follow-up in 84 patients [corrected] [published erratum appears in J Natl Med Assoc 1994; 86(6):432]. J Natl Med Assoc 1994; 86:125–128.

45. Mason EE, Ito C. Gastric bypass in obesity. Surg Clin North Am 1967; 47:1345–1351.

46. Mason EE, Ito C. Gastric bypass. Ann Surg 1969; 170: 329–339.

47. Alden JF. Gastric and jejunoileal bypass. A comparison in the treatment of morbid obesity. Arch Surg 1977; 112:799–806.

48. Griffen WO Jr, Young VL, Stevenson CC. A prospective comparison of gastric and jejunoileal bypass procedures for morbid obesity. Ann Surg 1977; 186:500–509.

49. Griffen WO Jr, Bivins BA, Bell RM, Jackson KA. Gastric bypass for morbid obesity. World J Surg 1981; 5:817–822.

50. Torres JC, Oca CF, Garrison RN. Gastric bypass: Roux-en-Y gastrojejunostomy from the lesser curvature. South Med J 1983; 76:1217–1221.

51. Torres JC, Oca C. Gastric bypass lesser curvature with distal Roux-en-Y. Bariatric Surg 1987; 5:10–15.

52. Fobi MA, Fleming AW. Vertical banded gastroplasty vs gastric bypass in the treatment of obesity. J Natl Med Assoc 1986; 78:1091–1098.

53. Scopinaro N, Gianetta E, Civalleri D, Bonalumi U, Bachi V. Bilio-pancreatic bypass for obesity. 1. An experimental study in dogs. Br J Surg 1979; 66:613–617.

54. Scopinaro N, Gianetta E, Civalleri D, Bonalumi U, Bachi V. Bilio-pancreatic bypass for obesity: II. Initial experience in man. Br J Surg 1979; 66:618–620.

55. Brolin RE, Kenler HA, Gorman JH, Cody RP. Long-limb gastric bypass in the superobese. A prospective randomized study. Ann Surg 1992; 21:387–395.

56. Jordan JH, Hocking MP, Rout WR, Woodward ER. Marginal ulcer following gastric bypass for morbid obesity. Am Surg 1991; 57:286–288.

57. Hess DS. Biliopancreatic diversion with duodenal switch procedure (abstract). Obes Surg 1994; 4:105.

58. Marceau P, Biron S, Bourque AE. Biliopancreatic diversion with a new type of gastrectomy. Obes Surg 1993; 3:29–36.

59. Baltasar A, Bou R, Cipagauta LA. 'Hybrid' bariatric surgery: biliopancreatic diversion and duodenal switch—preliminary experience. Obes Surg 1995; 5: 419–423.

60. Fried M, Peskova M. Gastric banding in the treatment of morbid obesity. Hepatogastroenterology 1997; 44: 582–587.

61. Belachew M, Legrand M, Vincenti VV, Deffechereux T, Jourdan JL, Monami B, Jacquet N. Laparoscopic placement of adjustable silicone gastric band in the treatment of morbid obesity: how to do it. Obes Surg 1995; 5:66–70.

62. Ballesta-Lopez C, Bastida-Vila X, Catarci M, Bettonica-Larranaga C, Zaraca F. Laparoscopic gastric banding for morbid obesity with expanded PTFE: technique and early results in the first 100 consecutive cases. Hepatogastroenterology 1998; 45:2447–2452.

63. Abu-Abeid S, Szold A. Results and complications of laparoscopic adjustable gastric banding: an early and intermediate experience. Obes Surg 1999; 9:188–190.

64. O'Brien PE, Brown WA, Smith A, McMurrick PJ, Stephens M. Prospective study of a laparoscopically placed, adjustable gastric band in the treatment of morbid obesity. Br J Surg 1999; 86:113–118.

65. Kunath U, Susewind M, Klein S, Hofmann T. Success

and failure in laparoscopic "gastric banding." A report of 3 years experience. Chirurg 1998; 69:180–185.

66. Hauri P, Steffen R, Ricklin T, Riedtmann HJ, Sendi P, Horber FF. Treatment of morbid obesity with the Swedish adjustable gastric band (SAGB): complication rate during a 12-month follow-up period. Surgery 2000; 127:484–488.

67. Dumont L, Mattys M, Mardirosoff C, Picard V, Alle JL, Massaut J. Hemodynamic changes during laparoscopic gastroplasty in morbidly obese patients. Obes Surg 1997; 7:326–331.

68. Dumont L, Mattys M, Mardirosoff C, Vervloesem N, Alle JL, Massaut J. Changes in pulmonary mechanics during laparoscopic gastroplasty in morbidly obese patients. Acta Anaesthesiol Scand 1997; 41:408–413.

69. Sugerman H, Windsor A, Bessos M, Wolfe L. Intra-abdominal pressure, sagittal abdominal diameter and obesity comorbidity. J Intern Med 1997; 241:71–79.

70. Lönroth H, Dalenbäck J, Haglind E, Josefsson K, Olbe L, Fagevik Olsen M, Lundell L. Vertical banded gastroplasty by laparoscopic technique in the treatment of morbid obesity. Surg Laparosc Endosc 1996; 6:102–107.

71. Lönroth H, Dalenbäck J, Haglind E, Lundell L. Laparoscopic gastric bypass. Another option in bariatric surgery. Surg Endosc 1996; 10:636–638.

72. Higa KD, Boone KB, Ho T. Complications of the laparoscopic Roux-en-Y gastric bypass: 1,040 patients—what have we learned? Obes Surg 2000; 10:509–513.

73. Schauer PR, Ikramuddin S, Gourash W, Ramanathan R, Luketich J. Outcomes after laparoscopic Roux-en-Y gastric bypass for morbid obesity. Ann Surg 2000; 232:515–529.

74. Ren CJ, Patterson E, Gagner M. Early results of laparoscopic biliopancreatic diversion with duodenal switch: a case series of 40 consecutive patients. Obes Surg 2000; 10:514–523; discussion 524.

75. Sundbom M, Gustavsson S. Hand-assisted laparoscopic Roux-en-y gastric bypass: aspects of surgical technique and early results. Obes Surg 2000; 10:420–427.

76. Lewis LA, Turnbull RB Jr, Page IH. Effects of jejuno-colic shunt on obesity, serum lipoproteins, lipids and electrolytes. Arch Intern Med 1996; 117:4–16.

77. Shibata HR, MacKenzie JR, Long RC. Metabolic effects of controlled jejunocolic bypass. Arch Surg 1967; 95:413–428.

78. Buckwalter JA. A prospective comparison of the jejunoileal and gastric bypass operations for morbid obesity. World J Surg 1977; 1:757–768.

79. Rucken Rd Jr, Goldenberg F, Varco RL, Buchwald H. Lipid effects of obesity operations. J Surg Res 1981; 30:229–235.

80. Deitel M, Bojm MA, Atin MD, Zakhary GS. Intestinal bypass and gastric partitioning for morbid obesity: a comparison. Can J Surg 1982; 25:283–289.

81. O'Leary JP. Gastrointestinal malabsorptive procedures. Am J Clin Nutr 1992; 55(suppl):567S–570S.

82. Laws HL, Piantadosi S. Superior gastric reduction procedure for morbid obesity: a prospective, randomized trial. Ann Surg 1981; 193:334–340.

83. Lechner GW, Callender AK. Subtotal gastric exclusion and gastric partitioning: a randomized prospective comparison of one hundred patients. Surgery 1981; 90: 637–644.

84. Lechner GW, Elliott DW. Comparison of weight loss after gastric exclusion and partitioning. Arch Surg 1983; 118:685–692.

85. Näslund I, Wickbom G, Christoffersson E, Ågren G. A prospective randomized comparison of gastric bypass and gastroplasty. Complications and early results. Acta Chir Scand 1986; 152:681–689.

86. Näslund I. Gastric bypass versus gastroplasty. A prospective study of differences in two surgical procedures for morbid obesity. Acta Chir Scand Suppl 1987; 536: 1–60.

87. Hall JC, Watts JM, O'Brien PE, Dunstan RE, Walsh JF, Slavotinek AH, Elmslie RG. Gastric surgery for morbid obesity. The Adelaide Study. Ann Surg 1990; 211:419–427.

88. Linner JH. Comparative effectiveness of gastric bypass and gastroplasty: a clinical study. Arch Surg 1982; 117: 695–700.

89. Backman L, Granström L. Initial (1-year) weight loss after gastric banding, gastroplasty or gastric bypass. Acta Chir Scand 1984; 150:63–67.

90. Sugerman HJ, Wolper JL. Failed gastroplasty for morbid obesity. Revised gastroplasty versus Roux-Y gastric bypass. Am J Surg 1984; 148:331–336.

91. Gleysteen JJ. Four-year weight loss Roux-Y gastric bypass: anastomotic reinforcement not additive. Gastroenterol Clin North Am 1987; 16:525–527.

92. Howard L, Malone M, Michalek A, Carter J, Alger S, Van Woert J. Gastric bypass and vertical banded gastroplasty—a prospective randomized comparison and 5-year follow-up. Obes Surg 1995; 5:55–60.

93. Sugerman HJ, Starkey JV, Birkenhauer R. A randomized prospective trial of gastric bypass versus vertical banded gastroplasty for morbid obesity and their effects on sweets versus non- sweets eaters. Ann Surg 1987; 205:613–624.

94. MacLean LD, Rhode BM, Sampalis J, Forse RA. Results of the surgical treatment of obesity. Am J Surg 1993; 165:155–160; discussion 160–162.

95. Mason EE, Doherty C, Maher JW, Scott DH, Rodriguez EM, Blommers TJ. Super obesity and gastric reduction procedures. Gastroenterol Clin North Am 1987; 16:495–502.

96. Sugerman HJ, Londrey GL, Kellum JM, Wolf L, Liszka T, Engle KM, Birkenhauer R, Starkey JV. Weight loss with vertical banded gastroplasty and Roux-Y gastric bypass for morbid obesity with selective versus random assignment. Am J Surg 1989; 157:93–102.

97. Lindroos AK. Lissner L, Sjöström L. Weight change

in relation to intake of sugar and sweet foods before and after weight reducing gastric surgery. Int J Obes Relat Metab Disord 1996; 20:634–643.

98. Flancbaum L, Choban PS, Bradley LR, Burge JC. Changes in measured resting energy expenditure after Roux-en-Y gastric bypass for clinically severe obesity. Surgery 1997; 122:943–949.

99. Kellum JM, Kuemmerle JF, O'Dorisio TM, Rayford P, Martin D, Engle K, Wolf L, Sugerman HJ. Gastrointestinal hormone responses to meals before and after gastric bypass and vertical banded gastroplasty. Ann Surg 1990; 211:763–770; discussion 770–771.

100. Mason EE. Ileal [correction of ilial] transposition and enteroglucagon/GLP-1 in obesity (and diabetic?) surgery. Obes Surg 1999; 9:223–228.

101. Orskov C, Poulsen SS, Moller M, Holst JJ. Glucagon-like peptide I receptors in the subfornical organ and the area postrema are accessible to circulating glucagon-like peptide I. Diabetes 1996; 45:832–835.

102. Date Y, Kojima M, Hosoda H, Sawaguchi A, Mondal MS, Suganuma T, Matsukura S, Kangawa K, Nakazato M. Ghrelin, a novel growth hormone-releasing acylated peptide, is synthesized in a distinct endocrine cell type in the gastrointestinal tracts of rats and humans. Endocrinology 2000; 141:4255–4261.

103. Kojima M, Hosoda H, Date Y, Nakazato M, Matsuo H, Kangawa K. Ghrelin is a growth-hormone-releasing acylated peptide from stomach. Nature 1999; 402: 656–660.

104. Shintani M, Ogawa Y, Ebihara K, Aizawa-Abe M, Miyanaga F, Takaya K, Hayashi T, Inoue G, Hosoda K, Kojima M, Kangawa K, Nakao K. Ghrelin, an endogenous growth hormone secretagogue, is a novel orexigenic peptide that antagonizes leptin action through the activation of hypothalamic neuropeptide Y/Y1 receptor pathway. Diabetes 2001; 50:227–232.

105. Tschop M, Smiley DL, Heiman ML. Ghrelin induces adiposity in rodents. Nature 2000; 407:908–913.

106. Tschop M, Weyer C, Tataranni PA, Devanarayan V, Ravussin E, Heiman ML. Circulating ghrelin levels are decreased in human obesity. Diabetes 2001; 50:707–709.

107. Andersen T, Backer OG, Astrup A, Quaade F. Horizontal or vertical banded gastroplasty after pretreatment with very-low-calorie formula diet: a randomized trial. Int J Obes 1987; 11:295–304.

108. Catona A, LaManna L, Forsell P. The Swedish adjustable gastric band: laparoscopic technique and preliminary results. Obes Surg 2000; 10:15–21.

109. Miller K, Hell E. Laparoscopic adjustable gastric banding: a prospective 4-year follow-up study. Obes Surg 1999; 9:183–187.

110. Berrevoet F, Pattyn P, Cardon A, de Ryck F, Hesse UJ, de Hemptinne B. Retrospective analysis of laparoscopic gastric banding technique: short-term and mid-term follow-up. Obes Surg 1999; 9:272–275.

111. Fried M, Peskova M, Kasalicky M. Assessment of the

outcome of laparoscopic nonadjustable gastric banding and stoma adjustable gastric banding: surgeon's and patient's view. Obes Surg 1998; 8:45–48.

112. Belachew M, Legrand M, Vincent V, Lismonde M, Le Docte N, Deschamps V. Laparoscopic adjustable gastric banding. World J Surg 1998; 22:955–963.

113. Forsell P, Hellers G. The Swedish adjustable gastric banding (SAGB) for morbid obesity: 9-year experience and a 4-year follow-up of patients operated with a new adjustable band. Obes Surg 1997; 7:345–351.

114. Doherty C, Maher JW, Heitshusen DS. An interval report on prospective investigation of adjustable silicone gastric banding devices for the treatment of severe obesity. Eur J Gastroenterol Hepatol 1999; 11:115–119.

115. DeMaria EJ, Sugerman HJ. A critical look at laparoscopic adjustable silicone gastric banding for surgical treatment of morbid obesity: does it measure up? Surg Endosc 2000; 14:697–699.

116. Chelala E, Cadiere GB, Favretti F, Himpens J, Vertruyen M, Bruyns J, Maroquin L, Lise M. Conversions and complications in 185 laparoscopic adjustable silicone gastric banding cases. Surg Endosc 1997; 11: 268–271.

117. Westling A, Bjurling K, Öhrvall M, Gustavsson S. Silicone-adjustable gastric banding: disappointing results. Obes Surg 1998; 8:467–474.

118. Scopinaro N, Gianetta E, Adami GF, Friedman D, Traverso E, Marinari GM, Cuneo S, Vitale B, Ballari F, Colombini M, Baschieri G, Bachi V. Biliopancreatic diversion for obesity at eighteen years. Surgery 1996; 119:261–268.

119. Scopinaro N, Adami GF, Marinari GM, Gianetta E, Traverso E, Friedman D, Camerini G, Baschieri G, Simonelli A. Biliopancreatic diversion. World J Surg 1998; 22:936–946.

120. Nanni G, Balduzzi GF, Capoluongo R, Scotti A, Rosso G, Botta C, Demichelis P, Daffara M, Coppo E. Biliopancreatic diversion: clinical experience. Obes Surg 1997; 7:26–29.

121. Noya G, Cossu ML, Coppola M, Tonolo G, Angius MF, Fais E, Ruggiu M. Biliopancreatic diversion for treatment of morbid obesity: experience in 50 cases. Obes Surg 1998; 8:61–66.

122. Totte E, Hendrickx L, Van Hee R. Biliopancreatic diversion for treatment of morbid obesity: experience in 180 consecutive cases. Obes Surg 1999; 9:161–165.

123. Friedman D, Cuneo S, Valenzano M, Marinari GM, Adami GF, Gianetta E, Traverso E, Scopinaro N. Pregnancies in an 18-Year Follow-up after Biliopancreatic Diversion. Obes Surg 1995; 5:308–313.

124. Adami GF, Meneghelli A, Scopinaro N. Night eating and binge eating disorder in obese patients. Int J Eat Disord 1999; 25:335–338.

125. Chapin BL, LeMar HJ Jr, Knodel DH, Carter PL. Secondary hyperparathyroidism following biliopancreatic diversion. Arch Surg 1996; 131:1048–1052; discussion 1053.

126. Brolin RE, Leung M. Survey of vitamin and mineral supplementation after gastric bypass and biliopancreatic diversion for morbid obesity. Obes Surg 1999; 9: 150–154.

127. Smets RM, Waeben M. Unusual combination of night blindness and optic neuropathy after biliopancreatic bypass. Bull Soc Belge Ophtalmol 1999; 271:93–96.

128. Quaranta L, Nascimbeni G, Semeraro F, Quaranta CA. Severe corneoconjuctival xerosis after biliopancreatic bypass for obesity (Scopinaro's operation). Am J Ophthalmol 1994; 118:817–818.

129. Clare MW. Equal biliopancreatic and alimentary limbs: an analysis of 106 cases over 5 years. Obes Surg 1993; 3:289–295.

130. Bajardi G, Ricevuto G, Mastrandrea G, Branca M, Rinaudo G, Cali F, Diliberti S, Lo Biundo N, Asti V. Surgical treatment of morbid obesity with biliopancreatic diversion and gastric banding: report on an 8-year experience involving 235 cases. Ann Chir 2000; 125: 155–162.

131. Murr MM, Balsiger BM, Kennedy FP, Mai JL, Sarr MG. Malabsorptive procedures for severe obesity: comparison of pancreaticobiliary bypass and very very long limb Roux-en-Y gastric bypass. J Gastrointest Surg 1999; 3:607–612.

132. Hess DS, Hess DW. Biliopancreatic diversion with a duodenal switch. Obes Surg 1998; 8:267–282.

133. Baltasar A, del Rio J, Escriva C, Arlandis F, Martinez R, Serra C. Preliminary results of the duodenal switch. Obes Surg 1997; 7:500–504.

134. Marceau P, Hould FS, Simard S, Lebel S, Bourque RA, Potvin M, Biron S. Biliopancreatic diversion with duodenal switch. World J Surg 1998; 22:947–954.

135. Rabkin RA. Distal gastric bypass/duodenal switch procedure, Roux-en-Y gastric bypass and biliopancreatic diversion in a community practice. Obes Surg 1998; 8: 53–59.

136. Näslund E, Freedman J, Lagergren J, Stockeld D, Granström L. Three-year results of laparoscopic vertical banded gastroplasty. Obes Surg 1999; 9:369–373.

137. Davila-Cervantes A, Ganci-Cerrud G, Gamino R, Gallegos-Martinez J, Gonzalez-Barranco J, Herrera MF. Open vs. laparoscopic vertical banded gastroplasty: a case control study with a 1-year follow-up. Obes Surg 2000; 10:409–412.

138. Juvin P, Marmuse JP, Delerme S, Lecomte P, Mantz J, Demetriou M, Desmonts JM. Post-operative course after conventional or laparoscopic gastroplasty in morbidly obese patients. Eur J Anaesthesiol 1999; 16:400–403.

139. De Luca M, de Werra C, Formato A, Formisano C, Loffredo A, Naddeo M, Forestieri P. Laparotomic vs laparoscopic lap-band: 4-year results with early and intermediate complications. Obes Surg 2000; 10:266–268.

140. Nguyen NT, Ho HS, Palmer LS, Wolfe BM. A comparison study of laparoscopic versus open gastric bypass for morbid obesity. J Am Coll Surg 2000; 191: 149–155; discussion 155–157.

141. Ashy AR, Merdad AA. A prospective study comparing vertical banded gastroplasty versus laparoscopic adjustable gastric banding in the treatment of morbid and super-obesity. Int Surg 1998; 83:108–110.

142. Suter M, Giusti V, Heraief E, Jayet C, Jayet A. Early results of laparoscopic gastric banding compared with open vertical banded gastroplasty. Obes Surg 1999; 9: 374–380.

143. Suter M, Bettschart V, Giusti V, Heraief E, Jayet A. A 3-year experience with laparoscopic gastric banding for obesity. Surg Endosc 2000; 14:532–536.

144. Wittgrove AC, Clark GW. Laparoscopic gastric bypass, Roux-en-Y- 500 patients: technique and results, with 3–60 month follow-up. Obes Surg 2000; 10:233–239.

145. The Danish Obesity Project: randomised trial of jejunoileal bypass versus medical treatment in morbid obesity. Lancet 1979; 2:1255–1258.

146. Stokholm KH, Nielsen PE, Quaade F. Correlation between initial blood pressure and blood pressure decrease after weight loss: a study in patients with jejunoileal bypass versus medical treatment for morbid obesity. Int J Obes 1982; 6:307–312.

147. Andersen T, Backer OG, Stokholm KH, Quaade F. Randomized trial of diet and gastroplasty compared with diet alone in morbid obesity. N Engl J Med 1984; 310:352–356.

148. Andersen T, Stokholm KH, Backer OG, Quaade F. Long-term (5-year) results after either horizontal gastroplasty or very- low-calorie diet for morbid obesity. Int J Obes 1988; 12:277–284.

149. Martin LF, Tan TL, Horn JR, Bixler EO, Kauffman GL, Becker DA, Hunter SM. Comparison of the costs associated with medical and surgical treatment of obesity. Surgery 1995; 118:599–606.

150. Sjöström L, Larsson B, Backman L, Bengtsson C, Bouchard C, Dahlgren S, Hallgren P, Jonsson E, Karlsson J, Lapidus L. Swedish obese subjects (SOS). Recruitment for an intervention study and a selected description of the obese state. Int J Obes Relat Metab Disord 1992; 16:465–479.

151. MacDonald KG Jr, Long SD, Swanson MS, Brown BM, Morris P, Dohm GL, Pories WJ. The gastric bypass operation reduces the progression and mortality of non-insulin-dependent diabetes mellitus. J Gastrointest Surg 1997; 1:213–220.

152. Dhabuwala A, Cannan RJ, Stubbs RS. Improvement in co-morbidities following weight loss from gastric bypass surgery. Obes Surg 2000; 10:428–435.

153. Monteforte MJ, Turkelson CM. Bariatric surgery for morbid obesity. Obes Surg 2000; 10:391–401.

154. Naef M, Sadowski C, deMarco D, Sabbioni M, Balsiger B, Laederach K, Burgi U, Buchler MW. [Mason vertical gastroplasty in treatment of morbid obesity.

Results of a prospective clinical study.]. Chirurg 2000; 71:448–455.

155. Cowan GS Jr, Buffington CK. Significant changes in blood pressure, glucose, and lipids with gastric bypass surgery. World J Surg 1998; 22:987–992.

156. Sugerman HJ, Felton WL III, Sismanis A, Kellum JM, DeMaria EJ, Sugerman EL. Gastric surgery for pseudotumor cerebri associated with severe obesity. Ann Surg 1999; 229:634–640. discussion 640–642.

157. Stieger R, Thurnheer M, Lange J. [Morbid obesity: 130 consecutive patients with laparoscopic gastric banding.] Schweiz Med Wochenschr 1998; 128:1239–1246.

158. Carson JL, Ruddy ME, Duff AE, Holmes NJ, Cody RP, Brolin RE. The effect of gastric bypass surgery on hypertension in morbidly obese patients. Arch Intern Med 1994; 154:193–200.

159. Foley EF, Benotti PN, Borlase BC, Hollingshead J, Blackburn GL. Impact of gastric restrictive surgery on hypertension in the morbidly obese. Am J Surg 1992; 163:294–297.

160. Wolf AM, Beisiegel U, Kortner B, Kuhlmann HW. Does gastric restriction surgery reduce the risks of metabolic diseases? Obes Surg 1998; 8:9–13.

161. Luyckx FH, Scheen AJ, Desaive C, Dewe W, Gielen JE, Lefebvre PJ. Effects of gastroplasty on body weight and related biological abnormalities in morbid obesity. Diabetes Metab 1998; 24:355–361.

162. Brolin RE, Kenler HA, Wilson AC, Kuo PT, Cody RP. Serum lipids after gastric bypass surgery for morbid obesity. Int J Obes 1990; 14:939–950.

163. Gleysteen JJ, Barboriak JJ, Sasse EA. Sustained coronary-risk-factor reduction after gastric bypass for morbid obesity. Am J Clin Nutr 1990; 51:774–778.

164. Wittgrove AC, Clark GW, Schubert KR. Laparoscopic gastric bypass, Roux-en-Y: technique and results in 75 patients with 3–30 months follow-up. Obes Surg 1996; 6:500–504.

165. Smith SC, Edwards CB, Goodman GN. Changes in diabetic management after Roux-en-Y gastric bypass. Obes Surg 1996; 6:345–348.

166. Pories WJ, Swanson MS, MacDonald KG, Long SB, Morris PG, Brown BM, Barakat HA, deRamon RA, Israel G, Dolezal JM. Who would have thought it? An operation proves to be the most effective therapy for adult-onset diabetes mellitus. Ann Surg 1995; 222:339–350. discussion 350–352.

167. Pories WJ, MacDonald KG Jr, Flickinger EG, Dohm GL, Sinha MK, Barakat HA, May HJ, Khazanie P, Swanson MS, Morgan E. Is type II diabetes mellitus (NIDDM) a surgical disease? Ann Surg 1992; 215:633–642; discussion 643.

168. Pories WJ, MacDonaldJr KG, Morgan EJ, Sinha MK, Dohm GL, Swanson MS, Barakat HA, Khazanie PG, Leggett-Frazier N, Long SD. Surgical treatment of obesity and its effect on diabetes: 10-y follow-up. Am J Clin Nutr 1992; 55(suppl):582S–585S.

169. Pories WJ, Caro JF, Flickinger EG, Meelheim HD, Swanson MS. The control of diabetes mellitus (NIDDM) in the morbidly obese with the Greenville gastric bypass. Ann Surg 1987; 206:316–323.

170. Noseda A, Kempenaers C, Kerkhofs M, Houben JJ, Linkowski P. Sleep apnea after 1 year domiciliary nasal-continuous positive airway pressure and attempted weight reduction. Potential for weaning from continuous positive airway pressure. Chest 1996; 109:138–143.

171. Pories WJ. Why does the gastric bypass control type 1992; 2:303–313.

172. Hickey MS, Pories WJ, MacDonald KG Jr, Cory KA, Dohm GL, Swanson MS, Israel RG, Barakat HA, Considine RV, Caro JF, Houmard JA. A new paradigm for type 2 diabetes mellitus: could it be a disease of the foregut? Ann Surg 1998; 227:637–643; discussion 643–644.

173. Burstein R, Epstein Y, Charuzi I, Suessholz A, Karnieli E, Shapiro Y. Glucose utilization in morbidly obese subjects before and after weight loss by gastric bypass operation. Int J Obes Relat Metab Disord 1995; 19:558–561.

174. Guichard-Rode S, Charrie A, Penet D, Teboul F, Thivolet C. Massive weight loss does not restore normal insulin secretory pulses in obese patients with type 2 (non-insulin-dependent) diabetes mellitus. Diabetes Metab 1997; 23:506–510.

175. Sjöström L. Follow-up rates in the NBSR and the SOS. NBSR Newslett 1992; 7:12–13.

176. Karason K, Lindroos AK, Stenlöf K, Sjöström L. Relief of cardiorespiratory symptoms and increased physical activity after surgically induced weight loss. Results from the SOS study. Arch Intern Med 2000; 160:1797–1802.

177. Narbro K, Ågren G, Jonsson E, Larsson B, Näslund I, Wedel H, Sjöström L. Sick leave and disability pension before and after treatment for obesity: a report from the Swedish Obese Subjects (SOS) study. Int J Obes Relat Metab Disord 1999; 23:619–624.

178. Narbro K, Ågren G, Jonsson E, Näslund I, Sjöström L, Peltonen M. Pharmaceutical costs in the obese: a comparison with a randomly slected population sample, and long-term changes after conventional and surgical treatment. The SOS intervention study. Submitted, 2001.

179. Ågren G, Narbro K, Jonsson E, Näslund I, Sjöström L, Peltonen M. Costs of inpatient care among the obese. A prospective study of surgically and conventionally treated patients in the Swedish Obese Subjects intervention study. Submitted, 2001.

180. Lindroos AK, Lissner L, Sjöström L. Validity and reproducibility of a self-administered dietary questionnaire in obese and non-obese subjects. Eur J Clin Nutr 1993; 47:461–481.

181. Lindroos AK, Lissner L, Sjöström L. Does degree of

obesity influence the validity of reported energy and protein intake? Results from the SOS dietary questionnaire. Eur J Clin Nutr 1999; 53:375–378.

182. Sjöström CD, Håkangård AC, Lissner L, Sjöström L. Body compartment and subcutaneous adipose tissue distribution—risk factor patterns in obese subjects. Obes Res 1995; 3:9–22.

183. Sjöström CD, Lissner L, Sjöström L. Relationships between changes in body composition and changes in cardiovascular risk factors: the SOS Intervention Study. Swedish Obese Subjects. Obes Res 1997; 5:519–530.

184. Wadden TA, Anderson DA, Foster GD. Two-year changes in lipids and lipoproteins associated with the maintenance of a 5% to 10% reduction in initial weight: some findings and some questions. Obes Res 1999; 7: 170–178.

185. Sjöström CD. Effects of surgically induced weight loss on cardiovascular risk factors (Ph.D. thesis). ISBN 91-628-3984-5. Göteborg: Göteborg University, 2000: 87.

186. Sjöström CD, Peltonen M, Sjöström L. Blood pressure and pulse pressure during long-term weight loss in the obese: the Swedish Obese Subjects (SOS) intervention study. Obes Res 2001; 9:188–195.

187. Pinkney JH, Sjöström CD, Gale EA. Should surgeons treat diabetes in severely obese people? Lancet 2001; 357:1357–1359.

188. Pamuk ER, Williamson DF, Serdula MK, Madans J, Byers TE. Weight loss and subsequent death in a cohort of U.S. adults. Ann Intern Med 1993; 119: 744–748.

189. Williamson DF, Pamuk E, Thun M, Flanders D, Byers T, Heath C. Prospective study of intentional weight loss and mortality in never-smoking overweight US white women aged 40–64 years [published erratum appears in Am J Epidemiol 1995; 1;142:369]. Am J Epidemiol 1995; 141:1128–1141.

190. Williamson DF, Pamuk E, Thun M, Flanders D, Heath C, Byers T. Prospective study of intentional weight loss and mortality in overweight men aged 40–64 years [abstr]. Obes Res 1997; 5(suppl):94.

191. Jacobson P, Lindroos AK, Sjöström CD, Sjöström L. Long-term changes in serum homocysteine following weight loss in the SOS study. Int J Obes 2000; 24(suppl 1):175.

192. Moghadasian MH, McManus BM, Frohlich JJ. Homocyst(e)ine and coronary artery disease. Clinical evidence and genetic and metabolic background [published erratum appears in Arch Intern Med 1998; 158: 662]. Arch Intern Med 1997; 157:2299–2308.

193. Karason K, Wallentin I, Larsson B, Sjöström L. Effects of obesity and weight loss on left ventricular mass and relative wall thickness: survey and intervention study. BMJ 1997; 315:912–916.

194. Karason K, Wallentin I, Larsson B, Sjöström L. Effects of obesity and weight loss on cardiac function and valvular performance. Obes Res 1998; 6:422–429.

195. Karason K, Mölgaard H, Wikstrand J, Sjöström L. Heart rate variability in obesity and the effect of weight loss. Am J Cardiol 1999; 83:1242–1247.

196. Karason K, Wikstrand J, Sjöström L, Wendelhag I. Weight loss and progression of early atherosclerosis in the carotid artery: a four-year controlled study of obese subjects. Int J Obes Relat Metab Disord 1999; 23:948–956.

197. Nichols WW, O'Rourke MF. McDonald's Blood Flow in Arteries. Philadelphia: Lea & Febiger, 1998.

198. Boutouyrie P, Bussy C, Lacolley P, Girerd X, Laloux B, Laurent S. Association between local pulse pressure, mean blood pressure, and large-artery remodeling. Circulation 1999; 100:1387–1393.

199. Franklin SS, Khan SA, Wong ND, Larson MG, Levy D. Is pulse pressure useful in predicting risk for coronary heart disease? The Framingham Heart Study. Circulation 1999; 100:354–360.

200. Grunstein RR, Stenlöf K, Hedner J, Sjöström L. Impact of obstructive sleep apnea and sleepiness on metabolic and cardiovascular risk factors in the Swedish Obese Subjects (SOS) study. Int J Obes Relat Metab Disord 1995; 19:410–418.

201. Grunstein RR, Stenlöf K, Hedner JA, Sjöström L. Impact of self-reported sleep-breathing disturbances on psychosocial performance in the Swedish Obese Subjects (SOS) Study. Sleep 1995; 18:635–643.

202. Stenlöf K, Grunstein R, Hedner J, Sjöström L. Energy expenditure in obstructive sleep apnea: effects of treatment with continuous positive airway pressure. Am J Physiol 1996; 271:E1036–E1043.

203. Karlsson J, Sjöström L, Sullivan M. Swedish Obese Subjects (SOS)—an intervention study of obesity. Measuring psychosocial factors and health by means of short-form questionnaires. Results from a method study. J Clin Epidemiol 1995; 48:817–823.

204. Stunkard AJ, Messick S. The three-factor eating questionnaire to measure dietary restraint, disinhibition and hunger. J Psychosom Res 1985; 29:71–83.

205. Karlsson J, Sjöström L, Sullivan M. Swedish obese subjects (SOS)—an intervention study of obesity. Two-year follow-up of health-related quality of life (HRQL) and eating behavior after gastric surgery for severe obesity. Int J Obes Relat Metab Disord 1998; 22:113–126.

206. Karlsson J, Persson LO, Sjöström L, Sullivan M. Psychometric properties and factor structure of the Three-Factor Eating Questionnaire (TFEQ) in obese men and women. Results from the Swedish Obese Subjects (SOS) study. Int J Obes Relat Metab Disord 2000; 24:1715–1725.

207. Narbro K, Jonsson E, Waaler H, Wedel H, Sjöström L. Economic consequencies of sick leave and disability pension in obese Swedes (abstr). Int J Obes 1994; 18 (suppl 2):14.

208. Sjöström L, Narbro K, Sjöström D. Costs and benefits when treating obesity. Int J Obes Relat Metab Disord 1995; 19(suppl 6):S9–S12.

209. Narbro K, Jonsson E, Larsson B, Waaler H, Wedel H, Sjöström L. Economic consequences of sick-leave and early retirement in obese Swedish women. Int J Obes Relat Metab Disord 1996; 20:895–903.

210. Narbro K, Ågren G, Näslund I, Sjöström L, Peltonen M. Decreased medication for diabetes and cardiovascular disease after weight loss (abstract). Int J Obes Relat Metab Disord 2000; 24(suppl 1):S42.

211. Ågren G, Narbro K, Näslund I, Sjöström L, Peltonen M. Long-term effects of weight loss on pharmaceutical costs in obese subjects. A report from the SOS intervention study. Submitted, 2001.

212. Narbro K, Sjöström L. Willingness to pay for obesity treatment. Int J Technol Assess Health Care 2000; 16: 50–59.

213. Lönroth H, Dalenbäck J. Other laparoscopic bariatric procedures. World J Surg 1998; 22:964–968.

214. Katz JN, Larson MG, Phillips CB, Fossel AH, Liang MH. Comparative measurement sensitivity of short and longer health status instruments. Med Care 1992; 30:917–925.

Index